NURSING PROCESS AND PRACTICE
IN THE COMMUNITY

NURSING PROCESS AND PRACTICE
IN THE COMMUNITY

Joan M. Cookfair, RN, MSN, EdD
Associate Professor
D'Youville College, Division of Nursing
Buffalo, New York

Illustrated

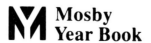

Mosby
Year Book

St. Louis   Baltimore   Boston   Chicago   London   Philadelphia   Sydney   Toronto

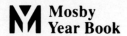
**Mosby
Year Book**

Dedicated to Publishing Excellence

Editor: **N. Darlene Como**
Developmental Editor: **Laurie Sparks**
Project Supervisor: **Barbara Bowes Merritt**
Production Editors: **Sylvia Barnard, Marilyn Stanaway**
Design: **Elizabeth Fett**

Printed in the United States of America

Mosby−Year Book, Inc.
11830 Westline Industrial Drive
St. Louis, MO 63146

Library of Congress Cataloging-in-Publication Data

Nursing process and practice in the community [edited by] Joan M.
   Cookfair.

     p.   cm.

    Includes bibliographical references and index.
    ISBN 0-8016-2581-5
    1. Community health nursing.   I. Cookfair, Joan M.
RT98.N89   1991
610.73′43—dc20   90-13560
                                      CIP

GW/D/D 9 8 7 6 5 4 3 2 1

Contributors

Patricia A. Anderson, RN, PhD
Assistant Professor
Division of Nursing
D'Youville College
Buffalo, New York

Carol Batra, RN, PhD
Professor
Chairperson, Division of Nursing
D'Youville College
Buffalo, New York

Elizabeth Johnson Blankenship, RN, BSN, CNA
Director of Nursing
Briarwood Nursing Center
Little Rock, Arkansas

Arthur S. Cookfair, BA, EdD
Adjunct Professor
Department of Chemistry
Canisius College
Buffalo, New York

Mary K. Dete, BSN, PHN
Vice President of Patient Services
Hospital Home Health Care Agency of California
Torrance, California

Janice Cooke Feigenbaum, RN, PhD
Associate Professor
Division of Nursing
D'Youville College
Buffalo, New York

Carole A. Gutt, RN, EdD
Associate Professor
Director of Graduate Program and Assistant Chairperson
D'Youville College
Buffalo, New York

Janet T. Ihlenfeld, RN, PhD
Associate Professor
Division of Nursing
D'Youville College
Buffalo, New York

Janet E. Jackson, RN, MS
Faculty, Department of Nursing
Bradley University
Peoria, Illinois

Linda M. Janelli, RNC, EdD
Assistant Professor of Nursing
State University of New York at Buffalo
Buffalo, New York

Patricia A. O'Hare, RN, DPH
Assistant Professor of Nursing
Georgetown University School of Nursing
Washington, D.C.

Therese M. Mudd, MAT
Case Manager
Opportunities Unlimited of Niagara Falls
Niagara Falls, New York

Robert J. Perelli, CJM, D.Min.
Founder, AIDS Family Services
D'Youville College
Buffalo, New York

Christine L. Rubadue, RN, MN
Associate Director for Operations
Division of Federal Employee Occupational Health
U.S. Public Health Service, Region X
Clinical Instructor
Department of Community Health Care Systems
University of Washington
Seattle, Washington

Mary K. Salazar, RN, MN
Acting Director, Occupational Health Nursing
Department of Community Health Care Systems
University of Washington
Seattle, Washington

June A. Schmele, RN, PhD
Associate Professor
College of Nursing
University of Oklahoma

Elizabeth Chenk, MSN, CRRNRNe
Vice President of Nursing
Heather Hill Inc.
Chardon, Ohio

Corinne Stuart, RN, MS
Associate Professor
School of Nursing
State University of New York at Buffalo
Buffalo, New York

Diana M. Stulc, RNL, MS
Health Care Coordinator
Infant Program
Robert Warner Rehabilitation Center
Children's Hospital of Buffalo
Buffalo, New York

Sandra L. Termini, RN, MS
Private Practice
Health Educator, Consultant
Buffalo, New York

Edward H. Weiss, RD, PhD
Associate Professor
Dietetics Program Director
D'Youville College
Buffalo, New York

William E. Wilkinson, RNC, DrPH, COHN
LEXIS Associate
Mead Data Central/College of Law
University of Arizona
Tucson, Arizona
Commander
U.S. Public Health Service Reserve

Foreword

The challenges inherent in the practice of community health nursing reflect the vast complexity and diversity comprising its history, evolution, and future needs. It is difficult to envision a text which can give students knowledge for today and the tools and concepts needed for tomorrow. This text is a welcome and much needed addition to the literature in community health nursing since it clearly addresses both these areas. The unique nursing theorist approach used allows educators and students to synthesize the foundations and accomplishments of the past and the fundamentals of contemporary practice into a blueprint for future directions.

Nursing process from the perspective of the *Betty Neuman Health Care Systems Model* is utilized as a framework for analyzing the health of target groups and of a community. The historical development of health care and the health care delivery system are presented in a cogent, relevant manner. The reader is then provided with parameters for integration of key concepts in health education, leadership, research, and accountability needed for community health nursing in today's society. A comprehensive overview of health interventions at primary, secondary, and tertiary levels is offered to assist in understanding the nurse's role in health promotion across the life span.

Knowledge of family structure and types of families is a necessary component in nursing's role in health promotion. Nursing actions within the family context are presented in an understandable and pragmatic manner. The new thrust toward home health care, the nurse's role in discharge planning and home coordination, and the use of modern technology in the home setting bring the text into the 1990s and beyond. The expanded role of the community health nurse in caring for the chronically ill client, the client in the workplace, and the client with a communicable disease including AIDS is done in a sensitive and challenging fashion. Illustrative examples and case studies are used throughout the text giving it a concrete dimension as well as a conceptual one.

The author and contributors have drawn on their vast backgrounds and experience to provide the perfect blend of technical and theoretical concepts while affording the reader the opportunity to learn, improve, and dream.

Leah L. Curtin states it succinctly, "In today's strained world among tomorrow's strange machines, people more than ever need to be touched to be restored, renewed, revived, and redeemed. Today, technology has brought us closer than ever before to the pain of living, so finally we have learned that health really does lie in restoring independence, not merely ministering to illness."

Carol A. Gutt, R.N., Ed.D.
Assistant Chairperson
Director of Graduate Program
Division of Nursing
D'Youville College
Buffalo, New York

Preface

Today, more than ever, community health is the cornerstone of health care delivery. In the U.S. the change to a prospective system of reimbursement based on DRG's has shortened hospital stays and increased the need for community-based health care. Clients cared for in the community now require a broad range of nursing services. Fiscal realities and social demands appear likely to mandate the continued growth of community-based care for the foreseeable future.

Many of today's nursing students will eventually go on to practice in the community. They must gain the knowledge and skills necessary to undertake varied community health nursing roles in diverse settings. This requires a firm education which includes both the essential concepts and practices which provide the foundation for contemporary community health nursing.

The preparation of students for practice in contemporary society must also include an awareness that they will need to adapt to an environment characterized by kaleidoscopic change. Today's absolutes often become tomorrow's controversy. Value systems that worked well a decade ago no longer resolve daily ethical dilemmas. "High tech" must be balanced with a conscious effort to maintain "high touch" by caring practitioners. A depleted economy forces nurses to make painful decisions daily about the allocation of services. Students must be prepared to cope with limitless uncertainty and frustration.

Nursing Process and Practice in the Community is an introductory text, written to provide baccalaureate nursing students with a basic foundation in community health nursing. It concisely presents the knowledge and skills essential to contemporary practice. Nursing process is used as a framework for practice. Discussion of the historical development of nursing and the emergence of nursing theory demonstrates the relationship between theory and practice. Research highlights and case studies are included throughout to reflect current developments and application of knowledge to practice.

The text is organized into seven units. Unit I describes historical events that have influenced the development of health care and the emergence of nursing theory. The current complexity of health care delivery systems is presented as well as the application of the nursing process to the community as a client.

Unit II lays the foundation for health promotion in the community by focusing on health education, research, leadership, and accountability. Concepts and strategies discussed include various models of health, the teaching/learning process, group processes, and leadership skills. Epidemiological concepts are described and applied to community health nursing. Various models of quality assurance are outlined.

Unit III supplies information that will assist the nurse in planning interventions across the life span at primary, secondary, and tertiary levels of prevention as well as giving an overview of various community health nursing roles. Erikson's developmental stages are incorporated throughout, showing that development is a lifelong process.

Unit IV focuses on the family as a unit of service and shows the importance of health promotion in both functional and dysfunctional families. Cultural diversity is discussed within the context of the family, further demonstrating the importance of the family in influencing an individual's health.

Unit V describes the changing picture of contemporary home health care, describing home care nursing, the nurse's role as a discharge planner, the challenge of high tech care in the home, and special concerns of chronically ill clients.

Unit VI describes specific practice roles and settings to introduce the student to the diversity present in the community health nursing role. Guidelines related to occupational health nursing are provided. Special concerns of high risk aggregates in the community are discussed. The subject of communicable disease is presented with an emphasis on prevention. The impact of AIDS is given a special focus. The nurse's role with developmentally disabled clients is described together with information to help the nurse act as a client advocate.

The emerging professional issues of the 1990s are addressed in unit VII. The nurse's role in the promotion and maintenance of health related to nutrition is discussed. Environmental hazards are described in terms of present and possible future problems. Legal and ethical concerns are outlined. Substance abuse and its effect on the community is examined. The final chapter discusses professional issues that the community health nurse can expect to encounter as we approach the twenty-first century.

To facilitate the teaching-learning process, a number of pedagogical aids are included in the text. Chapter objectives assist the student to identify essential content. Case studies demonstrate the application of concepts to practice. Research highlights are integrated throughout the text to illustrate the application of research to community health nursing practice. Chapter summaries and chapter highlights review and reinforce important content. Study questions challenge the student to integrate and apply content presented in the chapter. References provide resources for further study. A glossary of key terms used in the text facilitates understanding and using complex or unfamiliar terms.

The author and the contributors of this text view nursing and the emerging role of the community health nurse as an exciting challenge. We earnestly hope that we have conveyed our enthusiasm and our vision of the nurse of the future.

I would like to thank Janet Ihlenfeld for writing an excellent instructor's manual. I am grateful for the patience and assistance I received from Laurie Sparks as developmental editor. I would like to express my appreciation to my colleagues at D'Youville College for their help and suggestions and my family for their patience and support throughout this lengthy process. To the students, who contributed ideas, posed for photos, and provided the incentive for writing this text—thank you. I wish you well.

Joan M. Cookfair

Contents

UNIT I   Introduction to Community Health Nursing

1   Historical Overview of Community Health Nursing, 3
JOAN M. COOKFAIR
Antiquity, 4
The Middle Ages, 7
The Renaissance (1400 to 1700), 8
Contributors, 9
The Twentieth Century, 13
Nursing Theory and Community Health Nursing, 16
Public Health Nursing, 18
Summary, 19

2   Health Care Delivery Systems, 21
JOAN M. COOKFAIR
Beginnings of Health Departments in the United States, 22
Involvement in the Health Care System, 23
Components of the Health Care Delivery System, 25
Financing of Health Care, 29
Evaluation of the Current System, 30
Health Care Delivery Systems in Other Countries, 34
Summary, 35

3   The Nursing Process in the Community, 37
JOAN M. COOKFAIR
Definitions of Community, 39
The Nursing Process, 39
The Neuman Health Care Systems Model, 40
The Nursing Process Applied to a Community, 44
Case Study 1, 45
Case Study 2, 53
Summary, 58

UNIT II Strategies and Tools for Health Promotion

4 Health and Wellness in the Community, 65
CAROLE A. GUTT
Historical Development of the Wellness Movement, 66
Prominent Individuals in the Wellness/Health Movement, 68
Terms Used in the Wellness Movement, 70
Models of Wellness, 71
Assessment of Wellness Behaviors, 80
Wellness Components, 85
Summary, 93

5 Health Teaching in the Community, 96
JANET E. JACKSON and ELIZABETH JOHNSON BLANKENSHIP
Historical Background, 97
Legal Issues in Health Teaching, 99
Teaching/Learning Theories, 99
Types of Learning, 100
Principles of Teaching/Learning, 103
The Teaching/Learning Process and the Nursing Process, 105
Summary, 119

6 Working with Groups in the Community, 122
LINDA JANELLI
Definition of Group, 123
Functions of Groups, 124
Characteristics of Groups, 125
Group Development, 125
Role Differentiation, 127
Shared Leadership, 129
Social Power and Group Conflict, 129
Leadership Styles, 130
Motivational Theory, 131
Types of Groups, 132
Initiating a Small Group, 135
Summary, 135

7 Epidemiology, 138
JOAN M. COOKFAIR
Historical Evolution, 139
Epidemiological Concepts, 141
Types of Data Collection, 148
Methods Used in Epidemiological Research, 151
Application of Epidemiological Concepts to Community Health Nursing, 153
Summary, 154

8 Quality Assurance in Community Health Nursing, 156
JUNE A. SCHMELE
Environmental Context, 158
Quality, 163
Quality Assurance in Health Care, 164
Quality Assurance Methods, 175
Related Programs, 177
Quality Assurance Roles, 178
Research and Quality Assurance, 180
The Future of Quality Assurance, 180
Summary, 181

UNIT III The Individual in the Community

9 The Child from Birth to Five Years, 187
JANET T. INHLENFELD
Physical Growth and Development, 188
Cognitive Development, 188
Play, 190
Health Problems of Infants, Toddlers, and Preschoolers, 192
Health Promotion Activities, 194
Roles of the Community Health Nurse, 196
Summary, 204

10 The Child of Primary and Secondary School Age, 208
JOAN M. COOKFAIR
Physical Growth and Development of the Primary-School Child, 209
Physical Growth and Development of the Secondary-School Child
   (Adolescence), 213
Cognitive Development, 214
Personality Development, 214
Moral and Spiritual Development, 214
Major Causes of Mortality and Illness, 215
Mental Health, 220
The Community Health Nurse in the Schools, 221
Summary, 232

11 The Young and Middle-Aged Adult, 234
JOAN M. COOKFAIR
The Young Adult, 236
The Middle-Aged Adult, 247
Summary, 251

12 The Adult in Later Maturity, 253
JOAN M. COOKFAIR and PATRICIA A. ANDERSON
The Aging Process, 256
Developmental Tasks of Aging, 257
Psychosocial Theories of Aging, 261
Common Health Problems of Later Maturity, 261
Health Promotion in the Senior Citizen Center, 266
Other Community Resources, 269
The Fragile Elderly Person, 270
Spiritual Nursing Care, 270
Summary, 271

UNIT IV   The Family in the Community

13 The Family as a Unit of Service, 275
SANDRA L. TERMINI
What is a Family, 277
Types of Families, 277
The Evolving Family Structure, 278
Roles within the Family, 278
The Functional Family, 279
Adaptive Family Coping Patterns, 280
Conceptual Frameworks for Studying the Family, 282
Family Health, 284
Nursing Care of the Family, 284
The Family/Community System, 294
Summary, 296

14 The Family as a Bearer of Culture, 299
DIANA M. STULC
Culture and Families, 302
Cultural Assessment, 303
Culturally Diverse Families, 308
Using the Nursing Process to Provide Culturally Appropriate Care, 316
Summary, 318

15 The Dysfunctional Family, 321
JANICE COOKE FEIGENBAUM
Characteristics, 322
Assessment, 325
Nursing Diagnosis, 335
Planning and Intervention, 336
Implementation, 337
Evaluation, 342
Summary, 344

UNIT V Home Health Care

16 Home Health Service Agencies, 349
JOAN M. COOKFAIR
Clients who Require Home Care, 350
Professionals Involved in Planning Home Care, 351
Types of Agencies that Provide Home Care, 352
Financing of Home Health Services, 355
Logistical Aspects of Home Health Care, 356
Future Trends in Home Health Care, 365
Summary, 366

17 Discharge Planning, 368
PATRICIA A. O'HARE
Historical Perspective, 369
Current Perspectives, 370
The Process of Discharge Planning, 371
Components for Providing Continuity of Care, 374
Review of Critical Process Information, 375
Discharge Planning Roles, 378
Summary, 380

18 Home Health Care and Advanced Technology, 382
MARY K. DETE
Services and Service Models, 384
Team Members and Roles, 384
Planning for the Use of Advanced Technology in the Home, 386
Application of the Nursing Process, 404
Summary, 406

19 Home Health Care and Chronic Illness, 408
JOAN M. COOKFAIR
Definitions of Chronicity, 409
Effects of Chronic Illness on Stages of Personality Development, 410
Chronic Illness Across the Life Span, 411
Trajectory of Chronic Illness, 414
Nursing Process, 416
Current Issues in Home Care of the Chronically Ill, 416
Future Trends, 417
Summary, 417

UNIT VI Practice Roles and Settings

20 Occupational Health Nursing, 421
MARY K. SALAZAR, WILLIAM E. WILKINSON, and CHRISTINE L. RUBADUE
History, 423
Work-Related Injuries and Illness, 426

Maintenance of Health in the Workplace, 427
Major Categories of Hazards in the Workplace, 428
Roles and Functions of the Occupational Health Nurse, 434
Summary, 446

21 High-Risk Aggregates in the Community, 449
JOAN M. COOKFAIR
Infants at Risk, 450
The Prison Population, 453
The Homeless Population, 457
Summary, 461

22 Communicable Diseases, 463
ROBERT J. PERELLI and JOAN M. COOKFAIR
Application of Betty Neuman's Systems Model to the Concept of Immunity, 465
Epidemiological Triad, 465
Surveillance, 467
Prevention, 468
Common Communicable Diseases, 472
Summary, 482

23 Developmentally Disabled Persons in the Community, 485
THERESE M. MUDD and JOAN M. COOKFAIR
Role of the Community Health Nurse, 488
Definitions of Developmental Disability, 489
Selected Developmental Disabilities, 489
Historical Background, 495
Developmental Disabilities Throughout the Life Span, 495
Legal and Ethical Issues, 500
Summary, 505

UNIT VII Issues and Concerns in Community Health Nursing

24 Nutrition in the Community, 511
EDWARD H. WEISS
What is a Healthy Diet? 512
Dietary Recommendations for Most Persons, 513
Nutritional Needs Through the Life Span, 521
Use of the Nursing Process to Improve Nutritional Status and Promote Health, 532
Summary, 535

25 Environmental Concerns, 539
ARTHUR S. COOKFAIR
The Population Effect, 541
Waste Disposal and Dispersal, 543
Water Pollution, 552
Noise Pollution, 553

Air Pollution, 555
Radiation in the Environment, 558
Environmental Disasters, 560
Pollution in the Home, 561
Nursing Interventions, 565
Summary, 566

26 Substance Abuse, 569
ELIZABETH CHENK
Issues and Trends in Substance Abuse, 570
Scope of the Problem, 571
Theories of Causation, 571
Factors that Place Populations at Risk, 572
Common Substances of Abuse, 577
Chemical Dependency, 582
Use of the Nursing Process, 582
Summary, 589

27 Legal and Ethical Issues, 592
CORINNE T. STUART
Legal Issues, 594
Ethical Issues, 603
Summary, 610

28 Professional Issues: The Future of Community Health Nursing, 613
CAROL BATRA
The Metaparadigm of Nursing, 614
The Future of Community Health Nursing, 630
Summary, 632

Introduction to Community Health Nursing

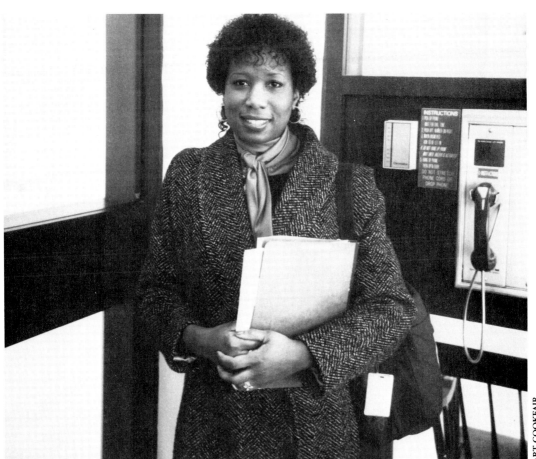

Sickness and suffering always have been part of the human experience, and from the very earliest times there have been men and women who have cared about the welfare of the afflicted. The first semblance of "nursing" probably was practiced by family members as they attempted to soothe and protect the ill and the injured. As knowledge accumulated and moral codes evolved, a class of dedicated individuals, who belonged mainly to religious orders, focused their energy on the alleviation of suffering and helping those in need of care. However, it was not until Florence Nightingale established a training school for nurses, at St. Thomas Hospital in London, that organized nursing became a reality. Early nursing leaders continued to respond to the needs of the sick and the poor in the community, and a sense of uniqueness about nursing as a profession began to develop.

In the United States the system for health care services to the community has become increasingly complex during the last few decades. This is due, in part, to the accelerating accumulation of information about the causes of ill health and disease and the rapid growth of sophisticated technology available to health care providers.

The health care delivery system in the United States is divided into the public and the private sectors. Federal regulations control the public sector; competition and limited funds are beginning to control the private sector. Furthermore, health care needs are not always met, which has led health care providers and legislators to explore a more effective and equitable method for the distribution of care to citizens of the United States. Other developed countries have less complicated systems for the delivery of health care, which is primarily controlled by the central government.

Nursing has begun to define itself as an autonomous profession. A body of theoretical knowledge is available that assists nurses to make decisions about their practice and to analyze objectively the needs of their clients. Community health nurses are using this knowledge to become more effective health care providers and advocates for their clients in the community setting.

Unit I describes historical events that have influenced the development of health care, the complexity of health care delivery systems, and an application of nursing theory to the analysis of the health of a community using nursing process as a framework.

Historical Overview of Community Health Nursing

JOAN M. COOKFAIR

Change is the process by which the future invades our lives, and it is important to look at it closely, not merely from the grand perspectives of history, but also from the vantage point of the living, breathing individuals who experience it.

ALVIN TOFFLER

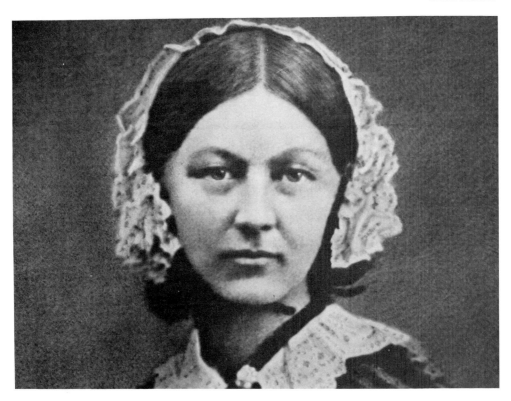

Courtesy of the Bettman Archives.

OBJECTIVES

At the conclusion of this chapter the student will be able to:
1. Define the key terms listed
2. Describe various historical events that have influenced the development of community health nursing
3. Identify selected individuals who have contributed to the development of community health nursing
4. Describe the development of organized public health
5. Describe selected nursing theories that can be applied to community health nursing
6. Define public health nursing and community health nursing
7. Describe the standards of the American Nurses' Association for community health nursing practice

KEY TERMS

American Nurses' Association
Community health nurse
Community health nursing
District nursing
Environment
Frontier Nursing Service
Health

Florence Nightingale
Nurse
Nursing Theory
Person
Public health
St. Vincent de Paul
Lillian Wald

Throughout the ages historical events and scientific discoveries have influenced societal attitudes toward the care of the sick and those who care for them. An understanding of the sequence of these events will enable nurses to better understand the way their profession developed and the impact of these events on the practice of nursing in the community today. Table 1-1 provides an outline of the historical events that have influenced nursing and medicine from ancient times until the last part of the nineteenth century.

ANTIQUITY

Even in the Neolithic Age, which began around 10,000 BC, people attempted to find ways to cure illness and stop death. Archaeologists have found artifacts that indicate a belief during this period that supernatural forces controlled life and death. Physical anthropologists have discovered remains that indicate a surgical procedure was performed, which consisted of boring a hole in the head (trephination), to let out evil spirits.

It was not until the Egyptians invented a method of writing (around 2000 BC) that records were kept concerning care of the sick. An ancient manuscript from that time period, the *Book of Surgery,* documented the observations of a court physician who made the following assessment concerning diagnosis and treatment (Lucas, 1953, p. 62):

> If thou examinist a man having a crushed vertebrae in his neck and thou findest that one vertebrae has fallen into the neck, while he is voiceless and cannot speak, his one vertebrae crushed into the next one; and shouldest thou find that he is unconscious of his two arms and legs because of this diagnosis, thou shouldest say concerning him, one having a crushed

TABLE 1-1 Historical events influencing the development of nursing and medicine

Time	Place	Historical event	Cultural event
Antiquity			
3000 BC	Egypt	Written records	System of diagnosis
2000 BC	Canaan	Old Testament	Standards of conduct and behavior
500 BC	Greece	Hippocrates' papers	Scientific method
Anno Domini *(AD)*			
First century	Jerusalem, Rome, Greece	New Testament	Spread of moral code
79	Rome	Pliny's Historia Naturalis (Natural History)	Record of medical practice
130	Greece	Galen's study of physiology	Scientific approach
200	Rome	Central distributing system for water	Sanitation
400	Rome	Fall of Western Roman Empire	Cultural decline
500	Byzantium	Written records	Preservation of knowledge
The Middle Ages			
500	Europe	Continuous warfare	Folklore, unscientific approach
1096-1149	Middle East	Crusades	Cultural exchange
1181-1286	Rome	St. Francis of Assisi's Order of Friars Minor	Organized care of sick
1224-1274	Rome	Thomas Aquinas' papers on cause and effect	Logical reasoning
1390-1400	Europe	Epidemics	Cultural decline
The Renaissance			
1400	Europe	Humanism	Emphasis on classics
1492	Western hemisphere	Columbus discovers America	Expansion of world view
1517	Europe	Protestant Reformation	Diminished influence of Catholic church
1530	Europe	Girolamo Fracastoro names syphilis	Beginning of germ theory
1576-1660	Belgium	Sisters of Charity	Hospices established
1591-1600	Europe	Beginnings of rationalistic approach	Scientific method
1628	England	William Harvey's study	Understanding of blood circulation
1646	England	Invention of microscope	Scientific research possible
1649	England	Watch with second hand	Ability to count pulse and respiration
Age of Enlightenment			
1749	England	Variolation (Jenner's discovery of vaccination)	Concept of prevention of disease
1781	Vienna	René Laënnec's invention of stethoscope	Ability to listen to heart and breath sounds

Continued.

TABLE 1-1   Historical events influencing the development of nursing and medicine—cont'd

Time	Place	Historical event	Cultural event
Nineteenth century: beginning of modern scientific age			
1852	France	Louis Pasteur's discovery of pasteurization	Prevention of growth of bacteria
1855	England	John Snow's discovery of mode of cholera transmission	Prevention of disease spread
1870	Germany	Robert Koch's germ theory	Prevention of disease
1870	Scotland	Joseph Lister's principle of antisepsis	Use of antiseptics

vertebrae in his neck, he is unconscious of his two arms and legs, he is speechless, he has an ailment not to be treated.

Record keeping and documentation increased knowledge about the care of the sick and helped spread this accumulated information. Evidence exists that medicines were prescribed in ancient times. The following remedy, also noted in the *Book of Surgery,* was prescribed for crying children (Lucas, 1953, p. 62):

> Pods of poppy plant
> Fly dirt which is on the wall
> Make it into one, strain, give for four days

One wonders how many children survived the cure.

The Hebrews

Around 2000 BC the Hebrew people kept written records and instructed as to what was safe to eat and drink. Considering the lack of refrigeration at that time and the prevalence of parasites the following advice was excellent:

> Ye are the children of the Lord your God
> Thou shalt not eat any abominable thing
> Ye shall not eat of them that chew the cud
>   as the camel, the hare or the swine
> Ye shall eat of all that are in the waters,
>   all that have fins and scales.
> All clean birds ye shall eat, but not
>   the vulture or his kind
> Ye shall not eat of anything that dieth of itself.
>
> DEUTERONOMY XII:7-21

One group of Hebrews, the Israelites, developed a moral code that greatly influenced the cultural environment of that time. The Ten Commandments, for example, continue to influence Judeo-Christian cultures today:

> THE TEN COMMANDMENTS
> You shall have no other gods before me.
> You shall not make for yourself a graven image. . . .
> You shall not take the name of the Lord your God in vain. . . .
> Observe the sabbath day. . . .
> Honor your father and your mother. . . .

You shall not kill.
Neither shall you commit adultery.
Neither shall you steal.
Neither shall you bear false witness against your neighbor.
Neither shall you covet your neighbor's wife. . . .

DEUTERONOMY V:7-21

The teachings of Jesus Christ, which form the basis of the Christian religion, emphasized empathy and concern for others. Jesus commanded his followers to "love thy neighbor as thyself" (Mark XII:31). This gentle approach to human relationships still influences the way that Christian religious groups, many of which still exist today, provide care to the sick.

Ancient Greece

The Greeks developed a society that took great interest in healing disease and preventing illness. This is evidenced in the writings of two of the famous Greek physicians who lived in ancient times.

Hippocrates, who is believed to have lived between 460 to 375 BC, documented his work with his associates, who were called the Guild of Healers. They studied anatomy and classified diseases. They encouraged rest, fresh air, diet, and cleanliness as prevention against disease (Lucas, 1953).

Galen, who lived in the second century AD, wrote numerous treatises on anatomy and physiology. He was the first person to write about the study of animals, and he documented his experiments with animals (*The Columbia Enclyclopedia*, vol 8, 1969).

Rome (79 AD to 476 AD)

The Roman culture made a major contribution to the advancement of sanitation. When the city of Pompeii was excavated, archaeologists found the Roman methods of water distribution and drainage systems to be quite sophisticated. The Romans also established hospitals and health organizations. One excavated hospital contained forty wards, vestibules, administration rooms, and apothecary shops (Lucas, 1953).

When the Western Roman Empire collapsed (476 AD), the eastern Byzantine section served as a keeper of the developed culture. The Byzantine empire preserved the scientific knowledge, moral codes, and works of art accumulated up to this time from invading Mongols and Turks (Lucas, 1953).

THE MIDDLE AGES
Western Civilization (500 AD to 1200 AD)

After the fall of Rome the Western world moved into the Dark Ages. Constant warfare and plague depleted energy and creative thought. Scientific and rational thought became eroded by folk practices. The Celts, Germans, and Slavs relied on spells and incantations to cure disease. The following example is taken from German folklore (Lucas, 1953, p. 280):

> Balder and Woden fared to a wood there was Balder's foal's foot sprained. Then charmed Woden as well he know how for bone sprain for blood sprain for limb sprain bone to bone, blood to blood, limb to limb as though they were glued.

Vestiges of this kind of folk remedy still surface in today's society, particularly when medical science has no effective treatment for an incurable disease and people feel hopeless and helpless as they did during the early Middle Ages.

The Crusades (1096 to 1149)

The early crusades, which took place over a 50-year period, were an attempt to rid the city of Jerusalem and the surrounding area of so-called infidels or people who did not believe in Jesus Christ. Knights and nobles from France and England journeyed from their homes to Palestine. Their adoption of some Greek and Arabic concepts of science is believed to have contributed to scientific thought in the Western world.

Religious Figures

St. Francis of Assisi (1181-1226) was a Christian monk who founded an order that included men and women, called brothers and sisters, who cared for the sick and helped the destitute. Some of the hospitals in the United States are still administered by the Franciscan order.

St. Thomas Aquinas (1225-1274), a Dominican monk, developed a concept of cause and effect, which resulted in a method of logical reasoning that is rational and linear in character. It led to a tendency to treat the body and the mind separately. Although nursing has taken a more holistic approach in recent years, this philosophical approach still is apparent in medical practice today.

Epidemics (1353 to 1400)

Bubonic plague (Black Death), typhus (the plague), smallpox, scarlet fever, and diphtheria occurred in epidemic proportion throughout Europe during the fourteenth century. In the year 1394 it is estimated that two thirds of the European population died during an outbreak of the Black Plague. This widespread occurrence of disease contributed to the lack of scientific development during the so-called Dark Ages.

THE RENAISSANCE (1400 to 1700)

From the fifteenth through the seventeenth centuries a period of "rebirth" occurred. A group called *the humanists* encouraged reading, art, and literature, and there was renewed interest in pursuing a scientific approach to curing illness and preventing disease. Furthermore, with the discovery of America by Christopher Columbus, much of the work by scientists such as Copernicus, Galileo, and Sir Isaac Newton was accepted. Copernicus' discovery that the earth was only part of a planetary system, Galileo's work in astronomy and physics, and Newton's proof of the laws of gravity stimulated reflection, scientific methods, and logical reasoning in other fields. The events of the Renaissance ushered in the Age of Enlightenment in the 1700s.

Seminal Figures

St. Vincent de Paul (1581-1660) founded the Sisters of Charity. His society of missioners and "dames de charité" went from cottage to cottage giving food, medicine, and care to the sick. He encouraged the brothers and sisters in the order to "help people help themselves" (Dolan, 1973).

William Harvey (1578-1657), an English physician and anatomist, discovered blood circulation. His book, *Anatomical Exercises and Motions of the Heart in Animals,* provided health professionals with information that helped them understand blood circulation in human beings.

Theodur Fliedner founded the deaconesses of Germany in the seventeenth century, who created hospices to provide care for the sick and destitute.

Edward Jenner (1749-1823), who proved that cowpox provided immunity against smallpox, laid the foundation for modern immunology as a science.

CONTRIBUTORS

Since before antiquity nurses have cared for the sick and attempted to heal or cure. Their role and their ability to influence health care always have depended on the cultural and the historical events of the time. Even in the Neolithic Age the older men and women in a tribe were looked on as healers and caretakers, and those individuals who seemed to have a talent for caretaking and a concern about the sick were consulted. This tradition continued through ancient times and the Middle Ages. The Brothers and Sisters of Mercy of the Franciscan order, founded in the twelfth century, are perhaps the first organized and longest-surviving group. A number of individuals have made significant contributions to the nursing profession, and their profiles are presented here.

Mother D'Youville (1701-1771)

In Montreal, Canada, Mother D'Youville founded an order called the Grey Nuns of the Sacred Heart. These women provided a home for orphans and unwed mothers. (See

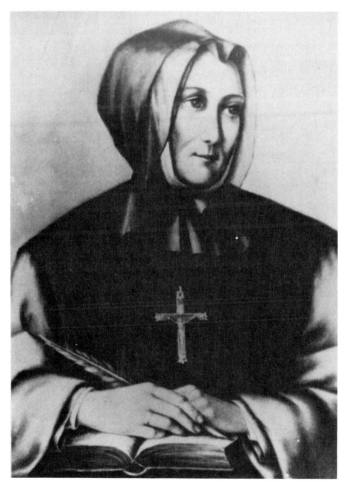

FIG. 1-1 Mother D'Youville (1701-1771), founder of the Grey Nuns of the Sacred Heart. The nuns visited the sick at home and provided a home for orphans and unwed mothers. *(Reprinted by permission of D'Youville College Archives, Buffalo, NY.)*

Fig. 1-1.) They also began a program that included visiting the sick in their homes. A branch of the order moved to Buffalo, New York, and continued ministering to the needs of the community. This group, which still exists, provides family care, job training, and education to community residents. The nuns started a school in Buffalo in 1908 that included a nursing school. Today this school offers programs that lead to baccalaureate and master of science degrees in nursing. Branches of the order exist in other parts of the world.

Florence Nightingale (1820-1910)

Florence Nightingale was employed as superintendent of the Home for Invalid Ladies in England until 1854. When England became involved in the Crimean War in 1853, she was asked to take a group of nurses to the war zone to care for the wounded.

Nightingale went to Scutari in the Crimea with 38 nurses. She reported that the barracks were "filthy, delapidated [sic] and had no sanitation" (Baly 1986, p. 5). The small group of nurses had to plan cooking arrangements, organize the hospital, and give care, at times, to four miles of patients (Baly 1986, p. 6) In addition, despite the lack of cooperation from the military physicians, the nurses' work made a measurable difference in the mortality rate from secondary infection and disease.

Nightingale believed that sanitation, ventilation, and the proper foods would prevent a good deal of sickness. She also believed that nursing was an art as well as a science. These beliefs were put into practice during her work in the Crimean War.

Nightingale's experience left her physically ill and emotionally drained, but she returned home a national heroine. A grateful English public collected a large sum of money, which was placed into a fund called *The Nightingale Fund,* for her use in supervising a hospital nursing school. She used it to establish a training school for nurses at St. Thomas Hospital in London. She never directly supervised the nurses nor taught them, but she set up the program and hired the staff that provided these functions. She also helped finance the Nurses Home near Liverpool Hospital, where nurses were trained to provide home nursing care, which became a model that was used to establish branches of the District Nursing Service throughout England. Nightingale insisted that in addition to nursing the patient, a home nurse should show the family how to achieve sanitary conditions, keep the patient's room healthy, and improvise appliances in the home for patient care (Baly 1986, p. 132). Florence Nightingale's ability to organize and influence the development of nursing had a profound effect on the profession, one that is still felt today.

Queen Victoria (1819-1901)

In 1887 Queen Victoria appropriated a large sum of money to found the Queen Victoria Jubilee Institute for nursing the poor and the sick in their homes. By the end of the century 539 nurses had formed the District Nursing Service, which was modeled after the Nightingale home nursing plan. These nurses, who lived in a nursing home and were responsible to a home supervisor, were trained in the hospitals for 1 year and then received 13 months of additional training in public health. Similar district nursing services were set up throughout the United Kingdom (Raveno, 1921).

Clara Barton (1821-1912)

Clara Barton was inspired by the work of Jean Henri Durant, who founded the International Red Cross in 1863. Its guidelines state that it mobilizes services to assist soldiers and civilians during time of war and assists civilians and soldiers who have been caused suffering during the war. In peacetime it helps individuals who have been affected by personal or community disaster. It maintains a Red Cross nursing reserve that could be called on in times of emergency (Griffin & Griffin, 1973).

Barton spent years studying the organization of the Red Cross in other countries. She returned to the United States and in 1881 persuaded government officials to organize the American Red Cross. She became its first president in 1882.

American Red Cross nurses served in their first war in Cuba during the Spanish-American confrontation in 1898. In 1900 the Red Cross received its first federal charter, with William Howard Taft proclaiming himself ex officio president of the organization (Griffin & Griffin, 1973).

Jane Delano (1862-1919)

In the late nineteenth century Jane Delano organized the American Red Cross Nursing Service and became president of the Associated Alumni of Nurses (later to be called the American Nurses' Association). As a result of her administrative experience she was asked, in 1909, to become superintendent of the Army Nurse Corps reserve. Her chief goal was to improve the quality of nurses who would be reserve members of the Corps. She succeeded in building up the reserve list to 3000 nurses before she resigned as superintendent in 1912 (Fitzpatrick, 1983). Her successors, Isabel McIsaac and Doris Thompson, continued her work.

Jane Delano, as head of nursing for the American Red Cross, and Doris Thompson, as superintendent of the Army Nurse Corps, organized base hospitals and staffed them with members of the Army Nurse Corps before and during World War I (Fitzpatrick, 1983). Their leadership and organizational abilities were responsible for saving many lives during the war.

Lillian Wald (1867-1940)

Lillian Wald was a prominent figure in the organization of public health in the United States. She graduated from the New York School of Nursing in 1891. Then she and a friend, Mary Brewster, rented a tenement in New York City and established a center called the Henry Street Settlement, where Wald employed nurses to work on a fee-for-service basis. Wald developed a detailed and comprehensive method of keeping records and statistics regarding the incidence and prevalence of disease in the neighborhoods in which the nurses worked. Her nurses taught families how to care for sick members, promote good hygiene, encourage prevention of disease, and raise healthy children (Fig. 1-2). They also were encouraged to delve into the social causes of the illnesses that affected families. The poor of New York City, for example, were victims of tuberculosis, cholera, scarlet fever, and diphtheria.

Lillian Wald worked closely with health administrators, physicians, and legislative officials. It was largely through her efforts that a Children's Bureau was formed to facilitate care of sick children in New York City. Wald also was instrumental in organizing the Town and Country Service of the American Red Cross. In addition, the nursing division of the Metropolitan Life Insurance Company was formed at her urging (Griffin and Griffin, 1965). Wald convinced the Metropolitan's executives that it was more economical to use the services of her nurses than to employ their own. She wrote of her experiences in *The House on Henry Street* and noted the many obstacles her nurses had to overcome to reach the families that needed home care.

Wald believed that public health nurses had to know more about teaching and prevention than did hospital nurses. She and her friend Mary Gardner were instrumental in organizing the National Organization for Public Health Nursing (NOPHN). The purpose

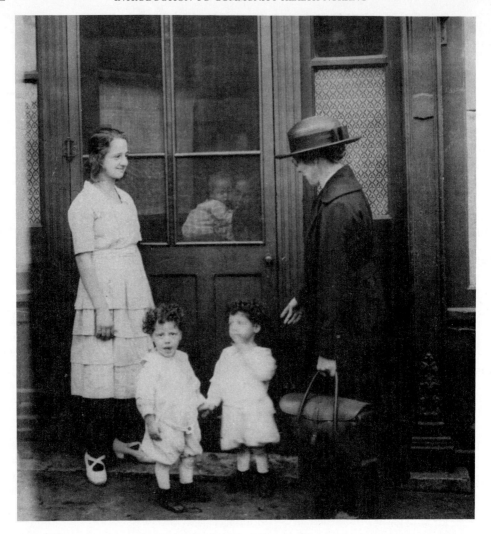

FIG. 1-2 Visiting nurse, circa 1900. *(Reprinted by permission of the Visiting Nursing Association of Western NY.)*

of the new society was to standardize public health efforts at a high level and coordinate all efforts in the field (Griffin & Griffin, 1973). The NOPHN stressed collaboration with physicians, legislators, and public health officials. Lillian Wald became its first president. This group, probably more than any other, influenced the development of organized public health nursing in this country until it was absorbed by the National League of Nurses in 1952, which also incorporated the following organizations: the National League for Nursing Education, the Association of Collegiate Schools of Nursing, the Joint Committee of Practical Nurses and Auxiliary Workers in Nursing Services, the Joint Committee on Careers in Nursing, and the National Accrediting Service. (Table 1-2 lists nursing organizations in the United States.)

TABLE 1-2 Development of nursing organizations in the United States

Year	Society	Purpose and function
1894	National League for Nursing Education	• To expand American Society of Superintendents of Training Schools • To establish minimum entrance requirements • To improve living and working conditions • To increase opportunities for postgraduate and specialized training
1900	American Red Cross	• To maintain a reserve list of nurses who can serve in war and disaster • To instruct the public in hygiene and care of the sick
1911	American Nurses' Association (ANA)	• To establish and maintain a code of ethics • To elevate standards of nursing education • To promote interests of the nursing profession
1912	National Organization of Public Health Nurses	• To standardize public health nursing • To coordinate efforts in the field
1952	National League for Nursing	• To expand NOPHN • To provide examination and related services for use in licensing professionals • To accredit educational programs for nurses • To promote continued study and educational curricula to meet changing needs • To define standards for organized nursing services and education
1952	Reorganized American Nurses' Association	• To work for continuing improvement of professional practice • To define functions and promote standards of professional nurse practice • To provide professional counseling • To serve as a national lobby for professional nurses • To implement the international exchange of nurses' program
1953	National Student Nurses' Association	• To represent student nurses • To provide counseling • To interact with ANA to promote improvement of professional practice

THE TWENTIETH CENTURY
World War I

American casualties in World War I numbered over 318,000: 50,280 were killed in battle, 62,000 died of disease, and 206,000 were wounded despite the work of the Army Nurse Corps and the American Red Cross. Nurses worked close to the battlefield under grueling conditions. They were exposed to danger from disease and shelling. At times the nurse-patient ratio was 1:50, and a total of 101 nurses died (Surgeon General, 1919).

There was a nursing shortage in the war zone and at home. In 1918 Annie Warburton Goodrich, who had worked with Lillian Wald at the Henry Street Settlement, recommended the establishment of an army school of nursing to supply hospitals with needed personnel. The budget to support the school was approved in June 1918, and Goodrich became dean of the Nursing Department of the United States Army. In 1921, 500 nurses were graduated from the school and entered the Army Nurse Corps.

Julia Stimson, director of the American Expeditionary Force during World War I, believed that the Army Nurse Corps should be a progressive organization. After the war she replaced Annie Goodrich as dean of the army nursing school and began advocating that nurses become teachers of health, a role she believed was part of the nurse's responsibility (Griffin & Griffin, 1973).

Post–World War I

The Army Nurse Corps had distinguished itself during the war and under the direction of Annie Goodrich and Julia Stimson had developed quite a sophisticated curriculum which included some theoretical knowledge as well as technical skills. It was not until 1920, however, that nurses were given relative rank in the army, although physicians continued to have supervisory status. The army nursing school was closed in 1932 as an economic measure by the government (Griffin & Griffin, 1973), and membership in the Army Nurse Corps declined until about 1940 when a second world war appeared unavoidable.

World War II

The United States did not enter World War II until December 1941. The Council for National Defense, however, was organized in 1940, with Julia Stimson as president. The organization immediately began to recruit nurses in preparation for the need another war would create. It was instrumental in forming the Cadet Nurse Corps. In World War I the army had its own nursing school. In World War II the government provided tuition, fees, uniforms, and stipends to interested young women to attend existing schools. Many nurses were graduated from this program and entered military service at home or abroad (Fitzpatrick, 1983).

During this war the mobile army surgical hospital was formed (MASH). Nurses helped convert transport planes to flying ambulances and organized the loading and unloading of the sick and wounded. After the ill and injured were placed on board, the nurses were responsible for their care. The nurses' excellent work is evidenced by a record of five deaths per 100,000 casualties.

Post–World War II

After the war army nurses benefited from the GI Bill of Rights, which awarded veterans funds for education. This opportunity encouraged some nurses to return to school to obtain baccalaureate degrees.

The Korean War

During the Korean War the mobile Army surgical hospitals operated only 8 to 10 miles from the front line. Rapid evacuation of the wounded by helicopter considerably decreased the mortality rate of the combat troops (Fitzpatrick, 1983).

The Vietnam War

During the Vietnam War the concept of mobile hospital units was changed because there were no front lines. Medical unit, self-contained and transportable (MUST) was an inflatable rubber shelter with necessary equipment contained in a compact unit. These units were delivered to the combat zone, to which soldiers were transported by helicopter. Four navy nurses sustained wounds in a bombing in Saigon, and one Army nurse was killed at an evacuation hospital at Chu Lai (Fitzpatrick, 1983).

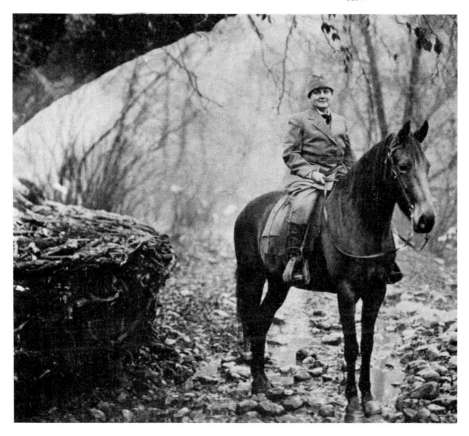

FIG. 1-3 Mary Breckinridge founded the Frontier Nursing Service in Lexington, Kentucky. *(Reprinted by permission of the Frontier Nursing Service, Wendover, KY.)*

The Frontier Nursing Service

Mary Breckinridge (Fig. 1-3) founded the Frontier Nursing Service (FNS) in Lexington, Kentucky, in 1925. The organization began as a small group whose purpose was to provide basic health care for mothers and babies in the hills of southeastern Kentucky. It soon became evident that it was impossible for a nurse to enter a home without providing care to the entire family. For example, a nurse would enter a home to check on an expectant mother and would be asked to give advice about a grandmother's leg ulcer. Soon Mary Breckinridge's nurses on horseback were providing a broad program of preventive and curative care for all family members. The program, after 62 years in operation in one of the poorest regions of the United States, is responsible for the delivery of more than 20,000 babies, with a loss of only 11 mothers in childbirth throughout its entire history.

Today the FNS includes a hospital that has a primary health clinic, four district nursing clinics, a home health agency, a dental clinic, and a school of midwifery (FNS Development Office).

Over the years the FNS has evolved into a model of decentralized health care in a rural setting. It is known worldwide as an exceptional example of family-centered health

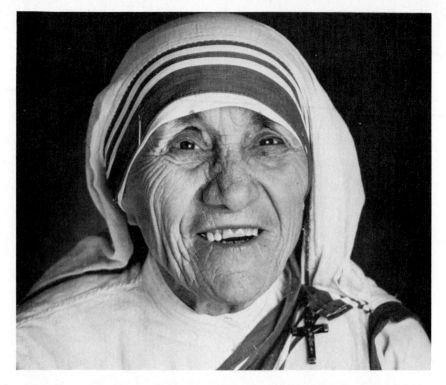

FIG. 1-4   Mother Teresa founded the Missionaries of Charity. They care for the sick and dying in India, Italy, Australia, Latin America, Holland, and New York City. *(Photo courtesy Michael Collopy.)*

care. Graduates from the school of midwifery at FNS have served all over the world, and each year professionals from other countries come to observe the program.

In the beginning nurses rode their horses through blizzards, fog, and floods on mountain paths and trails (Fig. 1-3). Today, nurses ride in Jeeps on roads that are at least passable. They still emphasize prevention and family care, which is consistent with the focus of public health nursing since Florence Nightingale's time when nurses began visiting the sick in the home. The family was then and remains now the unit of care for the public health nurse.

Mother Teresa

Mother Teresa (Fig. 1-4) is a world-renowned nurse from the religious community. In 1955 she founded the Missionaries of Charity. They minister to the needs of dying derelicts, abandoned children, and starving adults. Mother Teresa's work began in Calcutta and has spread to Rome, Australia, Latin America, Holland, and New York City.

NURSING THEORY AND COMMUNITY HEALTH NURSING

The development of a theory of nursing has helped to legitimize nursing as a profession. Nursing scholars have analyzed the nature and scope of nursing knowledge and practice in an attempt to define the role of the nurse and to explain its unique contribution to the individual person, to health, and to the environment. Nursing theory helps to guide practice, to stimulate research, and to upgrade professional education.

The Standards of Community Health Nursing Practice state that the nurse applies theoretical concepts to decision making in practice. Florence Nightingale recommended that the nurse be instrumental in manipulating the environment to improve health. In so doing, she influenced the development of the practice of nursing in the community in a very meaningful way.

This text focuses on the work of Betty Neuman as a basis for practice. Her broad concept of nurse, environment, health, and client encompasses the entire community within a systems framework. A client is viewed by Neuman as an interacting open system in total interface with both internal and environmental forces or stressors. The environment is the viable arena that has relevance to the life space of the system. The nurse's role is to keep the client system stable through accuracy both in assessment of effects and possible effects of environmental stressors and in assisting client adjustments required for an optimal wellness level (Neuman, 1989).

Neuman perceives nursing as "a unique profession that is concerned with all the variables affecting an individual's response to stress." The goal of nursing according to Neuman is "to facilitate for the client optimal wellness through retention, attainment or maintenance of client system stability." She views persons as dynamic composites of interrelationships among physiological, psychological, sociocultural, and developmental factors. Health is a condition in which all parts and subparts are in harmony with the whole of the client/client system (Neuman, 1989).

Other nursing theorists continue to contribute to nursing's knowledge base. This knowledge clarifies the nurse's role and provides the necessary groundwork on which to build an autonomous profession, clearly delineated as to its role in society and in the health care system. Table 1-3 outlines the concepts of selected nurse theorists who have influenced the development of community health nursing.

TABLE 1-3 Selected nursing theorists who have influenced the development of community health

Name	Time	Conceptual view of nurse's role
Florence Nightingale	1910	Nurse manipulates the environment to allow the patient time to recover.
Hildegard Peplau	1952	Nurse is involved in a therapeutic interpersonal process that makes health possible for individuals and communities.
Virginia Henderson	1955	Nurse assists the individual in activities contributing to health or its recovery (or to a peaceful death).
Dorothea Orem	1958	Nurse takes action to assist clients who have self-care deficits.
Faye Abdellah	1960	Nurse gives services to individuals, families, and societies.
Sister Callista Roy	1964	Nurse intervenes to facilitate the adaptation process of human beings.
Martha Rogers	1970	Nurse seeks to promote symphonic interaction between the environment and the human being.
Madeleine Leininger	1978	Nurse focuses on behaviors in individuals and groups toward promoting, maintaining, and recovering health, which have physical, psychocultural, and social significance for those assisted.
Dorothy Johnson	1980	Nurse is an external force acting to preserve the organization of the person's behavior.
Betty Neuman	1982	Nursing is a unique profession that is concerned with all the variables affecting an individual's response to stress.

PUBLIC HEALTH NURSING

Public health nursing was redefined by the American Public Health Association in 1980 to incorporate the impact of nursing theory on public health nursing practice (American Public Health Association, 1980, p. 4):

> Public health nursing synthesizes the body of knowledge from the public health sciences and professional nursing theories for the purpose of improving the health of the entire community. This goal lies at the heart of primary prevention and health promotion and is a foundation for public practice.

As all nurses begin to define their role in a broad way that focuses not only on the patient and the family but also on the effect of the total environment on the patient/ client and the family, they are becoming more involved in the community. For this reason, public health nurses now are being described as community health nurses.

In 1980 the American Nurses' Association (ANA) defined community health nursing as follows (p. 2):

> Community health nursing is a synthesis of nursing theory and public health practice applied to promoting and preserving the health of populations. Health promotion, health maintenance, health education and management, coordination, and continuity of care are utilized in a holistic approach to the management of the health care of individuals, families and groups in the community.

STANDARDS OF COMMUNITY HEALTH NURSING PRACTICE

Standard I: Theory

The nurse applies theoretical concepts as a basis for decisions in practice.

Standard II: Data collection

The nurse systematically collects data that are comprehensive and accurate.

Standard III: Diagnosis

The nurse analyzes data collected about the community, family, and individual to determine diagnoses.

Standard IV: Planning

At each level of prevention, the nurse develops plans that specify nursing actions unique to client needs.

Standard V: Intervention

The nurse, guided by the plan, intervenes to promote, maintain, or restore health, to prevent illness, and to effect rehabilitation.

Standard VI: Evaluation

The nurse evaluates responses of the community, family, and individual to interventions in order to determine progress toward goal achievement and to revise the data base, diagnoses, and plan.

Standard VII: Quality assurance and professional development

The nurse participates in peer review and other means of evaluation to assure quality of nursing practice. The nurse assumes responsibility for professional development and contributes to the professional growth of others.

Standard VIII: Interdisciplinary collaboration

The nurse collaborates with other health care providers, professionals, and community representatives in assessing, planning, implementing, and evaluating programs for community health.

Standard IX: Research

The nurse contributes to theory and practice in community health nursing through research.

Reprinted with permission from *Standards of community health nursing practice*, American Nurses' Association, © 1986, Kansas City, Mo.

This definition includes the following assumptions (ANA, pp. 2-4):

1. The health care system is complex.
2. Primary, secondary, and tertiary prevention are components of the health care system.
3. Nursing, as a subsystem of the health care system, is the product of education and practice based on research.
4. The provision of primary health care predominates in community health practice with lesser involvement in secondary and tertiary health care.

The ANA has set standards of community health nursing practice in an attempt to clarify the functions of the nurse's role (box on opposite page.)

SUMMARY

Throughout the ages historical events and the beliefs and activities of certain influential individuals have affected social attitudes toward the care of the sick and toward nursing.

Nursing as an organized profession began when Florence Nightingale started a training school for nurses at St. Thomas Hospital in London. Lillian Wald contributed greatly to the development of community health nursing in the United States by founding settlement houses.

Nursing theory has added a sense of professionalism to community health nursing practice. Defining the role of the nurse relative to a person, health, and environment has helped to delineate the nurse's role in society and in the health care delivery system.

Community health nursing is a synthesis of nursing theory and public health practice applied to promoting and preserving the health of populations. Community health nurses utilize a holistic approach in the management of the health care of individuals, families, and communities.

CHAPTER HIGHLIGHTS

- Historical events throughout antiquity, the Middle Ages, and modern times have influenced societal attitudes toward the care of the nurse and nursing.
- Thomas Aquinas developed the concept of cause and effect, a method of logical reasoning.
- The Age of Enlightenment was ushered in by the work of scientists such as Copernicus, Galileo, and Newton, who stimulated reflection, scientific methods, and logical reasoning.
- Florence Nightingale perceived the nurse's role to be the manipulation of the immediate environment to give the patient a chance to recover. Other nursing theorists attempted to define the role of the nurse relative to the individual person, to health, and to the environment.
- Public health nursing synthesizes the body of knowledge from the public health sciences and professional nursing theories for the purpose of improving the health of the entire community.
- Community health nursing synthesizes nursing theory and public health practice to promote and preserve the health of populations. Health promotion, health maintenance, and continuity of care are incorporated into a holistic approach to the management of the health care of individuals, families, and groups in the community.

STUDY QUESTIONS

1. Describe five historical events that have influenced the attitudes of society toward the care of the sick and nursing.

2. Describe Florence Nightingale's unique role in the development of community health nursing.
3. Discuss the impact of nursing theory on community health nursing.
4. Define community health nursing.
5. Describe the ANA Standards of Community Health Nursing Practice.

REFERENCES

American Nurses' Association, Division on Community Nursing. (1980). *A conceptual model of community health nursing* (ANA Pub No Ch-102 M, 5/80). Kansas City, MO: (Author) (2420 Pershing Rd, Kansas City, MO 64108).

American Public Health Association, Nursing Section (1980). *The definition and role of public health nursing in the delivery of health care.* Washington, DC: Author.

Baly, M. B. (1986). *Florence Nightingale and the nursing legacy.* Beckenham, UK: Croom Helm.

Breckenridge, M. (1981). *Wide neighborhoods.* Lexington, KY: The University Press of Kentucy.

Dolan, J. (1973) *Nursing in society.* New York: Saunders. D'Youville College Archives, Buffalo, NY. 14214.

Falco, S. (1980). *Nursing theories: The base for professional nursing practice.* Englewood Cliffs, NJ, Prentice-Hall.

Fitzpatrick, L. (1983). *Prologue to professionalism: A history of nursing.* London: Prentice-Hall International.

Frontier Nursing Service, Development Office, Wendover, KY 41775.

Giff, P. (1986). *Mother Teresa: Sister to the poor.* New York: 1986, Viking Penguin.

Griffin, G.J., & Griffin, J.K. (1973). *History and trends of professional nursing.* (7th ed.). St. Louis: Mosby.

Hall, J. & Weaver, B.R. (1986). *A systems approach to community health.* Philadelphia: Lippincott.

Henderson, V. (1966). *The nature of nursing: A definition and its implications for practice research and education.* New York: Macmillan.

King, I. (1981). *A theory of nursing: Systems, concepts, process.* New York: Wiley.

Leininger, M. (1984). *Care: The essence of nursing and health.* Thorofare, NJ: Slack.

Lucas, H.S. (1953). *A short history of civilization* (2nd ed.). New York: McGraw-Hill.

Marriner-Tomey A. (1989). *Nursing theorists and their work* (2nd ed.) St. Louis: Mosby.

Neuman, B. (1989). *The Neuman systems model* (2nd ed.). Norwalk, CT: Appleton & Lange.

Orem, D. (1985). *Nursing concepts of practice* (3rd ed.). New York: McGraw-Hill.

Peplau, H. (1952). *Interpersonal relationships in nursing.* New York: Putnam's Sons.

Ravenol, M. (1921). *A half century of public health.* New York: American Public Health Association.

Surgeon General of the United States. (1919). *Report of the surgeon general.* Washington, DC, United States Army Historical Unit.

Toffler, A. (1970) *Future shock.* New York: Random House.

The Visiting Nurses Association, 4230 Ridge Lea Road, Amherst, NY 14226.

Health Care Delivery Systems

JOAN M. COOKFAIR

A system can be defined as a complex of interacting elements.

LUDWIG VAN BERTALANFFY

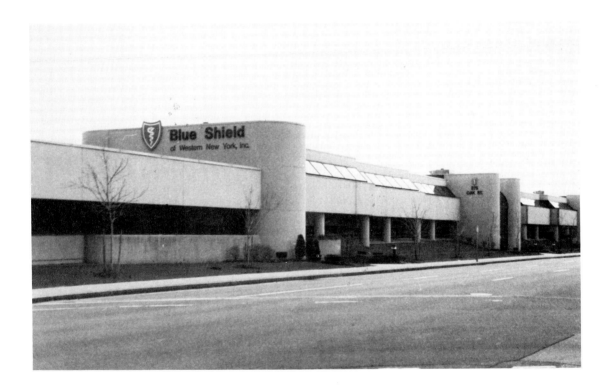

OBJECTIVES

At the conclusion of this chapter the student will be able to:

1. Define the key terms listed
2. Discuss the health care delivery system from a historical perspective
3. Identify the components of the health care delivery system in the United States
4. Describe types of health care financing in the United States
5. Identify selected problems in the health care delivery system and discuss proposed solutions
6. Describe the health care delivery systems in selected countries outside the United States

KEY TERMS

Accreditation

Diagnosis-related groups (DRGs)

Health maintenance organizations (HMOs)

Licensure

Medicaid

Medicare

Omnibus Budget Reconciliation Act

Private sector

Prospective payment system

Public sector

Social vulnerability index

One of the first attempts at providing organized health care in the United States was made by the Dutch East India Company in 1658 when it established a small company clinic in New York City. This "cottage hospital," which eventually became Bellevue Hospital, still exists today. Some other hospitals founded about that time were Philadelphia General Hospital, Charity Hospital in New Orleans, and the Boston Dispensary. The creation of these institutions for the sick precipitated the establishment of the American Medical Association in 1847 and the Nightingale School of Nursing in 1873. By 1890 there were fifteen schools of nursing in the United States. The Joint Commission for the Accreditation of Hospitals was formed in 1918, and the American Hospital Association was established in 1951 (Hawkins & Higgins, 1982).

BEGINNINGS OF HEALTH DEPARTMENTS IN THE UNITED STATES
Local Level

Epidemics in the United States in the eighteenth and nineteenth centuries led to the need for public health regulations. Efforts to fill this need led to the development of local health departments, many of which still exist today. Local health departments generally are responsible to city, town, or county governments.

State Level

State health departments became involved in health care when the Louisiana legislature established the first permanent state board of health in the United States in 1869. According to the Constitution, states have the power to enact and enforce laws to protect their populations.

INVOLVEMENT IN THE HEALTH CARE SYSTEM

The official entry of the federal government into the health care delivery system began in 1798 when an act of Congress established the Marine Hospital for the relief of sick and disabled seamen. The evolution of the role of the federal government can be traced through the laws passed by Congress over the past 200 years.

Federal involvement in health care was expanded in 1935 when the Social Security Act made provisions for old-age and survivors' assistance, child health care, and aid to crippled children. The Hill-Burton Act of 1946 provided money for upgrading and equipping public and private health institutions. The Nurse Training Act in 1964 provided direct support for students and schools of nursing. Medicaid was enacted in 1965 to provide health care to certain low-socioeconomic groups. Medicare provided care for those over 65. Between 1961 and 1968 Congress passed 138 laws influencing health care delivery. The Comprehensive Health Services amendment of 1966 created health planning agencies to coordinate health services. The Occupational Safety and Health Act was enacted by the Ninety-first Congress and signed into law by President Nixon on December 29, 1970. In 1972 state labor departments began actively enforcing the Act, and every employee in the country came under the jurisdiction of the Occupational Safety and Health Administration (OSHA), which charged employers with the responsibility of furnishing their employees with safe working conditions in a site free from recognized hazards that cause or are likely to cause death or serious physical harm (Hogan & Hogan, 1977).

The Health Maintenance Act (1973) authorized grant funding and loans to stimulate funding of health maintenance organizations. The National Health Planning and Resources Act (1974) promoted collaborative efforts among local, state, and federal agencies. By 1979 a network of 205 health service agencies had been designated by state governments and approved by the Department of Health, Education and Welfare (Hawkins and Higgins, 1982) (renamed the Department of Health and Human Services in 1979). These agencies functioned until 1987 when the Health Planning and Resources Act was repealed.

In 1982 the Omnibus Budget Reconciliation Act was enacted, which created large cuts in domestic programs (Jonas, 1986). The legislation reduced the allowable income for persons to qualify for Aid to Families with Dependent Children (AFDC). Furthermore, families ineligible for this aid were no longer automatically eligible for Medicaid.

In 1983 the Tax Equity and Responsibility Act established a cost-per-case basis for hospital payment and placed a ceiling on the rate of increase in hospital revenues that would be supported by the Medicare program. It mandated the prospective payment system for Medicare patients.

The 1983 amendments to the Social Security Act defined a set, preestablished payment fee for types of cases defined by diagnosis-related groups (DRGs). These groupings are divided into 23 major diagnostic categories, which are subdivided into 470 diagnostic groups. Each group is medically oriented, and the entire prospective payment system is based on a medical model.

In January 1989 the Medicare Catastrophic Coverage Act expanded the scope of Medicare benefits to include an unlimited hospital stay for covered services and 150 days in a skilled nursing facility. Hospice and psychiatric benefits also were increased. Many senior citizens, concerned about their inability to pay the increased income tax surcharge that would have funded it, lobbied successfully for its repeal in December of that year.

Table 2-1 outlines the history of federal legislation affecting the health care delivery system.

Local, state, and federal governments have contributed to the evolution of the health care delivery system in the United States. Professional associations, such as the American

TABLE 2-1 Federal legislation affecting the health care system	
Date	**Legislation**
1798	Bill to create the United States Marine Hospital (Marine Hospital Service) for sick and disabled seamen
1849	Indian Health Affairs assigned to Department of Interior
1906	Pure Food and Drugs Act
1912	Creation of Children's Bureau; Marine Hospital Service renamed Public Health Service
1922	Bill to provide monies for child health care and establish child and maternity centers
1935	Social Security Act
1944	Public Health Service Act extended to all National Institutes of Health; authority to award research grants to nonfederal establishments
1946	Hill-Burton legislation, which authorized federal assistance in the construction of hospitals and health centers, improved beds per population ratios, especially in rural areas; National Mental Health Act—National Institute of Mental Health created
1949	Establishment of a common system of 10 regional offices of the Federal Security Agency (later to become the nucleus of the Department of Health, Education and Welfare)
1953	Establishment of the Department of Health, Education and Welfare (DHEW) as a cabinet-status agency
1956	Authorization of the National Health Survey, a continuing interview and clinical appraisal of the health of Americans; Vocational Rehabilitation Act amendments; Housing and Urban Development Act; establishment of the National Library of Medicine
1958	Amendments to the 1906 Food, Drug, and Cosmetic Act requiring manufacturers of new food additives to submit evidence to the Food and Drug Administration (FDA) that a product's safety had been tested and established before marketing
1962	Organization of a Special Staff on Aging, later to become the Administration of Aging
1964	Nurse Training Act, aiding construction of new schools for nursing students and support for curriculum development; Economic Opportunity Act, creating the Office of Economic Opportunity (OEO)
1965	Medicare: medical health insurance for citizens 65 and older; Medicaid: medical assistance program for the indigent; Regional Medical Programs Act: regional cooperation in health care planning
1968	Vocational rehabilitation amendments extending appropriations for grants to states for services, innovation projects, and training
1970	Migrant health amendments, extending health services for migrant and other seasonal agricultural workers; creation of the Environmental Protection Agency (EPA), National Institute on Alcohol Abuse and Alcoholism, and the National Institute on Drug Abuse; Occupational Safety and Health Act (OSHA) (administered principally by the Department of Labor) to regulate and correct health hazards of the workplace
1971	National Cancer Act; Nurse Training Act: capitation grants to schools, support for advanced education; first federal law to reduce hazard of lead poisoning in children
1972	Social Security Act amendments: creating Professional Standards Review Organization (PSRO); further defined benefits under Medicaid and Medicare; important new benefits, including dialysis
1973	Health Maintenance Organization (HMO) Act: model for development of HMOs and funds for demonstration projects

Modified from *Nursing and the American health care delivery system* (pp. 59-63) ed. 3, by J. Hawkins and L. Higgins, 1989, New York: Tiresias Press.

TABLE 2-1 Federal legislation affecting health care system	
Date	**Legislation**
1974	National Health Planning and Resources Act
1976	National Health Consumer and Health Promotion Act; establishment of the Office of Health Information
1979	Nurse Training amendments; bill to create Department of Education (cabinet level) and to rename Health, Education and Welfare, the Department of Health and Human Services
1982	Omnibus Budget Reconciliation Act, which reduced the allowable income for families with dependent children to obtain aid
1983	Tax Equity and Fiscal Responsibility Act, which mandated prospective payment for Medicare patients; amendments to the Social Security Act defined a set of pre-established payment fees for types of cases divided into 23 diagnostic groupings

Nurses' Association, the American Medical Association, and the American Hospital Association, continue to influence and contribute to its development.

COMPONENTS OF THE HEALTH CARE DELIVERY SYSTEM
The Public Sector

The federal government. The federal government has the responsibility for the following aspects of health care: providing direct care for certain groups such as native Americans, military personnel, and veterans; and safeguarding the public health by regulating quarantines and immigration laws and the marketing of food, drugs, and products used in medical care. The government also should prevent environmental hazards; gives grants-in-aid to states, local areas, and individuals; and supports research (Hawkins & Higgins, 1982). The most important federal agency involved with health care is the Department of Health and Human Services, which is responsible for the administration of Social Security, social welfare, and related programs. The Surgeon General of the United States is the chief executive of this department. The health functions are administered by the US Public Health Service, which in turn works through several branches (Fig. 2-1) (Roemer, 1982).

A number of other agencies supervise the quality of health care in the United States. The Drug Enforcement Agency is responsible for dealing with all aspects of alcohol and drug abuse. The Health Services Administration oversees the financing of federal grants to state agencies, and the Centers for Disease Control have the responsibility for surveillance and prevention of disease. The Food and Drug Administration is authorized to monitor the safety and effectiveness of new drugs. The Health Resource Administration is concerned with such needs as adequate personnel for health care and hospital construction. The National Institutes of Health grant monies for research to universities and other centers for research.

State governments. Many state agencies are involved in the health care delivery system, with major responsibilities in the following areas (Hawkins & Higgins, 1982):

1. Control of licensure, vital statistics, medical laboratories, and fire and sanitation regulations and enforcement of OSHA regulations
2. Enforcement of third-party reimbursement, especially Medicaid
3. Policy influence on communicable disease control, data collection, and assessment

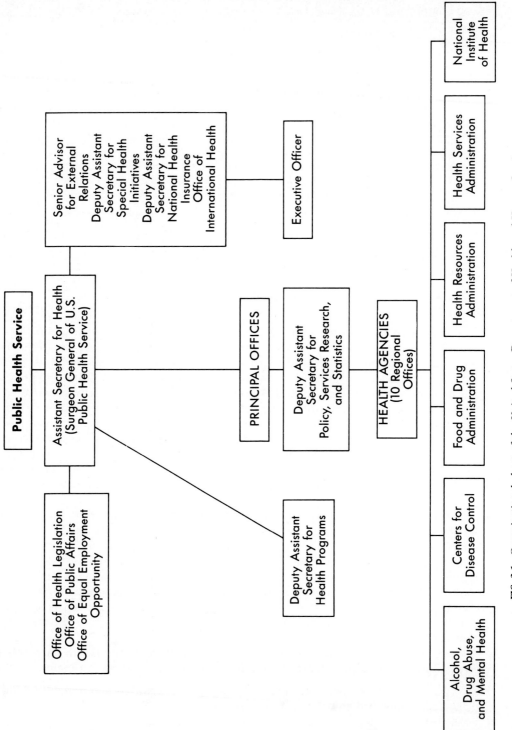

FIG. 2-1 Organizational chart of the United States Department of Health and Human Services.

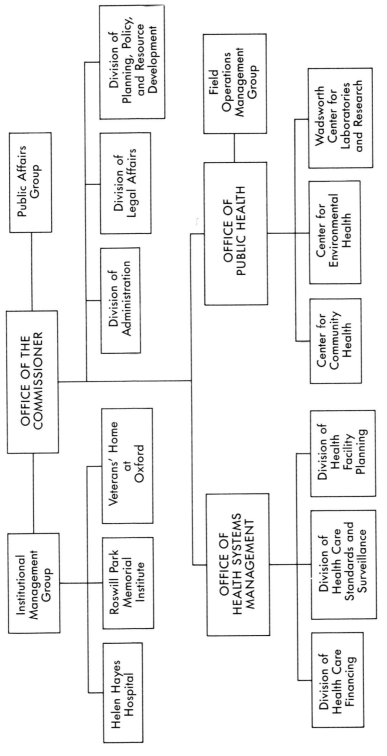

FIG. 2-2 Organizational chart of the New York State Department of Health. *(Reprinted with permission of the New York State Department of Health, Albany, NY.)*

4. Delivery of services, maternal and child care, public health nursing, keeping vital records, clinic services, etc.

An organizational chart of the New York State Department of Health is depicted in Fig. 2-2.

Local health departments. Local health departments focus on local regional needs. They usually provide immunization against infectious disease, direct environmental surveillance, and sponsor programs for maternal and infant child care. Fig. 2-3 depicts an organizational chart of a local health department in New York State.

The Private Sector

Physicians. Physicians in private practice provide care on a fee-for-service basis. They are paid directly by the patient or by third-party insurance. Physicians are largely responsible for setting fee levels.

Private hospitals. In the United States there are more than 6000 proprietary, for-profit hospitals and convalescent homes. They cater to upper- and middle-income clients and, unless there is an emergency situation, may refer to a public hospital those unable to pay. Physicians may wield considerable power in these institutions because the hospitals depend on the physicians' good will to obtain clients.

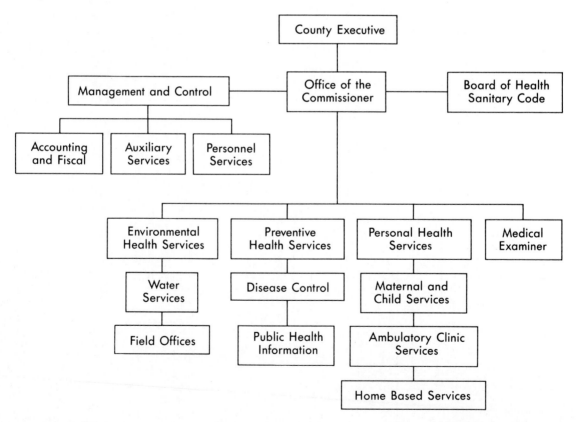

FIG. 2-3 Organizational chart of the Erie County Health Department. *(Reprinted by permission of the Erie County Health Department, Buffalo, NY.)*

Outpatient services. Most private hospitals offer care to ambulatory clients, although some provide this service through emergency rooms rather than through hospital-based outpatient clinics.

FINANCING OF HEALTH CARE
Medicare and Medicaid

Medicaid and Medicare benefits became available in 1965. Those persons eligible for Medicare benefits fit into two categories: (1) persons 65 years of age and older who are eligible for Social Security benefits and (2) disabled persons younger than 65 years who meet certain criteria for disability under Social Security regulations and have been disabled for more than 24 months (Stewart, 1979). A comparison of Medicaid and Medicare benefits is shown in Table 2-2.

Blue Cross

In the 1930s the American Hospital Association's bill to allow subscribers to enroll in a hospital prepayment plan was adopted by the New York State legislature. This payment plan arose out of the need for hospitals and physicians to be guaranteed an income after the depression of the 1930s. It was meant to provide payment for services for eligible persons who were financially able to enroll in a group plan. Blue Cross insurance, which initially was allied with the American Hospital Association, formally separated from the Association in 1972.

Blue Shield

Blue Shield also was created in the 1930s. Initially associated with the American Medical Association, it now is a separate entity. Blue Cross and Blue Shield insurance is purchased through group plans in the workplace or privately by individual persons who can afford it.

Health Maintenance Organizations

A health maintenance organization (HMO) is a prepaid health cooperative with an emphasis on prevention and health maintenance. Individual persons enroll in an organization

TABLE 2-2 Comparison of Medicare and Medicaid Benefits

	Medicaid (Title XIX)	Medicare (Title XVIII)
Description	Medical welfare for the disabled, the elderly, and families in need	Federal health insurance for the aged (65 yr and older)
Administration	Administered by welfare bureaus: federal, state, and local	Administered by Social Security Administration
Financing	Cost sharing: federal, state, and local	Financed by Social Security tax (Part B by monthly premium payments)
Eligibility	Left to state's means test (some 9 million below poverty level ineligible)	Virtually all (more than 90%) persons 65 yr and older
Services provided	Services delineated	Services delineated
Provider restrictions	Choice of provider physicians who accept Medicaid	Free choice of provider physicians

Modified from *Nursing and the American health care delivery system* (p. 106) ed. 3, by J. Hawkins and L. Higgins, 1989, New York: Tiresias Press.

that meets most of their health care needs. All HMOs, however, have common components:

1. They assume contractual responsibility for a stated range of health care services, including inhospital and ambulatory care.
2. They serve a voluntary population.
3. There is a fixed annual or monthly payment.
4. The HMO assumes some financial risk or gain.
5. In contrast with physicians in private practice, physicians employed by HMOs receive a fixed salary.

Independent Insurance Plans

Some profit-making insurance companies (e.g., Aetna and Metropolitan Life) sell supplemental major medical and cash payment policies that help defray costs not covered by other insurance policies. Prudential and the American Association of Retired Persons, for example, have developed a long-term care health care package for older citizens whose primary coverage is through Medicare only (Hays, 1989).

EVALUATION OF THE CURRENT SYSTEM
Problems

Most Americans believe that all persons have a right to equal access to health care; however, there is a marked decline in access for those who cannot pay. This lack is emphasized by the fact that Medicaid payments are based on a medical diagnosis of an illness. Thus preventive health care seldom is available to the indigent, which is not likely to change under the present system. Increasing the level of charity care will not solve the problem unless it includes health promotion and prevention in the community.

A further complication is the increase in technologic advances, which has created a gray area in terms of life and death issues. The use of this technology to prolong life is costly and controversial. Legislative action to define life in terms of function and not just heartbeat and brain wave has been proposed to allow the nonuse or withdrawal of life support systems for the terminally or chronically ill. Such a legal definition would reduce the fear of malpractice suits and would allow a dignified and comfortable death. This is, of course, a controversial area.

An example of the confusion and controversy that exists in the legal system is the Cruzan case. Nancy Cruzan was injured in an automobile accident 7 years ago. Ms. Cruzan was an active young woman prior to her accident and now remains in a vegetative state. Her parents, after watching her slowly deteriorate, never regaining consciousness, and being totally dependent on a feeding tube for her nourishment, petitioned the courts for authorization to remove her feeding tube. A lower court granted the petition. The Missouri Supreme Court reversed that ruling, and the case was then appealed to the United States Supreme Court. Their decision was to deny the Cruzans' petition based on the lack of stronger evidence of intent on the part of the patient. (Gibbs, 1990, Wetmiel, 1990).

Possible Solutions

Limiting malpractice claim awards might decrease the cost of health care, inasmuch as many physicians have raised fees to cover the high cost of malpractice insurance and are more likely to perform expensive tests in an effort to practice "defensive medicine." One possible solution might be to reevaluate the effectiveness of the DRG as the criterion for payment and replace it with another method.

TABLE 2-3 Factors and variables used in the social vulnerability index

Factors	Variable
Social pathology	Percentage of households receiving Aid for Families with Dependent Children (ADFC)
	Female head of household with children under 18 as a percentage of total families
Economic well being	Percentage of persons below poverty level
	Median family income
Education	Median school years completed by persons more than 25 years of age
	Median cost of education per pupil
	Percentage of free lunches
Health access	Hospital beds per 1,000 population
	Number of total physicians per 10,000 population
	Number of primary care physicians per 10,000 population
Health status	Infant mortality per 1,000 live births
	Percentage of low birth weight infants (2500 g)
	Teen pregnancy (ages 10-19) per 1,000 female population

From "Creation of a social vulnerability index for justice in health planning" by A. Dever et al., 1988; *Family & Community Health*, 10(4), p. 28. Copyright 1988 by Aspen Publishers. Reprinted with permission.

Reevaluating the advantages of establishing national health insurance might lead to ensuring health care for all citizens in the future.

An article in *Family & Community Health* suggests the use of a social vulnerability index to determine areas most in need of assistance. Use of such a tool could help to target types of assistance needed. (Table 2-3). A field study in the state of Georgia was performed with the use of this social vulnerability index (Figs. 2-4 and 2-5). Results were obtained relative to five factors: social pathology, economic well-being, level of education, health care access, and health status. Studies such as this could pinpoint areas of need and assure taxpayers that tax dollars were being used in a prudent manner in areas that are at highest risk for disease and disability.

Also proposed was a new conceptual model that recognizes the need to assess social vulnerability in the planning of health care. The authors argue that various disease patterns that go beyond infectious diseases, that is, chronic disease patterns, require a change in life style to promote wellness. The model, shown in Fig. 2-6, includes a life-style component, which is directed toward values and dilemmas that either impair or create social justice. Included is a recognition of the change to a service and information transfer society, which recognizes a need for collective caring, an allusion to the accelerating rates of change in the society, increased technology, information overload, and stress. The model shows that the population is aging and lists social illnesses, such as drug abuse, infections that result from life-style, and violence, caused by certain disease patterns. Finally, the authors present their perceptions of ethical dilemmas and the need for social justice in health planning (Dever et al. 1988).

Need for Cost Containment

Health care costs have risen rapidly over the past several years and are expected to continue to rise. For example, according to the Health Care Financing Administration (HCFA), the national health expenditures were $500.3 billion in 1987, which is 11.1%

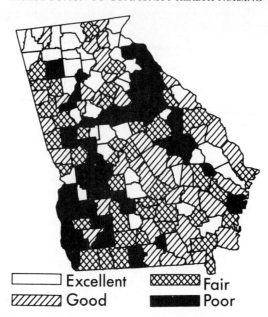

FIG. 2-4 Grades of health status in counties of Georgia. *(From "Creation of a social vulnerability index for justice in health planning" by G.E.A. Dever, M. Sciegaj, T. Wade, and T. Lofton, 1988,* Family & Community Health, *10(4), p. 31. Copyright 1988 by Aspen Publishers, Inc. Reprinted by permission.)*

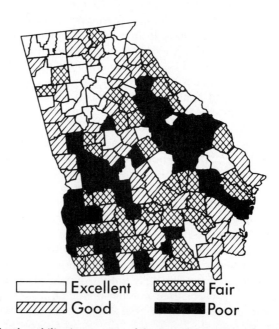

FIG. 2-5 Index of social vulnerability in counties of Georgia. *(From "Creation of a social vulnerability index for justice in health planning" by G.E.A. Dever, M. Sciegaj, T. Wade, and T. Lofton, 1988,* Family & Community Health, *10(4), p. 31. Copyright 1988 by Aspen Publishers, Inc. Reprinted by permission.)*

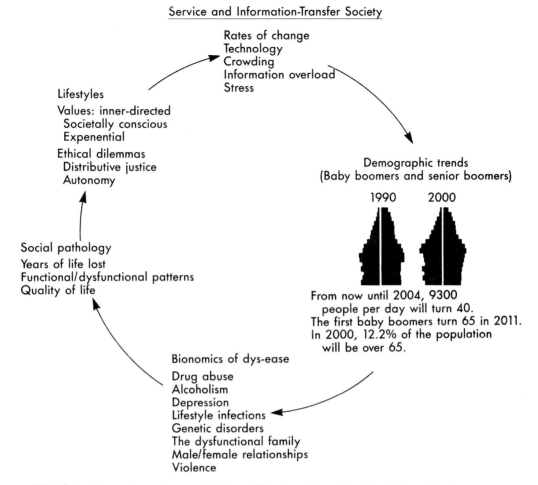

Service and Information-Transfer Society

Rates of change
Technology
Crowding
Information overload
Stress

Lifestyles
Values: inner-directed
    Societally conscious
    Expenential
Ethical dilemmas
    Distributive justice
    Autonomy

Demographic trends
(Baby boomers and senior boomers)

1990   2000

From now until 2004, 9300
    people per day will turn 40.
The first baby boomers turn 65 in 2011.
In 2000, 12.2% of the population
    will be over 65.

Social pathology
Years of life lost
Functional/dysfunctional patterns
Quality of life

Bionomics of dys-ease
Drug abuse
Alcoholism
Depression
Lifestyle infections
Genetic disorders
The dysfunctional family
Male/female relationships
Violence

FIG. 2-6 Social transformation model. *(From "Creation of a social vulnerability index for justice in health planning" by G.E.A. Dever, M. Sciegaj, T. Wade, and T. Lofton, 1988, Family & Community Health, 10(4), p. 24. Copyright 1988 by Aspen Publishers, Inc. Reprinted by permission.)*

of the gross national product (GNP). This sum reflected an increase of 9.8% over 1986. The projection for the year 2000 is that health care expenditures will reach $1.5 trillion, which is 15% of the GNP. In 1986 the resource allocation for each person in the United States was approximately $1837. Of these funds 60% were from private sources (either out-of-pocket or private health insurance). Local, state, and federal governmental expenditures, most of which were for Medicare (Title XVIII) or Medicaid (Title XIX) benefits, comprised the remaining 40%.

The response of providers, consumers, and legislators has been one of intense concern for the high price of health care, which sometimes has resulted in a preoccupation with cost almost to the exclusion of all else. It would seem that the major issue is one of balance between cost and quality.

Several theories have been advanced to explain the dramatic increase in the cost of care. Originally, payment systems were designed to encourage the expansion of the delivery system and the patient's access to it (Anderson, 1984). No attempt was made to contain costs. The growth of expensive technology increased institutional costs in a general way. The cost of new equipment spilled over into maintenance costs and daily patient care. The reduction in out-of-pocket cost to the client because of insurance coverage made the consumer less critical of physicians' fees. Clients also did not question extensive laboratory tests and the prolonging of life at any cost for any reason, such as supporting life systems for the preservation of organs for transplantation. Medicare and Medicaid criteria for reimbursement encouraged some agencies to hire services and invest in equipment they otherwise might not have purchased.

Under the DRG system, hospitals cut operating costs by slowing their purchase of new technologically advanced equipment. It is predicted by some that increased cost sharing by the patient may reduce spending and utilization of ancillary services (Jonas, 1986). Emphasis on ambulatory care also may decrease cost. Many hospitals are making outpatient surgery available, which of course decreases the cost of the procedure to both patient and insurer.

HEALTH CARE DELIVERY SYSTEMS IN OTHER COUNTRIES

The United Kingdom instituted the National Health Service in 1948, which provides health care to all. Canada has funded complete medical and hospital care through federal and provincial taxes since 1961. In 1955 compulsory universal health insurance was founded in Sweden to cover all citizens. China has a unique system of health care that uses paramedics in rural areas; general health care, both rural and urban, is covered by government funding (Hawkins & Higgins, 1982).

Because Canada is close to the United States, both in proximity and culture, a comparison of the two health care systems is appropriate. In 1964 the Royal Commission of Health Services recommended the institution of a universal and comprehensive health scheme for Canada (Fry & Ferndale, 1972). The Canadian parliament passed the Medical Care Act in 1966, which provides for federal contributions to provincial plans for health care.

The provinces have jurisdiction over some aspects of health care. However, the federal Hospital and Diagnostic Services Act of 1957, which provides hospital insurance and laboratory services, combined with the Medical Care Act, financed services throughout Canada to registered Indians and Eskimos, certain categories of seamen, immigrants, and members of the armed forces. The Act now covers more than 99% of Canada's population. Although some outpatient services are included, care in tuberculosis hospitals or hospitals for the mentally ill is not included. Some of the provinces pay these costs. Health departments at the local and provincial level are concerned mainly with environmental health and disease prevention.

Canada has a philosophical commitment to the well being of its people, which it implements by providing health services. The Medical Care Act and the Hospital and Diagnostic Services Act have contributed greatly toward implementing that goal. The health care delivery system in Canada still is in a state of transition, and the cost of health care is high. However, it does not have the complex system of third-party payment methods that exists in the States. In many cases government-sponsored medical care in Canada is supplemented by private insurance to cover dental care and prescribed drugs. The Royal Commission on Health Services has recommended extending the Medical Care Act to provide extended services in the future (Fry & Ferndale, 1972).

SUMMARY

The health care delivery system in the United States has evolved gradually and has been strongly influenced by both the public and the private sectors. Federal legislation has molded much of the system, as have physicians and other private interest groups.

The components of the health care delivery system in the United States include federal, state, and local health departments in the public sector. The private sector includes physicians in private practice and many proprietary agencies.

Expensive technology, increased life expectancy, and heightened consumer awareness have contributed to a rise in health care costs, and many consumers express the need for cost containment.

Health care is not evenly distributed in the United States. Lower socioeconomic groups receive less in the way of health prevention and promotion. On the other hand, the United Kingdom, Canada, Sweden, and China provide health care to their populations through national health insurance.

CHAPTER HIGHLIGHTS

- Since the 1798 bill to create the U.S. Marine Hospital Service for sick and disabled seamen, the federal government has taken an active role in providing direct care for certain groups such as native Americans, military personnel, and veterans, as well as regulating quarantines, immigration laws, and the marketing of food and drugs and preventing environmental hazards.
- State health departments control licensure, collect vital statistics, enforce third-party payment, influence communicable disease control, and deliver selected types of service.
- Local health departments provide immunizations against infectious disease, perform environmental surveillance, and sponsor programs for maternal and infant child care.
- Financing for health care in the public sector has been regulated through legislation (Medicare and Medicaid) that focuses primarily on indigent and elderly populations and is medically oriented.
- The private sector is composed of physicians in private practice, private hospitals, and private outpatient services. Financing for the private sector is available through Blue Cross and Blue Shield, health maintenance organizations, and other independent insurance plans.
- Other developed countries differ from the United States in terms of the financing of health care. The United Kingdom's National Health Service has been in effect since 1948. Canada provides complete medical and hospital care, as do Sweden and China.
- The cost of health care has risen dramatically over the past decade because of increased technology and consumer demands for quality care.

STUDY QUESTIONS

1. Discuss the effect of federal legislation on the health care delivery system in the United States.
2. Identify which clients are eligible for Medicare and Medicaid. What is the difference between the two?
3. Describe methods of financing health care in the United Kingdom, Canada, Sweden, and China.

4. Describe the reasons for the escalation of the cost in health care in the United States today.

REFERENCES

Anderson, A. (1984). *Health care in the 1990s*. American College of Hospital Administrators, Chicago, Ill., Arthur Anderson & Co.

Bertalanffy, L. V. (1968). *General systems theory*. New York: George Braziller.

Dever, A., & Sciegej, M., Wade, T., & Lofton, T. (1988). Creation of a social vulnerability index for justice in health planning. *Family & Community Health, 10*(4), 23-32.

Fry, J., & Ferndale, W. A. J. (1972). *International medical care*. Oxford and Lancaster: Medical and Technical Pub. Co.

Gibbs, N. (1990) Love and let die, *Time Magazine*, March 19.

Hawkins, J., & Higgins, L. (1982). *Nursing care and the American health care delivery system*. New York City: 1982, Tiresias Press Inc.

Hays, A. (1989). Paying for long-term care. *Geriatric Nursing (London), 10*(1), p. 20.

Hogan, R. B., & Hogan, R. B. (1977). *Occupational Safety and Health Act*. New York: Matthew Bender.

Jonas, S. (1986). *Health care delivery in the United States*. New York: Springer.

Legislative update. (1988, Winter). *Health Care Financing Review, 10*(2), p. 131.

Roemer, M. (1982). *An introduction to the US health care system*. New York: Springer.

Sofaer, S. (1988). Community health planning in the United States: A postmortem. *Family & Community Health, 10*(4), 1-12. Aspen Publishing Co.

Stewart J. (1979). Home Health Care, St. Louis, CV Mosby.

Wetmiel, S. (1990). Life support issue centers on patients clear wish, not the family desires, *Wall Street Journal*, June 26.

The Nursing Process in the Community

JOAN M. COOKFAIR

*We must now emphatically refuse to deal with single components,
but instead relate to the concept of wholeness.*

BETTY NEUMAN

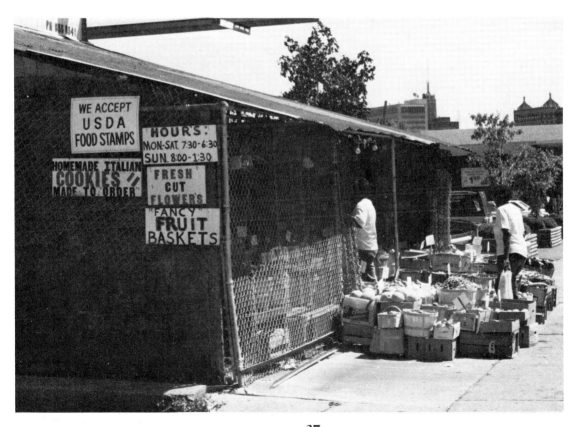

OBJECTIVES

At the conclusion of this chapter the student will be able to:
1. Define the key terms listed
2. Describe selected concepts of the Neuman health care systems model
3. Describe the use of nursing process in a community
4. Describe selected concepts of the Neuman systems theory and integrate them into the nursing process
5. Compare a community with a low level of wellness to a community with a high level of wellness

KEY TERMS

Aggregate

Basic core

Community

Community assessment

Community health nurse

Flexible line of defense

Health

Lines of resistance

Nursing process

Primary prevention

Secondary prevention

Stressors

Target group

Tertiary prevention

As nurses prepare to meet the challenges of the 1990s, it is clear that the role of the community health nurse is becoming more complex. A perception of the community as an interactive system helps enable a community health nurse to plan, implement, and evaluate effective health care.

The American Public Health Association (APHA), in reference to public health nursing, emphasizes the community as a whole rather than individual health care (APHA, 1980). In a publication of the American Nurses' Association (ANA) entitled *A Conceptual Model of Community Health Nursing,* community health nursing is defined as health promotion, health maintenance, health education, management, and coordination and continuity of care that is implemented in terms of a holistic approach to the management of the health care of individuals, families, and groups in the community (ANA, 1985). Both the APHA and the ANA emphasize that effective community nursing services should be based on an orderly assessment and analysis of community needs.

One director general of the World Health Organization (WHO), Halfdon Mühler, has focused attention on nurses as an especially important group in regard to WHO's goal of "health for all by the year 2000." In 1985 Muhler wrote:

> Nurses lead the way. If the millions of nurses in a thousand different places articulate the same ideas and convictions about primary health care, and come together as one force, then they could act as a powerhouse for change.

Health is defined by the WHO as the absence of disease. Most nurses take a more holistic view. Health is described by one nursing theorist, Betty Neuman (1989), as being equated with optimal system stability, that is, the best possible state for an individual, group, or community at any given time.

DEFINITIONS OF COMMUNITY

According to a dictionary definition, community means the people living in a specific area. This is consistent with the definition of a community as a place. This focus fits an epidemiological approach, which might include an assessment of demographical data such as morbidity and mortality statistics within a specific area of assessment.

The community also can be defined as a *social system*. This implies some type of interaction. People interact formally or informally within the broad community structure. They form networks that operate externally or internally for the benefit of the people in the community.

A group that constitutes a community because of common interests of its members is called a *community of interest*. This would include religious groups and ethnic groups (Tinkham, Voorkies, and McCarthy, 1984).

A community may be viewed as a practice setting, a target of service, or a small group within a larger community (Neuman, 1989). A nurse who identifies one of these components as a client of interest for investigation then proceeds to collect data. For example, a nurse who is conducting an investigation concerning the number of infants who died during the first year of birth will collect infant mortality statistics from local records. However, the nurse who wishes to investigate the number of upper respiratory infections experienced by senior students in a nursing program before examinations will have to collect the statistics through health records and interviews. The identified community in this example is senior students in a specified college setting. In the first instance the client is the practice setting; in the second, the client is the population of senior students in a specified college setting.

When decisions have been made as to the identified client and the method of data collection, client system boundaries, that is, limitations, must be set (Neuman, 1989). Client system boundaries may be determined by a geopolitical boundary, such as the practice setting within a specific census tract, or the boundary may be determined by the target group to be focused on, such as senior students in specified institution.

Once the client of interest has been identified, the method of data collection decided upon, and the boundaries for data collection determined, the nurse can proceed with assessment and determine a framework for practice. A useful framework in formulating a nursing diagnosis and facilitating higher levels of wellness for the identified clients is the nursing process.

THE NURSING PROCESS

Nursing leaders in the 1960s developed a scientific approach to nursing called *the nursing process*. According to Yura and Walsh (1983) the four components of the nursing process are assessment, planning, implementation, and evaluation. These components are defined as follows:

1. *Assessment:* Assessing is the act of collecting data about a situation for the purpose of diagnosing a client's actual or potential health problems.
2. *Planning:* Careful planning and thoughtful goal setting should occur here. The nurse must validate the plan with the data assessment.
3. *Implementation:* During this phase the nurse implements and completes the actions necessary to carry out the plan.

4. *Evaluation:* Appraisal of the client's behavioral changes as a result of the actions taken or the lack of change.

Some authors contend that the nursing process consists of five sequential steps: assessment, diagnosis, planning, intervention and evaluation. The nursing diagnosis is the outcome of the assessment. (Muecke, 1984).

According to the ANA, a nursing diagnosis is a description of the human response to an actual or potentail health problem (ANA, 1980).

THE NEUMAN HEALTH CARE SYSTEMS MODEL

Betty Neuman presents a nursing process that encompasses three steps or categories: nursing diagnosis, nursing goals, and nursing outcomes. The first step assumes the assessment as an integral part of the nursing diagnosis. The nursing goals include plans and interventions. The nursing outcomes include evaluation. Nursing process as used by Neuman is less of a linear progression and more of a systems approach.

Neuman has developed a model that demonstrates her approach to patient problems (1989, p. 79). This model uses a systems approach to patient problems (Fig. 3-1). It is a total-client approach that considers all the factors that can affect a client: physiological, psychosocial, sociocultural, and developmental. *Health* is viewed as a condition in which all parts and subparts are in harmony. Disharmony reduces the wellness state. *Environment* is believed to be all those factors that affect or are affected by the person or that influence that person's wellness state or normal line of defense.

Normal line of defense is an adaptive state that has been developed by an individual or community over time. This state is considered normal for that individual or community. Surrounding the normal state in the model is a broken circle that represents the *flexible line of defense.* This represents a protective buffer that can change. It can strengthen and help prevent stressors from breaking through the normal line of defense. On the other hand, undernutrition, lack of sleep, can weaken this line of defense and penetrate the normal line of defense. This may threaten the line of resistance.

Lines of resistance are the individual's internal factors that help to defend against a stressor. For example, the body's innate immune response would be the last line of defense against a stressor's breaking through to the *basic core:* the energy resource that enables the individual to fight against a stressor, for example, normal temperature, genetic structure, or ego structure.

In Neuman's system *primary prevention* is aimed at reducing the possibility of encounters with stressors and strengthening the flexible line of defense. *Secondary prevention* relates to early case finding and treatment of symptoms. *Tertiary prevention* focuses on readaptation, education to prevent further occurrences, and maintenance of stability. Fig. 3-2 demonstrates Neuman's format for primary, secondary, and tertiary interventions.

Nurses who are beginning a community assessment might find it helpful to use Neuman's approach to view the community as a client. This approach, which is illustrated in a model by Anderson, McFarlane, and Helton (Fig. 3-3), expands Neuman's systems model, which is based on the nursing process as a framework, to activate her view of the community as a system that affects target groups. This concept is based on the nursing process as a framework. Health services, government, the availability of fire fighters and police education, housing, recreation, environment, and employment are assessed. The population is assessed, and the impact of stressors that affect its health status is analyzed. The interventions are planned at primary, secondary, and tertiary levels. Evaluation of the health plan is included. Eight interacting subsystems are included: health and safety,

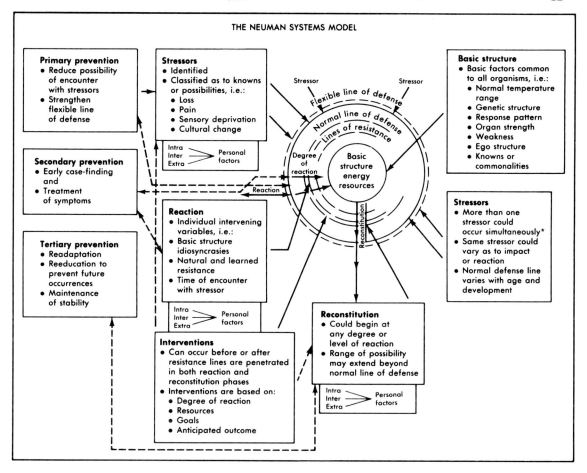

FIG. 3-1 The Neuman systems model. *(Courtesy Betty Neumann, Ph. D.)*

sociocultural, education, communication and transportation, recreation, economics, law and politics, and religion (Anderson, McFarlane and Helton). This model is useful in identifying high-risk aggregates in a community. As with any systems model, the nurse must avoid collecting irrelevant data in the assessment process. Although all data may have an indirect connection in terms of this model, information may be outside the nurses's range of influence.

For simplicity and clarity a community assessment may need only to incorporate selected concepts from the Neuman model (Neuman, 1989). In the community, *basic structure* includes all the variables that keep the community functioning as a unit. The *normal line of defense* may be the coordinated efforts of the city mayor, city council, and the health department. *The flexible line of defense* might be a special nutrition program for low-income pregnant women that suddenly could be discontinued (Neuman, 1989).

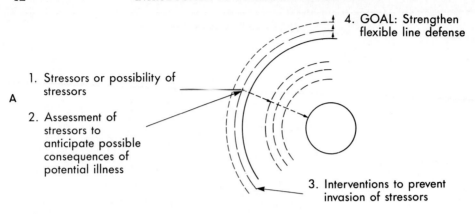

A

1. Stressors or possibility of stressors

2. Assessment of stressors to anticipate possible consequences of potential illness

4. GOAL: Strengthen flexible line defense

3. Interventions to prevent invasion of stressors

Format for primary prevention/intervention mode

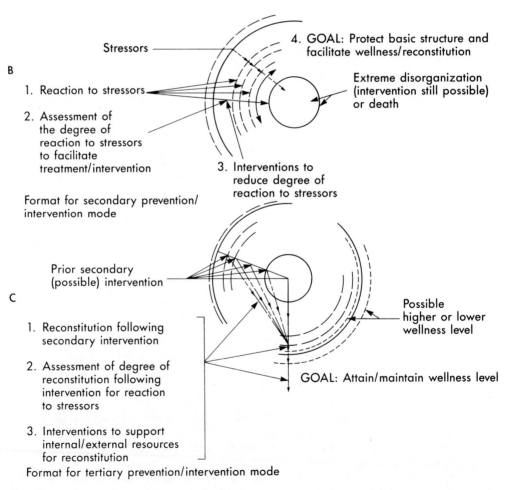

B

Stressors

1. Reaction to stressors

2. Assessment of the degree of reaction to stressors to facilitate treatment/intervention

4. GOAL: Protect basic structure and facilitate wellness/reconstitution

Extreme disorganization (intervention still possible) or death

3. Interventions to reduce degree of reaction to stressors

Format for secondary prevention/intervention mode

C

Prior secondary (possible) intervention

1. Reconstitution following secondary intervention

2. Assessment of degree of reconstitution following intervention for reaction to stressors

3. Interventions to support internal/external resources for reconstitution

Possible higher or lower wellness level

GOAL: Attain/maintain wellness level

Format for tertiary prevention/intervention mode

FIG. 3-2 A, Primary prevention/intervention mode. **B,** Secondary prevention/intervention mode. **C,** Tertiary prevention/intervention mode. *(Courtesy Betty Neuman, Ph. D.)*

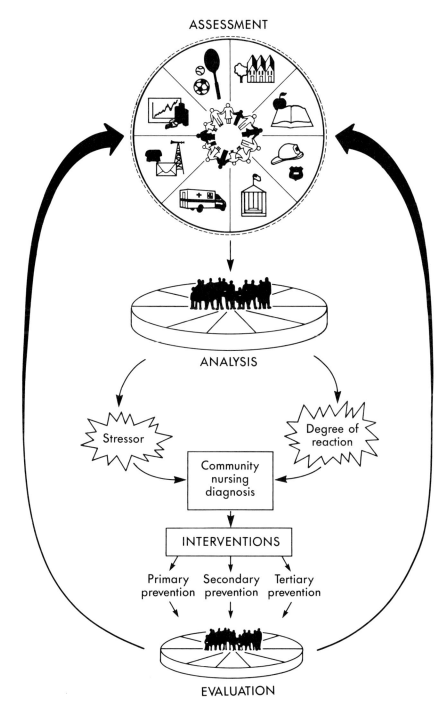

FIG. 3-3 The community-as-client model. *(From "Community as client: A model for practice" by E. Anderson, J. McFarlane, and A. Helton, 1986, Nursing Outlook, 5, p. 22. Copyright 1986 by American Journal of Nursing Co. Reprinted by permission.)*

It is possible that a community may have health problems that require intervention at primary, secondary and/or tertiary levels. On the basis of Neuman's terminology, primary prevention in a community would be aimed at strengthening the flexible line of defense; secondary prevention would be directed toward protecting the basic structure; and the tertiary prevention would be directed toward promoting maximum wellness in a target group or practice setting already identified as having a compromised level of wellness. The nurse may find it helpful to refer to the Client Community Assessment Guide (Appendix 3-1) in applying Neuman's model.

THE NURSING PROCESS APPLIED TO A COMMUNITY

One hundred nursing students in a baccalaureate program were asked by local community leaders to assess the health of a selected urban community close to their school and to prioritize the needs of that community. The students based their definition of health on that in Neuman's health care systems model:

> "Health or wellness is the condition in which all parts and subparts (variables) are in harmony with the whole of man" (Neuman, 1989, p. 9).

For purposes of the assessment the students were guided by the following considerations: The community was defined by geographical boundaries (the environment to be evaluated) and was limited to one census tract within the city. This census tract provided the statistical data and the study population. The students used nursing process to conduct their assessment and organized the information in the following manner:

   I. Assessment
     A. Community boundaries
     B. Statistical data
     C. Education
     D. Economy/occupations
     E. Environment
     F. Community resources
     G. Vital statistics
     H. Morbidity data
     I. Health resources
     J. Other
  II. Community diagnosis
 III. Nursing goals (plans and interventions)
 IV. Nursing outcomes (evaluation)

The case study that follows is a compilation of the nursing students' work.

CASE STUDY 1

Assessment
The community boundaries

The community was located in a low-income urban area. Its boundaries were established within a specific census tract that encompassed approximately 4 square miles.

Demographical data

Students collected statistical data from the 1980 census taken by the local county government and interviewed approximately 250 families and some community leaders. The total population was 5329 and, according to statistics, was fairly stable. Estimates of newcomers during the previous 5 years was 16.6%. Slightly fewer than half the residents were white: the remaining population was mostly black or Hispanic. The age and ethnic distribution of the population is described in Table 3-1. According to local officials some native Americans refused to participate in the census because they considered themselves members of the Indian nation. It was therefore believed that more native Americans resided in the area than the statistics indicated. The 1980 census tract information indicated that there were 780 households headed by woman in this community

Education

The distribution of children who attended school the year before the assessment is recorded in Table 3-2. The level of education in the community showed that fewer than half of all adults older than 25 years had any high school education. A very small group (6%) had finished college.

Economy/occupations

The average income was low; more than half the families had an annual income below $5000. Many were receiving public assistance. Of the adults older than 16 years, 26% were unemployed (Table 3-3). The majority of the labor force, those individuals age 16 years and older, were employed in clerical positions or service jobs. A small group (16%) was engaged in lower-level managerial positions.

Environment

The area is located in a temperate climate that has very harsh winters, sometimes accompanied by deep snow. Summers are warm and pleasant; spring and fall are cold and damp. There are few trees and flowers, and the living quarters are crowded close together. The neighborhood is in an urban area, bordered on one side by a main street leading to a downtown shopping section, a middle-income housing district on the other side, and lower-income housing districts on the other two sides. Houses generally are run down and in need of repair (Fig. 3-4). Many fences are broken and yards untended. Playgrounds are not visible because of broken equipment (Fig. 3-5).

Three of the families interviewed said that they kept their children in the yard and away from the playground because it was a "drug drop." Another drug drop, according to neighbors, was the corner in front of the local day-care center. Residents voiced concern about the lack of police surveillance in spite of a high incidence of crime in the area. They complained that the city fire department was slow to answer calls for assistance and that snow removal in the wintertime often took much longer than it did in surrounding neighborhoods.

Students reported communication difficult because many of the residents of the community did not speak English and the students did not speak Spanish, which was the primary language in house after house where students attempted to obtain information from residents.

TABLE 3-1 Age and race distribution of community studied

Yr	Age distribution No.	%	Race	Ethnic distribution No.	%
<5	614	11.5	White	1131	21.2
5-9	615	11.5	Black	1783	33.5
10-14	551	10.3	Indian	241	4.5
15-19	612	11.5	Hispanic	1935	36.3
25-34	892	16.8	Other	239	4.5
35-44	529	9.9	TOTAL	5329	100.0
45-54	573	10.8			
55-64	600	11.3			
65-74	343	6.4			
TOTAL	5329	100			

TABLE 3-2 Children attending school in the community

Type of school	No.	%
Nursery	144	5.9
Kindergarten	153	6.3
Elementary (1-8)	1789	73.9
High school (9-12)	336	13.9
TOTAL	2422	100

TABLE 3-3 Income levels in the community

Earnings	No.	%
Below $5000	1207	55.2
$5000-7499	395	18.1
$7500-9999	238	10.9
$10,000-14,999	345	15.8
TOTAL	2185	100.0

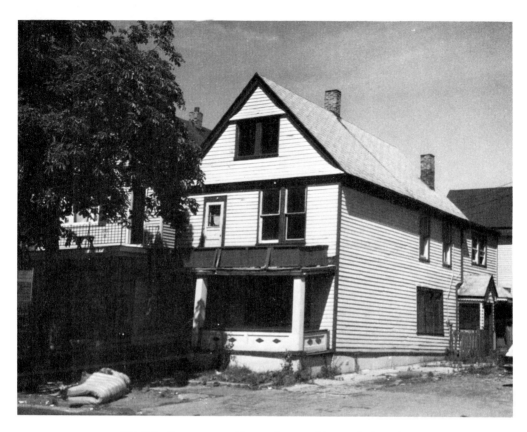

FIG. 3-4 Houses generally run down and in need of repair.

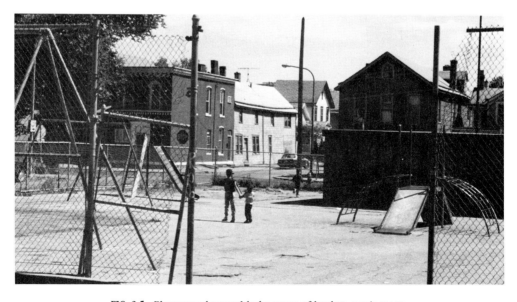

FIG. 3-5 Playground unusable because of broken equipment.

CASE STUDY 1—cont'd

Dogs and cats roamed the streets in great number. Some people said they needed the dogs for protection and the cats to keep the rat population down. According to residents, there was no attempt made by local authorities to enforce a leash law or to impound dogs that roamed free.

Some area residents were concerned about individuals attracted to the area by a neighborhood food pantry. Students expressed feelings of anxiety when they walked past some groups of men who stood around and talked in front of stores and on street corners and were verbally abusive to them.

Community resources

The area is governed by the city, and the local councilman seemed aware of the needs of the residents. When students interviewed him, however, he did not have a plan to respond to those needs. Among the resources were a library, a city college, and a hospital that were available to neighborhood residents by public transportation. A local newspaper enhanced a sense of community.

Vital statistics

Statistics from the 1980 census tract survey concerning infant mortality were compared with city, county, and state norms (Table 3-4).

Local records showed that between the years 1978 and 1982 the incidence of neonatal death was 3.9 times higher than in the surrounding county. The incidence of post neonatal death was 3.6 times higher.

Morbidity data

Data were not available for the census tract studied.

TABLE 3-4 Infant mortality statistics	
Area	No. deaths/1000
Local neighborhood	25.4
City	15.2
County	11.7
State	10.5

CASE STUDY 1—cont'd

Health resources

Students reported that there was one private physician in the area and that an ambulatory care clinic and a large county hospital were available by bus.

Community diagnosis

After analyzing the data, the students prioritized the elements of the community diagnosis in the following manner:

1. Potential weakness in the flexible line of defense of the community related to low income and unemployment
2. Potential weakness in the flexible line of defense related to communication difficulties (language barrier)
3. Potential hazard to normal line of defense related to state of community health, for example, infant mortality
4. Potential hazard to lines of resistance related to hazardous and inaccessible playground in the community (Fig. 3-5)
5. Potential weakness in the lines of resistance resulting from unsafe environment in the community, for example, abandoned housing, drug traffic, increased crime rate
6. Potential penetration of the basic structure of the community related to high infant mortality

Nursing goals

Students planned interventions at primary, secondary, and tertiary levels and integrated their plans into Neuman's model. Fig. 3-6 illustrates assessment, nursing diagnosis, goals, interventions, and expected outcomes at all three levels.

Nursing outcomes

The students' evaluative outcome projected that the infant morality rate would decrease over a 3-year period. The students also concluded that a community health nurse could provide health education through the schools and a Puerto Rican community center and could encourage the use of an ambulatory care clinic for prenatal care. There also could be an attempt to raise the level of awareness of public officials as to the plight of this community by making the students' research available to them.

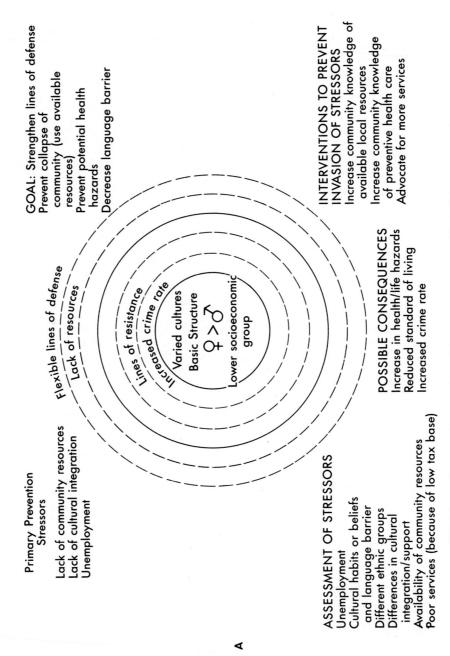

GOAL: Strengthen lines of defense
Prevent collapse of community (use available resources)
Prevent potential health hazards
Decrease language barrier

INTERVENTIONS TO PREVENT INVASION OF STRESSORS
Increase community knowledge of available local resources
Increase community knowledge of preventive health care
Advocate for more services

Flexible lines of defense
Lack of resources

Lines of resistance
Increased crime rate

Varied cultures
Basic Structure
♀ > ♂
Lower socioeconomic group

POSSIBLE CONSEQUENCES
Increase in health/life hazards
Reduced standard of living
Increased crime rate

Primary Prevention
Stressors
Lack of community resources
Lack of cultural integration
Unemployment

ASSESSMENT OF STRESSORS
Unemployment
Cultural habits or beliefs and language barrier
Different ethnic groups
Differences in cultural integration/support
Availability of community resources
Poor services (because of low tax base)

A

FIG. 3-6 Application of Neuman's model to a community at risk. A, Primary prevention.

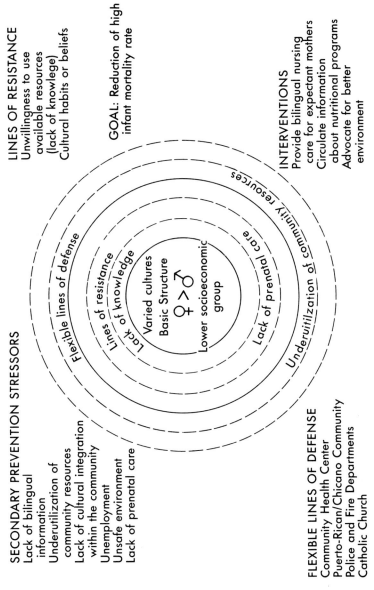

LINES OF RESISTANCE
Unwillingness to use
   available resources
   (lack of knowlege)
Cultural habits or beliefs

GOAL: Reduction of high
infant mortality rate

INTERVENTIONS
Provide bilingual nursing
   care for expectant mothers
Circulate information
   about nutritional programs
Advocate for better
   environment

SECONDARY PREVENTION STRESSORS
Lack of bilingual
   information
Underutilization of
   community resources
Lack of cultural integration
   within the community
Unemployment
Unsafe environment
Lack of prenatal care

FLEXIBLE LINES OF DEFENSE
Community Health Center
Puerto-Rican/Chicano Community
Police and Fire Departments
Catholic Church

FIG. 3-6, cont'd Application of Neuman's model to a community at risk. **B**, Secondary prevention.

B

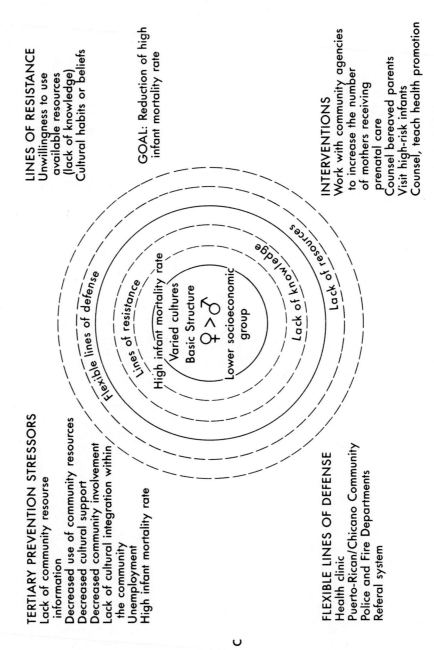

LINES OF RESISTANCE
Unwillingness to use
available resources
(lack of knowledge)
Cultural habits or beliefs

GOAL: Reduction of high
infant mortality rate

INTERVENTIONS
Work with community agencies
to increase the number
of mothers receiving
prenatal care
Counsel bereaved parents
Visit high-risk infants
Counsel, teach health promotion

TERTIARY PREVENTION STRESSORS
Lack of community resourse
information
Decreased use of community resources
Decreased cultural support
Decreased community involvement
Lack of cultural integration within
the community
Unemployment
High infant mortality rate

FLEXIBLE LINES OF DEFENSE
Health clinic
Puerto-Rican/Chicano Community
Police and Fire Departments
Referal system

C

FIG. 3-6, cont'd Application of Neuman's model to a community at risk. C, Tertiary prevention.

CASE STUDY 2

Another group of students conducted an assessment of the health of a suburban community as a course requirement. They used the same definition of community as that used by the students in case study 1 and confined their study to one census tract.

Assessment
Community boundaries

The community was located in an upper middle-class suburban area. The boundaries were within a single census tract spread over an area of about 8 square miles that included a small park. The total population of the census tract was 5110.

Demographical data

The statistical data were obtained primarily from the most recent census (about 2 years previously) taken by the county government and from information on record at the county court house and at the local school district office.

The population (5110) of the community has been increasing steadily for about 5 years. The residents were predominantly white (97%); 73% of the population was older than 18 years and 12% was older than 65 years. The most recent census information indicated that there were fewer than 100 households headed by women.

Education

Exact statistics concerning education were not readily available because the boundaries of the census tract did not coincide with the boundaries of the local school districts. It was established, however, that there were approximately 2250 students in the tract, including about 180 kindergarten students, 1800 elementary students, and 280 secondary school students. Approximately 75% of the adults older than 25 years were high school graduates, and approximately 25% had completed at least 4 years of college.

Economy/occupations

There was a high percentage of white collar workers in the community, and the average family income level was more than $20,000. Unemployment was low at the time of the study (about 6%), and many households had two incomes.

Environment

The community was located in a temperate climate (the same as that of the community of case study 1), with harsh winters, cool, damp springs and falls, and warm, pleasant summers. The area was well kept, the houses neat and well maintained. No garbage or trash was observed except that which was placed at the curb on garbage pick-up days (Fig. 3-7). The residential streets were characterized by well-kept lawns, neat flower gardens, and young trees. The residents interviewed all spoke English and voiced no concern about public services. A leash law was enforced to keep pets off the streets.

Community resources

The community included a library, two nearby hospitals, many private physicians, and a senior citizens' center. The community was within a township, and members of the town board seemed to be firmly committed to working on the problems of the community. A playground recently had been donated by a local community group for area children (Fig. 3-8).

Continued.

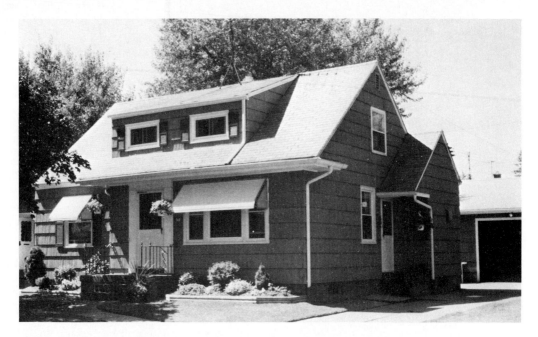

FIG. 3-7 Houses and yards clean and well maintained.

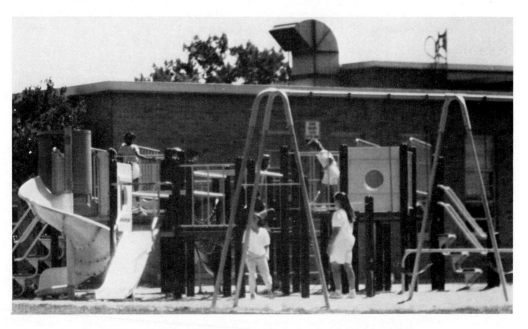

FIG. 3-8 Playground with new equipment is used by area children.

CASE STUDY 2—cont'd

Vital statistics

Infant mortality in this suburban community was 7.3 per 1000 compared with 15.2 per 1000 in the nearby city and 11.7 per 1000 in the surrounding county. The community was predominantly white (about 97%).

Morbidity data

Data were not available. However, interviews with several local physicians indicated that the leading and possibly major causes of mortality in the community were cardiovascular disease and malignant neoplasms in the over-65 population.

Health resources

Health resources were ample and included a number of private physicians, a well-baby clinic, and two private nearby hospitals.

Community diagnosis

Students judged this area as having a strong normal line of defense, adequate flexible lines of defense, and a high level of wellness. They hypothesized that lines of resistance could be compromised in the over-65 population (12%) because of aging and a consequent lowering of immunity to selected disease states. Their community diagnosis consisted of the following analysis:

1. Alteration of lines of resistance in a specific target group (older than 65 years) to cardiovascular disease and malignant neoplasm as a part of the aging process
2. Potential high risk of cardiovascular disease and malignant neoplasm

Nursing goals and outcomes

The students' goals focused on primary and secondary prevention in terms of Neuman's health care systems model (Fig. 3-9). Their projected outcome was that knowledge of method of prevention of cardiovascular disease and malignant neoplasms and early diagnosis of altered health states would decrease the incidence of cardiovascular disease and malignant neoplasms in the target population (persons older than 65 years).

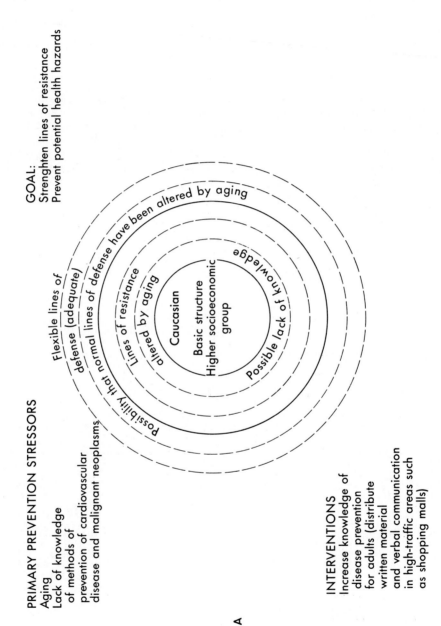

PRIMARY PREVENTION STRESSORS
Aging
Lack of knowledge
of methods of
prevention of cardiovascular
disease and malignant neoplasms

GOAL:
Strenghten lines of resistance
Prevent potential health hazards

INTERVENTIONS
Increase knowledge of
disease prevention
for adults (distribute
written material
and verbal communication
in high-traffic areas such
as shopping malls)

A

FIG. 3-9 Application of Neuman's model to a healthy community. **A,** Primary prevention.

SECONDARY PREVENTION STRESSORS
Potential for hypertension
and early malignant
neoplasm in aging
population

GOAL: Prevent health problem
through early treatment
by appropriate referral

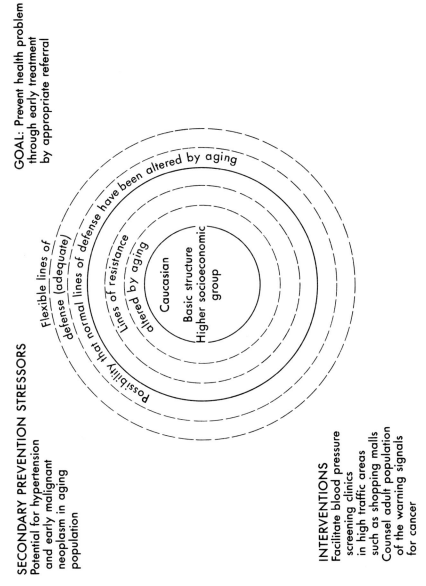

Flexible lines of
defense (adequate)
Possibility that normal lines of defense have been altered by aging
Lines of resistance
altered by aging
Caucasian
Basic structure
Higher socioeconomic
group

INTERVENTIONS
Facilitate blood pressure
screening clinics
in high traffic areas
such as shopping malls
Counsel adult population
of the warning signals
for cancer

B

FIG. 3-9, cont'd   Application of Neuman's model to a healthy community. **B**, Secondary prevention.

SUMMARY

A view of the community as an interactive system emphasizes the concept of holistic nursing practice. Use of nursing process to assess the health or wellness of a client population enables the nurse to objectively analyze data related to that population and to make an accurate nursing diagnosis. Nursing interventions planned at primary, secondary, and tertiary levels should include the establishment of criteria for evaluating the effectiveness of those interventions to promote optimum system stability in the community.

CHAPTER HIGHLIGHTS

- Community health nursing is defined as health promotion, health maintenance, health education, management, and coordination and continuity of care that is implemented in terms of a holistic approach to the management of the health care of individuals, families, and groups in the community (ANA, 1985).
- According to Neuman, health is equated with open system stability, that is, the best possible state for an individual, a group, or a community at any given time.
- A community can be defined as the people living in a geographic area, a social system, a group of people with a common interest, or a target population of service.
- The nursing process is a scientific approach to nursing, which consists of 5 components: assessment, nursing diagnosis, planning, implementation, and evaluation.
- Neuman views the nursing process as having three steps: nursing diagnosis, nursing goals, and nursing outcomes.
- Neuman's health care systems model utilizes a total client approach that considers all factors that may affect a client: physiological, psychological, sociocultural, or developmental.
- Primary prevention consists of nursing intervention that makes individuals aware of potential health problems.
- Secondary prevention consists of nursing interventions aimed at identifying and correcting health problems before they occur.
- Tertiary prevention consists of nursing interventions that facilitate rehabilitation or are helpful in a palliative way to an individual or community.

STUDY QUESTIONS

1. Define and discuss two definitions of community.
2. Describe what Neuman means by the flexible line of defense, the normal line of defense, the lines of resistance, and the basic core.
3. List and describe steps in the nursing process.
4. Describe primary, secondary, and tertiary prevention.
5. How would a nurse use Neuman's adaptation of the nursing process to study a community? Give examples of each step in the process.

APPENDIX 3-1
The Neuman Community-Client Assessment Guide*

Aggregate client	Geopolitical client
Intrasystem	**Intrasystem**
System boundary—client defined	Same as for aggregate client
Physiological	*Physiological*
1. Physical assessment as appropriate	Same as for aggregate client
2. Specific maturational stage data, for example, Apgar scores of newborns	
Psychological	*Psychological*
1. Emotional health of aggregate members: prevalence of isolation and depression, divorce and crime rates	1. Emotional health of community
2. Communication patterns: response patterns to feedback from other systems	2. Same as for aggregate client
Developmental	*Developmental*
1. Maturational stage of aggregate	1. Maturational stage of community
2. Age range and median of aggregate	2. Age range and median of population
Sociocultural	*Sociocultural*
1. Demographic characteristics: sex, age, education level, income, and ethnicity	Same as for aggregate client
2. Health beliefs: immunization levels, child-rearing practices	
3. Life-styles, including risk-taking behaviors	
4. Consumer participation in community programs	
Spiritual	*Spiritual*
Religious affiliation	Same as for aggregate client
	Client perceptions
	Perceived problems
	Perceived solutions
Intersystem	**Intersystem**
Primary care-giver system	System boundary—geographical or political
Health and safety	*Health and safety*
1. Personnel: number, education, and experience	1. Health indicators: morbidity, life expectancy, etc.
2. Case load of personnel	2. Resource allocation and utilization

From *The Neuman systems model* (2nd ed., pp. 371-373) by B. Neuman, 1989, Norwalk, CT: Appleton & Lange.
*The list of assessment data and examples of the type of data collected serve only as a guide and are not exhaustive.

APPENDIX 3-1
The Neuman Community-Client Assessment Guide—cont'd

Aggregate client	Geopolitical client

Health and safety

3. Occupational health programs
4. Agency programs and clientele served:
   —Services to strengthen families
   —Services for special groups
5. Environmental conditions and safety hazards within the building

Health and safety

3. Facilities: hospitals, health department, outpatient clinics
4. Safety services:
   —Official services, such as police, fire
   —Volunteer services, such as block parent, neighborhood watch
5. Sanitation services, such as garbage and sewage disposal
6. Case loads of professionals
7. Environmental conditions and safety hazards:
   —Air, water, soil inspection
   —Abandoned or unkempt buildings, trash and garbage, broken sidewalks

Sociocultural

1. Ethnic composition of personnel and languages
2. Membership in associations and professional organizations

Sociocultural

1. Culture composition of population and languages spoken
2. Guiding values
3. Positions and roles
4. Associations and clubs
5. Services to strengthen families, such as preschool and senior day care
6. Services for special groups, such as handicapped and new immigrant

Education

1. Education level and experience of personnel
2. Continuing education for employees: journal subscriptions, in-service education

Education

1. Personnel: education level of residents
2. Facilities: universities, colleges, schools, libraries
3. Personnel: number, education, and experience

Communication and transportation

1. Communication patterns within agencies: formal and informal system
2. Communication methods to intrasystem and extrasystems: pamphlets, posters, home visits, and mass media
3. Accessibility:
   —Location: accessibility and acceptability
   —Hours of service
   —Cultural interpretation and translation services

Communication and transportation

Same as for aggregate client

APPENDIX 3-1
The Neuman Community-Client Assessment Guide—cont'd

Aggregate client	Geopolitical client
Recreation	*Recreation*
1. Facilities: lunchrooms, lounges, etc.	1. Facilities: schools, library, museums, ice rinks, etc.
2. Activities: planned and informal	2. Personnel: number, education, and experience
	3. Programs: adult, children, and special needs
	4. Accessibility
Economics	*Economics*
1. Resources: funding, personnel, buildings, equipment, supplies	1. Employment: employment status and income levels of residents
2. Health and welfare benefits for employees: health and dental insurance, pension plans, etc.	2. Income assistance: percentage of the population
3. Paid continuing education programs	3. Education levels, literacy rate
	4. Housing: quality and types
	5. Industry and occupational health programs
Law and politics	*Law and politics*
1. Policy formulation: decision and problem-solving patterns	1. Power: sanctions and making legislation as they relate to health of community
2. Positions and roles	
3. Contracts	
Religion	*Religion*
1. Agency philosophy	1. Number and types of churches
2. Beliefs and values of employees	2. Church programs and activities
	Client perceptions
	Perceived problems
	Perceived solutions
Extrasystem description	*Extrasystem description*
Same as the geopolitical intersystem	System boundary: location, climate, urban or rural, topography, square miles
	—Population: number per square mile, mobility
	—History
Subsystem data	*Subsystem data*
Same as the geopolitical intersystem	Collect data selectively about subsystems at a federal level or state or provincial level, or both, as it pertains specifically to the needs of the geopolitical community

REFERENCES

Anderson E., McFarlane, J., & Helton, A. (1986). Community-as-client: A model for practice. *Nursing Outlook 34* (5), 220-224.

American Nurses' Association Council of Community Health Nurses. (1980). *A conceptual model for community health nursing* (ANA Publication No. CH-102M 5/80). Kansas City, MO 64108: Author 2420 Pershing Rd., Kansas City, MO 64108).

American Nurses' Association (ANA), (1980b). Nursing, a social policy statement, Kansas City, Mo.

American Public Health Association, Division of Nursing. (1980). *The definition and role of public health nursing in the delivery of health care.* Washington, DC: Author.

Dzimian, J., Schoelkopf, N., Spalti, K., Waldowski, L., & Zimmerman, M. *Community project,* Class of 1987 Unpublished manuscript, D'Youville College, Buffalo, NY.

Griffith-Kenney, J., & Christensen, P. (1986). *Nursing process: Application of theories, frameworks, and models.* St. Louis: Mosby.

Muecke, M. (1984). Community health diagnosis in nursing. *Public Health Nursing,* 1(1), 24.

Neuman, B. (1989). The Neuman systems model. (2nd ed.). Norwalk, CT: Appleton & Lange.

Smith, J. (1988). Public health and the quality of life. *Family Community Health,* 10(4), 49-57.

Tinkham, C., Voorkies, E., & McCarthy, N. (1984). *Community health nursing.* Norwalk, CT: Appleton Century-Crofts.

Yura, H. & Walsh, M. (1983) *Nursing process (4th ed.).* New York: Appleton & Lange, 131-132.

World Health Organization, Regional Office for Europe. (1985). *Targets for health for all two thousand: Targets in support of the European strategy for health for all.* Copenhagen: WHO.

UNIT II

Strategies and Tools for Health Promotion

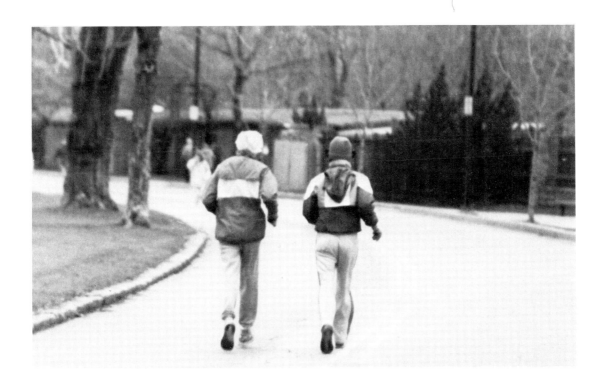

Promoting health and wellness is an integral part of the role of the nurse in the community. Chapter 4 presents a number of conceptual models that will assist the nurse in that role. In addition, teaching strategies and an overview of the teaching/learning process are described in Chapter 5. Chapter 6 outlines the importance of group process and effective leadership in promoting health.

Chapter 7 details the epidemiological model for nursing practice and describes various concepts that the community health nurse can use to assess the health of aggregates and large groups of people in the community. The epidemiological research process is described, and examples are provided for the application of that process to nursing practice.

The evaluative component of community health nursing practice is becoming increasingly important. Chapter 8 outlines various models that may be used in the evaluative process. Cost containment and consumer advocacy cannot be maintained without the implementation of quality assurance measures.

Health education, leadership, research, and accountability are essential components of contemporary community health nursing. This unit provides a background for the integration of these components into the nurse's role.

Health and Wellness in the Community

CAROLE A. GUTT

There will either be an increase in wellness or a depressed, deprived, depleted and short-lived society which will not be recognizable. We can't continue to survive living the way we do, physically, economically, and environmentally. Since there are too many survivors among us, wellness must and will prevail.

DONALD B. ARDELL

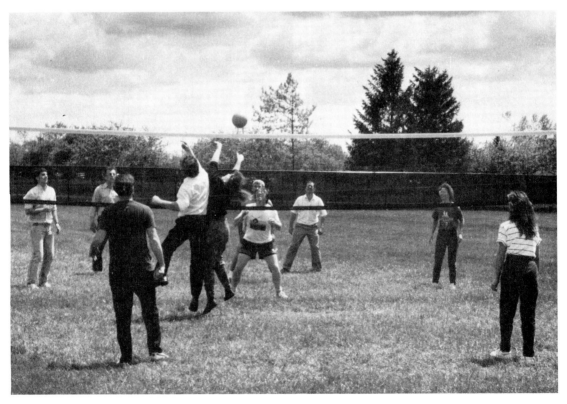

OBJECTIVES

At the conclusion of this chapter the student will be able to:
1. Define the key terms listed
2. Describe the historical development of the wellness movement in the United States
3. Identify individuals who have contributed to the development of the wellness movement
4. Differentiate among wellness, disease prevention, health education, medical self-care, health promotion, and holistic health
5. Describe selected wellness models that can be applied to community health nursing
6. Integrate concepts of teaching/learning with selected wellness models
7. Discuss the components of wellness
8. Discuss the role of the community health nurse in wellness education

KEY TERMS

Disease prevention	Life-style assessment questionnaire
Environmental sensitivity	Medical self-care
Health	Nutrition
Health behavior contract	Physical fitness
Health education	Rosenstock's health belief model
Health promotion	Self-efficacy model
Holistic health	Wellness
Inner harmony	

HISTORICAL DEVELOPMENT OF THE WELLNESS MOVEMENT

The Roman philosopher Seneca, who died 65 AD, said more than 1900 years ago, "Man does not die, he kills himself." The growing public awareness of wellness as a concept is related to several contributing factors and movements that occurred in the late 1970s. These trends came together as a force and shaped the climate and nature of the wellness movement.

Until the late 1970s the approach to health was curative rather than preventive. At that time several landmark publications brought to the public's attention the need to emphasize preventive aspects of health. In 1975 several prominent American foundations pooled their resources and published a two-volume collection of works by prominent persons in the medical field, which reflected growing concern with the status quo of the health care delivery system at that time and the need for sweeping reforms to include wellness concepts and changes in life-style. These works were John Knowles's *Doing Better and Feeling Worse* (1977) and *Future Directions in Health Care. Dietary goals,* a report issued by the Senate Select Committee on Nutrition and Human Needs (1977), showed a direct link between diet and disease and called for major adjustments in American dietary patterns, including marked decreases in consumption of meat, dairy products, sugar, and salt.

In 1979 the American Hospital Association (AHA) issued a policy statement entitled "Hospitals' Responsibility for Health Promotion." As a result, several American hospitals established health promotion and wellness programs. These programs became a routine extension of hospital-based care in the 1980s; however, at the time of the AHA report the concept was relatively unknown and innovative.

Perhaps the most well-known and significant report in terms of impact was the 1979 document entitled *Healthy People* issued by the secretary of the Department of Health, Education and Welfare (now the Department of Health and Human Services). *Healthy People* stressed that many of the illnesses prevalent in our society could be avoided by a change in life-style and environment. A shift from high-technology, medical-model, and acute hospital-based care was urged, with emphasis on health promotion and disease prevention.

A major contributing factor in the development of the wellness movement of the 1970s was the cost crisis that occurred in health care. Americans suddenly found that medical bills were soaring to unheard-of heights. There were annual increases in health care spending both at the federal governmental level in terms of the percentage of the gross national product being consumed for health care and personal individual expenses. Large corporations and businesses found that employees' medical costs, coupled with rising inflation rates, were cutting into their profit margins, necessitating increased costs to their customers. Financial motivation proved to be a powerful impetus for companies to look at ways to improve the health of their employees before they became ill. Direct benefits to companies were measurable in terms of reduced absenteeism and turnover and improved employee morale. Cures are costly, and sustaining chronic illnesses with resulting disability proved overwhelming for many companies. Wellness measures with life-style–related interventions were cost effective and easy to design and implement not only in the workplace but also in school and community settings.

Blue Shield of Northern California initiated what was perhaps the first practical application of these concepts when it issued the "Stay Well Plan" in 1978. Employees of the Mendocino school district were the target population of the plan. They were offered classes on a variety of topics related to health and self-care. They also were offered financial incentives if they used less than $500 of medical care benefits in 1 year. The district saved considerable monies in insurance premiums, and Blue Shield was able to decrease its premium rates as a result of the program.

Consumer consciousness came to play a vital role in the development of the wellness movement. The media became increasingly involved with dissemination of health information to the public. At the same time the public began to emphasize its desire to care for its own minor medical needs. American consumers wanted to take an active part in the control of their own health needs rather than having those needs dictated by health professionals. This public interest in self-treatment has been referred to as the "third wave of health" by some prominent health educators. Coupled with a growing consumer consciousness was a heightened mind-body awareness resulting from political, ideological, and sociological changes that occurred in this country after the Vietnam War. The "baby boom" generation had reached young adulthood and placed an awesome burden on the health care delivery system. This segment of the population, which began to approach middle age in the 1980s, is beginning to fall prey to many of the life-style–related diseases first noted in the 1970s. For example, individuals who have been sedentary and obese as young adults will be at greater risk for heart disease as they age. The influence of Eastern philosophies and psychological theories of self-actualization also was evident as consumers of health care began to seek holistic alternatives to the scientific models of care to which they had been accustomed.

During this same time frame, several other shifts were occurring in society. The women's movement became a strong political and personal force in this country. Its proponents urged women to question their medical care and assume personal responsibility for their own health needs. Ecologists also began to give loud public voice to concerns related to environmental effects on health. Physical fitness became almost an obsession with large segments of the American population. This was due in part to published results of studies on the growing incidence of coronary heart disease in this country. Americans were urged to jog, do aerobics, and eat natural, healthful foods. The quality of life was seen as something that the health consumer could and should control. Researchers began to supply health care deliverers with findings relevant to the impact of improved life-styles on health and the quality of life. The 1970 Framingham study on risk factors and heart disease formed the baseline for many of our current health hazard appraisal instruments. Also in 1970, the surgeon general's report on smoking and health provided the first definitive link between smoking and various diseases of both a chronic and lethal nature. Several organizations played a key role in the wellness movement, including the President's Council on Physical Fitness and Sports, the Society for Prospective Medicine, the American Federation of Fitness Directors in Business, and chapters of the Young Men's Christian Association throughout the country. It is important to note that none of these factors operated in isolation. It was the dovetailing and meshing of the various forces that produced the wellness/health movement of today (Ardell, 1985).

PROMINENT INDIVIDUALS IN THE WELLNESS/HEALTH MOVEMENT

Halpert L. Dunn was perhaps the most notable visionary in the early wellness movement. In 1961 he published his landmark work entitled *High-Level Wellness,* the first publication to significantly influence health professionals and introduce them to the total concept of wellness. Dunn stressed the need for mind/body/spirit connections and their importance to total well being. He repeatedly stressed the need for valued purposes in life and the necessity of personal satisfaction in the maintenance of a healthy state. Health, according to Dunn, was much more than nonillness, which was the traditional view of health until this time.

Belloc and Breslow (1972) studied the effect of health care skills on life expectancy and quality of life. Their results showed that individuals who observed six to seven basic practices could expect to live longer lives. These practices included moderate use of alcohol or abstinence, daily breakfast, three regular meals daily, moderate weight, nonsmoking, 7 to 8 hours of sleep daily, and moderate exercise twice weekly.

John Travis, one of Dunn's earliest followers, developed a health/wellness model (1977) that compared traditional views of health to a self-responsibility model. The illness-wellness continuum is used frequently by wellness-oriented practitioners (Fig. 4-1). At one end of the continuum is the treatment model, which moves along the continuum and stops at a neutral point in the middle. At this point there is no discernible illness or wellness. The model for self-responsibility goes beyond this point and encompasses education, growth, and self-actualization, with the achievement of high-level wellness at the other end of the continuum. Travis' *The Wellness Workbook for Helping Professionals,* published in 1987, still is used extensively today in wellness courses throughout the country.

Another book, Donald Ardell's *High-Level Wellness: An Alternative to Doctors, Drugs and Disease* also was published in 1977. This work provided a framework and an ethic that were to guide most future programs in wellness. Ardell outlined five dimensions of wellness that need to be considered by practitioners in the development of wellness approaches and programs: self-responsibility, nutritional awareness, stress management,

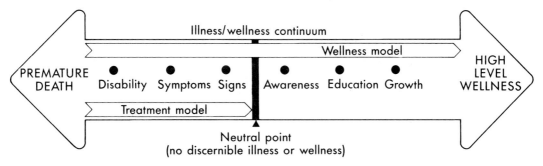

FIG. 4-1 Travis' illness/wellness continuum. *(From* The wellness workbook *by J. W. Travis and R. S. Ryan, 1981, Berkeley, CA: Ten Speed Press. Copyright 1981 by Ten Speed Press. Reprinted by permission.)*

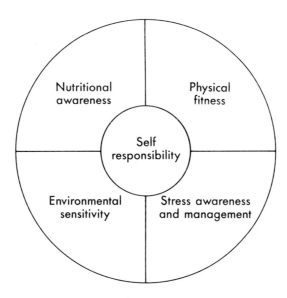

FIG. 4-2 Ardell's wellness model. *(From* 14 Days to a wellness lifestyle *by D. Ardell, 1982, San Rafael, CA: New World Library. Copyright 1982 by New World Library. Reprinted by permission.)*

physical fitness, and environmental sensitivity. Self-responsibility is depicted as the center of the other dimensions. It is crucial to the development and implementation of well-related behaviors in the other four spheres (Fig. 4-2).

William Hettler, while serving as the head of the student health service at the University of Wisconsin during the 1970s, developed the first student-led wellness model. This model is used extensively in colleges and universities throughout the country. His efforts led to the inception of the annual wellness festivals held at Stevens Point, Wisconsin, which were instrumental in dissemination of wellness-promoting activities nationwide (Ardell, 1985).

Certainly numerous other individuals contributed to the development of the wellness movement as it has come to be called, but the individuals named here defined the foundations and key concepts of wellness.

TERMS USED IN THE WELLNESS MOVEMENT

Students who read on the topic of wellness might easily become confused by the vast spectrum of terminology that describes wellness and its related concepts. Very often these terms are used interchangeably, which increases the general confusion.

Health itself has been defined in a variety of ways and from differing perspectives. The first definition of health to deviate from a purely biological orientation was that issued by the World Health Organization in 1947. It defined health as "a state of complete physical, mental, and social well-being and not merely the absence of disease or infirmity." The importance of this definition was its inclusion of psychosocial considerations. Halpert Dunn's definition of health is considered conclusive: "health is an integrated method of functioning which is oriented toward maximizing the potential of which the individual is capable, within the environment where he is functioning" (Dunn, 1961, p. 5). Donald Ardell integrated concepts of health, wellness, and prevention and defined what he called high-level wellness as "a life-style—focused approach designed for the purpose of pursuing the highest level of health within one's capability. A wellness life-style is dynamic or everchanging as the individual evolves throughout life. It is an integrated life-style in that it incorporates some approach or aspect of each wellness dimension" (Ardell, 1977, p. 65).

Rene Dubos, philosopher and microbiologist, defined health from an ecological perspective as an expression of fitness to the environment, that is, as a state of adaptedness. It is the condition of the whole person engaged in effective and fruitful interaction with the physical and social environment. Health then represents freedom from physical and mental discomfort (Dubos, 1965). The well-known social critic, Ivan Illich, defined health as "the intensity with which individuals cope with their internal states and their environmental conditions" (1977, p.271).

Several nursing theorists also have presented views on health. Betty Neuman, Parse, and Pender are considered to be among the foremost health theorists in nursing. These three theorists view the individual holistically and perceive health as a process that reflects person-environment relationships. Persons are seen not as passive receivers of health care or respondents to their environments but rather as self-determining beings in continuous interaction with their environment, with resultant positive and negative consequences. Pender defines health as "the actualization of the person's potential through goal-directed behavior, competent self-care and satisfying relationships with others while adjustments are made as needed to maintain structural integrity and harmony within the environment" (Pender, 1987, p. 27). The following terms are seen frequently in wellness-related literature and are defined here for clarity.

Disease prevention encompasses those activities that contain or actually prevent the spread of disease. It includes primary, secondary, and tertiary levels of prevention.

Health promotion refers to a wide variety of activities, including risk-reduction classes (e.g., weight loss and stop-smoking clinics), testing, health hazard assessments, jogging and other fitness activities, and physical examination. Health-promotion activities are examples of primary prevention (Ardell, 1985).

Health education focuses on risk reduction and alleviation of problems through retraining of attitudes and behavior. It assists persons with medical concerns and problems to function and cope more effectively.

Holistic health emphasizes the mind-body connection in health and illness, personal responsibility, and a balanced life-style. In this approach, fitness, stress management, and nutrition, along with other aspects of optimal functioning, are integrated into a total approach. Nondrug, nonsurgical interventions for the treatment of illness conditions are stressed in holistic health.

Medical self-care stresses personal responsibility for health by teaching appropriate levels of self-sufficiency with self-monitoring of blood pressure, diet, exercise, and routine health-related procedures such as breast and pelvic examinations.

Wellness is defined as "an integrated method of functioning which is oriented toward maximizing the potential of which the individual is capable. It requires that the individual maintain a continuum of balance and purposeful direction within the environment where he is functioning" (Dunn, 1977, pp. 5-6). It includes a conscious and deliberate approach to an advanced state of physical, psychological, and spiritual health and is a dynamic, fluctuating state of being.

In addition to basic definitions of wellness-related terms as they are used in nursing literature, it is important to understand the various approaches to wellness. These approaches often are referred to as *conceptual frameworks* or *models.* These terms mean that a viewpoint or structure is presented by an expert in the field of wellness, which provides a way of viewing wellness or understanding how best to present the concepts to the client.

MODELS OF WELLNESS
Health Belief Model

A frequently used model in the development of wellness programs is the health belief model developed by Rosenstock (Becker, Haefner, Kasl, Kirscht, Maiman, & Rosenstock, 1977). This model attempts to explain why and under what conditions persons take action to prevent, detect, or comply with treatment. The model asserts that the decision to undertake preventive health measures is influenced by an individual's perception of personal susceptibility to a particular condition and the severity of consequences if that condition develops. Motivation to take action to promote health or to prevent disease is based on how strongly the individual believes that the following statements apply to him or her (Becker, 1974):

1. I am personally susceptible to the disease.
2. The illness would affect my life in a significant way.
3. Taking action would reduce my susceptibility or, if the illness occurred, would reduce its severity.
4. Taking action would not require me to endure significant financial strain, inconvenience, pain, or embarrassment.
5. Disease can be present even in the absence of apparent illness or symptoms.

Together these perceptions produce a readiness that will result in the desired behavior when there is an appropriate cue to action, a lack of barriers, and belief of the usefulness of the action. Consider the wellness behavior of breast self-examination. A woman's estimated probability that she will encounter breast cancer constitutes perceived susceptibility. Given an appropriate cue (exposure to the media) and the lack of significant barriers (fear, embarrassment, or a lack of knowledge), a woman would find the value of breast self-examination enhanced by the recognition that she is susceptible to breast cancer, by her perception of the severity of the negative aspects of breast cancer, and by the belief that performing breast self-examination is useful. According to the health belief model the woman who is most likely to carry out the behavior of breast self-examination in the prescribed way will be one who believes that she is especially vulnerable to breast cancer (Calnan & Rutter, 1986).

Rosenstock's model includes two variables, a psychological state of readiness to take action and the extent to which a particular action is believed to be beneficial. Rosenstock

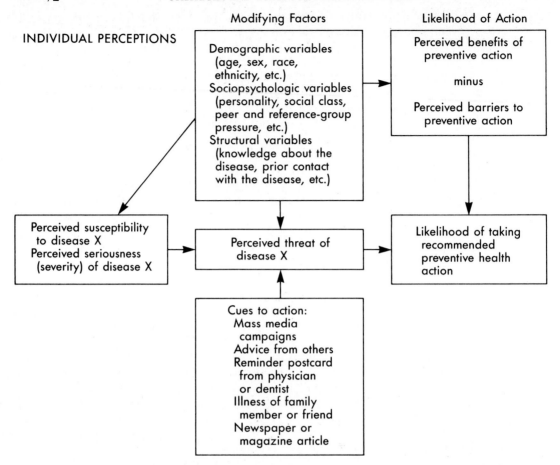

FIG. 4-3 Rosenstock's health belief model. *(From Becker MD, "Selected psychosocial models and correlates of individual health-related behaviors" by M.D. Becker, D. P. Haefner, S. V. Kasl, J.P. Kirscht, L.A. Maiman, and I.M. Rosenstock, 1977,* Medical Care, *15(5), p. 24. Copyright 1977 by ——— . Reprinted by permission.)*

defined the state of readiness as the person's perceived susceptibility to a condition and the perceived seriousness of that condition (Fig. 4-3). Previous research has established a relationship between perceived susceptibility and preventive health behaviors.

The health belief model was tested by Larson et al (1979) by studying the relationship of certain health beliefs and values to the influenza vaccination and the effect of a postcard reminder concerning vaccination dates. The persons who followed up and received the vaccine believed vaccination to be more efficacious than did those who remained unvaccinated. In addition, those individuals who were not vaccinated were less satisfied with their medical care generally; they also considered the vaccine to be more expensive than did those who were vaccinated. The study indicated that persons who perceive the benefits of a preventive behavior as outweighing the barriers usually have a higher health value orientation and thus undertake the preventive behavior (Larson, Bergman, Herdricht, Alvin, & Schneeweiss, 1979).

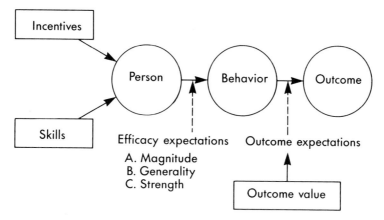

FIG. 4-4 The self-efficacy model. *(Modified from "Self-efficacy and weight control* [11] *by S.M. Desmond and J.H. Price, 1988,* Health Education, *19(1), 13 [Modified from A. Bandura, 1977,* Psychological Review, *84(2), p. 191.])*

The Self-Efficacy Model

Recent work in the field of wellness has suggested that the health belief model would be enhanced by the addition of concepts from the self-efficacy model (Desmond & Price, 1988). Bandura's theory of self-efficacy looks at whether an individual will initiate a healthy behavior and how long that person will maintain that behavior and/or strive to achieve it (Bandura, 1977). Use of the perceived self-efficacy model is an effective vehicle for bringing about desired behavior changes in a specific area of life-style (Fig. 4-4). A person's belief regarding (1) ability to perform a specific health-related behavior and (2) the probability that the performed behavior will lead to the anticipated outcome directly affect its performance or lack of it.

Consider the case of Jack M, who decides it would be healthy to embark on an exercise regimen. Jack's physician suggests that he attend aerobic classes three times a week. Although Jack knows that his work schedule prohibits attendance at such a class three times a week on a consistent basis, he agrees to try to meet this goal. During the first week Jack regularly attended the classes. His second week's attendance drops to twice a week. The classes are rigorous and tiring, and Jack has difficulty keeping up with the fast tempo. The only perceivable outcome at this point is increased stress from trying to meet the proposed attendance schedule and sore, aching muscles. By the end of 1 month Jack no longer is attending the classes and has decided that maybe he really does not need to exercise after all. Thus this client's *efficacy expectations* (i.e., what he hopes to achieve—in this case improved health) were incongruent with his outcome expectations (sore muscles and stress).

Efficacy expectations vary in magnitude, generality, and strength, which, combined, affect performance. *Magnitude* refers to the difficulty level of the involved tasks and the person's belief regarding ability to perform them. The individual's perception of whether the expected behavior relates to only one specific situation or to a variety of situations is referred to as *generality* of self-efficacy. *Strength* of efficacy expectation relates to the individual's resoluteness of belief in the ability to perform the health-related behavior. Sources of efficacy expectations include the way the individual accomplishes the performed task, observance of successful performance of the task by others, verbal persuasion to convince the individual that he or she can perform the behavior, and emotional arousal to convince the client of his or her ability to complete the task (Desmond & Price, 1988).

Consider again Jack's situation regarding the need for an exercise program. Taking into account his rigorous work schedule and lack of conditioning at the time, the occupational health nurse at his work setting suggests that Jack begin his exercise program by walking for 15 minutes daily during his lunch hour for a 2-week period. She also suggests that Jack walk with another person in the company who has been involved in a walking program for 1 month. Jack begins walking and achieves success. His co-worker encourages him and stresses how much better he feels since embarking on the walking program. Jack then decides he would like to engage in some other type of exercise program to develop and tone other body muscle groups.

The nurse suggests stopping at a local gymnasium twice a week, one of the days to be a weekend day when Jack would have no work commitments. This particular facility designs individual exercise programs after assessing preexercise tone levels, age, and ability to work with weights and toning machines. It opens early in the morning and Jack schedules his weekday visits on Wednesdays at 7 AM, which is a lighter day for him in terms of workload. The nurse and Jack discuss specific benefits he wishes to see from his exercise program and how certain he is that he can carry out his new goals. Jack finds that his lunchtime walking program and the twice-weekly individually tailored program at the local gym meet his needs for an exercise regimen. He also feels that he is able to accomplish his goals, and he continues to receive encouragement and support from the occupational nurse, his walking partner, and the staff members of the exercise facility he has chosen. Jack's efficacy expectations and outcome expectations are congruent this time, and he is successful in maintaining his exercise program over a specified period of time.

Contracting

The health behavior contract is another useful approach for achieving behavior changes in the wellness area. A health behavior contract is a formal written agreement between the nurse and the client, which is designed to systematically change a behavior within the client's life-style (Fig. 4-5). Important components of behavior contracts include short- and long-term goals, measurable behaviors, planning for steps needed to achieve the goal, and consideration of positive and negative factors that may affect goal achievement. A self-care contract should provide rewards and punishments and indicate a target date for reevaluation of goal achievement. Behavior contracts have been shown to improve goal-setting abilities and awareness of behavior cues. Clients also can be assisted to substitute positive health practices for negative ones (Kittleson & Hageman-Rigney, 1988). Health-behavior contracts stress self-responsibility and the need to take control of one's health and life-style management.

Social Support

Most wellness models include some reference to the importance of social support for achievement of wellness behavioral changes. Effective models contain two components: a direct support component and a modeling component. Supportiveness is the degree to which respondents perceive others in their environment as actively supporting or helping them in their efforts to change health-related behaviors. Modeling refers to the degree of personal involvement of significant others in the individual's health-related efforts. Early research findings suggest that change is affected both by social supports that help the person stay motivated and by the modeling of positive health-related behaviors on the

NURSE-CLIENT CONTRACT/AGREEMENT

Statement of health goal: _____ Nutritional planning for weight control _____

I _____ Jean Jones _____ promise to _____ Maintain a dietary _____
         (Client)

_____ intake log of all foods eaten daily _____
         (Client responsibility)

for a period of_____ one week _____ , whereupon,

_____ Cheryl Jenkins _____ will provide _____ a copy of _____
         (Nurse)

Ann Smith's book, Nutrition and Weight Control _____
         (Nurse responsibility)

on _____ Friday, January 7, 1989 _____ to me.
         (Date)

If I do not fulfill the terms of this contract in total, I
understand that the designated reward will be withheld.

Signed: _____
         (Client)

_____
         (Date)

_____
         (Nurse)

_____

FIG. 4-5 Nurse-client contract/agreement:

part of others in that person's environment (Robbins & Slavin, 1988). Therefore it is suggested that a health-support index be used in wellness programs to assess the degree of support persons receive from their social environments.

Individuals of course rarely function in isolation in our society; they are viewed instead as part of a system. Thus the "Heart Smart" cardiovascular health program (Johnson, Nicklas, Arbeit, Franklin, & Berenson, 1988) has developed a family health-promotion model that incorporates and relates many of the aforementioned models and concepts to the family setting. The program seeks to modify cardiovascular risk factors in parents and children through alterations in behavior in the areas of diet, exercise, and stress management. Major components of the maintenance program are intrafamily and interfamily social support, personal self-management, and reinforcement of the cardiovascular health program.

Contact with program participants was maintained by telephone, mail, or personal contact over a 5-year period. Designers of the program sought to help families maintain changes in the previously cited areas for the purpose of improving cardiovascular health. Based on the success of such groups as Weight Watchers and Alcoholics Anonymous, Heart Smart's family health promotion program enlisted participants to carry the message to new members, to share their experiences, and to offer support personally or by telephone contact. Personal self-management was achieved by teaching adults and children to become in essence their own counselors. The participants kept eating behavior and exercise logs and were responsible for self-observation and monitoring. Clients were taught stimulus control principles and were urged to reward themselves for weekly self-monitoring. Self-evaluation was based on comparison of behavioral records and individual goals. Self-reinforcement was provided through reciprocal contracts and rewards during the maintenance phase. The overall effectiveness of the Heart Smart maintenance model was monitored by physiological assessments and self-reported behaviors. Fig. 4-6 shows an example of a data collection timeline used in the program.

**The "Heart Smart" Family Health
Promotion Maintenance Data
Collection Timeline**

Weekly
24-hour food records (self-monitored)
Exercise log (self-monitored)
Behavioral records (self-monitored)

Monthly
Grocery receipts (self-monitored)
Weight

Quarterly
Blood pressure
Group 24-hour dietary recalls

Semiannually
Risk factor screening (including venipuncture and urine collection)

Annually
Paper-and-pencil questionnaires

FIG. 4-6 Data collection time line. (From *"A comprehensive model for maintenance of family health behaviors: the heart smart family health promotion program" by C. Johnson et al., 1988,* Family and Community Health, *11(1), p. 6, with permission of Aspen Publishers, Inc., copyright 1988.)*

The MATCH Model

The models presented thus far have viewed wellness and health promotion from a personal and family perspective. A great deal of controversy surrounds the area of focus for health/wellness educational efforts. A multilevel intervention approach has been proposed (Simons-Morton, D.G., Simons-Morton, B.G., Parcel, G.S., & Bunker, J.F.,1988), which is useful in influencing both personal preventive services and community preventive services. The multilevel approaches toward community health (MATCH) model conceptualizes intervention directed at individual, organizational, and governmental levels (Fig. 4-7). Individual health is affected through personal behaviors, whereas organizations affect the health of their members through policies and practices. A government affects its electorate's health by public action and legislation. Thus community health intervention can consist of "(1) influencing individuals to reduce personal risk factors for disease and (2) influencing organizations and governments to reduce environmental risk factors for disease and to facilitate positive influences on personal behaviors and physiology" (Simons-Morton, D.G., Simons-Morton, B.G., Parcel, G.S., & Bunker, J.F., 1988, p. 27).

Phase I of the MATCH model consists of the selection of health goals for the target population. The target population is in this instance those persons whose health is of concern. It can be an individual client, a group, or an identified community. Appropriate health goals are selected for the target population.

In Phase II appropriate interventions are planned to achieve the health goals in the target population through environmental and personal change. An example of intervention at the individual level is reduction in the personal disease risk factors of individual participants. Organizational-level objectives include changes in or establishment of organizational policies or programs, and government-level objectives include changes in or establishment of local, state, or federal governmental policies, programs, and legislation.

Individual target populations are family groups as well as the individual members themselves. Organizational-level target populations include decision makers and persons of influence in the targeted organization. Governmental-level target populations include leaders and persons of power and influence in the targeted governmental entity.

Phase III involves several steps. These include development and implementation of the interventions selected in Phase II, development and testing of needed materials, hiring of additional personnel, scheduling meeting or class sites, and conducting interventions. Phase IV evaluates the achievement of health goals and intervention objectives from Phases I and II.

Consider the example of coronary artery disease. To decrease the prevalence and severity of this health problem in the community, nurses who use the MATCH model might consider influencing the process at all three levels (Simons-Morton, D.G., Simons-Morton, B.G., Parcel, G.S., & Bunker, J.F., 1988, pp. 31-32), as follows:

> ... *individuals* to eat foods that are low in fat and salt, to do aerobic exercise on a regular basis, and to not smoke, *organizations* to provide low-fat and low-salt selections for food purchase, to establish exercise facilities, and to implement smoking restriction policies, and *governments* to fund research on dietary practices to lower CHD [coronary heart disease] risk, to provide food commodities that meet dietary recommendations to lower CHD risk, to initiate community education campaigns, and to pass ordinances, laws, and regulations restricting smoking in public places.

This model is unique in that it involves health and education professionals, as well as others, in intervention efforts to improve the health of the population. Laypersons, institutions, and political action groups all can make a significant contribution.

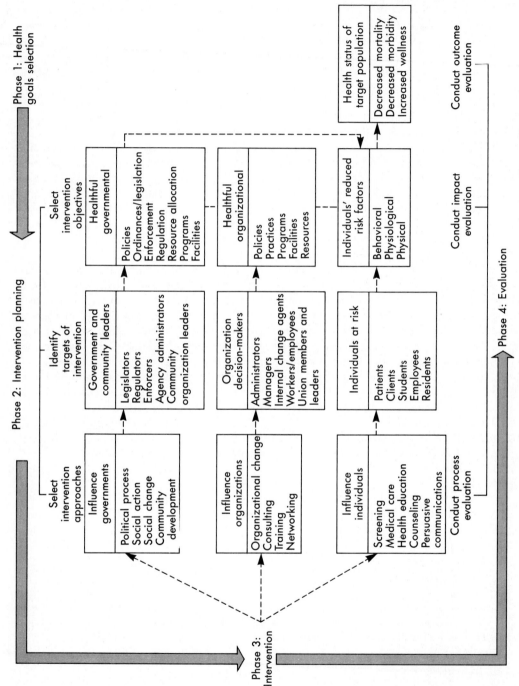

FIG. 4-7 The MATCH model for community health intervention. (*From "Influencing personal and environmental conditions for community health: A multi-level intervention model" by D.G. Simons-Morton, B.G. Simons-Morton, G.S. Parcel, J.F.Bunker, August 1988, Family & Community Health, 11(2), p. 29. Copyright 1988 by Aspen Publishers, Inc. Reprinted by permission.*)

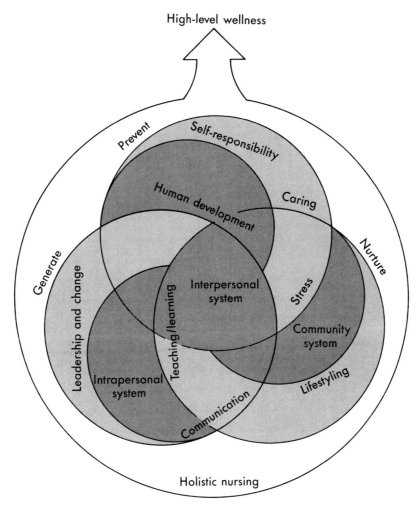

FIG. 4-8 The holistic nursing model. *(From* Holistic nursing *(p. 24) by B. Blattner, 1981, Englewood Cliffs, NJ: Prentice-Hall. Copyright 1981 by Prentice-Hall. Reprinted by permission.)*

The Holistic Nursing Perspective

Another wellness model reflects the holistic nursing perspective (Blattner, 1981). This model (Fig. 4-8) has many interlocking circles, half-circles, and eclipses that show the relationships and connectedness of the systems and their relationship to the holistic nursing process. Central to the figure are three circles that represent nurturant, generative, and preventive nursing interventions. The nine areas that require processing to achieve wellness are self-responsibility, caring, stress, life-style, human development, problem solving, communication, teaching-learning and leadership, and change. Superimposed on these areas are the intrapersonal, interpersonal, and community systems. Intrapersonal encompasses the nurse/client relationship, interpersonal involves groups such as families, and community denotes organizations or persons with common interests. High-level wellness is achieved through the nine life processes within these three systems.

ASSESSMENT OF WELLNESS BEHAVIORS

Nurses first must understand their own wellness practices and philosophies if they are to be effective teachers and models of wellness. Self-assessment of life-style beliefs and behaviors is a good starting point. Several tools for wellness life-style assessment have been developed that require only a short time for completion, (Fig. 4-9). Complete the questionnaire and determine your own "wellness score." What deficits and strengths did you find? How might this affect your ability to effectively teach wellness concepts to your clients?

Completion of a life-style assessment questionnaire by clients enables them to look objectively at their wellness practices and assess positive as well as negative areas. For total accuracy of responses the client should be allowed to complete the questionnaire without interference. Clients generally find this exercise interesting and often revealing. It is important to recognize that a client's ability to incorporate wellness concepts into personal beliefs and behaviors is governed by many factors, including a positive self-concept and attitude, a holistic perspective on health, cultural beliefs, and self-discipline. The ability to make wellness choices depends in part on the client's flexibility and capacity for change.

Values

Values play a key role in wellness choices because they affect motivation, thought, affect, and behavior. For a value to be internalized as a wellness behavior, the client must choose the value freely from among several alternatives. The outcomes of the various alternatives must have been considered in a deliberate fashion. The selected value must be prized or cherished and made known to others. Clients then must be willing to act upon the value and incorporate it into life-style practices. Consider the nurse who counsels the hypertensive client about the hazards of smoking but smokes two packs of cigarettes per day. An inconsistent message is given to the client, which indicates that the nurse advocates choosing the value of nonsmoking but does not prize it or act upon it. Individuals who have determined what is important in their lives (choosing a value) tend to make responsible decisions regarding their life-style (acting upon the value). Nurses who work with clients cannot prescribe wellness activities and choices for a client but must maintain an open, supportive, and nonjudgmental attitude. Nurses should serve as catalysts to help clients move toward self-responsibility in a wellness life-style (Gutt, 1983).

Motivation

Motivation is a crucial element in understanding why a client will accept and practice a wellness behavior. Clients first must become aware of things as they are, then as they might be. Strategies for bridging the gap must be devised, and the client must believe in his or her ability to carry out the strategies. This incorporates both the self-efficacy model and the health belief model. The client's social support and locus of control also must be considered in motivation assessment. Social support can be material or psychological support. It can include the expectations that the support group places on the client. The locus of control can be internal or external. Internally controlled individuals believe that their actions control outcomes in their lives. Externally controlled individuals believe that their outcomes are determined by others (Blattner, 1981).

Numerous strategies can be used by the nurse in working with clients to achieve

SELF TEST FOR HEALTH STYLE

Directions

This is not a pass-fail test. Its purpose is simply to tell you how well you are doing in staying healthy. The behaviors covered in the test are recommended for most Americans. Some of them may not apply to persons with certain chronic diseases or handicaps. Such persons may require special instructions from their physician or other health professional.

The test has six sections: smoking, alochol and drugs, nutrition, exercise and fitness, stress control, and safety. Complete one section at a time by circling the number corresponding to the answer that best describes your behavior (2 for "Almost always", 1 for "Sometimes", and 0 for "Almost never"). Then add the numbers you have circled to determine your score for that section. Write the score on the line provided at the end of each section. The highest score you can get for each section is 10.

Cigarette smoking	Almost always	Sometimes	Almost never
If you never smoke, enter a score of 10 for this section and go to the next section.			
1. I avoid smoking cigarettes.	2	1	0
2. I smoke only low-tar and nicotine cigarettes, or I smoke a pipe or cigars.	2	1	0

Smoking score: _____

Alcohol and drugs	Almost always	Sometimes	Almost never
1. I avoid drinking alcoholic beverages, or I drink no more than one or two drinks a day.	4	1	0
2. I avoid using alcohol or other drugs (especially illegal drugs) as a way of handling stressful situations or the problems in my life.	2	1	0
3. I am careful not to drink alcohol when taking certain medicines (for example, medicine for sleeping, pain, colds, and allergies) or when pregnant.	2	1	0
4. I read and follow the label directions when using prescribed and over-the-counter drugs.	2	1	0

Alcohol and drugs score: _____

Eating habits	Almost always	Sometimes	Almost never
1. I eat a variety of foods each day, such as fruits and vegetables, whole grain breads and cereals, lean meats, dairy products, dry peas and beans, and nuts and seeds.	4	1	0
2. I limit the amount of fat, saturated fat, and cholesterol I eat (including fat on meats, eggs, butter, cream, shortenings, and organ meats, such as liver).	2	1	0
3. I limit the amount of salt I eat by cooking with only small amounts, not adding salt at the table, and avoiding salty snacks.	2	1	0
4. I avoid eating too much sugar (especially frequent snacks of sticky candy or soft drinks).	2	1	0

Eating habits score: _____

Continued.

FIG. 4-9 Self-test for health style. *(From U.S. Department of Health and Human Services, Office of Health Information, Health Promotion, and Physical Fitness and Sports Medicine. Washington, DC: U.S. Government Printing Office.)*

Exercise/fitness	Almost always	Sometimes	Almost never
1. I maintain a desired weight, avoiding overweight and underweight.	3	1	0
2. I do vigorous exercises for 15-30 minutes at least three times a week (examples: running, swimming, brisk walking).	3	1	0
3. I do exercises that enhance my muscle tone for 15-30 minutes at least three times a week (examples: yoga and calisthenics).	2	1	0
4. I use part of my leisure time participating in individual, family, or team activities (such as gardening, bowling, golf, and baseball) that increase my level of fitness.	2	1	0

Exercise/fitness score: _____

Stress control	Almost always	Sometimes	Almost never
1. I have a job or do other work that I enjoy.	2	1	0
2. I find it easy to relax and express my feelings freely.	2	1	0
3. I recognize early, and prepare for, events or situations likely to be stressful for me.	2	1	0
4. I have close friends, relatives, or others whom I can talk to about personal matters and call on for help when needed.	2	1	0
5. I participate in group activities (such as church and community organizational activites) or hobbies that I enjoy.	2	1	0

Stress control score: _____

Safety	Almost always	Sometimes	Almost never
1. I wear a seat belt while riding in a car.	2	1	0
2. I avoid driving while under the influence of alcohol and other drugs.	2	1	0
3. I obey traffic rules and the speed limit when driving.	2	1	0
4. I am careful when using potentially harmful products or substances (such as household cleaners, poisons, and electrical devices).	2	1	0
5. I avoid smoking in bed.	2	1	0

Safety score: _____

FIG. 4-9, cont'd. Self-test for health style.

Your healthstyle scores

After you have figured your scores for each of the six sections, circle the number in each column that matches your score for that section of the test.

Cigarette smoking	Alcohol and drugs	Eating habits	Exercise and fitness	Stress control	Safety
10	10	10	10	10	10
9	9	9	9	9	9
8	8	8	8	8	8
7	7	7	7	7	7
6	6	6	6	6	6
5	5	5	5	5	5
4	4	4	4	4	4
3	3	3	3	3	3
2	2	2	2	2	2
1	1	1	1	1	1
0	0	0	0	0	0

Remember, there is no total score for this test. Consider each section separately. You are trying to identify aspects of your lifestyle that you can improve in order to be healthier and to reduce the risk of illness. So let's see what your scores reveal.

Scores of 9 and 10: Excellent! Your answers show that you are aware of the importance of this area to your health. More importantly, you are putting your knowledge to work for you by practicing good health habits. As long as you continue to do so, this area should not pose a serious health risk. It's likely that you are setting an example for your family and friends to follow. Since you got a very high score on this part of the test, you may want to consider other areas where your scores indicate room for improvement.

Scores 6 to 8: Your health practices in this area are good, but there is room for improvement. Look again at the items you answered with a "Sometimes" or "Almost Never." What changes can you make to improve your score? Even a small change can often help you achieve better health.

Scores of 3 to 5: Your health risks are showing! Would you like more information about the risks you are facing and about why it is important for you to change these behaviors? Perhaps you need help in deciding how to make successfully the changes you desire. In either case, help is available.

Scores 0 to 2: Obviously, you were concerned enough about your health to take the test, but your answers show that you may be taking serious and unnecessary risks with your health. Perhaps you are not aware of the risks and what to do about them. You can easily get the information and help you need to improve, if you wish. The next step is up to you.

FIG. 4-9, cont'd.　Self-test for health style.

	Positive Beliefs and Attitudes	Negative Beliefs and Attitudes
Adequate supports	Category 1 Teaching strategies	Category 2 Teaching Strategies
Adequate supports	Structured to facilitate affective, cognitive, psycho-motor learning. Discuss important points first and repeat. Present clearly and concisely in logical categories. Aim printed material at learner reading level. If denying, give basic survival information. If client focuses on the prob-lem, give him detailed information.	Focus on consciousness-raising techniques. Use nurse/client discussions to explore feelings. Form self-help groups with clients having similar problems. Use values clarification. Use behavior modification techniques by identifying a list of rewards ahead of time and giving temporary artificial rewards for healthy behavior. Identify cues for healthy and unhealthy behaviors. Keep a log or diary for several days to identify cues.
Inadequate supports	Category 3 Teaching Strategies	Category 4 Teaching Strategies
Inadequate supports	Increase social support and cognitive strengthening. Provide family and friends with important information and encourage involvement with therapy regime discus-sions and value clarification sessions. Use assertiveness training, relaxation and imagery. If clients have external locus of control, involve them with com-munity agencies and self-help groups. If clients have internal locus of control, utilize problem-solving and goal-setting approaches.	Utilize foot in the door strategies and aim for the minimal behavior change needed to accomplish the goal with a positive result. Provide simple regimens with basic goal-setting. Give rewards and rein-forcements for healthy behaviors. Break goals into subsets mov-ing from simple to complex. Utilize written versus verbal contracts.

FIG. 4-10 Integrated health belief and social support model. *(Modified from* Holistic nursing: A handbook for practice *p. 140, by B. Dossey, L. Keegan, C. E. Guzetta, and L. G. Kolkmeier, 1988, Rockville, MD: Aspen. Copyright 1988 by Aspen Publishers, Inc. Reprinted with permission.)*

wellness goals (Dossey, Keegan, Guzzetta, & Kolkmeier, 1988). The client's health beliefs (positive or negative) and social support (adequate or absent) are assessed, and the client is placed in one of four categories. Specific teaching strategies are then chosen to implement wellness learning and behaviors depending on the category in which the client falls. Not all strategies are useful in each of the categories, which may account for a client's lack of adherence to a wellness program. Fig. 4-10 presents a diagrammatic interpretation of these categories and strategies that the nurse can use in wellness education.

Consideration of client value systems, locus of control, social support, and motivation is necessary for the successful development and implementation of individual or group wellness programs.

WELLNESS COMPONENTS
Physical Fitness

Today's sedentary life-style, with its dependency on high technology, is a deterrence to active use of the body and the total self in either the workplace or home setting. The wellness movement stressed a total body-mind integration, and as a result, many Americans began to exercise on a regular basis. Several benefits were noted. Among them were increased longevity and prevention of several life-style—related diseases such as diabetes, obesity, and coronary heart disease. Other benefits, more noticeable on a daily basis, included better sleep habits, decreased stress, improved posture and energy, and a general sense of well being.

Physical fitness programs include several types of movement. Aerobic exercise targets the heart, blood vessels, and lungs; it is achieved through such activity as dancing, swimming, jogging, cycling, rowing, and aerobic walking. It is important to engage in this type of exercise at least three times a week. (Fig. 4-11 illustrates two types of exercise that are beneficial and inexpensive.) The exercise activity should include a 5-minute warm-up period, sustained exercise for at least 20 to 30 minutes, and a cool-down period of 5 minutes. To achieve maximum benefit from aerobic exercise, participants must attain and maintain what is known as the *target heart rate* (THR). To calculate the THR, the person's

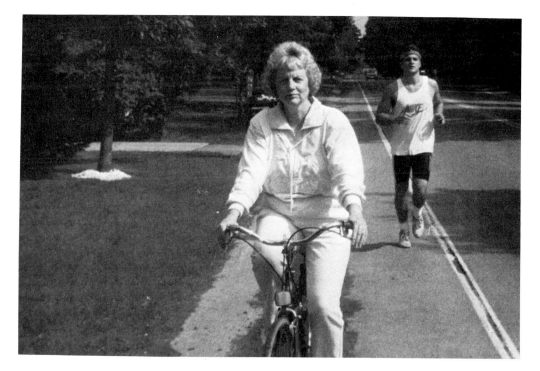

FIG. 4-11 Exercise activities can be varied to suit the age and fitness levels of the individual. Note the middle-aged adult riding the bicycle, while in the background a young adult is seen jogging for fitness.

age is subtracted from 220. This number is then called the maximum heart rate (MHR) and is multiplied by 60% to 85%, depending on age and general condition. Older or extremely sedentary persons would use the 60% figure to calculate their THR. Younger, reasonably fit persons would multiply by 75%. Individuals who already participate in a regular, vigorous exercise plan would use 85% of the MHR to calculate their target rate. For example, consider Mary M, aged 62 years, a recently retired office worker who feels she would like to go to Jazzercise sessions at the YWCA with her friend Judy now that she has more leisure time. *Mary had not before participated in any type of exercise program.* The following calculation provides Mary's THR:

$$
\begin{array}{ll}
220 & \\
-\,62 & \text{(Mary's age)} \\
=158 & \text{(MHR)} \\
\times\ \ 65\% & \text{(appropriate for Mary's age and condition)} \\
=102.70,\ \text{or}\ 103 & \text{(Mary's THR)}
\end{array}
$$

The pulse rate must be checked frequently during the exercise session to be sure that the THR is being sustained for the entire half-hour period.

Yoga and stretching exercises can be used to improve flexibility and to enhance a regular exercise regimen. These types of exercises should be done slowly and gradually to achieve maximum range of motion.

Exercises to increase muscle strength and endurance are termed *isotonic and iso-kinetic.* Calisthenics and weightlifting programs frequently involve this type of exercise.

Isometric exercise produces a contraction of muscle groupings, with little or no joint movement. Unlike aerobic exercise, it does not affect the heart and lungs.

Nurses frequently are asked to counsel clients about wellness exercise programs. Clients should be advised to learn what types of programs are available in their areas. Consultation with a physician or exercise physiologist is advised if the client is older than 35 years of age or has a handicapping or chronic condition. Age 35 generally is used as a parameter for the middle-adulthood grouping. Clients must be assisted to establish long- and short-term goals and a specific schedule and timetable for the exercise program. It is important to evaluate any type of exercise program monthly to determine results, problems, and client satisfaction. The saying "no pain—no gain" is untrue; exercise should be enjoyable as well as beneficial. The client who feels pain while exercising should proceed with caution because injuries can result.

Fitness programs now are part of many nursery school activities and senior citizen programs. Fitness for everyone is the goal. Looking good should include not only the external manifestations of fitness, such as slimness and muscle development, but also the condition of the internal organs, particularly the cardiovascular system. More specific information on physical fitness can be found in any comprehensive wellness or health education text.

Nutrition

Good nutrition management is an essential component of a wellness life-style and therefore an inherent element of any wellness program, individual or group. It is necessary for individuals to nurture the body through dietary intake; however, recent discoveries in the field of nutrition indicate that caloric consumption cannot be the only guiding factor in dietary selection. It has been found that the amounts of salt, sugar, fiber, and saturated fats that an individual consumes relate directly to the prevention or the incidence of

A Guide to Good Eating

Milk group	Meat group
3 or more glasses milk—children	2 or more servings
(Small glasses for some children under 8)	Meats, fish, poultry, eggs, or cheese—with dry beans, peas, nuts as alternates
4 or more glasses—teenagers	
2 or more glasses—adults	
Cheese, ice cream and other milk-made foods can supply part of the milk	
Vegetables and fruits	**Breads and cereals**
4 or more servings	4 or more servings
Include dark green or yellow vegetables; citrus fruit or tomatoes	Enriched or whole grain Added milk improves nutritional values

FIG. 4-12 The four basic food groups. *(From* Guide to Good Eating, *1988. Courtesy National Dairy Council.)*

several diseases. These include diabetes, cancer, ulcers, heart disease, hypertension, and stroke. Knowledge of basic dietary principles to maintain ideal body weight and to assist in the maintenance of a prudent diet can be the key to improved energy, better health, and longer life span.

In the U.S. government publication *Dietary Goals for the United States* (1977) a Senate subcommittee looked at the issue of nutrition and its links to health and established seven basic dietary goals for the remainder of this century.

Four basic food groups (Fig. 4-12) have been identified as being necessary to wellness, and recommended amounts from each group should be included in the daily diet. Varying food within the groups also is urged because each has different nutritional value; for example, cauliflower differs from lettuce or peas even though all are vegetables.

Clients must receive health teaching regarding the need to eat foods that are as free as possible from excessive processing and chemical contamination. They should be encouraged to exclude foods from the diet that contain excessive additives, toxins, chemicals, and preservatives. Consumers must become label conscious, carefully screening lists of ingredients and recognizing misleading statements. The food we eat is exposed to multiple processes to enhance the shelf life of the product and at times its appearance. Clients need to be made aware of the hazards of food irradiation, meat and poultry supplementation, and chemical additives and preservatives. Irradiation causes depletion of vitamins A, C, E, and B complex and creates radioactive trace chemicals in the treated food. Some sources suggest that these elements may over time have carcinogenic properties. Hormones and antibiotics are given to farm animals and poultry to increase size and weight and therefore market value. The long-range effects of these procedures is unknown. Chemical additives are found in many foods to enhance color and taste. Again, the long-range effects of many of these dyes and flavor enhancers over time is unclear. Nurses need to be aware of these issues and be prepared to act as client advocates if necessary (Dossey, Keegan, Guzzetta, & Kolkmeier, 1988).

An important wellness consideration in the nutrition component is that of weight. Although Americans are eating more, they are not necessarily eating better. A successful weight-control program views psychological factors, environmental concerns, and genetics in assessing the client's weight gain. Additional factors in assessment are family history of obesity, situational factors that trigger eating, and psychological components of eating patterns. A dietary log that tracks what is eaten daily and weekly, as well as the circumstances, helps clients analyze factors relevant to their eating patterns. Caution is needed to avoid diets in which fewer than 1000 calories are allowed, which are deficient in essential vitamins or minerals, or which actually may contain hidden sources of fat. Fad diets come and go as quickly as the weather changes. Most are not effective for sustained weight loss and may, in fact, be harmful to health. The greatest success in achieving and maintaining weight loss occurs through a combination of a nutritionally balanced food plan and behavior-modification techniques in a self-help setting. The importance of support groups, be they friends, co-workers, or family cannot be overemphasized in long-term maintenance of weight loss (Swinford & Webster, 1989).

All weight-loss programs should incorporate exercise if they are to be effective. Here it is important to assess the client's age, fitness level, and existing health state to ensure that too rigorous an exercise program is not chosen. For some individuals, exercises to tone tissue and muscle may be accomplished through isometrics or low-impact aerobics without posing any hazards to health.

Clients can be referred to nutrition counselors, weight-loss support groups, and a variety of literature sources for additional information regarding nutritional and dietary concerns as they relate to wellness.

Inner Harmony

The ability to feel, think, and act well depends in great part on the ability to partake in the banquet of life. In contemporary society individuals are continually subjected to time, role, and social stressors that can affect the best-planned physical wellness program. The loss of family interaction and support, friends with whom to share positive and negative events, and the ability to laugh and enjoy takes its toll over time. The inability to cope with stressors in one's personal and extrapersonal environment often leads to symptoms of anxiety and stress.

Stress can manifest itself in a variety of domains. Clients may complain of insomnia, fatigue, irritability, anger, depression, hyperactivity, lack of concentration, forgetfulness, changes in eating habits, frequent tears, and impulsive behaviors. Physical symptoms abound and can include headaches, diarrhea, tics, backache, teeth grinding, shortness of breath, heart pounding, and vertigo.

The Social Readjustment Rating Scale (Fig. 4-13), which is an assessment tool to evaluate the statistical probability of contracting an illness, is based on stressors or change experienced by clients during the previous year. It is important to note that happy or

	Social Readjustment Rating Scale		
Rank	Event	Value	Score
1	Death of a spouse	100	_____
2	Divorce	73	_____
3	Marital separation	65	_____
4	Jail term	63	_____
5	Death of a close family member	63	_____
6	Personal injury or illness	53	_____
7	Marriage	50	_____
8	Fired from work	47	_____
9	Marital reconciliation	45	_____
10	Retirement	45	_____
11	Change in family member's health	44	_____
12	Pregnancy	40	_____
13	Sex difficulties	39	_____
14	Addition to family	39	_____
15	Business readjustment	39	_____
16	Change in financial status	38	_____
17	Death of a close friend	37	_____
18	Change to different line of work	36	_____
19	Change in number of marital arguments	35	_____
20	Mortgage or loan over $10,000	31	_____
21	Foreclosure of mortgage or loan	30	_____
22	Change in work responsibilities	29	_____
23	Son or daughter leaving home	29	_____
24	Trouble with-in-laws	29	_____
25	Outstanding personal achievement	28	_____
26	Spouse begins or stops work	26	_____
27	Starting or finishing school	26	_____
28	Change in living conditions	25	_____
29	Revision of personal habits	24	_____
30	Trouble with boss	23	_____
31	Change in work hours, conditions	20	_____
32	Change in residence	20	_____
33	Change in schools	20	_____
34	Change in recreational habits	19	_____
35	Change in church activities	19	_____
36	Change in social activities	18	_____
37	Mortgage or loan under $10,000	17	_____
38	Change in sleeping habits	16	_____
39	Change in number of family gatherings	15	_____
40	Change in eating habits	15	_____
41	Vacation	13	_____
42	Christmas season	12	_____
43	Minor violation of the law	11	_____

Score of less than 150: 37% chance of illness during the next two years.

Score of 150-300: 51% chance of illness during the next two years.

Score of more than 300: 80% chance of illness during the next two years.

FIG. 4-13 The Social Readjustment Rating Scale. *(From "Social Readjustment Rating Scale" by T. H. Holmes and R. H. Rahe, 1967,* Journal of Psychosomatic Research, 11, *p. 213. Copyright 1967 by Pergamon Press, Ltd. Reprinted by permission.)*

joyful events such as a new job or a wedding are changes that also are accompanied by a certain degree of stress. Individual scores are totaled, and ranges provide guidelines for the probability of illness occurring in the next 2 years. Quite often, clients are amazed at their scores and unaware of the cumulative effect of the many changes in their lives.

Coping strategies to produce relaxation and to assist in stress management must begin with awareness of stress, identification of specific stressors or stressful situations, and an evaluation of usual coping methods. Life-style behaviors must be scrutinized to ensure that adequate rest, nutrition, and physical activity are part of the daily routine. A regular exercise program is helpful in relieving stress and anxiety. Clients who participate in such activity on a regular basis state that missing the activity makes a definite difference in their attitude and coping in stressful situations.

A variety of other techniques and exercises are available to aid in achievement of inner harmony.

Progressive relaxation is a simple technique that can be done anywhere and at any time, particularly when one feels tension mounting. Through a combination of deep breathing and alternate tensing and relaxation of body muscle groups, clients can be taught to rid themselves of excess stress. A comfortable position is assumed, and muscle groups are first contracted, held, and then relaxed, progressing from the toes up through the neck and face muscles. Soothing music can be used in accompaniment to the exercise. Participants usually find the exercise helpful as an escape valve for excess tension.

Biofeedback is a technique that provides ongoing input to the client about internal physiological responses (generally believed to be good indicators of stress) such as pulse, temperature, blood pressure, and muscle tension. This is accompanied by placing a type of electronic monitoring device on the client and providing a meter reading of tension levels. With practice, clients can learn to monitor and control their specific body responses when they are under stress.

Meditation is useful to many clients in the achievement or maintenance of a non-stressful state. It involves assuming a comfortable, relaxed position, freeing the body of extraneous thoughts, and concentrating on the inner mind and spirit through low, soft repetition of a mantra or chant. Words used as mantras are such resonant phrases as *om* and *lum*. A 10- to 15-minute period is needed to free the body of excess pressures and to achieve a true meditative state.

Hypnosis has of late come into prominence as a useful tool in specific client management areas such as smoking cessation and pain control. Self-hypnosis has been found helpful in increasing the ability to cope with stressors. One way clients can use self-hypnosis is through audiotapes specifically geared to their individual relaxation or life-style intervention needs.

Imagery, also known as visualization, is an excellent coping strategy for dealing with stress. Memories, dreams, or fantasies experienced by clients can be used to focus the client's experience. Relaxing or soothing music can be used as a background to the imagery exercise. Clients assume a comfortable position, engage in deep breathing to relax, and imagine a place or time that holds positive or beautiful memories, for example, a favorite beach. They then are asked to visualize the sounds, sights, and smells associated with that experience; for example, a beach would include hearing the waves, tasting the sea spray, and smelling the sea breezes. The exercise is carried out for a 10- to 15-minute period, with a gradual awakening or return to the real world. Imagery "minibreaks," which often are useful to defuse a stressful workday and to assist in coping, can be practiced for a 3- to 5-minute period if more time is not available.

Humor is gaining prominence as an inexpensive and accessible way to deal with tension. It has long been said that "laughter is the best medicine." Muscle tension decreases after laughter. The cardiovascular system also shows positive effects from laughter. Humor makes everything look better and often opens new avenues of communication. Nurses can use positive humor in client/nurse situations and in their own stressful work climates. Clients undergoing chemotherapy, with its accompanying hair loss, have used laughter at their own appearance during support group sessions to diminish their stress levels during treatment (Swinford & Webster, 1989).

Environmental Sensitivity

Environmental sensitivity is an integral dimension of wellness. Historically, nurses played key roles in environmental consciousness and improvement of living conditions for their clients/patients. Today this role again is becoming increasingly important, with concerns about chemical contamination, air pollution, and radiation noted daily in the media. Human beings are in constant interaction with their environment, both immediate and global, yet have little ability to control the myriad of negative factors that exist in that environment.

A person's immediate environment usually consists of home and workplace. In the workplace prolonged exposure to noise levels above 75 decibels has been shown to cause hearing loss and cardiovascular changes. Inharmonic sound (random, unstructured noise), although it may not be excessively loud, can cause restlessness and irritability. These exposures over time take their toll on the human body systems. Noise problems are seen not only in factory settings but in white-collar environments where typewriters, telephones, and office machinery all become cumulative culprits.

Air pollution occurs through contamination from vehicles and machines, as well as cigarette smoke. Sidestream smoke from breathing air contaminated by family members' or co-workers' smoke has been found to be as hazardous to health as actual mainstream smoking. Kidney disease, respiratory diseases, and cancer have been linked to air pollution and pose a grave environmental concern. Automobile exhaust fumes and by-products of industrial manufacturing contribute greatly to the "dust domes" seen in many major cities. Work environments also have proved hazardous. Prolonged exposure to workplace chemicals, asbestos, and trace fibers used for insulation have fostered the "sick building syndrome." When workers employed in these settings began to complain of symptoms of malaise, headaches, rash, and upper respiratory irritation, investigation showed links to workplace pollutants (Dossey, Keegan, Guzzetta, & Kolkmeier, 1988).

Throughout the nation there are waste dumps, in which toxic substances of a carcinogenic nature are stockpiled, and many citizen advocacy groups have begun to lobby actively for their removal. An example of one such waste site is the now infamous Love Canal area in Niagara Falls, New York, which had served as a waste dump for the many chemical companies located in that city. Chapter 27 contains a detailed discussion of the problems related to toxic waste dumps and the role of the nurse in helping families living in such areas.

Nurses, as professional health care workers, must act as advocates for clients in issues relevant to environmental concerns. This role includes informing clients about these hazards and urging self-responsibility in monitoring environmental health. Fig. 4-14 presents a complete overview of the many sources of risk to clients from the environment.

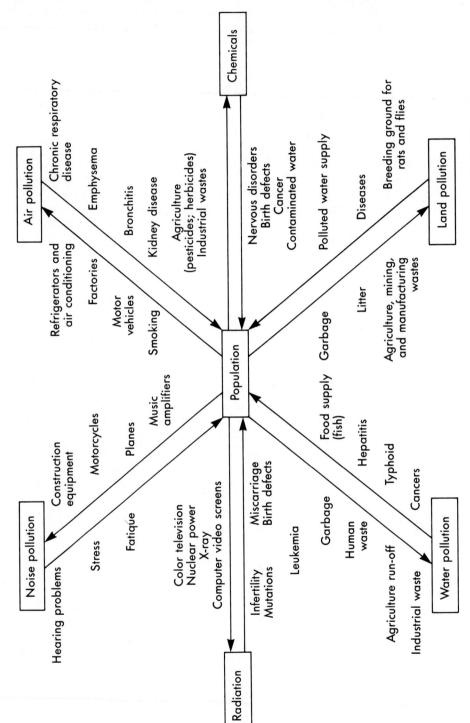

FIG. 4-14 Environmental hazards. (*From "Ecominnea; A strategy for teaching environmental health" by K.L. Rotter 1989, 17(4) pp. 26-27. Copyright 1989 by Association for the Advancement of Health Education. Reprinted by permission.*)

SUMMARY

The new focus on nursing practice in a variety of nonhospital settings and roles has placed nurses in a unique position as wellness advocates. Nurses have accessibility to clients in community settings and the ability to serve as models and teachers of the wellness dimensions. The role of nursing in wellness promotion goes beyond the provision of services related to medical and technical care. The focus should be on *health* services and prevention, not illness services. Nurses must gain the skills needed to assist clients in the development and practice of self-help and self-care techniques to empower them to achieve positive health behaviors and coping skills needed for optimal wellness. The nursing arts and skills must encompass information dissemination, communication, and advocacy. Nurses must become active in multidisciplinary, community roles, in policy-making, and in the creation of a wellness-oriented health care delivery system. Nurses have provided the very best care possible for the dying. Nursing's challenge for the future means refocusing priorities to provide the very best wellness education for the living (Magiacas, 1988).

CHAPTER HIGHLIGHTS

- Several landmark publications alerted the public to the need for preventive health care, including *Dietary Goals, Hospitals' Responsibility for Health Promotion, Healthy People, Doing Better and Feeling Worse,* and *Future Directions in Health Care.*
- The rapidly rising costs of health care in the 1970s motivated employers and insurance companies to find ways to cut costs through prevention of illness and disability.
- Individuals who contributed to the wellness movement include Halpert L. Dunn, John Travis, Donald Ardell, and William Hettler.
- *Health* has been defined in a variety of ways. Recent definitions incorporate concepts of well being and psychosocial aspects, as well as absence of disease.
- The concept of wellness refers to maximizing an individual's ability to function. It is a dynamic, fluctuating state of being.
- According to Rosenstock's health belief model, an individual's decision to perform a health action is determined by perceptions of susceptibility to an illness, severity of the illness, and personal threat of the illness.
- The self-efficacy model is a useful tool for bringing about desired behavioral changes in a specific area of life-style. The more likely a behavior is perceived as leading to a desired outcome, the more likely it is to be performed.
- A contract between the nurse and client stresses the need for the individual to take responsibility for health and life-style management.
- The multilevel approaches toward community health (MATCH) model is useful in implementing changes at the levels of individual, community, and government.
- Blattner's wellness model is based on the holistic nursing perspective and the processes needed to achieve wellness.
- Self-assessment of life-style beliefs and behaviors enables clients to assess their positive and negative health behaviors.
- Nurses cannot prescribe wellness activities for a client but should serve as catalysts to help clients move toward self-responsibility.
- Regular exercise is beneficial in helping to prevent many chronic diseases, as well as in promoting a general sense of well being.
- Aerobic exercise raises the heart rate and benefits the heart, blood vessels, and lungs.

- Good nutrition is an integral component of health promotion.
- Contemporary society contains many stresses that can be manifested in a variety of physical symptoms. Effective stress management strategies are necessary to achieve high-level wellness.
- Strategies to produce relaxation and improve stress include progressive relaxation, biofeedback, meditation, hypnosis, imagery (or visualization), and humor.
- Environmental hazards that can negatively affect health include air pollution, chemicals, noise pollution, and toxic waste.
- Community health nurses can play a key role in health promotion. To do so, they must develop skills in information dissemination, communication, and advocacy.

STUDY QUESTIONS

1. Discuss two factors that contributed to the wellness movement during the 1970s. As a result of each, what changes occurred in health care?
2. Define and differentiate between the following terms: (a) health promotion and illness prevention, (b) health and wellness.
3. How could a nurse use the MATCH model to reduce the incidence of smoking and its related diseases? Give examples of interventions at each of the three levels, and discuss the role of the nurse in each.

REFERENCES

American Hospital Association, Center for Promotion, *Hospital's responsibility for health promotion* Chicago, IL.: Author.

Ardell, D. B. (1977). *High level wellness: An alternative to doctors, drugs and disease.* Emmaus, PA: Rodale Press.

Ardell, D. B. (1982). *14 days to a wellness lifestyle.* Mill Valley, CA: Whatever Publishing.

Ardell, D. B. (1985). The history and future of wellness. *Health Values, 9,* 37-56.

Bandura, A. (1977). Self-efficacy: Toward a unifying theory of behavioral change. *Psychological Review, 84(2),* 191-215.

Becker, M. H. (Ed.). (1974). *The health belief model and personal health behavior.* Thorofare, NJ: Charles B. Black.

Becker, M. H., Haefrer, D. P., Kasl, S. V., Kirscht, J.P., Maiman, L.A. & Rosenstock, I.M. (1977). Selected psychosocial models and correlates of individual health-related behaviors. *Medical Care, 15 (5),* 24-26.

Belloc, N. B., & Breslow, L. (1972). Relationship of physical health status and health practices. *Preventive Medicine, 1,* 409-421.

Blattner, B. (1981). *Holistic nursing.* Englewood Cliffs, NJ: Prentice-Hall.

Blue Cross Association. (1977). The Rockefeller Foundation and the Health Policy Program at the University of California (San Francisco): *The proceedings of the conference on future directions in health care: the dimensions of medicine,* Chicago, IL: Author.

Calnan, M. & Rutler, D.R. (1986). Do health beliefs predict health behavior? an analysis of breast self-examination. *Social Science Medicine, 22 (6),* 673-678.

Desmond, S.M. & Price, J.H. (1988). Self-efficacy and weight control, *Health Education,* February/March, *19 (1),* 12-21.

Dossey, B., Keegan, L., Guzzetta, C. E., & Kolkmeier, L. G. (1988). *Holistic nursing: A handbook for practice.* Rockville, MD: Aspen Publishers.

Dubos, R. (1965). *Man adapting.* New Haven, CT: Yale University Press.

Dunn, H. L. (1961). *High level wellness.* Arlington, VA: R. W. Beatty.

Gutt, C. (1963). *Wellness discovery curriculum and instructor guide.* Buffalo, NY: Greater Buffalo Chapter American Red Cross.

Illich, I. (1977). *Medical nemesis.* New York: Bantam Books.

Institute of Medicine. (1978). *Perspectives of health promotion and disease prevention in the U.S.* Washington, DC: National Academy of Sciences.

Johnson, C., Nicklas, T., Arbeit, M., Franklin, F., & Berenson, G. (1988). A comprehensive model for maintenance of family health behaviors: The "Heart Smart" family health promotion program. *Family & Community Health,* May, *11 (1),* 1-7.

Kittleson, M. J., & Hageman-Rigney, B. (1988). Wellness and behavior contracting. *Health Education,* April/May, *19 (2),* 8-11.

Knowles, J. H. (Ed.). (1977). *Doing better and feeling worse.* New York: Norton.

Larson, E.B., Bergaman, J., Herdricht, F., Alvin, B.L. & Schneeweiss, R. (1982). Do postcard reminders improve influenza compliance? prospective trial of different postcard cues. *Medical Care,* June, *20 (6),* 639-648.

Maglacas, A. (1988). Health for all: Nursing's role. *Nursing Outlook,* March/April, 66-71.

National Heart, Lung, and Blood Institute. (1970). *National cooperative pooling project.* Bethesda, MD: Author.

Neuman, B. N. (1989). The Neuman Systems model (2nd ed.). Norwalk, CT: Appleton & Lange.

Orem, D. (1985). *Nursing: Concepts of practice* (3rd ed.) New York: McGraw-Hill.

Parse, R.R. (1981) *Man-living health: a theory of nursing.* New York: John Wiley, 25-36.

Pender, N. J. (1987). *Health promotion in nursing practice* (2nd ed.). East Norwalk, CT: Appleton-Century-Crofts.

Public Health Service. (1981) *Health style: A self-test.* U.S. Department of Health and Human Services, Office of Disease Prevention and Health Information, Health Promotion, Physical Fitness and Sports Medicine. (Publication No. 81010877). Washington DC: U.S. Government Printing Office.

Public Health Service. (1979). *Healthy people: The surgeon general's report on health promotion and disease prevention* (DHHS Publication No. 79-55071). Washington, DC: U.S. Government Printing Office.

Redeker, N. (1988). Health beliefs and adherence in chronic illness. *Image,* 20, 31-34.

Robbins, S., & Slavin, L. (1988). A measure of social support for health-related behavior change. *Health Education,* June/July, *19 (3),* 36-39.

Rosenstock, I.M. (1966). Why people use health services. *Milbank Memorial Fund Quarterly, July 44,* 94-127.

Senate Select Committee on Nutrition and Human Needs. (1977). *Dietary goals for the United States.* (Publication No. 052-070-03913-2). Washington, DC: U.S. Government Printing Office.

Simons-Morton, D.G., Simons-Morton, B.G., Parcel, G.S., & Bunker, J.F. (1988). Influencing personal and environmental conditions for community health: A multi-level intervention model. *Family & Community Health,* August *11 (2)* 29.

Swinford, P. and Webster, J.: *Promoting wellness: A nurse's handbook,* Rockville, MD, 1989, Aspen Publishers.

Travis, J.W. (1977): *The wellness workbook for helping professionals.* Mill Valley, CA. Wellness Associates.

Travis, J.W. & Ryan, R.S. (1981). The Wellness Workbook. Berkeley, CA: Ten Speed Press.

Williamson, J. and Danaher, K. (1978): *Self-care in health,* London, Croom Helm.

World Health Organization: Constitution of the World Health Organization, *Chronicles of WHO,* 1-2, 1947.

Health Teaching in the Community

JANET E. JACKSON and ELIZABETH JOHNSON BLANKENSHIP

Things are experienced but not in such a way that they are composed into an experience if there is distraction and dispersion in what we observe and what we think.

JOHN DEWEY

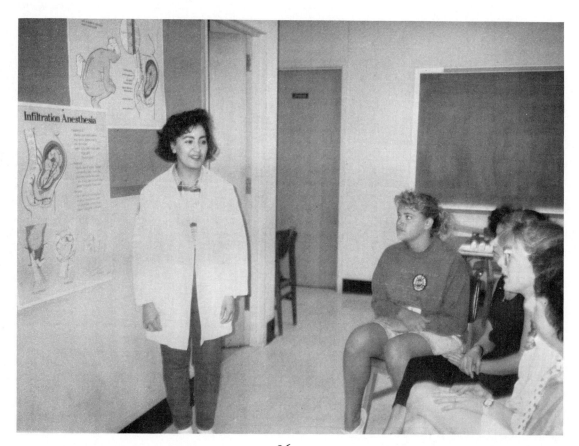

OBJECTIVES

At the conclusion of this chapter the student will be able to:

1. Define the key terms listed
2. Discuss the differences between teaching and learning
3. Review the development of client teaching throughout the history of nursing
4. Discuss the legal implications of health teaching in the community
5. Identify principles of health teaching
6. Relate the teaching/learning process to the nursing process
7. Identify the areas of assessment related to health teaching
8. Discuss the use of various teaching methods and audiovisual materials
9. Identify guidelines that assist in the implementation of the teaching plan
10. Recognize common barriers, problems, and mistakes
11. Explore methods of evaluating the teaching plan and the teacher

KEY TERMS

Affective domain	Intrinsic motivation
Assessment	Learning
Client teaching	Objective
Cognitive domain	PRECEDE model
Compliance	Psychomotor domain
Educational need	Readiness to learn
Extrinsic motivation	Teaching/learning process
Goal	Teaching situation
Health belief model	

According to the American Nurses' Association (ANA) and the American Public Health Association (APHA), community health nursing focuses on the prevention of illness and the promotion and maintenance of health. To accomplish these goals the community health nurse directs practice in two areas. The first area is the direct care given to individuals, families, and groups within a community. The second area is the concern for the health of the total population and the community health problems and issues that affect individuals, families, and groups. In both areas of practice the community health nurse uses nursing interventions that involve client education, counseling, advocacy, and the management of care. To effect these interventions the nurse must possess knowledge of concepts such as family-centered care, principles of teaching/learning, and assessment skills. The community health nurse takes on many roles, such as communicator, educator, and community advocate (Peters, 1989).

HISTORICAL BACKGROUND

In considering the role of health educator it is important to look at the historical background and legal issues related to health teaching. The value placed on health, the right to health care, and the right to know how to attain better health care all have become very important to the consumer.

This need for knowledge regarding one's health is not new to nurses. Nurses have been providing health teaching to their clients as early as the midnineteenth century. The public health nurses and the visiting nurses both in England and in the United States who were caring for clients in their homes recognized the great need for health teaching. In 1918 the National League of Nursing specified the need to include preventive care and health teaching in nursing curricula. The incorporation of teaching/learning principles now can be found in almost all nursing curricula.

Whether the client is an individual, a family, or a group, education is a basic community health nursing intervention. In the past several years the demand for health education in the community has greatly increased. Consumers of health care actively seek health education in many areas to maintain and improve their health. In addition, the rapidly growing field of home health care has been included in the realm of community health nursing and greatly increases the need for client education.

Historically and currently, community health nursing focuses on health promotion and disease prevention, whereas home care nursing focuses on individuals who are experiencing disease or infirmity (Humphrey, 1988). The nurse who is involved in home care is able to gain access to families that often are in great need of health education concerning care for an ill family member. A survey of 35 home health agencies indicated that 83% reported seeing clients whose conditions were more acute and less stable than in the past, including some clients discharged directly home from intensive care units

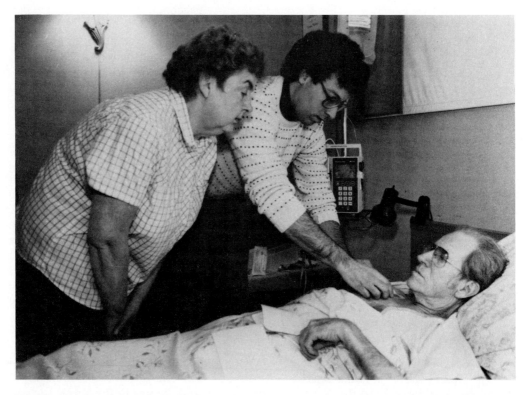

FIG. 5-1 The use of advanced equipment in the home has increased the need for client teaching. *(By permission of Visiting Nurses' Association of Buffalo, NY.)*

(Hardy, 1989). All these factors point to the increasing need for client education. The community health nurse may be teaching classes on nutrition to teenaged mothers or teaching a spouse how to manage complicated equipment in the home (Fig. 5-1). Whatever the setting the nurse is not only asked but expected to provide client teaching as part of daily practice.

Client education may be provided at the primary, secondary, or tertiary level of prevention. Education programs often encompass all three levels. For example, a class related to cardiovascular disease might include clients who are trying to avoid heart disease (primary prevention), clients who have angina and are trying to change their life-styles (secondary prevention), and clients who have had a myocardial infarction and are trying to achieve optimal health (tertiary prevention). Similarly, the levels of prevention also would be considered in teaching the client about the home care.

It becomes evident that the role of educator is a dominant one for community health nurses; education is an integral component of practice. The nurse must therefore become familiar with the teaching/learning process, which is the only way to ensure effective teaching. The following discussion of health teaching and the teaching/learning process encompasses the traditional setting of community health nursing and also the area of home care. Within these areas the community health nurse has the opportunity and challenge to meet the needs of clients through health teaching (Peters, 1989).

LEGAL ISSUES IN HEALTH TEACHING

With the development of nurse practice acts, nurses now are held accountable for their practice by law. The purpose of the practice acts is to protect the lay public from incompetent practitioners by means of establishing licensing procedures and defining the practice of nursing. Some state practice acts are ambiguous, but many are highly specific and include health teaching as a component of nursing practice.

Helen Creighton, a leading authority on legal issues in nursing, has identified a list of legal issues in home care. These include adequately prepared nurses, a thoroughly documented assessment, appropriate nursing judgment related to the assessment, use of appropriate terminology in documentation, complete documentation of all activities, adequate supervision of staff, and the inclusion of client education. She also indicates that nurses in the home cannot assume that teaching was carried out in the hospital; often the information from the hospital must be reinforced or retaught.

The American Hospital Association prepared a document entitled "A Patient's Bill of Rights" in 1975. The goal of this document was to ensure high-quality care. Although written for the hospital, these rights apply equally to care in the client's home. The document establishes that clients have a right to knowledge concerning their condition, the health care delivery system, the immediate environment, and skills needed to care for self-care.

TEACHING/LEARNING THEORIES

The literature abounds with descriptions of theories and definitions of teaching and learning. Some define teaching as a process that facilitates learning, which results when a behavioral change occurs (Chatham & Knapp, 1982). Others define teaching as activities by which the teacher helps the student learn, as the process of facilitating learning, and as a deliberate action that is undertaken to help another person learn to do something (Narrow, 1979; Redman, 1988). Learning is said to have occurred when a person becomes capable of doing something he or she could not do before. To take it one step further, the person who has learned will be able to explain, discuss, demonstrate, or make something by using a set of ideas (Stanton, 1985). Rankin & Duffy (1983) describe client teaching as an act in which the nurse becomes involved in assisting clients to become active members of the health care team and to make informed choices regarding the quality of their life. It also enables clients to learn things that may help them live a longer and/or fuller life and to reach an optimal level of health.

A learning theory is "a systematic integrated outlook in regard to the nature of the process whereby people relate to their environments in such a way as to enhance their ability to use both themselves and their environment more effectively" (Bigge, 1982, p. 3).

Before the twentieth century most Western learning theories were based on learning as a mental discipline. Early theorists believed the learner has a substantive mind separate from the body. Different points of view developed. Some saw the mind as innately bad and in need of correction and advocated the use of strict discipline. This theory was called theistic mental discipline. Others described the mind as neutral and in need of exercise, which formed the basis of the humanistic mental discipline theory. The third was the natural unfoldment or self-actualization theory, based on the belief that the mind was good and should unfold naturally. The last of the mental discipline theories, termed apperception theory, viewed the mind as passive and neutral. It encouraged the process of new ideas associating themselves with old ones.

A new category of learning theories was developed in the twentieth century; these are classified as stimulus-response theories. The stimulus-response bond theory states that certain stimuli, with conditioning, evoke certain response patterns. In the coreinforcement theory, desired responses depend on the learner's innate reflexive drives to accomplish the desired response after conditioning. Reinforcement theory states that the desired response will be elicited by the use of successive, systematic changes in the learner's environment to enhance the probability of desired responses.

More contemporary theories are those cognitive theories of Gestalt psychology which emphasizes an holistic approach to learning. These theories assume that human beings are neither good nor bad, that they simply interact with their environment and that learning is related to perception. The insight theory views learning as a process in which the learner develops new insights or changes old ones. Goal insight theory is similar to insight theory but suggests that teachers assist learners in higher level insights as they begin to form and attain conceptual thought processes. The cognitive field theory states that the learner has purpose and is problem centered. The learner still is assisted to gain new insights. Today these theories are the most popular.

Learning theories provide the framework for the development of a philosophy of teaching. Theories help the nurse to sort out beliefs regarding the teaching/learning process; thus the knowledge base increases and teaching should improve.

TYPES OF LEARNING

The nurse should become familiar with the different types or domains of learning (Bloom, 1969): (1) cognitive learning, (2) affective learning, and (3) psychomotor learning.

Cognitive Learning

The cognitive domain deals with "recall or recognition of knowledge and the development of intellectual abilities and skills" (Bloom, 1969, p. 7). It involves the mind and thinking processes. Six major categories comprise a hierarchical classification of behavior, with the simplest being first.

Knowledge. This is the lowest level and involves recall. Nurses often call upon this behavior. For example, the nurse teaches clients the signs and symptoms of congestive heart failure or hyperglycemia. The client who can identify the signs and symptoms of hyperglycemia has reached this level.

Comprehension. This level of learning combines remembering with understanding. Nurses want their clients to understand why it is important to possess certain health behaviors. The client who learns the signs and symptoms of hyperglycemia should understand how medication and life-style affect blood glucose levels. It certainly is a level the nurse would like to see the client reach.

Application. In the third level of cognitive learning, learners can take material they understand and apply it to theoretical and actual situations. The test of application is a transfer of understanding into practice. In teaching a client about a diet, application would be seen when the client displayed a food diary that reflects knowledge of a diet to help control blood glucose levels.

Analysis. This stage requires the mastery of knowledge, comprehension, and application. To analyze, the learner must break information into parts, understand the relationships among parts, and distinguish among elements. This level of learning leads to problem solving. In community health nursing this level often is promoted as clients are encouraged to use analytical methodology. An example of this would be a person with newly diagnosed diabetes explaining the relationship among diet, insulin, activity, and blood glucose.

Synthesis. Synthesis is the ability to form elements into a unified whole. It brings all the previous levels of cognitive learning to the stage of developing a plan. Through assistance and encouragement from the nurse, the client can formulate a plan. By answering a question such as "What do you think you can do to keep your blood glucose in a normal range?" the client demonstrates synthesis.

Evaluation. The highest level of cognitive learning occurs when the learner uses appropriate criteria to judge the value of ideas, procedures, and methods. The client must compare one situation with another or judge a health behavior in relation to set standards. Through evaluation of daily blood glucose levels the client can decide if the new actions are meeting set goals. This level enables the client to examine closely the newly found health behavior, judge its adequacy, and decide if there is need for improvement.

Measuring cognitive learning is not difficult. It can be seen easily in the client's actions. It is important to recognize the client's cognitive abilities and plan the teaching accordingly. The nurse and the client's behaviors will vary depending on the client's cognitive level.

Affective Learning

The affective domain deals with "changes in interest, attitudes, values, and the development of appreciations, and adequate adjustment" (Bloom, 1969, p. 7). Through health teaching nurses promote healthier behavior patterns. The acceptance of these patterns may depend on how they are communicated to the client. Past reference has indicated the importance of health beliefs in relation to health teaching. Nurses can greatly influence a client's attitudes and values. They also must be aware of their own values and attitudes, which may not concur with those of the client.

Affective learning occurs on several levels as learners respond with varying degrees of involvement and commitment (Spradley, 1985). At the first level the learner is receptive. He or she listens, pays attention, and shows awareness of what is going on. At the second level the learner is responsive, showing some willingness to read or respond to what is being taught. The third level is valuing. The client finds value in the information being taught. The information is accepted, and the client may make a commitment to changing behavior. At the fourth level the client internalizes or conceptualizes an idea or value. The information that is learned is put into practice. The last level is that of adoption. The learner now takes the information learned and adopts a behavior consistent with what was taught.

It is difficult to measure affective learning. It is also difficult to change values and attitudes. However, through cognitive learning the client often will experience affective learning as well.

Psychomotor Learning

The psychomotor domain includes observable performance of skills that require some degree of neuromuscular coordination. The skill will vary depending on the task to be learned. The psychomotor skills taught to community health nursing clients are numerous. Bathing infants, breast self-examination, self-injection, food preparation, catheter irrigation, tracheostomy care, central line care, crutch walking, and dressing changes are a few examples.

For psychomotor learning to take place, the learner must first have the necessary ability. A client with diabetes and Parkinson's disease may not have the manual dexterity to perform insulin self-injections. Clients with limited intelligence should not be expected to learn complex skills. The learner also must have a sensory image of how to carry out a skill; that is, the client must be able to visualize a procedure to perform it in a logical sequence. A sensory image is obtained through demonstration of a task. The client also must have the opportunity to practice the skill. Through repetition of a task, the client will achieve mastery of the skill.

In addition to these theories there are two models that relate directly to health teaching. These are the PRECEDE model and the health belief model.

The PRECEDE model is a health education planning model (Green, 1980). PRECEDE stands for *p*redisposing, *r*einforcing, and *e*nabling *c*auses in *e*ducational *d*iagnosis and *e*valuation (Fig. 5-2). The model indicates that certain environmental factors motivate the individual to exhibit certain health behaviors. It is based on the theory that because health and health behavior are determined by several factors, efforts to change behaviors must be multidimensional. The model works by means of a process in which the individual considers the desired outcomes and works back to the original cause. The model is applied by means of the following seven steps:

1. Consider the quality of life of the group or person involved.
2. Identify specific health problems and choose the one deserving the most attention.
3. Identify specific health-related behaviors that appear to be causing the health problem.
4. Categorize factors that have direct impact on the behavior selected:
   - Predisposing factors: attitudes, beliefs, values, and perceptions that may facilitate or hinder motivation
   - Enabling factors: barriers created by outside forces
   - Reinforcing factors: related to feedback that the learner receives from others, be it positive or negative
5. Decide which factors will be the focus of intervention.
6. Select interventions and assess problems that may arise.
7. Evaluate.

The health belief model is discussed in detail in Chapter 4.

PRECEDE Model

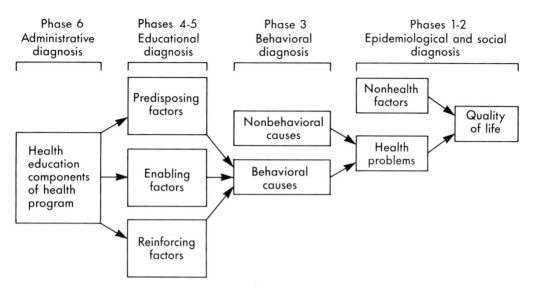

FIG. 5-2 The PRECEDE model. *(From* Health education planning: A diagnostic approach *(pp 14,15) by L.W. Green, M.W. Kreuter, S.G. Deeds, and K.B. Partridge, 1980, Palo Alto, CA: Mayfield. © 1980 by Mayfield Publishing Company. Reprinted by permission.)*

Both these models indicate the importance of the relationship among motivation, the learning process, and compliance. The nurse may do an excellent job of teaching a client, but if the client was not motivated to learn or change behavior, very little is accomplished, noncompliance may result.

PRINCIPLES OF TEACHING/LEARNING

Nurses in the community are expected to teach on a daily basis as part of their practice. To do this nurses must have a solid knowledge base, not only of theories and models of the teaching/learning process but of general principles of teaching/learning. Nurses recognize certain cues from the client that indicate a need to learn. When nurses respond to that cue, they are teaching. Teaching may be simple or complex; it may take a short time or many days to complete. Client teaching requires great involvement by both the nurse and the client (Jackson & Johnson, 1988). The nurse's knowledge of teaching/learning principles will enhance the teaching relationship established with each individual, family, or group.

The primary goal of teaching is learning. This holds true for health teaching also, but there are other goals to consider: those of promoting health, preventing illness, and coping with illness (Narrow, 1979). To reach these goals of health teaching the nurse should take into consideration the following principles (Dugas, 1972):

- Learning is more effective when it is a response to a felt need of the learner.
- Active participation on the part of the learner is essential if learning is to take place.
- Learning is made easier when the material to be learned is related to what the learner already knows.
- Learning is facilitated when the material to be learned is meaningful to the learner.

TABLE 5-1 Superior conditions of learning and principles of teaching

Conditions of learning	Principles of teaching
The learners feel a need to learn.	1. The teacher exposes students to new possibilities for self-fulfillment. 2. The teacher helps each student clarify his own aspirations for improved behavior. 3. The teacher helps each student diagnose the gap between his aspiration and his present level of performance. 4. The teacher helps the students identify the life problems they experience because of the gaps in their personal equipment.
The learning environment is characterized by physical comfort, mutual trust and respect, mutual helpfulness, freedom of expression, and acceptance of differences.	5. The teacher provides physical conditions that are comfortable (as to seating, smoking, temperature, ventilation, lighting, decoration) and conducive to interaction (preferably, no person sitting behind another person). 6. The teacher accepts each student as a person of worth and respects his feelings and ideas. 7. The teacher seeks to build relationships of mutual trust and helpfulness among the students by encouraging cooperative activities and refraining from inducing competitiveness and judgementalness. [sic] 8. The teacher exposes his own feelings and contributes his resources as a colearner in the spirit of mutual inquiry.
The learners perceive the goals of a learning experience to be their goals.	9. The teacher involves the students in a mutual process of formulating learning objectives in which the needs of the students, of the institution, of the teacher, of the subject matter, and of the society are taken into account.
The learners accept a share of the responsibility for planning and operating a learning experience, and therefore have a feeling of commitment toward it.	10. The teacher shares his thinking about options available in the designing of learning experiences and the selection of materials and methods and involves the students in deciding among these options jointly.
The learners participate actively in the learning process.	11. The teacher helps the students to organize themselves (project groups, learning-teaching teams, independent study, etc.) to share responsbility in the process of mutual inquiry.
The learning process is related to and makes use of the experience of the learners.	12. The teacher helps the students exploit their own experiences as resources for learning through the use of such techniques as discussion, role playing, case method, etc. 13. The teacher gears the presentation of his own resources to the levels of experience of his particular students. 14. The teacher helps the students to apply new learnings to their experience, and thus to make the learnings more meaningful and integrated.
The learners have a sense of progress toward their goals.	15. The teacher involves the students in developing mutually acceptable criteria and methods for measuring progress toward the learning objectives. 16. The teacher helps the students develop and apply procedures for self-evaluation according to these criteria.

From *The modern practice of adult education: From pedagogy to andragogy, revised and updated* (pp. 57-58) by M. S. Knowles, 1980, Engelwood Cliffs, N.J.: Prentice Hall, Inc. Reprinted by permission.

- Learning is retained longer when it is put into immediate use than when its application is delayed.
- Periodic plateaus occur in learning.
- Learning must be reinforced.
- Learning is made easier when the learner is aware of his or her progress.

Table 5-1 reiterates some of these principles but suggests the existence of superior conditions of learning and related principles of teaching.

The nurse also must look closely at the client. Whether the client is a group or an individual in the home, the person or persons who are learning often are adults. Adults bring to educational activities different self-images, experiences, and goals than do children. Knowles (1984, p. 174,175), considered the father of adult education, offers the following guidelines in teaching adults:

- Adults prefer learning activities based on active involvement and the problems they encounter in their everyday work environment.
- Adults tend to withdraw from learning situations that are potentially humiliating and detrimental to their self-concept.
- Adults possess a large reservoir of life and work experiences and desire opportunities to capitalize on and share their knowledge.
- Adults possess a variety of individual learning styles and rates.
- Adults have many compelling and conflicting demands on their time and thought processes.

Of course the community nurse will deal with clients other than adults. Often the client may be a child or group of children. Teaching/learning related to such groups will be discussed later in the chapter.

THE TEACHING/LEARNING PROCESS AND THE NURSING PROCESS

Community health nurses function as a primary source for health teaching. Their knowledge, opportunities for teaching, and the nature of the client-nurse relationship enable them to assume this role. As nurses use their knowledge of teaching/learning principles, they should consider the following questions (Jackson & Johnson, 1988):

- What factors influence readiness to learn?
- Does the client want to learn?
- How important is it that the client learn?
- What should the client learn?
- What does the client want to learn?
- What is the best way to teach the information?
- What can you do to increase the likelihood that your client will learn what you taught?
- How can you tell when a person has learned something?

These questions can be answered by means of the nurse's understanding of the teaching/learning process.

The nursing process is the foundation of nursing practice. It is an orderly sequence of steps that include assessment, diagnosis, planning, implementation, and evaluation. The nursing process can provide a framework in which a nurse can develop, plan, and carry out teaching plans. By employing knowledge of the nursing process and teaching/learning principles, the nurse can provide client education in such a way that both the nurse and

THE TEACHING/LEARNING PROCESS AND THE NURSING PROCESS

1. Assessment
   a. The need
   b. The learner
      • Ability to learn
      • Readiness to learn
      • Attitude and motivation
   c. The teaching situation
   d. The teacher
2. Diagnosis
   a. Identify the problem
   b. Establish a diagnosis
3. Planning
   a. Establish a plan of teaching
   b. Formulate learning objectives
   c. Develop contracts
   d. Select teaching methods and audiovisual materials
4. Implementation
   a. Carry out teaching
   b. Recognize obstacles
5. Evaluation
   a. Teaching effectiveness
   b. Teaching ability

Modified from *Patient education in home care* (p. 20) by J. Jackson and E. Johnson, 1988, Rockville, MD: Aspen Publishers, Inc., copyright 1988. Reprinted by permission.

client will grow in a cooperative relationship (Jackson & Johnson, 1988). The teaching/learning process and the nursing process fit very easily together, providing an excellent framework for developing and effecting a teaching plan. The five steps of the nursing process and how the teaching/learning process fits into the process are described in the box. Each of the steps would be used in developing a teaching plan.

Assessment

To formulate a teaching plan a thorough educational assessment must be performed. This includes assessment of the need, the learner, the teaching situation, and the teacher. All these areas are vital to a complete assessment of educational needs.

The educational need. Before the assessment is begun, the resources available to provide the needed information should be examined. Table 5-2 describes sources that can be used.

The following list presents four classifications of educational needs (Atwood & Ellis, 1971):

1. A real need is one that is based on a deficiency that actually exists.
2. An educational need is one that can be met by a learning experience.
3. A real educational need indicates that specific skills, knowledge, and attitudes are required to assist the client in attaining a more desirable condition.
4. A felt need is recognized as important by the learner.

TABLE 5-2 Informational resources related to educational need

Source	Information provided
Client	Attitude toward learning
	Motivation, values, beliefs
	Interest and readiness to learn
	Medical, social, cultural, and educational background
	Activities of daily living
	Routine coping mechanisms
	Likely areas of noncompliance
	Support systems
	Comprehension level
Family or significant other	Insight into past experience
	Reinforcement of information obtained from client
Client's chart	Medical diagnosis and prognosis
	Current treatment regimen
	Client's response to treatment
	Teaching that has been done and client response
Nursing care plan	Identification of unique individual characteristics of client
	Goals of the present illness
	Daily life-style modifications
	Nursing interventions and response
Other health care professionals	New client information
	Coordination of teaching efforts
	Information already taught and client's response
Standardized teaching plans for specific diagnosis; literature regarding teaching content for specific diagnosis	Help in formulation of the teaching plan
	Provide knowledge for the teacher
	Access to available resources dealing with the content to be taught

It is important to recognize educational needs because they determine the specific content to be taught. Even though clients often will identify their needs, the nurse must be able to recognize needs not perceived by the client and to question suspect health practices. Ten areas to consider in assessing the client's educational needs are normal body functions, health problems and diagnosis, medication prescribed, diet, activity limitations, diagnostic tests, preventive and/or health promotion activities, community resources, financial resources, and future plans for the use of the health care system (Chatham & Knapp, 1982).

Often the teaching is related to the client's prescribed medical regimen. In assessing the client's educational needs in this area, the nurse should consider the following questions: Why is it done? Who does it? When is it done? How long does it take? What is the cost? What is the client required to do? Can the client do it?

The areas of health teaching are vast, reflecting the client's many different educational needs. In assessing these needs, the client, family, and teachers should consider certain questions (Chatham & Knapp, 1982):

1. What should the patient know about his or her health condition(s), testing, treatments, prognosis?
2. What skills should the patient be able to perform to implement prescribed and recommended therapeutic or rehabilitative interventions?

3. What attitudes should the patient possess to adopt and integrate health-related skills and practices into his or her daily life?

4. What long-term health practices should the patient incorporate into his or her life-style?

5. What resources does the patient need to accomplish all the above?

Many different questions and areas are considered in the assessment of educational needs. Identification of educational needs is vital to the assessment. Once these are established, the nurse can move on to assessment of the learner.

The learner. In community health practice the learner may be a community, a group, or an individual. The individual may be a child or an adult. The learner also may be the spouse, parent, or significant other. Whoever the learner is, three areas to consider are (1) readiness to learn, (2) ability to learn, and (3) attitude and motivation.

Readiness to learn. The nurse implements a well-organized teaching plan, yet the client does not learn. The client is not ready to learn. Assessment of the client's readiness will save much time in the teaching/learning process. Client readiness greatly influences teaching effectiveness.

Readiness to learn is described as the state of being both willing and able to use health teaching (Narrow, 1979). There are two types of learner readiness: emotional readiness, which is described as motivation or willingness, and experiential readiness, which includes the client's background of experiences, skills, attitudes, and ability to learn (Redman, 1988).

Many factors influence a client's readiness to learn. Among them are comfort, energy, capability, and motivation. A client's health or lack of health also can influence readiness. A client who is anxious or in pain certainly is not ready to learn. The nurse must consider the client's physical and psychological comfort, emotions, and level of energy. The client's developmental stage also is important: "The teachable moment for adults is when the content and skills to be taught are consistent with the developmental tasks" (Stanhope & Lancaster, 1988, p. 190). Because of the multiplicity of influences on learning, it is imperative that the nurse know the client and recognize the effect of these factors on learning.

Ability to learn. The ability to learn can be easily assessed; it can be observed, tested, and measured. Ability is influenced by many factors, including age, maturation, previous learning, physical and mental health, and the environment. If the client has physical or intellectual disabilities, these must be recognized. A client who has hemiplegia cannot be expected to accomplish a psychomotor task that requires the use of both hands. Strength, coordination, dexterity, and the senses must be taken in account. Mathematics, reading, and verbal skills must be assessed. Printed material should not be used as a teaching tool if the client's reading skills are poor. (Readability of learning material is discussed later in the chapter.) Previous experience and past learning must be assessed. The client's ability provides a basis for formulating the teaching plan related to the client's needs.

Attitude and motivation. The client's attitudes toward learning and health are paramount in learning the information presented. Motivation too is a major determinant of client learning. In relation to health teaching, it is essential that the learner wants to learn and perceives the importance of the activity before actually participating (Dracup & Meleis, 1982). The health belief model and the PRECEDE model are based on the importance of both attitudes and motivation.

There are two types of motivation: intrinsic and extrinsic. Intrinsic motivation is defined as values, attitudes, perceptions, and/or unmet needs. Extrinsic motivation comes from outside forces such as family pressure, environmental factors, and/or changes in life-style. A client can possess an abundance of knowledge but, if motivation is lacking, rarely will comply (Cohen, 1979). Clients must recognize the need for information and be mentally and physically ready before they can be motivated (Falvo, 1985).

Motivation moves people to action. The desire to know and understand, get well, return to work, avoid complications, please others, and manage their own care are all factors that can motivate clients to learn. What motivates is unique to each client, and any motivation to learn is a valid one.

All these aspects of assessment—the need, learner readiness, ability, and motivation— are necessary components of an educational assessment. The nurse must be knowledgeable and adept in all aspects. Although the client is the most important component of assessment, a complete assessment also includes the teaching situation and the teacher.

The teaching situation. The nurse should provide an environment that is conducive to learning. Three aspects of the environment must be assessed: the physical environment, the interpersonal environment, and the external environment.

The physical environment is the actual room where teaching occurs. The room should have comfortable physical surroundings, minimal distractions, and provide a comfortable setting for both client and teacher. It would be foolish to attempt to help a mother with breast-feeding in a room where Grandma is visiting with the next-door neighbor and three children are playing. Although there are times when control over the environment is impossible, the nurse must carefully and judiciously choose where the teaching will take place whenever possible.

The interpersonal environment is one over which the nurse has control. A trusting, caring relationship, with mutual respect, should be developed. Active listening is important. A rapport must be established for teaching to be effective. The nurse must listen, make eye contact, ask for the client's opinion, avoid reading or writing while the client is talking, and check with the client for clarification of what is understood. All these actions can foster a positive interpersonal environment.

The external environment includes the resources and support that are available to the educational process, for example, available specialists or consultants, time, money and materials, administrative support, collegial support, physician support, and familial support.

The nurse may question the need for physician support, believing that she or he is capable of identifying the client's educational needs. If, however, the client is being seen in the home and the visit is eligible for Medicare reimbursement, then the nursing service must be approved or ordered by a physician. Support from all the aforementioned areas allows for a more effective learning experience.

The teacher. All too often assessment of the teacher is ignored. Teaching is an integral component of nursing practice and a responsibility of each nurse. However, is every nurse capable of teaching? Nurses must carefully examine their own beliefs concerning the teaching/learning process (Jackson & Johnson, 1988), and all nurses should work to develop better teaching skills.

Four factors are considered in assessing the ability to teach: energy, attitude, knowledge, and skill. The act of teaching takes great energy and can be very time-consuming. The nurse's attitude should be considered in relation to teaching, the client, and the subject matter. The nurse's knowledge base should be examined. Knowledge of the topic to be taught is necessary to facilitate learning. Last, the nurse should possess skills that reflect teaching/learning principles and should be knowledgeable about content. All nurses who assume the role of teacher should evaluate themselves in these areas. The nurse who supervises other nurses who teach must also evaluate their teaching ability. Once the assessment is completed, the process continues to the next step, that of establishing the diagnosis.

Diagnosis

Nursing diagnosis can be defined in various ways. It is the end of the assessment. It can be accomplished when an actual or potential client problem that the nurse can legally treat is identified (Yuro & Walsch, 1983).

Although some might think that a nursing diagnosis is not relevant in developing a teaching plan, one of the 72 diagnostic categories is that of knowledge deficit. Carpenito (1987) describes collaborative problems as physiological complications that have resulted or may result from pathophysiological and treatment-related situations. Hyperglycemia would be a collaborative problem for a client with diabetes. Almost all the collaborative problems identified by Carpenito are associated with the nursing diagnosis "knowledge deficit." This emphasizes how important client teaching is in nursing. The diagnosis of knowledge deficit (Table 5-3) can easily be used in teaching plans. The problem (knowl-

---

TABLE 5-3 Diagnostic category of knowledge deficit

Definition	The state in which the individual experiences deficiency in cognitive knowledge or psychomotor skills necessary for management of a health problem
Defining characteristics	
Major (must be present)	Verbalizes a deficiency in knowledge or skill/requests information; expresses "inaccurate" perception of health status; does not correctly perform a desired or prescribed health behavior
Minor (may be present)	Lack of integration of treatment plan into daily activities; exhibits or expresses psychological alteration (eg., anxiety, depression) resulting from misinformation or lack of information
Etiological, contributing, and risk factors	
Pathophysiological	Any existing or new medical condition, regardless of the severity of the illness
Treatment-related	Lack of previous exposure; complex regimen
Situational (personal and environmental)	Lack of exposure to the experience; language differences; information misinterpretation; personal characteristics: lack of motivation, lack of education or readiness, ineffective coping patterns (e.g., anxiety, depression, nonproductive denial of situation, avoidance coping)
Maturational	Lack of education of age-related factors; examples include children: sexuality and sexual development, safety hazards, substance abuse, nutrition; adolescents: same as for children, automobile safety practices, substance abuse (alcohol, other drugs, tobacco), health maintenance practices; adults: parenthood, sexual function, safety practices, health maintenance practices; elderly: effects of aging, sensory deficits

From *Handbook of nursing diagnosis* (2nd ed., pp. 65-67), by L. Carpenito, 1987, Philadelphia: Lippincott. Copyright 1987 by J.B. Lippincott Co. Reprinted by permission.

edge deficit) and the factors that contribute to the problem (e.g., dietary management of a low-sodium diet) are identified. This diagnosis would be stated as knowledge deficit related to inability to manage a low-sodium diet. From the diagnosis a teaching plan can be developed. Knowledge deficit may not always be identified as the problem, but many times it is. Many other nursing diagnoses may indicate the need for client teaching by including statements such as ineffective coping related to knowledge deficit, alterations in parenting related to knowledge deficit, etc.

Planning

With the assessment completed and a diagnosis established the nurse prepares a teaching plan in collaboration with the client. The family and client must be involved in this part of the process. The questions of what, how, where, and when must be answered.

Writing objectives. At this point learning objectives should be established. In nursing the term *goals* often is used in planning patient care; in planning teaching it is more common to use *learning objective*. Learning objectives serve the following functions:

- To identify activities regarding content and methods to be used
- To inform the patient of what is expected
- To provide a basis for evaluation
- To promote continuity of the teaching activities when more than one discipline is involved
- To enable the setting of priorities regarding information the patient needs
- To provide a guide for patient teaching that ultimately should save time

Each of the following factors should be included in the writing of learning objectives:

- Behaviors the patient is expected to accomplish as a result of the teaching
- Objectives that are client-centered, including what the client will do
- A clear, concise statement that includes an action verb and the criterion for measurement

Objectives should be written in behavioral terms and categorized into the three domains of learning: cognitive, affective, and psychomotor. Examples of verbs related to the cognitive domain that can be used in writing objectives follow:

Knowledge: count, define, identify, list, report
Comprehension: compare, distinguish, describe, discuss, explain
Application: apply, demonstrate, practice, relate, utilize
Analysis: analyze, differentiate, distinguish, question, summarize
Synthesis: assemble, design, formulate, organize, plan
Evaluation: assess, determine, evaluate, measure, recommend

Developing contracts. The number of objectives depends on the individual needs of each client. From the assessment data the nurse and the client may set priorities related to the objectives. This is a time when a client-nurse contract may be developed. Fig. 5-3 provides an example of a written contract, and Table 5-4 illustrates characteristics and examples of good client contracts. A contract usually specifies what is to be learned, how long it will take to learn, how the learning will be evaluated, and possibly a reward. Contracting is believed to strengthen the involvement and responsibility of the learner and therefore increase the likelihood of effective teaching (Fig. 5-4).

TABLE 5-4 Good patient contracts: characteristics and examples			
Characteristics of a good patient contract	Questions health professionals can ask to help patient set an achievable goal	Sample contract: Mr. Dixon, 47, is an obese businessman, who had a heart attack 4 months ago. His goals:	Sample contract: Ms. Waverly, 56, is a plump woman with angina pectoris, who finds she snacks constantly. Her goals:
Realistic	Does goal seem possible? Have you ever had regular exercise? Sound reasonable at this time?	Walk the dog.	Lose weight.
Measurable	How often can you do this? What will show you have done this?	Walk the dog around the lake for 30 minutes.	Lose 5 pounds.
Positive	What goals are you working toward? What are you going to do for yourself? What strengths can you build on?	I will do this following exercise . . .	I will lose weight by a. Eating three meals b. Sitting down to eat c. An evening snack of an apple or other fruit
Time-dated	When can you start this? What will you do in the next 2 weeks?	Walk the dog each night before supper for the next 2 weeks.	Lose 5 pounds by the end of the month, which is my birthday.
Written	Could I write down your ideas? Would you write down these goals we are discussing?	Will walk dog 30 minutes around a lake before supper—2 weeks.	I'll lose 5 pounds by my birthday. 1. Eat three meals a day 2. Sit down 3. Fruit snack at bedtime
Rewardable	If you make this effort, what reward could you give yourself?	New walking shoes if I accomplish my goal.	A long-distance telephone call to my sister.
Evaluated	How can I help you evaluate your goals? Can you share your goals with anyone?	I'll come back in to see you to report progress in 2 weeks.	I'll ask my sister to work on these goals with me. I will send you a postcard the first of next month with my results.

Date _____ _____

Health-care contract

Contract goal: (Specific outcome to be attained)

I, (client's name), agree to (detailed description of required behaviors, time and frequency limitations) in return for (positive reinforcements contingent upon completion of required behaviors; timing and mode of delivery of reinforcements).

I, (provider's name), agree to (detailed description of required behaviors, time and frequency limitations).

(Optional) I, (significant other's name), agree to (detailed description of required behaviors, time and frequency limitations).

(Optional) Aversive consequences: (Negative reinforcements for failure to meet minimum behavioral requirements).

(Optional) Bonuses: (Additional positive reinforcements for exceeding minimum contact requirements).

We will review the terms of this agreement, and will make any desired modifications, on (date). We hereby agree to abide by the terms of the contract described above.

Signed:(Client) _____ _____
Signed:(Significant other, if relevant) _____
Signed:(Provider) _____
Contract effective from (Date) _____
to (Date) _____

FIG. 5-3 Example of a client contract. *(From N.K. Jany, M.H. Becker, and P.E. Hartman, 1984,* Patient Education and Counseling, *(5[4], p. 178.) Copyright 1984 by Elsevier Scientific Publishers Ireland Ltd. Reprinted by permission.)*

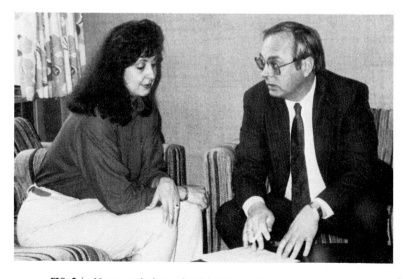

FIG. 5-4 Nurse and client should review the contract together.

TABLE 5-5 Summary of instructional methods

Instructor-centered	Interactive	Individualized
Lecture	**Class discussion**	**Programmed instruction**
Students are passive	Class size must be small	Most effective at lower learning
Efficient for lower learning	May be time-consuming	levels
levels and large classes	Encourages student involvement	Very structured
		Students work at own pace
		Students receive extensive feed-
		back
Questioning	**Discussion groups**	**Modularized instruction**
Monitors students learning	Class size should be small	Can be time-consuming
Encourages student involvement	Students participate	Very flexible formats
May cause anxiety for some	Effective for high cognitive and	Students work at own pace
	affective learning levels	
Demonstration	**Peer teaching**	**Independent projects**
Illustrates an application of a	Requires careful planning and	Most appropriate at higher
skill or concept	monitoring	learning levels
Students are passive	Utilizes differences in student	Can be time-consuming
	expertise	Students are actively involved in
	Encourages student involvement	learning
	Group projects	**Computerized instruction**
	Requires careful planning,	May involve considerable
	including evaluation tech-	instructor-time or expense
	niques	Can be very flexible
	Useful at higher learning levels	Students work at own pace
	Encourages active student par-	Students may be involved in
	ticipation	varying activities

Experiential learning methods

Field or clinical	Laboratory	Role playing	Simulations and games	Drill
Occurs in natural setting during performance	Requires careful planning and evaluation	Effective in affective and psychomotor domains	Provide practice of specific skills	Most appropriate at lower learning levels
Students are actively involved	Students actively involved in a realistic setting	Provides "safe" experiences	Produces anxiety for some students	Provides active practice
Management and evaluation may be difficult		Active student participation	Active student participation	May not be motivating for some students

From "Selecting instructional strategies," by C. Weston and P. A. Cranton, 1986, *Journal of Higher Education, 57(3)*, p. 263,264. Copyright 1986 by The Ohio State University Press. Reprinted with permission. All rights reserved.

Selecting teaching methods and audiovisual materials. During the planning stage the nurse must choose a teaching method or methods and educational materials needed to carry out the teaching plan. The choices should coincide with the stated objectives. Consideration must be given as to whether the nurse is teaching a group or an individual and the characteristics of the learner. Table 5-5 describes various teaching methods. Teaching methods can be matched with the domains and levels of learning (Table 5-6).

When making home visits, the nurse most often will be instructing one or a few individuals, but many times in the community the nurse will be instructing larger groups. Group instruction offers many advantages. It is economical, groups of learners can be reached with one teaching plan, it offers structured time, and usually allows for planning of content in advance. Common teaching methods used with groups include role playing, lecture, discussions, demonstrations, and case studies. Groups also can benefit the learner. They provide security and the opportunity to share experiences, resources, and to learn from one another (Stanhope & Lancaster, 1988). The nurse's role in working with groups is discussed in detail in Chapter 6.

TABLE 5-6 Matching domain and level of learning to appropriate methods

Domain and level	Method
Cognitive domain	
Knowledge	Lecture, programmed instruction, drill and practice
Comprehension	Lecture, modularized instruction, programmed instruction
Application	Discussion, simulations and games, CAI,* modularized instruction, field experiences, laboratory
Analysis	Discussion, independent/group projects, simulations, field experience, role-playing, laboratory
Synthesis	Independent/group projects, field experience, role-playing, laboratory
Evaluation	Independent/group projects, field experience, laboratory
Affective domain	
Receiving	Lecture, discussion, modularized instruction, field experience
Responding	Discussion, simulations, modularized instruction, role-playing, field experience
Valuing	Discussion, independent/group projects, simulations, role-playing, field experience
Organization	Discussion, independent/group projects, field experience
Characterization by a value	Independent projects, field experience
Psychomotor domain	
Perception	Demonstration (lecture), drill and practice
Set	Demonstration (lecture), drill and practice
Guided response	Peer teaching, games, role-playing, field experience, drill and practice
Mechanism	Games, role-playing, field experience, drill and practice
Complex overt response	Games, field experience
Adaptation	Independent projects, games, field experience
Origination	Independent projects, games, field experience

From "Selecting Instructional strategies" by C. Weston and P.A. Cranton, 1986, *Journal of Higher Education,* 57, p. 278. Copyright 1986 by The Ohio State University Press. Reprinted with permission. All rights reserved.
*CAI: Computer-assisted instruction

The nurse must select educational materials according to the client's needs and abilities. Audiovisual materials include printed material, films, videotapes, audiotapes, records, and slides. All materials should be viewed and evaluated before they are used. The following questions should be considered in the evaluation of audiovisual materials:

What is the readability factor (if printed material)?
Is the material incorrect or contradictory of other sources being used?
Is it beyond the level of understanding of the client?
Is the quality good?
Did the client find the audiovisual helpful?

The nurse should determine if the material actually will add to teaching effectiveness or will just take up valuable time.

If printed material is chosen, the literacy level of the client must be considered. If reading ability is not assessed, the nurse can easily embarrass the client or be unaware of why learning did not take place. The client's ability to comprehend the material is essential to client learning.

Many formulas can be used to measure readability. These include the Fry formula, the Flesch formula, and the Fog formula. These formulas are based on word and sentence length. The Fry formula can determine the level of materials from grade one through college. It must be used on passages of 300 words or more. The Flesch formula can determine the level of material between grade five through college completion. The Fog formula tests levels of material between grade four and college. Both the Flesch and the Fog are useful for short brochures and pamphlets because they can be used with only 100 words. The nurse should practice using these formulas and decide which is preferred. All printed materials should be closely evaluated and chosen according to the client's capabilities.

Implementation

The nurse who presents the plan of teaching should be knowledgeable in terms of content, and assessment of the learner's abilities should always be kept in mind. The more often the nurse takes the responsibility for teaching, the more the ability to teach and self-confidence will increase. When implementing the teaching plan, the nurse should take the following actions:

- Provide a conducive learning environment.
- Communicate the importance of learning.
- Communicate enjoyment in teaching the material.
- Express enthusiasm and concern through voice and body language.
- Take time and avoid rushing the client.
- Praise the client frequently and note progress.
- Repeat information often.
- Show flexibility, adjusting learning goals as necessary.
- Let the client share what he or she knows about the subject.
- Reinforce all information presented.
- Reward if beneficial.
- Try to allow the client to use the information learned without delay.

Obstacles to implementation. Obstacles to implementation include barriers, problems, and mistakes. These are common problems that can occur with the most organized teaching plan. Being aware of them can help when they actually are encountered in practice.

Barriers. Barriers are external problems that frequently are encountered, such as lack of administrative support, lack of time, poor resources, conflict with other disciplines, and inadequate teaching skills. Lack of administrative support can lead to almost all the other barriers listed. Administration and nursing personnel must share the same philosophy of health teaching and believe it to be beneficial and necessary. Nurses often are called on to demonstrate that health teaching is cost effective.

Lack of resources such as staff and audiovisual materials can be frustrating. Nursing staff is essential; however, audiovisual materials often are helpful but not always necessary. Both resources depend on financial assets.

Lack of time is related to inadequate staffing, high client load, and poor organization. The nurse must recognize the amount of time needed for health teaching and arrange the schedule accordingly. If staffing or high client load is the problem, administrative personnel should be informed.

A client also may be seen by other professionals such as a physical or an occupational therapist. Thus a lack of coordination of teaching activities can occur and cause conflict. Teaching activities should be coordinated by means of team conferences when necessary.

The last barrier is that of inadequate teaching skills. The effectiveness of teaching certainly depends on how well the material is taught. The nurse is responsible for health teaching and should update and seek knowledge when needed.

Problems. Some problems the nurse may encounter relate to client situations such as a wide age range, noncompliance, and terminal illness. These problems occur in the community, in group settings, or in the home.

The client's age presents various problems. Adult learning characteristics, discussed earlier in the chapter, also apply to the elderly client. There are, however, special considerations. In teaching elderly persons, information should sometimes be presented at a slower rate. The client should be evaluated carefully for sensory deprivation related to aging. The nurse also should be alert to decreased capacity related to cerebral changes.

When the client is a child, the nurse should make the teaching plan flexible and creative, schedule short sessions, and consider the child's developmental stage and cognitive level. Incorporating play into the plan usually is helpful. Parental involvement depends on the age of the child. With a small child the parents should be included whereas with adolescents it may be best to not include them; the nurse and client must make this decision on a case-by-case basis. Adolescent knowledge must be assessed carefully inasmuch as adolescents often imply that they are knowledgeable when they are not.

Noncompliance always is a potential problem when teaching is involved. Noncompliance occurs frequently. Cohen (1979) estimated that only one third of chronically ill clients adhere to their therapeutic regimens; one third are noncompliant because they adhere to a misunderstood regimen; and one third choose to be noncompliant. The community setting may contribute to noncompliance, especially in the home setting. Clients who have been compliant in the hospital often forget the regimen when they go home and return to old habits. The nurse possibly can increase client compliance by the following actions:

- Establishing a caring relationship
- Assessing the client's beliefs and values concerning health
- Encouraging the client to question what is being done

TABLE 5-7 Common mistakes in the teaching/learning process

Assessment	This step has already been identified as one of the most important components of the teaching/learning process. Poor and ineffective assessments lead to a poor and inadequate teaching plan. Always confirm information obtained. Many times, illiterate patients end up with printed teaching material. Always reassess.
Failure to negotiate goals	One often forgets that the goals established are (or should have been) the patient's goals. The nurse may have goals, but patient goals should be given priority. Recognize when the goals need to be renegotiated. Unrealistic goals lead to noncompliance.
Territoriality and duplication	Nurses can become very possessive of their patients and may want to be the only person available to them. They also feel personally responsible for the patient's teaching. One must remember that the patient is ultimately responsible for his behavior. Duplication of information often happens when the patient goes from the hospital to home and if the home health nurse changes. This can be solved with patient care conferences and good documentation of patient teaching.
Patient overload	Too often, too much material is presented at one time. Shorter sessions are usually helpful in preventing this, and they allow the patient to synthesize and formulate questions. Be alert to the patient yawning, fidgeting, or being unable to answer questions. These may indicate overload and the need for a break in teaching.
Poor timing of patient teaching	The nurse must consider the patient's schedule, physical comfort, and stress level. Very little learning can take place if the patient is in pain or anxious about something.
Poor use of media	Never use materials that have not been reviewed. This can lead to ineffective teaching and even very embarrassing moments. Know your material. Also, never rely solely on media for teaching.
Recognition of patient's background	There are times when the nurse seems to have forgotten the information gained from the assessment. Asking a patient who has financial problems to follow an expensive dietary regimen is unreasonable. The patient's ethnic, educational, and financial background is sometimes not remembered. The nurse too often teaches from previous background.
Making assumptions	Making assumptions is very easy to do but can be detrimental to effective teaching. The following nevers should be remembered: • Never assume that a patient understands the disease or prescribed treatment even if it has been diagnosed for some time. • Never assume that a patient knows why a prescription drug is taken. • Never assume because a patient is from a different socioeconomic, ethnic, or educational background that he will not be motivated or able to learn. • Never assume that because a patient has been noncompliant in the past that he will continue to be. • Never make assumptions!
Poor documentation	This is surely a very common mistake and a very important aspect of patient teaching, especially in home health.

From *Patient education in home care,* (pp. 43-44) by J. Jackson and E. Johnson, 1988, Rockville, MD: Aspen. Copyright 1988 by Aspen Publishers, Inc. Reprinted by permission.

- Reinforcing the benefits of the prescribed regimen
- Praising the client frequently
- Offering realistic expectations

Mistakes. Many mistakes can occur during the teaching/learning process, the most common of which are identified in Table 5-7.

The obstacles discussed can be encountered in many areas of health teaching. Through awareness the nurse can work to prevent them and minimize disruptions in the teaching/learning process.

Evaluation

Evaluating teacher effectiveness often is the most neglected component of the teaching/learning process. The worth of teaching can be known only through evaluation of two areas: (1) teaching effectiveness and (2) teacher performance.

If behavioral objectives were written, what the client learned can be evaluated. This can be accomplished through written tests, laboratory data, return demonstrations, compliance, and/or a follow-up questionnaire. Teacher performance can be evaluated through videotaping a teaching session or having a colleague present during teaching. Peer evaluation should be based on mutual trust and respect. The client also can evaluate the teacher through written or direct feedback.

If the teaching was deemed unsuccessful, the reasons for this are analyzed and the process begins again. It cannot be assumed that teaching was effective and that learning took place. The teaching/learning process is not complete until evaluation of the teaching and the learning takes place.

SUMMARY

Client teaching is an integral component of nursing practice. It should be included in daily practice. The community setting abounds with opportunities for client teaching. The clients may be a group or individuals, but whoever the clients, they bring to the teaching/learning situation a variety of life experiences, educational experiences, and emotional experiences. All these must be considered. Through use of the nursing process the nurse can develop teaching plans that are specific to each client. Each time the nurse teaches, teaching skills are further developed. One must work at becoming a good teacher. The act of teaching becomes an art only when the process is incorporated into daily practice.

CHAPTER HIGHLIGHTS

- Education is a basic community health nursing intervention. In the past several years the demand for health education has increased greatly.
- Teaching is a process that facilitates learning. Health teaching is an act in which a client is assisted to become an active member of the health team and to reach an optimal level of health.
- When learning occurs, there usually is a resultant change in behavior. The learner will be able to explain, discuss, demonstrate, or make something by using a new set of ideas.
- Types of learning theories include mental discipline theories, stimulus-response theories, and cognitive theories.
- The three types of learning are cognitive learning, affective learning, and psychomotor learning.

- The PRECEDE model and health belief model are useful in helping nurses to plan and carry out health teaching.
- Learning is most likely to occur when the learner perceives a need to learn, when he or she participates actively in the learning process, when the material to be learned is relevant, when it is reinforced, and when the new knowledge is put to immediate use.
- Motivation moves people to action and is paramount to learning. Intrinsic motivation comes from within the individual whereas extrinsic motivation comes from outside sources.
- The teaching/learning process can be related to the nursing process by means of the steps of assessment, diagnosis, planning, implementation, and evaluation.
- An educational assessment includes assessment of the educational need, the learner, the teaching situation, and the teacher.
- A nursing diagnosis of knowledge deficit indicates a need for client teaching.
- During the planning stage, objectives are formulated and teaching methods and materials are selected. A client contract may be developed at this time.
- The nurse carries out the teaching plan during the implementation stage.
- Obstacles to implementation of the teaching plan include external barriers, client problems, and mistakes in teaching.
- Noncompliance occurs when the client does not adhere to the medical regimen or when the client is insufficiently motivated.
- The evaluation stage includes evaluation of teaching effectiveness and teaching performance.

STUDY QUESTIONS

1. Discuss opportunities for teaching within community health nursing.
2. Identify five principles of adult learning and ways to use them in practice.
3. Explain the steps of the teaching/learning process in relation to the nursing process.
4. Describe teaching tools that could be used if a client were illiterate.
5. Discuss the importance of compliance in the teaching/learning process and how the nurse can facilitate compliance.

REFERENCES

American Hospital Association. (1972). *A patient's bill of rights.* Chicago: Author.

American Nurses' Association. (1980). *A conceptual model of community health nursing.* Kansas City, MO: Author.

American Public Health Association. (1981). *The definition and role of public health nursing in the delivery of health care.* Washington, DC: Author.

Atwood, H., & Ellis, J. (1971). Concept of need: An analysis for adult education. *Adult Leadership, 19,* 210-212.

Becker, M. H. (1974). *The health belief model and personal health behaviors.* Thorofare, NJ: Charles B. Black.

Bigge, M. (1982). *Learning theories for teachers.* New York: Harper & Row.

Bloom, B. S. (ed.). (1969). *Taxonomy of educational objectives: The classification of educational goals.* *Handbook I: Cognitive domain.* New York and London: Longman.

Carpenito, L. J. (1987). *Nursing diagnosis: Application to clinical practice.* Philadelphia: Lippincott.

Chatham, M., & Knapp, L. (1982). *Patient education handbook.* Bowie, MD: Brady.

Cohen S. (ed.). (1979). *New directions in patient compliance.* Lexington, MA: Lexington Books.

Creighton, H. (1987). Legal implication of home health care. *Nursing Management, 18*(2), 14-17.

Dewey, J. (1958). *Art as experience.* New York: Capricorn Books, G. P. Putnam's Sons.

Dracup, K., & Meleis, A. (1982). Compliance: An interactionist's approach. *Nursing Research, January/February 31*(1), 31-36.

Dugas, B. (1972). *Introduction to patient care* (2nd ed.). Philadelphia: Saunders.

Falvo, D. (1985). *Effective patient education*. Rockville, MD: Aspen.

Flesch, R. (1974). *The art of readable writing*. New York: Harper & Row.

Fry, E. (1968). A readability formula that saves time. Journal of Reading, 11, 514.

Green, L., Kreuter, M., Deeds, S., & Partridge, K. (1980). *Health education planning: A diagnostic approach*. Palo Alto, CA: Mayfield.

Gunning, R. (1952). *The Fog formula: the technique of clear writing*. New York, McGraw Hill Book Co.

Hardy, C. (1989). Patient-centered high technology care. *Holistic Nursing Practice, 3(2)*, 46-53.

Humphrey, C. (1988). The home as a setting for care. *Nursing Clinics of North America, 23*, 305-314.

Jackson, J., & Johnson, E. (1988). *Patient education in home care*. Rockville, MD: Aspen.

Knowles, M. (1978). *The adult learner: A neglected species* (2nd ed.). Houston, Gulf Publishing.

Narrow, B. W. (1979). *Patient teaching in nursing practice*. New York: John Wiley.

Peters, D. (1989). A concept of nursing discharge. *Holistic Nursing Practice, 3(2)*, 18-25.

Rankin, S., & Duffy, K. (1983). *Patient education: Issues, principles, and guidelines*. Philadelphia: Lippincott.

Redman, B. K. (1988). *The process of patient education* (6th ed.). St. Louis: Mosby.

Spradley, B. W. (1985). *Community health nursing* (2nd ed.). Boston: Little, Brown & Co.

Stanhope, M., & Lancaster, J. (1988). *Community health nursing*. St. Louis: Mosby.

Stanton, M. Patient and health education: lessons from the marketplace. Nursing Management, 16(4):26-30, 1985.

Weston, C. & Cranton, P.A. (1986). Selecting instructional strategies. *Journal of Higher Education, May/June 57(3)*, Ohio State University Press.

Yura, H. & Walsh, M.B. (1983). *The Nursing Process: Assessing* planning, implementing, evaluating. (4th ed.). Norwalk, CT: Appleton—Century-Crofts.

Working with Groups in the Community

LINDA JANELLI

A group is an open system composed of three or more people held together by a common interest or bond.

RUTH M. TAPPEN

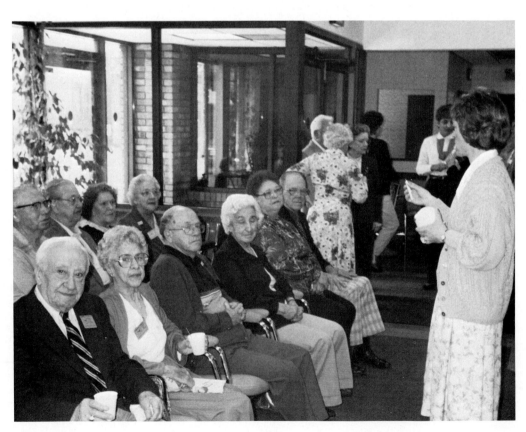

OBJECTIVES

At the conclusion of this chapter the student will be able to:

1. Define the key terms listed
2. Identify the three basic characteristics found in most groups
3. Describe the five stages of group development (forming, storming, norming, performing, and adjourning) and state how they differ from one another
4. Identify at least two task roles, two social roles, and two individual roles that could emerge from a group situation
5. Assess those elements that can contribute to the effectiveness of a group leader
6. Distinguish among the three major leadership styles: autocratic, democratic, and laissez faire
7. Explain how Herzberg's motivational factors can affect the group process
8. Explain the purposes of community, support, and educational groups and the potential role of the community health nurse in each one

KEY TERMS

Adjourning

Autocratic leadership

Community development group

Conflict

Democratic leadership

Educational group

Forming

Group

Individual roles

Laissez-faire leadership

Maintenance roles

Motivational theory

Norming

Performing

Power

Relationships

Shared leadership

Storming

Support group

Task roles

This chapter deals with types of groups, group development, negotiating the group process, identifying leadership styles, and the use of groups by helping professionals to promote health. Community health nurses often have the opportunity to work with three kinds of groups: *community development groups, support groups,* and *educational groups.* Each of these is formed to meet a specific community or individual need. Before examination of these groups and the community health nurse's role within each, it is important to explore first what a group is and how it is formed.

DEFINITION OF GROUP

The term *group* is defined in a variety of ways; however, the following definition is particularly appropriate to nursing: "A group is an open system composed of three or more people held together by a common interest or bond. The individuals who make up the group are its subsystems" (Tappen, 1983, p. 149).

It is believed that a minimum of three individuals constitute a group because only then can the complex relationships develop that characterize a group. A triad, or three-person group, permits four relationships. A group of four permits eleven possible relationships (Fig. 6-1). In a three-person group a power relationship can develop between

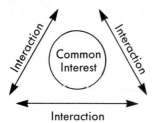

FIG. 6-1 A group of three permits four possible relationships, and a group of four permits eleven possible relationships.

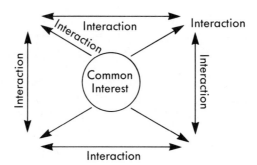

two of its members to win their position over the lone third member. In a dyad (a relationship between two individuals) a power relationship of this sort cannot exist. There is some evidence that suggests that larger groups produce lower member satisfaction. This lower level of satisfaction may be related to the time available for members to participate. However, the larger the size of the group the greater the availability of the resources among members (Hare, 1952).

FUNCTIONS OF GROUPS

Some of the basic functions of a community can be provided to its members through group formation. These functions include safety and security, mutual support, networking for distribution of resources, socialization, and a sense of belonging. Safety and security refer to protection of community members from crime, natural disasters, and threats against their physical safety. Groups that meet these needs include volunteer rescue squads, the American Red Cross, and neighborhood crime-watch groups.

Other groups may provide mutual support such as physical or psychological support during a crisis situation. Examples of such groups are Alcoholic Anonymous, Friendly Visitors, or Parents Without Partners. Communities provide networks for the distribution of resources, whether in the form of exchange of information or materials or services through groups such as the Salvation Army, the Cystic Fibrosis Association, and religious charity organizations.

Communities also provide opportunities for socialization by which values, beliefs, and attitudes can be shared. Community groups of this type include Kiwanis clubs, Chamber of Commerce groups, nutrition centers, and community Y. Furthermore, groups can provide an individual with a sense of belonging and an opportunity to contribute, for example, participation as a hospital or nursing home volunteer or as a member of a political action group.

Most of us have participated in one group or another, whether a school committee, a social club, or a religious organization. Perhaps you may have noticed that some groups you were involved with functioned better than others. Was this because of the leaders, the group members, the tasks involved, or a combination of all three factors? By the conclusion of this chapter you should be better prepared to understand the dynamics that can contribute to a group's effectiveness.

CHARACTERISTICS OF GROUPS

There is a difference between a group of individuals waiting at a bus stop and a group of nurses who meet each month as part of an honor society. The latter example is that of a formal group. Formal groups usually have three basic characteristics. Not all groups, however, serve the same function; thus not every group possesses each of the following characteristics:

Structure or organization. Individuals who compose a group have different functions. For example, one person in the group may be the leader; one may be a task master (concerned with how to best tackle the problem); one may be the maintainer (maintains good and harmonious working relationships); yet another may be the joker.

Shared goals. Members of a group work together to accomplish a shared goal that could not be achieved by individuals working alone. They may come together to solve a problem, to produce something, to reach a decision, or to enjoy one another's company.

Common sense of identity. Members of a group have a sense of belonging and feel the distinctiveness of their group compared with other groups.

Many similarities exist between small groups and the larger society. The group has rules and traditions, as well as a hierarchy of leaders and followers. The environment of the group affects it, and the group must change and adapt to survive. Last, groups, like societies, also have periods of difficulty and transition and may decline (Llewelyn & Fielding, 1982).

GROUP DEVELOPMENT

The manner in which all groups grow throughout their "life" refers to group development. According to Tuckman and Jensen (1977) there are five stages of group development: forming, storming, norming, performing, and adjourning. These stages of group development can be compared to the steps of the nursing process (assessing, analyzing, planning, implementing, and evaluating).

Stage 1: Forming (Assessing)

Forming is the process in which the group assembles and comes together as a group. Discovery takes place as individuals examine their backgrounds, attitudes, and personal style. Similar to the assessment component of the nursing process individuals are gathering information about each other. Typically, during this stage individuals exercise their best behavior to create a good impression. There usually is a great deal of stress during this time because members are not clear what the group will be like nor what will be expected of them. Communication within the group usually is formal and polite, and members tend to talk only about safe topics such as the weather or traffic. Even though uncomfortable feelings may exist, there generally is an underlying perception of optimism within the group. By the end of this stage, members have a sense of common identity and begin to define the boundary between the group and the environment.

Stage 2: Storming (Analyzing)

Storming can be an uncomfortable stage because there is conflict between the needs of the individuals in the group and the needs of the group as a whole. Bargaining begins in which members jockey for positions within the group. Individual members explore what they might be able to contribute to the group. This stage represents the analysis portion of the nursing process because it is at this point that the members review information obtained in the forming stage. The weak organizational structure developed in the first stage may have to be reworked. As the name implies, the group climate is unstable and emotional. Communication can become openly hostile and angry. Some group members may even leave the group altogether. Individual differences among group members may become more apparent and may lead to the development of subgroups or fractions. Power struggles also may occur in which two or more people may try to compete for the leadership position.

Stage 3: Norming (Planning)

Eventually, if the group members are able to satisfactorily resolve their individual differences, then norming will take place. At this time group "norms" or rules for participation are established. These norms must be established if the group is to form a cohesive unit. During this stage the group develops ways of achieving its goals, deciding who will do what and how it is to be done. Members begin to feel more relaxed, more a part of the group. They have made a decision to remain with the group and have begun to redefine their positions in the group. The group climate is characterized by more relatedness among members and therefore more purposeful and constructive action. This stage is comparable to the planning aspect of the nursing process in which ideas are generated in an attempt to solve the problem. The group begins to mature, with discussions focusing on suggestions and ideas, with a movement away from conflicts. Decisions now are made in a more democratic manner.

Stage 4: Performing (Implementing)

Once the norming stage is completed, the group can begin to work on the task at hand. The group can function as a unit, be productive, and work well together. Like the implementation phase of the nursing process various strategies are tested. This is the most enjoyable stage because the group has achieved consensus on its purposes and objectives. Each member feels a part of the group and knows what behavior is expected of him or her. The climate is one of openness in which members are cooperative and relaxed. Differences among group members still exist, but the mature group can deal with individuality and disagreement. Conflicts that arise can be resolved through negotiation, and feedback within the group is constructive.

Stage 5: Adjourning (Evaluating)

In this final stage the group comes to some kind of closure. A summary or an evaluation of the group takes place to determine if the original purposes were met. Similar to the evaluation phase of the nursing process the objectives are reexamined with the possibility of having to develop new strategies. If the group does not achieve complete closure, members may leave feeling dissatisfied. The adjourning stage may be characterized by

ROLES WITHIN GROUPS

Task roles

Initiator/energizer: proposes new ideas or tasks to the group

Information giver: provides facts from personal knowledge or experience that might assist the group in its deliberations

Opinion seeker: seeks clarification by asking for opinions, judgments, or feelings of other group members

Disagreer: points out problems with the information given; presents different points of view

Elaborator: expands on existing information or suggestions being made

Evaluator: critically evaluates ideas and proposals for their practicality and effectiveness

Social/maintenance roles

Encourager: offers praise to those who have made contributions and demonstrates acceptance of ideas and suggestions

Gatekeeper: attempts to obtain contributions from other members; may suggest ways to ensure that all members have an opportunity to speak

Normkeeper: expresses standards or guidelines for the group to use in its deliberations

Harmonizer: mediates conflicts and disagreements through humor, conciliation, and mediation

Consensus taker: states opinions and decisions made by the group to test group's agreement or disagreement

Expressor: describes feelings and reactions held by group members

Individual roles

Aggressor: criticizes others and makes hostile remarks

Blocker: can obstruct progress made by the group by being negative and unreasonable

Recognition seeker: uses the group as a personal audience and behaviorally calls attention to himself or herself

Monopolizer: talks often and long, thereby preventing others from participating

Definitions from "Task roles and social roles in problem-solving groups" by R.F. Bales, in *Readings in Social Psychology* (3rd ed.) by E.E. Maccoby, T.M. Newcomb, and E.L. Hartley, 1958, New York: Holt, Reinhart & Winston; and "Functional roles of group members" by P. Sheats, 1948, *Journal of Social Issues, 4*, pp. 41-49.

ambivalent feelings in which members are pleased that the tasks are completed but at the same time feel sad that the group is ending. Some groups may feel threatened by this stage and thus either avoid it or rush through it.

ROLE DIFFERENTIATION

Bales (1958) in his study of role differentiation suggests that there are two major specialist roles within all groups. He refers to these as task roles and socioemotional or maintenance roles. The individual identified as a task specialist is one who is interested in one or more of the aspects of getting the job done. The task specialist exhibits behavior that contributes to the completion of a group task. The socioemotional specialist attempts to keep the group working together in harmony by relieving tension with a joke. This specialist also will make peace after conflicts and, in addition, will control the more assertive group members so that the less confident can be heard.

An addition to Bales' work involves a third specialist role referred to as individual functions (Benne & Sheats, 1948). This third role includes those roles that serve individual members' own needs rather than those of the group as a whole. These three specialist roles complement each other. Those groups that are the most effective have members with different specialties. The box on p. 127 provides a summary of several examples of different roles within groups.

THE GROUP LEADER

An effective group leader is one who can influence others to work harmoniously and productively to attain the goals of the group. A group leader also is aware of the group's total resource potential and how to use it.

Four qualities are necessary in an effective group leader (Sampson & Marthas, 1981; Tappen, 1983). These are the ability to set goals, the ability to think critically, the ability to help the group become aware of its own resources, and the ability to motivate and initiate action.

Ability to Set Goals

A leader becomes involved in three types of goals: individual-level or personal goals, group-level goals, and organization-level goals. For example, Sue attends a morning meeting to discuss the discharging of a patient. Sue's personal goal is that the meeting concludes so that she does not miss her lunch appointment. Group-level goals often can be different from individual goals. The group may be more interested in discussing weekend plans than interventions for the patient's discharge. Finally, organizational goals also can affect the leader's action. In this case the organization is anxious not only to have the patient discharged but to be able to provide continuity of care. The group leader can be instrumental in helping group members find common ground in making compromises and in formulating clear and common goals.

Ability to Think Critically

A group leader is one who not only has knowledge about a problem but is able to analyze it rather than just complain about it. Possessing knowledge about nursing gives the leader credibility and self-confidence when working with others. The leader also needs to be aware of behavior and what motivates individual group members. In the previous example the group leader can help members "brainstorm" in identifying possible community resources that can assist the patient at home.

Ability to Help the Group Become Aware of Its Own Resources

The leader recognizes the strengths that individual members bring to the group and how they can best be used. In the discharge planning example, the leader attempted to match each member's talents with necessary tasks. Joan, the occupational therapist, was assigned to explore which structure modifications might be needed in the patient's home, whereas Betty, the physical therapist, was assigned to teach the patient transfer techniques.

Ability to Motivate and Initiate Action

The leader has to be able not only to listen to group members but also to encourage the flow of information. The leader may notice, for example, that a group member has not made any contributions to the discussion. Rather than assuming that the individual is bored or unconcerned, the leader could attempt to bring him or her into the conversation. A group with a good idea or suggestion may not be a productive group without a leader who can guide and help members see their ideas come to life. The leader facilitates openness to ideas that may be new and different so that the group does not become immobilized by conflict.

SHARED LEADERSHIP

The same elements that make an effective leader also apply to situations that involve shared leadership. Although some leaders prefer to work alone, others enjoy sharing leadership responsibility. For example, a community health nurse and a physician might co-lead a group by contributing their individual perspectives on the health problem under discussion.

There are both advantages and disadvantages of shared leadership. Some of the advantages include the following:

1. The novice group leader can learn from the more experienced leader through observation and role modeling.
2. The group can benefit in seeing co-leaders communicate, cooperate, and disagree in an effective manner.
3. After each group meeting, co-leaders can share their perceptions and provide feedback to each other on the group process.

Shared leadership is more complex than leadership by one individual, which can result in some of the following disadvantages:

1. Group members can play one leader against the other, just as a child can go first to the mother, then to the father, when denied a request.
2. One leader may be perceived by group members as having more authority or power, which can lead to tension between the leaders.
3. Shared leadership may be less efficient because leaders must share responsibility for decision making.

SOCIAL POWER AND GROUP CONFLICT

Social power and conflict are two additional concepts that the community health nurse needs to examine to enhance his or her leadership ability. Social power can be defined as the exercise of actual or potential power to influence another person's behavior, whether that individual wants it changed or not (Cartwright & Zander, 1968). Although social power is not evenly distributed to all group members, everyone has some power. The occupant of the group leader position often is given added social power. French and Raven (1968) have distinguished five types of social power: attraction power, reward power, coercive power, legitimate power, and expert power.

Attraction power refers to a "liking" relationship; that is, a person who is liked in a group has more power than a person who is disliked. *Reward power* is based on the ability of a group member to provide rewards to other members. The reward can be in the form of money or information. *Coercive power* is the ability of one person to inflict harm on another by threatening public embarrassment, loss of prestige, or loss of popularity. The belief that one person has the right to dictate the behavior of another person is referred to as *legitimate power.* Finally, *expert power* is based on an individual's education, skills, and experience. It may be helpful for the community health nurse to assess the social power of a group, especially if the goal is to bring about change. The nurse, for example, can use expert power to encourage group members to follow directions on health matters.

Group conflict is almost an inevitable process, but it is not necessarily harmful because it can stimulate creativity and growth. A group leader should attempt neither to avoid nor to stimulate conflict but rather to try to manage it.

There are many potential sources of conflict, including value and cultural differences among group members; conflict of loyalties within and outside of the group; power struggles; dislike of members for one another; and involvement in the group task itself. A group leader can take some preventive steps before conflicts arise by encouraging an atmosphere in which individual differences are considered normal. Open communication among group members is another measure that can be helpful in preventing conflict. Conflicts also can be reduced when leaders attempt to meet the needs of group members. Once a conflict has developed, the leader can help group members analyze the conflict to determine its source so that solutions can be generated (Tappan, 1983).

LEADERSHIP STYLES

Just as there are different characteristics or qualities that can be used to describe a leader, there also are differences in leadership styles. Some leaders seek opinions from members whereas others demand their obedience. The best-known researchers on leadership styles are Lewin, Lippitt, and White (1939). In the late 1930s they observed four groups of 10-year-old boys who came together in groups to participate in hobbies. Three distinct leadership styles emerged: autocratic, democratic, and laissez faire.

Autocratic

The autocratic or authoritarian approach is based on the premise "I am the leader, and this is the law" (Smith, 1980). This approach focuses on a leader-centered rather than member-centered style. Decisions are arrived at by the leader who also dictates the tasks and activities that are to be completed. Under an autocratic leader the work usually is accomplished in a smooth manner, but very little creativity and autonomy are permitted. The group members generally are dependent on the leader. Research by Lippitt and associates indicates that members of autocratically run groups do not initiate work without the presence of the leader. In emergency or crisis situations autocratic leadership may be appropriate because during these situations clear directions need to be given.

Democratic

Another leadership style is the democratic approach, which is based on the premise that "we are all equal, and whatever happens, happens" (Smith, 1980). The democratic leader allows members of the group to be active in the development of policies and goal setting. The democratic leader, rather than selling an approach, adopts a problem-solving pattern to help group members develop their own views and perspectives. Unlike the autocratic leader the democratic leader guides rather than directs. Control within the group is shared, and each group member is encouraged to participate in the process. Although the democratic approach is not as efficient as the autocratic style, it is believed to work well with groups that need to work closely and cooperatively for a long period of time, such as in health care. The democratic leadership style increases group cohesiveness and group involvement.

Laissez Faire

The laissez-faire leadership style is based on the belief that the group is self-directing within the limits of rules and guidelines. The leader's approach is "I am here if you need me" (Smith, 1980). In this style of leading the group members are given complete freedom

TABLE 6-1 Differences in leadership style

Leadership style	Advantages	Disadvantages	Appropriate use
Autocratic: all policy determined by leader	Work accomplished in a smooth and efficient manner	Allows little creativity; group members are dependent on leader	Emergency or crisis situation
Democratic: all policies a matter of group discussion	Control of the group is shared; group cohesiveness is increased	Not as efficient as autocratic style	Health care groups
Lassiez faire: complete nonparticipation of leader	Members are given complete independence in making decisions	Low productivity and efficiency	Groups that are highly motivated and self-directed

to make their own decisions. The laissez-faire leader provides little if any direction, guidance, or encouragement. Members in laissez-faire groups may work independently of each other and may very well be working at cross-purposes with little cooperation. Under a laissez-faire leader, work often is completed inefficiently or productivity is low. Generally, laissez-faire leadership style is viewed as inappropriate because it is inefficient. However, it may be a valid leadership approach with a group that is highly motivated and self-directed (Lewin, Lippitt, & White, 1939; Sampson & Marthas, 1981; Shaw, 1981). Table 6-1 summarizes the differences among the three leadership styles.

Whether a leader chooses to use the autocratic, democratic, or laissez-faire approach often is influenced by the situation. The characteristics and style of an effective leader will be fluid and will change as the situation demands. The following example demonstrates how one community health nurse chose her leadership style on the basis of the situation and the group's orientation. A community health nurse who worked primarily in a section of a city with an elderly population became aware of the lack of support services for women who had a history of psychiatric problems. Initially, the community health nurse used an autocratic approach in convening the meetings, and she chose the agenda. She also decided that the group would be called the "Chit-Chat Club" in an attempt to lessen the stigma attached to the meetings. The nurse also stipulated that the group would meet for 1 hour each week. As the weeks progressed, the nurse assumed a more democratic approach by encouraging the women to decide the topics or activities they wished to pursue. One week the group wanted to visit a wax museum so that they could reminisce about the "good old days," and another week they wanted to discuss how to handle stress. Over time the women began to support each other and no longer required the community health nurse to act as the leader.

MOTIVATIONAL THEORY

Leadership obviously is a complex process that involves specific qualities and patterns. In addition to possessing certain characteristics, an effective leader has to have some understanding about the factors that motivate individuals so that they feel satisfied and productive as group members.

One of the most widely used frameworks for exploring motivation at all organizational levels is the motivation maintenance theory (Herzberg, Mausner, & Synderman, 1959). This theory identifies five major "dissatisfiers": company policy and administration, supervision, salary, interpersonal relations, and working conditions. These factors are termed *hygiene factors* because of their similarity to the principles of medical hygiene; they have a preventive rather than a curative potential. For example, interpersonal relations among group members are not directly related to the group's task; however, these relationships can affect the environment or condition under which the group must function. According to the motivation maintenance theory a second group of factors, identified as "satisfiers," includes satisfying job content, task achievement, responsibility for a task, and professional achievement. These satisfiers are termed *motivators* because they provide impetus to superior performance.

Three principles of the motivational theory are applicable to groups. Regardless of how much recognition and status are provided, hygiene factors need to be reasonably satisfied or the productivity of group members will be diminished. The second principle is based on the premise that the talents and abilities of most individuals are not fully used and that many persons want to undertake new responsibilities. Therefore individual enrichment is likely to lead to a highly motivated group member. The third principle relates to developing goals or objectives, or both, that are not only clear to group members but will spur them to higher levels of productivity. This principle becomes important in the delegation of tasks. When tasks are assigned to group members, the significance of the task, as well as the reasons why an individual or group has been selected to complete the project, should be explained (Veninga, 1982).

Motivational theory emphasizes the humanistic side of leadership. It takes into consideration the needs of group members in order to enhance the group's productivity.

TYPES OF GROUPS

As already indicated, nurses are expected to understand group process and to be able to function competently both as group participants and as group leaders. Nurses who function in community settings may become involved in one of three types of groups: community development groups, support or self-help groups, and educational groups.

Community Development Groups

Community development groups are special groups that come together to support advocacy. Advocacy is action that is designed to help individuals who feel powerless to acquire and use power to make social systems more responsive to their needs. Community development groups may be formed for persons all along the age continuum. A Parent-Teacher Association (PTA) may be formed to ensure that teenagers are informed about acquired immunodeficiency syndrome (AIDS) and its transmission. A group of senior citizens may join together to form a Gray Panthers organization, the purpose of which may be to educate older adults about their rights regarding rent control.

An example of a successful community development group is presented in the box on the opposite page.

Support, or Self-Help, Groups

Many support groups in the United States have been formed to meet a variety of needs for both the layperson and the professional. Support, or self-help groups, may be composed of persons of all ages. The groups usually are self-regulating, with an emphasis on peer cohesiveness rather than formal structure (Burnside, 1984). The members often provide specific help in handling members' problems or conditions that require attention.

Four categories of support, or self-help, groups can be categorized as follows (Levy, 1976):

1. *Behavioral control.* The focus is on behavior modification and includes such groups as Alcoholics Anonymous, Weight Watchers, and Gamblers Anonymous.
2. *Stress, coping, and support.* Members share a common condition or life experience, for example, in such groups as arthritis clubs, Reach for Recovery, and the Parents' Association for Retarded Children.
3. *Survival oriented.* These groups advocate self-reliance and individual responsibility and include such groups at the National Organization for Women, Latch Key Programs, and the American Association of Retired Persons.
4. *Personal growth or self-actualization.* Groups that fit into this category provide socialization and promote self-expression for persons with common life values, for example, golden agers clubs, Big Brothers/Big Sisters, and the Young Women's Christian Association and Young Men's Christian Association.

The support group approach has been used in addressing teenage pregnancy. This type of group can provide a supportive milieu that offers socialization, education, discussion, and problem solving. Pregnant teenagers often have many psychological problems that can be ignored in an impersonal clinic atmosphere. Teenaged girls are at greater risk for the development of complications such as pregnancy-induced hypertension (PIH) and premature delivery because they still are maturing themselves. Many pregnant teenagers lack knowledge concerning the significance of symptoms, which causes them to delay seeking medical intervention. The community health nurse is in a good position to establish a support group for pregnant teenagers. The group could be scheduled while patients are waiting in the clinic to see the physician. The nurse, however, also would need to work closely with the clinic staff members to obtain their support by acquainting them with the goals of the group (Everett, 1980). Individuals isolated from social or emotional resources may benefit from the establishment of a newly organized support group that promotes their health and self-esteem.

Educational Groups

Although community development and support groups can provide an exchange of information, this exchange is the main focus of educational groups. Educational groups provide opportunities for continuing education in the area of preventive health. Fig. 6-3

COMMUNITY DEVELOPMENT GROUP SUCCESSFUL IN NUTRITION CENTER CONFLICT

Three years ago in a small urban community a neighborhood nutrition center was to be closed for budgetary reasons. The nutrition center had operated in the basement of a church for more than 7 years. The older participants were able to walk from their homes and apartments. They felt comfortable in attending because the center was an established part of the neighborhood. They were confused and angry over the closure, which would force them to travel greater distances and require the use of public transportation.

A few of the older adults formed a community development group to decide on the best course of action. The manager of the nutrition center and the nurse provided support and feedback to the group. Strategies were established, such as circulating a written petition, writing letters to city councilmen and letters to the editor, and inviting councilmen for whom the participants had voted to visit the nutrition center. With a local election soon approaching, the final strategy proved to be the best. The nutrition center is still flourishing and meeting the needs of the local neighborhood.

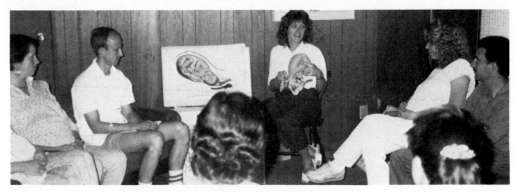

FIG. 6-2 Example of an educational group. The nurse uses a model and pictures to illustrate labor and delivery to a group of expectant parents.

shows a nurse leading a prenatal class. With the growing concern for relevant and meaningful instruction in health care, community nurses will find themselves being asked to lead such a group. Nurses in community settings also may be asked to provide educational material to other nurses and health care workers on such topics as discharge planning, community resources, and the use of high technology equipment in home care.

The leader of educational groups often takes on the role of teacher, but this does not mean that the leader has to dominate the session. The educational group leader can present some basic facts about the topic and then encourage group members to participate by stating their opinions and ideas or by asking questions.

There are several advantages to health teaching in groups. One advantage is that it is more cost effective than one-on-one teaching. A second advantage is that a group setting stimulates an organized presentation, which means more consistency in information giving. Finally, group teaching can affect and alter attitudes and behavior toward health practices. As group members begin to share personal experiences and discuss realistic approaches to health problems, they may modify their attitudes.

For the community health nurse involved in an educational group—whether the group's focus is prenatal instruction, chronic lung obstruction, or stress reduction—the principles are the same. The leader first must assess the characteristics and the needs of the population before the program is begun. Realistic and appropriate objectives need to be selected for the group. Finally, there is a need to evaluate the educational process either formally by questionnaires or tests or informally by observations and interviews (Lewis, 1984).

The community health nurse working in an area with many older adults may choose to use the group approach to provide health information. A senior citizen apartment complex may have an appropriate space for such health conferences. The nurse can survey the older adults to determine topics of greatest interest and most convenient times. Posters advertising the conferences could provide helpful reminders to the participants. Titles of the conferences should be simple but also attention grabbing, such as "Meet your Feet," "Drug Use and Misuse," "Fitness For Fun," and "Are You Losing Your Senses?" Given the opportunity, older adults are eager to learn what they can do to enhance their health.

INITIATING A SMALL GROUP

The community health nurse may have noticed an increase in his or her caseload of patients with a particular disease process. The nurse decides that instituting an educational or a support group would not only enhance the members' knowledge of the disease but would provide mutual support to combat feelings of isolation. The group might be a Better Breathers Club for those with chronic obstructive pulmonary disease, a stroke club for those with cerebral vascular accidents, or a Reach for Recovery group for women who have had mastectomies. Regardless of the group the nurse leader must complete three important tasks before the first meeting.

The first task involves administrative issues such as finding a place to hold the meeting, one that is convenient to the group. Finding a meeting place may require the nurse to negotiate with a hospital, school, or church administrator. There may be resistance from the administrator or from small community agencies, which requires time and energy to resolve. The nurse may have to persuade administrators as well as agency personnel that he or she can function as a group leader. Resistance can be decreased if the nurse is prepared to present specific objectives for the group experience.

The second task in establishing a group requires making decisions about the group itself. The nurse needs to decide who will comprise the group. Will the group consist of patients with acute or chronic illness? Will family members be included? What will the group size be? These are all important decisions that must be made before the initial meeting. It has been recommended that the group size be maintained at four to twelve members if the objectives are interaction and group cohesiveness. The nurse leader also needs to decide on how often the group will meet, at what time, and the length of each meeting. Answers to these questions depend on the composition of the group and its purposes. For some educational groups it may be beneficial to have established the total number of group sessions on the basis of the topics to be presented.

Preparing the prospective group members is the third task of the community health nurse. When possible it is best for the nurse to speak to each potential member individually. In this way the leader can prepare the member with information concerning what to expect from the group sessions. Later, written materials such as a summary of the content and topics to be covered can be sent (Clark, 1987). Beginning any small group takes persistence, energy, and collaboration on the part of the nurse leader, but the members' response often makes the effort worthwhile.

SUMMARY

Nurses have many opportunities to work with groups in the community. The different types of groups with which nurses may work are community development groups, support groups, and educational groups. There are three different types of leadership styles, and each may be appropriate at different times or with different types of groups.

Some groups develop according to a five-stage process that is similar to the nursing process. As the members of a group work together, the individual members take on specialized roles within the group.

Group work can be demanding because of the complex relationships that may develop among the members. The group leader must be aware of these relationships. Thus development of leadership skills is essential to the process of group work.

CHAPTER HIGHLIGHTS

- A group is an open system composed of three or more persons held together by a common interest or bond. A minimum of three individuals is needed to allow the development of the complex relationships that characterize a group.
- Some functions of groups include safety and security, mutual support, networking for distribution of resources, socialization, and a sense of belonging.
- Characteristics common to most groups include a typical structure or organization, shared goals, and a common sense of identity.
- The five stages of group development are forming, storming, norming, performing, and adjourning. These steps parallel the five steps of the nursing process.
- The major specialist roles within groups are task roles, social/maintenance roles, and individual roles.
- Effective group leadership requires the ability to set goals, think critically, help the group become aware of its own resources, motivate others, and initiate action.
- Shared leadership in a group has both advantages and disadvantages. Although it may be more effective in some groups, it also may be more complex and less efficient.
- Social power is the ability to influence another person's behavior. The five types of social power are attraction power, reward power, coercive power, legitimate power, and expert power.
- The three leadership styles are autocratic, democratic, and laissez faire. The leader's choice of leadership style is influenced by the situation and may change as the group progresses in its work.
- Herzberg's motivational theory, as applied to groups, takes into consideration that the needs of group members must be satisfied to enhance the group's productivity.
- Community health nurses may become involved with community development groups, self-help or support groups, or educational groups.

STUDY QUESTIONS

1. Describe three types of groups. For each, what is the role of the nurse?
2. Identify two major roles of individuals in groups.
3. Describe three leadership styles. For each, give an example of when and where it could be used appropriately.
4. Discuss Herzberg's motivational theory. How is it applicable to working with groups?

REFERENCES

Bales, R.F. (1959). Task roles and social roles in problem solving groups. In E.E. Maccoby, T.M. Newcomb, and E.L. Hartley (Eds.), *Readings in Social Psychology* (3rd ed). New York: Holt, Rinehart, & Winston.

Benne, K., & Sheats, P. (1948). Functional roles of group members. *Journal of Social Issues, 4,* 41-49.

Burnside, I. (1984). *Working with the elderly* (2nd ed.). Monterey, CA: Wadsworth Health Sciences.

Cartwright, D., & Zander, A. (Eds.). (1968). Group dynamics (3rd ed.). New York: Harper & Row.

Clark, C. (1987). *The nurse as group leader* (2nd ed.). New York: Springer.

Everett, M. (1980). Group work in the prenatal clinic. *Health and Social Work, 5,* 71-74.

French, J., & Raven, B. (1968). The bases of social power. In D. Cartwright and A. Zander (Eds.), *Group dynamics* (3rd ed.). New York: Harper & Row.

Hare, P.A. (1952). A study of interactions and consensus in different sized groups. *American Sociology Review, 17,* 261-267.

Herzberg, F., Mausner, B., & Synderman, B. (1959). *The motivation to work.* New York: Wiley.

Kohnke, M.F. (1982). *Advocacy: Risk and reality,* St. Louis: Mosby.

Levy, L. (1976). Self-help groups: Types and psychological process. *Journal of Applied Behavioral Sciences, 12,* 310-322.

Lewin, K., Lippitt, R., & White, R. (1939). Patterns of aggressive behavior in experimentally created "social climates." *Journal of Social Psychology, 10,* 271-299.

Lewis, S. (1984). Teaching patient groups. *Nursing Management, 15* (5), 49-56.

Llewelyn, S., & Fielding, G. (1982). Group dynamics: Forming, storming, norming and performing, Pt. 1. *Nursing Mirror, 155,* (July 21), 14-16.

Sampson, E., & Marthas, M. (1981). *Group process for the health professions,* (2nd ed.). New York: Wiley.

Shaw, M. (1981). *Group dynamics — The psychology of small group behavior* (3rd ed.). New York: McGraw-Hill.

Smith, L. (1980). Finding your leadership style in groups. *American Journal of Nursing, 80,* 1301-1303.

Tappen, R. (1983). *Nursing leadership: Concepts and practice.* Philadelphia: Davis.

Tuckman, B., & Jensen, M. (1977). Stages of small group development revisited. *Group and Organization Studies, 2,* 419.

Veninga, R. (1982). *The human side of health administration,* Englewood Cliffs, NJ: Prentice-Hall.

Epidemiology

JOAN M. COOKFAIR

Environment is that viable arena that has relevance to the life space of the system, including a created environment.

BETTY NEUMAN

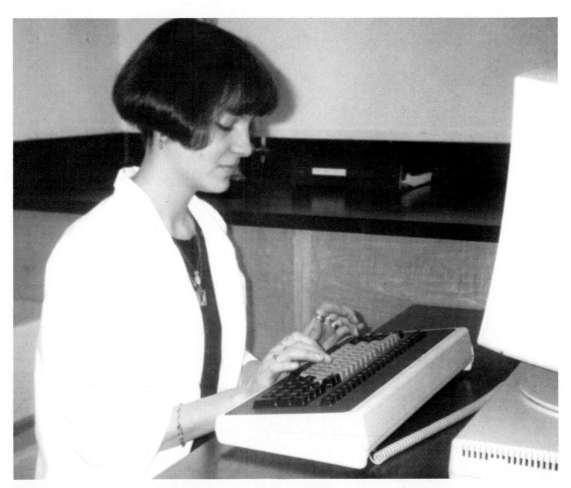

OBJECTIVES

At the conclusion of this chapter the student will be able to:
1. Define the key terms listed
2. Describe the historical evolution of epidemiology
3. Describe epidemiological concepts
4. Describe methods of collecting data
5. Describe methods of study used in epidemiological research
6. Identify selected epidemiological studies
7. Describe the application of epidemiology to community health nursing practice

KEY TERMS

Analytical studies	Natural history of disease
Causality	Person
Cohort study	Place
Cross-sectional study	Prevalence
Descriptive survey	Prospective study
Epidemiology	Rates
Incidence	Relative numbers
Method of transmission	Reservoir of infection
Morbidity	Retrospective study
Mortality	Time

Epidemiology, a field of science, is concerned with factors and conditions that determine the occurrence and distribution of health, disease, defect, disability, and death among groups of individuals (Leavell & Clark, 1965). Epidemiologists study patterns and trends in human populations relative to time, place, and individual persons for the purpose of preventing disease and maintaining and promoting health.

HISTORICAL EVOLUTION

The theory that the environment influences the spread of infectious disease dates back to the fifth century BC. During that period Hippocrates, in his book *Airs, Waters, and Places,* specified that for proper medical investigation one must take into account the seasons, the water supply, the orientation of the city and its topography, and the customs and occupations of the population under observation (Smith, 1941).

The practice of isolating persons with contagious diseases, first begun in antiquity, continues today. Those with active leprosy still are isolated although they no longer are ostracized. Prudent precautions still are recommended to prevent the spread of infectious disease even though they are not as drastic as the measures taken in London in the sixteenth century to fight the threat of plague. At that time town officials shut up the houses where the plague was found, confining well persons in the home with the sick and posting watchers at the door to prevent escape.

Bubonic plague, which is caused by a bacillus, occurs primarily in rodents, in whom the infection may be subacute or chronic. It is spread to human beings by the bite of an infected flea from the rodent (Merck, 1982). Called the *Black Death* during the Middle

Ages, it swept over Europe in the fourteenth century and killed half the population of London. In some instances the dead were left unburied because no one remained to bury them. The disease was almost always fatal. It was not surprising, therefore, that people were frightened and often reacted violently against the mere mention of the word *plague.* Although myth and superstition surrounded the cause of the disease, one fact emerged: it was contagious.

Gradually the concept of contagion began to spread. Parish clerks and village priests kept records, called *bills of mortality,* about deaths that occurred in London and Hampshire. In the seventeenth century John Gaunt, a pioneer in the field of epidemiology, began to look carefully at these statistics and to draw inferences from them, including the relationship between urban-rural differences and acute and chronic illness. His work, *Natural and Political Observations,* published in 1692, presented a strong case for the accurate recording of vital statistics to provide a base for similar studies (Lilienfeld, 1980).

Another pioneer in the science of epidemiology was Dr. William Farr, who was in charge of a General Register office established in England in 1837. Farr compiled statistical data about morbidity (illness) and mortality (death) and drew epidemiological inferences about the effect of inadequate sanitation and overcrowding on the spread of disease.

Florence Nightingale patterned her reports to superiors on the health conditions of the military during the Crimean War in the 1850s after Farr's work by presenting detailed statistics and their implications. On the basis of these reports she acquired funding to implement changes, which significantly reduced the mortality rate of British troops in hospitals (Cohen, 1984). Nightingale continued to use an epidemiological model in her early work to demonstrate the role of environment in health and its relevance to disease patterns (Stanhope & Lancaster, 1988).

John Snow, a contemporary of Farr's, collected data, based on the source of the water supply used by the victims, concerning the incidence (number of cases reported) of cholera. His results clearly indicated that the cholera rates of houses in London supplied by one water company were eight and nine times higher than in other neighborhoods, and Snow's findings greatly influenced the control of the disease. This logical ordering of events and empirical reasoning to identify the source of infection occurred many years before Pasteur formulated the germ theory of disease and Koch discovered the bacillus that caused cholera, *Vibrio cholerae* (Lilienfeld, 1980). Snow, however, had isolated an indirect cause, and improved sanitation of the water supply reduced the incidence of cholera long before the direct cause was known.

A contemporary example of the effectiveness of ongoing statistical surveillance concerns the outbreak of *Pneumocystis carinii* pneumonia and Kaposi's sarcoma reported to the Centers for Disease Control (CDC) between 1980 to 1982, including an unprecedented number (216) by January 13 of 1982 in New York City and California. All of the cases were in male homosexuals and drug addicts. A study of 81 male homosexuals demonstrated that they had symptoms of depressed immunity although they were not clinically ill. Conclusions began to be drawn that this phenomenon was associated with homosexual behavior long before the HIV virus was isolated. (The New England Journal of Medicine, 1982).

A gradual shift of focus has occurred in the field of epidemiology from an emphasis on the causes of infectious disease to an attempt to isolate factors that may have contributed to the development of disease. Studies done to determine cause and effect relationships related to the following events are examples of this approach.

- The surgeon general's report on smoking and health
- Legionnaires' disease

- Saccharin and breast cancer
- Bovine flu vaccination and Guillain-Barré syndrome
- Tampons and toxic shock syndrome
- Passive smoking
- Agent Orange

Information concerning the factors and events that led to toxic shock syndrome enabled health professionals to educate women about the proper use of tampons long before the causative agent was determined. Thus women could avoid the event and lessen their risk.

EPIDEMIOLOGICAL CONCEPTS

Several concepts have been developed that nurse epidemiologists can use in the community. An understanding of these concepts is necessary if the nurse is to apply them to community health nursing practice.

The Natural History of Disease

Leavell and Clark (1965) developed a concept that outlines the natural history of disease in human beings (Fig. 7-1).

During the prepathogenetic period, interactions may occur between the host-agent and environment that increase an individual's susceptibility to disease. For example, smoking increases an individual's risk for lung disease. Health education before the event (smoking) may prevent an individual from smoking and thus minimize the risk of a lung disease such as emphysema. If, during early pathogenesis a smoker with a chronic cough can be encouraged to prevent further sequelae by quitting smoking, disease progression still may be altered. Should a pathologic condition such as emphysema develop, rehabilitation or limitation of disability still is possible if the smoker is encouraged to cease smoking and make maximum use of remaining capabilities.

Primary, secondary, and tertiary prevention

Primary prevention is the prevention of disease by altering susceptibility or reducing exposure of susceptible individuals. It is accomplished by health promotion (teaching and advocacy) or specific protection (immunizations and altered environment).

Secondary prevention is the early detection and treatment of disease by such techniques as case finding, screening surveys, and prevention of spread of communicable disease.

Tertiary prevention is the alleviation of disability that results from disease and the attempt to restore effective functioning. It can be achieved by means of rehabilitation or palliative methods if rehabilitation is impossible.

Table 7-1 applies the Leavell and Clark model to the community by planning interventions to prevent acquired immunodeficiency syndrome (AIDS) at primary, secondary, and tertiary levels.

Causality

Reference was made earlier in the chapter to the detection of causal relationships between factors and events. Detecting causal relationships may be the key to interrupting a chain of events that can lead to disease or disability. Before an association can be ascertained, however, all other possible associations must be eliminated. There must be evidence that the existing factor increases or decreases the likelihood that an event may occur. To achieve validity studies should be repeated with unrelated population groups. All possible

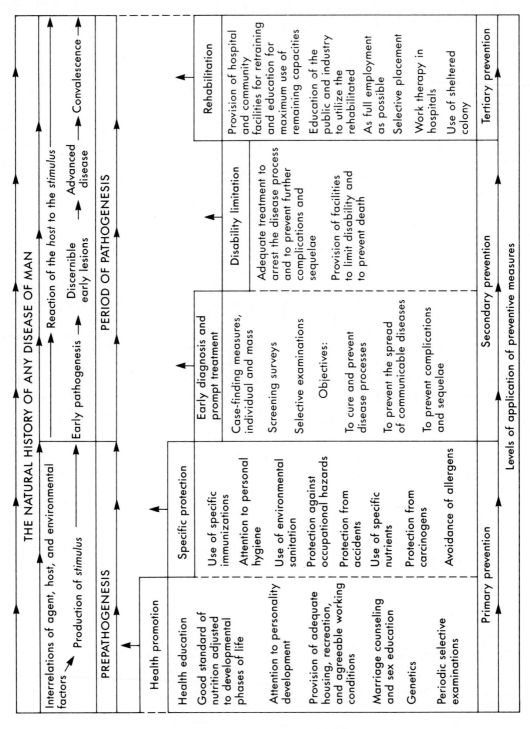

FIG. 7-1 Levels of application of preventive measures in the natural history of disease. *(From Preventive medicine for the doctor in his community: An epidemiologic approach by H. R. Leavell and E. G. Clark, 1965, New York: McGraw Hill. Copyright 1965 by McGraw Hill. Reprinted by permission.)*

TABLE 7-1 Prepathogenesis and pathogenesis of acquired immunodeficiency syndrome

Prepathogenesis: interrelationships among agent, host, and environment before disease occurs	Period of pathogenesis: course of disease in human beings		
Primary prevention: health promotion*	**Secondary prevention**		**Tertiary prevention**
	Early diagnosis and treatment: HIV positive (latent stage)	**Disability and limitation: onset of clinical symptoms of AIDS**	**Rehabilitative/palliative: onset of opportunistic infections known as disease indicators**

1. Encourage education of children as early as possible about the manner in which the HIV virus is transferred.
2. Screen all blood products for presence of HIV.
3. Educate IV drug abusers about danger of sharing needles.
4. Teach safer sexual practices:
   a. avoid sexual practices that injure mucosal tissue
   b. limit partners
   c. use condoms
   d. consider abstinence
5. Educate health care workers to use universal precautions recommended by the CDC
	Men:
	1. Avoid infections.
	2. Have regular check-ups.
	3. Avoid passing infection.
	4. Get adequate rest, nutrition, exercise.
	5. Maintain full employment, confidentiality.
	Women: (in addition to above)
	1. Avoid pregnancy.
	2. If pregnant, request cesarean section.
	3. Do not breast-feed.
	Child:
	1. Encourage medical supervision.
	2. Avoid infection.
	3. Maintain quality of life.
	4. Check status of parents.
		1. Encourage compliance with medical regimen.
		2. Make patient aware of side effects.
		3. Encourage employment as long as possible.
		4. Provide counseling for client and family.
		5. Take appropriate precautions for any opportunistic infection involved.
		6. Teach/use good hand washing.
		7. Teach/use needle precaution.
		8. Teach/use universal precautions.
		9. Use gloves during contact with body fluids.
		10. Use bleach such as Clorox for spills and clothes washing, etc.
			1. Counsel patients and family.
			2. Maintain medical regimen.
			3. Maintain quality of life by continuing employment as long as possible, maintaining nutrition, and limiting discomfort.
			4. Teach/use needle precaution.
			5. Teach/use universal precautions.
			6. Use gloves during contact with body fluids.
			7. Use bleach such as Clorox for cleanup as previously (No. 10).

Modified from (p. 21) by H. Leavell and E. Clark. (1965). *The natural history of disease in man.* New York: McGraw Hill.

AIDS, Acquired immunodeficiency syndrome; *HIV,* human immunodeficiency virus; *IV,* intravenous.

*No specific protection (no vaccine available).

relevant variables must be eliminated. For example, in the 1964 surgeon general's report regarding smoking and health outcomes, a framework of causality was established by the use of the following criteria to assess the causal relationship (Mausner, 1974):

1. *Correctness of temporality.* Exposure to the suspected factor under study occurred before the specific event being studied.
2. *Strength of association.* The larger the ratio the greater the likelihood that the factor affects the outcome. This association required statistical measurement by means of a relative risk ratio.
3. *Specificity of association.* It must be possible to predict the occurrence of one variable in relation to the extent or occurrence of another.
4. *Consistency of association.* The association found in one study must persist in other studies with other populations.
5. *Dose-response relationship.* With increasing levels of exposure to the factor, a corresponding increase of occurrence of disease is found.
6. *Biological plausibility.* There must be a reasonable biological explanation for the occurrence of event, one that coincides with current knowledge about the factor and the disease or disability.

The following information about a possible causal relationship between maternal smoking and infant mortality summarizes the results of accumulated data.

1. *Correctness of temporality.* Many investigators documented evidence that fetal and neonatal mortality is significantly higher for children born to smokers than for children born to nonsmokers.
2. *Consistency of association.* The results of many studies about the relationship between smoking and birth weight were examined, and they demonstrated a strong association between maternal cigarette smoking and delivery of infants of low birth weight. Babies born to mothers who smoke are, on the average, 200 gm lighter than babies born to women who do not smoke.
3. *Biological plausibility.* Available evidence shows that cigarette smokers' infants tend to be smaller for gestational age rather than gestationally premature.
4. *Specificity of association.* Infants of smokers have lower birth weights than do infants of nonsmokers. When a variety of known or suspected factors (e.g., age, parity, previous pregnancy history, and prenatal visits) that also exert an influence on birth weight have been controlled, cigarette smoking always has been shown to be related to low birth weight.
5. *Dose-response relationship.* The more cigarettes a woman smokes, the greater the reduction in birth weight.
6. *Consistency of association.* The association has been shown in many countries among different cultures and in different geographical settings. In addition, the infants of smokers experience an accelerated growth rate during the first 6 months after delivery compared with infants of nonsmokers. Data from experiments in animals also have documented that exposure to tobacco smoke results in the delivery of offspring of low birth weight (Spradley, 1985).

All six criteria were used to assess the possible cause-and-effect relationship between maternal smoking and infant mortality in the summative report.

The web of causation. Disease and disability can be caused by one factor or multiple factors. MacMahon and Pugh (1970) developed a concept they termed *chains of causation.* Multiple minor events can lead to illness. Identification of these events might

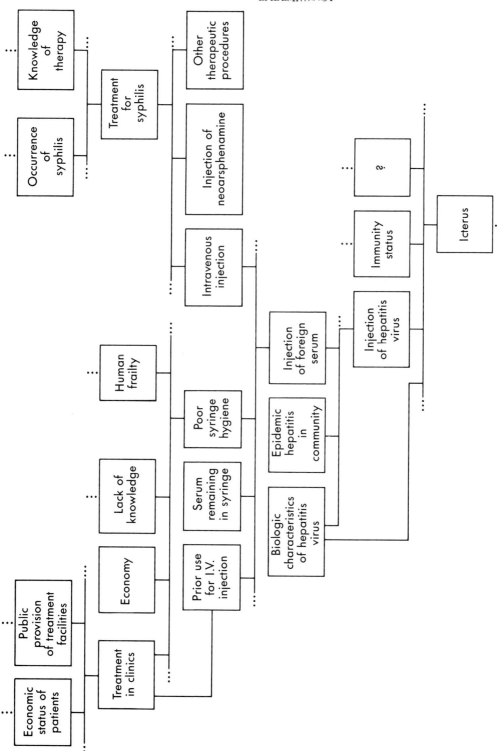

FIG. 7-2 The web of causation. *(From* Epidemiology: Principles and methods *by B. MacMahon and T. Pugh (1970), Boston: Little, Brown & Co. Reprinted by permission.)*

enable the health professional to break the chain and prevent death or disability. For example, Fig. 7-2 depicts the chain of events that could lead to icterus in a susceptible host. If the possible variables included every event that had ever affected the individual, they might show that a complex genealogy of prior events resulted in a web of causation.

In some instances a specific factor, which may be animate or inanimate, must be present to cause disease. Epidemiologists call this factor an *agent.* An agent does not cause disease unless (1) it connects with a susceptible host and (2) the host is susceptible to the agent when the contact is made.

The epidemiological triangle. The epidemiological triangle, used in some epidemiological studies, depicts three factors that must be present for an event to occur (Fig. 7-3): agent, host, and environment. A causative *agent* must be present for a disease to occur. The second factor is a susceptible *host,* a living species capable of being affected by the agent. The third factor, a conducive *environment,* is anything external to the specific agent or host that may cause transmission of the disease.

In Philadelphia in the summer of 1976 there were 24 deaths and more than 200 persons became seriously ill as a result of an outbreak of *Legionella pneumophila.* This unexplained epidemic affected participants of an American Legion convention who had stayed in the same hotel. The agent in this case was an airborne bacteria, and outbreaks such as this one have been traced to air-conditioning systems. Susceptible hosts frequently have depressed immunity. Fig. 7-4 shows the related factors that were collected by investigators. Elimination of one of the factors (host, agent, or environment) would have prevented the outbreak of Legionnaires' disease. If the men had not attended the convention, they would not have become ill. If the agent had not been present, illness would not have occurred. If the air conditioning system had not been operating, the disease would not have been transmitted.

The wheel model. Another model used to visualize this type of phenomenon is the wheel model of human-environmental interactions (Fig. 7-5). The hub of the wheel is the host, which has a unique genetic core. The surrounding environment is biological, social, or physical. The size of any of its components depends on the disease being studied. For a hereditary disease such as Tay-Sachs disease, the genetic core is prominent. In a disease such as AIDS the host's immune state and the social and biological environments are larger (Mausner, 1974).

Reservoirs of Infection

Reservoirs are defined as living organisms or inanimate objects (such as soil) that harbor an infectious agent (Mausner, 1974). Some reservoirs are specific to some infectious agents. Common cycles are described in Fig. 7-6.

Most viral and bacterial diseases are transmitted from one human being to another. Bovine tuberculosis, rabies, and brucellosis are known as zoonoses or infectious diseases transmissible from vertebrate animals to human beings.

Method of Transmission of Infection

Any mechanism whereby an infectious agent is spread through the environment to members of a population is called the method of transmission. It can be either direct or indirect. An example of direct transmission is the transfer of the AIDS virus through the body fluid of one person to that of another. By contrast, indirect transmission can be carried without human contact. For example, *Salmonella* organisms are carried by contaminated

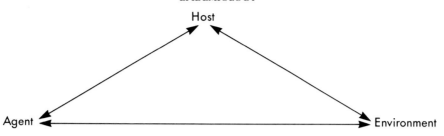

FIG. 7-3 The epidemiological triangle.

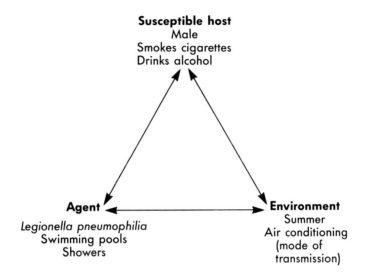

FIG. 7-4 The epidemiological triangle applied to the 1976 outbreak of Legionnaires' disease.

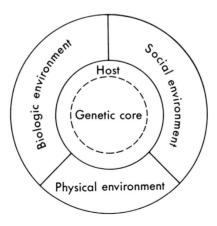

FIG. 7-5 The wheel model of human-environmental interactions. *From* Epidemiology *(2nd ed.) by J. Mausner (1974). Philadelphia, WB Saunders Co.*

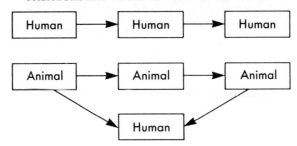

FIG. 7-6 Reservoirs of infection. A disease may be transmitted from one human being to another, or it may be transmitted from animals to human beings.

water, and *Rickettsia* organisms are carried by a tick. *L. pneumophilia* is carried by the air.

Immunity

The concept of resistance to infectious disease is related to the concept of immunity. Artificial active immunity to specific diseases can be acquired by immunizing susceptible individuals with live attenuated toxins. For example, childhood diseases such as mumps, rubella, diphtheria, and pertussis can be prevented through immunization. Temporary artificial passive immunity by gamma globulin administration can protect persons exposed to certain diseases, such as infectious hepatitis. Active natural immunity to some diseases is acquired by having the disease, such as varicella (chicken pox). For a limited period after birth, passive natural immunity to certain diseases the mother may have had is transferred to the child across the placental barrier during the last trimester of pregnancy. Herd immunity refers to the resistance of a group or population to the invasion or spread of an infectious agent.

TYPES OF DATA COLLECTION
Person

Although there are an almost infinite number of variables to characterize people, three demographical characteristics are basic: age, sex, and ethnic group (Mausner, 1974). Age is an important variable. Causes of mortality and morbidity frequently are selective and relative to age, both in individuals and in communities. For example, the incidence of cancer is higher in persons older than 50 years of age. The sex of the individual under study also is an important factor; for example, the mortality rate from ischemic heart disease is significantly higher in men than it is in women, whereas women are at a much greater risk for breast cancer. Ethnic factors are significant, particularly in screening for specific health problems among groups. Black persons, for instance, are at greater risk for sickle cell anemia; on the other hand, cystic fibrosis occurs primarily among the white population.

Place

Placing an event enables researchers to identify populations at risk in specific geographical areas and to target health care plans toward a specific problem. Diseases that depend on specific environmental conditions can be considered *place* diseases. For example, malaria usually is not found in cold, dry climates; it is vector-borne and depends on a hot moist climate to facilitate the mode of transmission.

Time

Recording events relative to time facilitates prediction of future health problems in a population and evaluation of the effectivensss of an implemented health plan. Events recorded on an annual basis can demonstrate short-term health trends in a population. Comparisons of events over time can highlight long-term changes or secular trends. For example, the National Center for Health Statistics released a statistical report in 1978 that described the mortality rates from 1900 to 1976. Of particular interest was the decrease in mortality from infectious diseases. Study of these rates could have a significant impact on health planning in the United States.

Rates

To predict trends and measure the occurrence and distribution of health in a population or community, epidemiological investigations frequently relate cases to a population base. Statements often consist of fractions or *rates,* where the *numerator* is the number of people with the factor being measured and where the *denominator* is the population in the area at the same time (Mausner, 1974):

$$\text{Rate} = \frac{\text{No. of cases or deaths in a time period}}{\text{Population at risk in a time period}}$$

The level of wellness in a population or community often can be assessed by obtaining statistical data about the number of deaths from specific causes (mortality) and the number of illnesses from specific causes (morbidity). For example, the infant mortality rate is a predictor of the general health of a community because the health of the mother, accessibility of prenatal care, other socioeconomic conditions, and the level of education all contribute to the mortality rate of infants in a community. The study described in Chapter 3 compared an infant mortality rate of 7.3 per 1000 live births in one neighborhood to an infant mortality rate of 25.4 per 1000 live births in another neighborhood. Further study confirmed the lack of wellness in the area with the higher infant mortality rate.

Relative Numbers

The infant mortality rate usually is calculated on a calendar-year basis. The number of deaths (deaths before 1 year of age) during the year is divided by the number of live births (infants born alive) during that year. To compare one population or community with another a constant or relative number is used, usually 1000:

$$\frac{\text{Infant mortality}}{\text{rate}} = \frac{\text{No. of deaths under 1 year of age}}{\text{No. of live births in same year}} \times 1000$$

Illness rates (morbidity) usually are calculated in terms of incidence and prevalence. The *incidence* of a disease refers to the number of *new* cases that occur in a selected population during a specified period of time, usually 1 year:

$$\text{Incidence rate} = \frac{\text{No. of new cases of specified illness}}{\text{Estimated midinterval population at risk}} \times 1000$$

The prevalence rate refers to the number of *new* and *old* cases in a population during a specified period of time, usually 1 year:

$$\text{Prevalence rate} = \frac{\text{No. of current old and new cases of specified illness}}{\text{Estimated midinterval population at risk}} \times 1000$$

The midyear population estimate is used because the population at risk cannot be determined accurately. It is possible, however, to place some parameters on the estimated population at risk. For example, when calculating the fertility rate in a population it is customary to include only women of usual childbearing age in the population risk:

$$\text{Fertility rates} = \frac{\text{No. of live births}}{\begin{array}{c}\text{No. of women}\\\text{aged 15 to 44 years midyear}\end{array}} \times 1000$$

In diseases that are age specific in terms of virulence and pathogenicity, it is possible to study an at-risk age group and set parameters on the population at risk to be studied. For example, the incidence of mortality from pertussis is rare after the child is 2 years of age, and it seldom is serious in older children. The mortality rate from this illness can therefore be estimated with the use of an age-specific formula such as the following:

$$\text{Age-specified death rate} = \frac{\text{No. of deaths from pertussis}}{\text{No. of children under age 2 in population}} \times 1000$$

Other common rates used as health indicators in a population follow:

$$\text{Birth rate} = \frac{\text{No. of live births}}{\text{Estimated midyear population}} \times 1000$$

$$\text{Maternal nortality rate} = \frac{\text{No. of deaths from puerperal causes}}{\text{No. of women giving birth}} \times 1000$$

$$\text{Neonatal mortality rate} = \frac{\text{No. of deaths of neonates under 28 days of age}}{\text{No. of live births}} \times 1000$$

Mortality in populations generally is compared by means of a larger constant (100,000) because of the large numbers of people:

$$\text{Crude death rate} = \frac{\text{No. of deaths during 1 year}}{\text{Average midyear population at risk}} \times 100,000$$

$$\text{Case-specific rate} = \frac{\text{No. of deaths from stated cause}}{\text{Population at risk midyear}} \times 100,000$$

Relative Risk

To determine if a relationship exists between a health condition and a suspected factor, it is necessary to compare its risk in populations *exposed* to the factor with populations *not exposed* to the factor.

$$\text{Relative risk} = \frac{\text{Incidence rate among those exposed}}{\text{Incidence rate among nonexposed}} \times 1000$$

For example, a comparison of the virtual absence of cervical carcinoma in nuns with its high incidence among prostitutes suggests that sexual activity probably is an important risk factor in the development of that disease (Gagnon, 1950).

Rates can be compared to illustrate risk factors by determining the ratio of one group to another, for example (Higgs & Gustafson, 1985, p. 40):

$$\frac{\text{Smoker lung cancer rate:}\quad 188/100,000}{\text{Nonsmoker lung cancer rate:}\quad 19/100,000} = \text{Ratio } 9.9:1$$

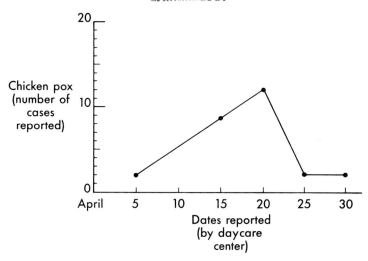

FIG. 7-7 A frequency distribution may be used to record the pattern of incidence of a disease over time.

Measures of Disease Frequency

Researchers can describe an event in terms of percentages and numbers to formulate a measure of disease frequency. Hypothetically, a day-care center reports three cases of chickenpox on April 5, eight cases on April 15, 12 on April 20, and three each on April 25 and April 30 (Fig. 7-7). It is possible to plot the pattern of the incidence of the disease and to draw conclusions and make predictions about the pattern of its occurrence. If for several years this pattern repeated itself every spring, then it is possible that chickenpox (varicella) is seasonal and endemic, which is in fact the case. A rate of frequency can be established if the number of cases is divided by the population at risk and multiplied by a relative number for example:

$$\frac{26 \text{ cases of chickenpox during April}}{52 \text{ children at risk during April}} \times 1000$$

The chickenpox rate in that day-care center is 500 per 1000 population. With the use of this calculation it is possible to compare the incidence of chickenpox in this population to the incidence of chickenpox in other populations. A summary of the tables used to calculate rates is found in the box on p. 152.

METHODS USED IN EPIDEMIOLOGICAL RESEARCH
Descriptive Surveys

Hypotheses or assumptions that evolve from collected data and surveys regarding the incidence and prevalence of disease or disability in populations logically can lead to further study. Variables identified as having some association with a selected event may suggest a possible causal relationship. For example, many studies have identified tobacco as a factor connected with lung cancer. A hypothesis could relate these descriptive surveys by stating simply that tobacco contributes to the development of lung cancer. Studies that examine the smoking habits of individuals within a population both retrospectively and prospectively then might prove or disprove the link of tobacco to lung cancer. A logical progression from large descriptive surveys to specific analytical types of research

COMMONLY USED FORMULAS

$$\text{Rate} = \frac{\text{No. of cases or deaths in a time period}}{\text{Population at risk in a time period}}$$

$$\text{Infant mortality rate} = \frac{\text{No. of deaths under 1 year of age}}{\text{No. of live births in same year}} \times 1000$$

$$\text{Incidence rate} = \frac{\text{No. of new caes of specified illness}}{\text{Estimated midinterval population at risk}} \times 1000$$

$$\text{Prevalence rate} = \frac{\text{No. of old and new cases of specified illness}}{\text{Estimated midinterval population at risk}} \times 1000$$

$$\text{Fertility rate} = \frac{\text{No. of live births}}{\text{No. of women aged 15-44 midyear}} \times 1000$$

$$\text{Age specified death rate} = \frac{\text{No. of deaths from pertussis}}{\text{No. of children under age 2 in population}} \times 1000$$

$$\text{Birth rate} = \frac{\text{No. of live births}}{\text{Estimated midyear population}} \times 1000$$

$$\text{Crude death rate} = \frac{\text{No. of deaths during 1 year}}{\text{Average midyear population at risk}} \times 100,000$$

$$\text{Maternal mortality rate} = \frac{\text{No. of deaths from puerperal causes}}{\text{No. of women giving birth}} \times 1000$$

$$\text{Neonatal mortality rate} = \frac{\text{No. of deaths of neonates under 28 days of age}}{\text{No. of live births}} \times 100,000$$

$$\text{Case-specific rate} = \frac{\text{No. of deaths from stated cause}}{\text{Population at risk midyear}} \times 100,000$$

$$\text{Relative risk} = \frac{\text{Incidence rate among those exposed}}{\text{Incidence rate among nonexposed}} \times 1000$$

proceeds through (1) descriptive survey (data collection and analysis), (2) formulation of hypothesis, (3) analytical study to test hypothesis; and (4) analysis of results.

Analytical Studies

If a descriptive survey identifies a possible causal relationship, a researcher can formulate a hypothesis and proceed to test it or can conduct some further analysis to determine its validity. Several types of analytical studies are discussed here.

Cross-sectional. An additional form of observational study is the cross-sectional study. Risk factors and disease for a population are recorded at one specific point in time. For example, a national health survey recorded the level of cholesterol in persons with coronary heart disease and individuals with no heart disease. A causal relationship was hypothesized because individuals with coronary heart disease had higher cholesterol readings than those who had no disease. This type of study may or may not lead to further analysis.

Case control. Another analytical study design is the case-control study. With the use of this approach a group of individuals having a particular disease are identified and compared with a second (control) group that does not have the disease. An attempt is made to determine a relationship, such as the frequency of exposure to some factor suspected of causing the disease. These studies may be retrospective (historical data) or prospective (data collected for a given period of time from a starting point).

Ecological. Analytical studies also may be carried out on an ecological level. Ecological studies compare aggregate data for entire populations; that is, the etiological factor for individuals is not established. For example, lung disease rates for the population of regions with heavy air pollution might be compared with the rates for populations of regions with low air pollution.

Experimental. If, as a result of a previous study, a specific factor is suspected of being causally related to a health problem common to a group of individuals, a study sample may be chosen from individuals exposed to the causal factor. The causal factor then is taken away from one study group and not from the other, and the two groups are compared over time. In another experimental approach, a group of individuals with a common health problem may be separated and treated differently for comparison purposes. For example, a consenting group of clients with AIDS agreed to participate in an experimental trial to test the drug zidovudine (formerly AZT). Some received the drug, and some received a placebo. The effects of the drug in controlling the progression of the disease then could be monitored. After a 6-month trial it became evident that the group receiving the drug had fewer symptoms than the group receiving the placebo. The effectiveness of zidovudine in slowing the progress of AIDS was established.

Analytical studies can indicate a cause-and-effect relationship, disprove it, or generate a hypothesis for further study.

APPLICATION OF EPIDEMIOLOGICAL CONCEPTS TO COMMUNITY HEALTH NURSING

The community health nurse can participate in the epidemiological process in a number of ways. First, a *case study* of an individual with a disease or disability can be conducted. That person's immediate environment, including the family, can be assessed, followed by an extended assessment of the community in which the individual is located. Other factors to consider are those that historically or presently affect that person's health. This is the simplest form of field activity.

Second, *field investigations* can be conducted by the nurse by careful recording of objective data. Information about variables that contribute to injuries, mental disorders, food poisonings, and other conditions can be collected in this way and inferences made as to causal relationships.

The *field survey,* which seeks to determine the frequency of a disease at a specified time or to examine total disease in an entire population, provides the nurse with an opportunity to contribute as a member of a team. Examples include national health surveys, tuberculin testing surveys, and chronic disease studies (Corrigan, 1961).

Applied epidemiology can assist the community health nurse to integrate the scientific method into practice. Most field investigations are team efforts conducted through health departments. However, increasing numbers of nurses are conducting individual research with the use of epidemiological methodology to determine the cause and effect of certain disease factors in individuals, families, and population groups.

SUMMARY

Community health nurses can use concepts of epidemiology to improve the health of their communities. By studying and understanding the patterns of disease, steps can be taken to prevent and slow the spread of disease in individuals, families, and community. Epidemiological concepts can be applied at the primary, secondary, or tertiary levels of prevention.

Several epidemiological models describe the cause-and-effect relationship between pathogens and disease. A disease can be caused by a single factor or by multiple factors; transmission may be either direct or indirect.

The use of epidemiological studies throughout history has shown a shift in types of disease prevalent in society. Although infectious disease was the cause of most illness and death early in the twentieth century, chronic illness and disability is more prevalent in today's society.

CHAPTER HIGHLIGHTS

- Epidemiology is a field of science concerned with various factors and conditions that determine the occurrence and distribution of health, disease, and defect and disability among groups of individuals.
- The science of epidemiology has evolved over a long period of time. John Gaunt was a pioneer in the field in seventeenth-century England, followed by William Farr in the nineteenth century.
- Concepts used in the field of epidemiology that might assist the nurse include the natural history of disease in human beings, levels of prevention, causality, the web of causation, the epidemiological triangle, the wheel model, reservoirs of infection, and immunity.
- Methods of collecting data used by epidemiologists include descriptive studies (person, place, and time), rates, relative numbers, relative risk, and frequency distributions.
- The process of epidemiological research includes analysis of data collected, formulation of hypothesis, an analytical study to test the hypothesis, and an analysis of the results. The results may lead to further study to determine cause-and-effect relationships.
- Community health nurses can apply epidemiological concepts to practice.

STUDY QUESTIONS

1. Define epidemiology.
2. Describe the components of the epidemiological triangle.
3. Discuss the epidemiological evidence concerning the causal relationship between maternal smoking and infant mortality reported by the U.S. Department of Health and Human Services, Education and Welfare in 1980.
4. Calculate the infant mortality rate in a community that recorded 25 infant deaths and 1275 live births during the same period.

REFERENCES

Adams, F. (1886). *The genuine works of Hippocrates* (translated from Greek). New York: William Ward.

Anderson, E. & McFarlane, J. (1988). *Community as client: Application of nursing process.* Philadelphia: Lippincott.

Berkow, R. (1982). *The Merck manual of diagnosis and therapy* (14th ed.). Rahway, NJ: Merck.

Cohen, I. (1984). Florence Nightingale. *Scientific American, 20(3),* 128, 133.

Corrigan, M. (1961). *Epidemiology in nursing.* Washington, DC: The Catholic University of America Press.

Friedman, G.D. (1950). *Primer of epidemiology* (2nd ed.). New York: McGraw-Hill.

Gagnon, F. (1950). *Contributions to the study of etiology and prevention of cancer of the cervix or uterus.* American Journal of Obstetrics and Gynecology, 60, 516.

Grant, M. (1975). *Handbook of community health* (2nd ed). Philadelphia: Lea & Febiger.

Higgs, Z., & Gustafson, D. (1985). *Community as a client: Assessment and diagnosis.* Philadelphia: Davis.

Kornfeld, H., Stawe, R., Lange, M., Reddy, M., & Greich, M. (1982). T. lymphocyte subpopulations in homosexual men. *The New England Journal of Medicine, 307(12),* 728-729.

Leavell, H.R., & Clark E.G. (1965). *Preventive medicine for the doctor in his community: An epidemiologic approach* (3rd ed.). New York: McGraw-Hill.

Lilienfeld, A., & Lilienfeld, D. (1980). *Foundations of epidemiology.* New York: Oxford University Press.

Mausner, J.S. (1974). *Epidemiology* (2nd ed). Philadelphia: Saunders.

MacMahon, B. & Pugh, T. (1970). *Epidemiology: Principles and methods.* Boston: Little, Brown & Co.

Peterman, T., Drotman, P., & Curran, J. (1985). *Epidemiology of acquired immunodeficiency syndrome (AIDS).* Epidemiologic Reviews, 7, 1-16.

Public Health Service. (1979). *Healthy people: The surgeon general's report on health promotion and disease prevention* (DHEW [PHS] Publication No. 79-5507). Washington, DC: U.S. Government Printing Office.

Rothman, K. (1986). *Modern epidemiology.* Boston: Little Brown & Co.

Smith, G. (1941). *Plague on us.* London: Oxford University Press.

Spradley, B.W. (1985). *Community health nursing concepts and practice* (2nd ed.). Boston: Little, Brown & Co.

Stanhope, M., & Lancaster, J. (1988). *Community health nursing.* St. Louis: Mosby.

U.S. Department of Health and Human Services, Public Health Service, National Institutes of Health. (1977). *The Framingham study: An epidemiological investigation of cardiovascular disease* (Section 32, Publication No. [NIH] 77-1247). Washington, DC: U.S. Government Printing Office.

U.S. Department of Health Education and Welfare, Public Health Service, Office on Smoking and Health. (1980). *The health consequences of smoking for women: A report of the surgeon general.* Washington, DC: U.S. Government Printing Office.

Valanis, B. (1986). *Epidemiology in nursing and health care.* Norwalk, CT: Appleton-Century-Crofts.

Quality Assurance in Community Health Nursing

JUNE A. SCHMELE

The nursing process is dynamic in that evaluation of outcomes either confirms goals or serves as a basis for formulation of new goals.

BETTY NEUMAN

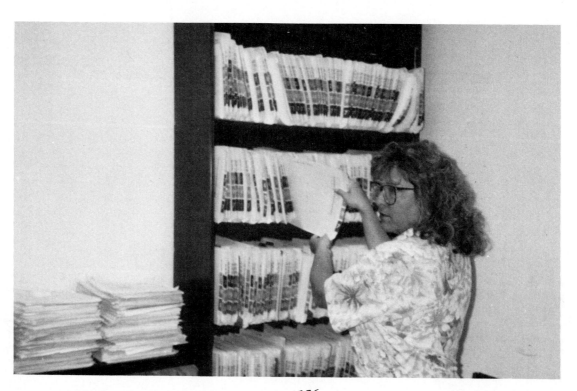

OBJECTIVES

At the conclusion of this chapter the student will be able to:
1. Define the key terms listed
2. Discuss the societal context that influences the quality of care
3. Identify selected models of quality assurance
4. Discuss selected methods of quality assurance
5. Define the steps of the quality assurance process of the American Nurses' Association
6. Use the quality assurance process of the American Nurses' Association in selected situations
7. Discuss selected programs that are related to quality assurance
8. Describe the role of the community health nurse in quality assurance
9. Relate the processes of quality assurance and research
10. Describe future health care trends and issues that will have an impact on quality assurance in the community

KEY TERMS

Accountability	Program evaluation
Accreditation	Quality
Certification	Quality assurance
Concurrent audit	Retrospective audit
Criteria	Risk management
Licensure	Standard
Outcome	Structure
Process	Utilization review

In the very broadest sense the definition of quality assurance (QA) includes all clinical and management functions that are directed toward the improvement of the delivery of desirable health care. In the strictest sense quality assurance is defined as a systematic planned approach directed toward the improvement of care. The common element in both these definitions is that the goal of QA is the improvement of health care. For the most part this chapter deals with this more specific approach to QA, as well as its application in the community by the nurse generalist. According to the American Nurses' Association (ANA, 1968a, p. 4):

> The community health nurse generalist, prepared in nursing at the baccalaureate level, provides care primarily to individuals, families, and groups in a wide range of primary care settings with an understanding of the values and concepts of population-based practice. The generalist participates in implementation of community-wide assessment and in the planning, implementation, and evaluation of health programs and services.

In this chapter an effort will be made to integrate the ANA position on community health nursing.

I wish to acknowledge Margo Wickersham, RN, BSN, for assistance in the preparation of this chapter and Mary Ann McClellan, RN, MN, PNP, for consultation in community health nursing.

Throughout the literature one does not find a consistent common use of words and ideas relevant to QA. Some of the major problems in the implementation of QA programs relate to semantic differences in key words and ideas. For the successful implementation of any QA program, it is essential that terms be made explicitly clear. This is not to imply the correctness or incorrectness of any particular usage but only to emphasize that there must be common usage within a specific agency. Common usage is essential for the establishment of a sound QA program. Therefore this chapter makes an effort to clarify definitions and ideas.

ENVIRONMENTAL CONTEXT
Historical

In a discussion of the historical perspectives of QA, most authors point out that Florence Nightingale herself is credited with some of the earliest and most significant contributions made during the mid-1800s. In her 1859 *Notes on Nursing* Nightingale published what is essentially a set of measures dealing with caring for the sick. Typical measures were such things as "to keep the air as pure as possible" and "to insure the cleanliness of all utensils and equipment used for and by the patient" (Nightingale, 1969, p. vi). Bull, in her succinct summary (1985) of the historical development of QA, credits Florence Nightingale with the use of outcome quality measures such as recovery and mortality rates. Nightingale is well known for recording statistics and collecting data concerning the sick for whom she cared. For example, during the Crimean War the mortality rate dropped from 32% to 2% within 6 months after the arrival of Nightingale and her nurses (Bull, 1985).

In England in 1908 the title of an article by Groves, "A Plea for Uniform Registration of Operation Results," illustrated a new direction in QA. Groves determined that there were variations in mortality rates after surgery and that there was a need to keep track of this information. Groves is credited with the development of a system of comparing hospital outcome data by following up on certain disease conditions to determine the outcomes of care (Bull, 1985).

In 1910 Abraham Flexner developed standards to survey the quality of medical schools. This survey led to the publication of the Flexner report, which revealed many inadequacies and resulted in the closure of many American medical schools (Sledin, 1984).

During this same period, nurse licensing laws were being passed throughout the country. By 1912 there were 33 states with nurse practice acts, as well as 38 states with state nurse associations (Christy, 1971).

Codman, a surgeon, is credited with developing the "End-Result Idea" in 1914. He proposed that patients be checked 1 year after surgery to determine the results of their surgery. He insisted on formal, published reports so that comparisons could be made. His work culminated in 1918 in the organization known as the American College of Surgeons' Hospital Standardized Program. This organization was the forerunner of the Joint Commission on the Accreditation of Hospitals (now the Joint Commission on Accreditation of Healthcare Organizations) (Codman, 1914).

In 1933 the classic work of Lee and Jones, *The Fundamentals of Good Medical Care,* was published. It is recognized for the development of key principles that defined good medical care. These principles were incorporated into the standards dealing with such areas as prevention of disease, coordination of holistic care, and the cooperative role of patients in their own care. These standards appear to be as relevant today as they were in the early 1930s.

In 1946 the legislation known as the Hill-Burton Act provided funding for the construction and expansion of hospitals in the United States (Shaffer, 1984). The standard of accessibility of care emerged with the passage of this act.

One of the events that had a major impact on QA was the development of the Joint Commission on the Accreditation of Hospitals, which was formed in 1951 for purposes of carrying out institutional accreditation and ultimately improving the quality of care. This accrediting body was formed under the joint sponsorship of the American College of Surgeons, the American College of Physicians, the American Medical Association, and the Canadian Medical Association. In 1959 Canada established its own accreditation system apart from the Joint Commission (Jonas & Rosenburg, 1986).

In 1961 the National League for Nursing (NLN) developed accreditation standards and criteria for home health agencies and community health services. The American Public Health Association (APHA) collaborated in the early development of this accreditation process. The current NLN accreditation requirements reflect the trend away from assessing structure (resources) and process (activities) toward the assessment of outcomes (results) (NLN, 1987).

Since the 1960s, Donabedian, a physician, has been one of the most respected and often quoted experts in the field of health care QA. His classic and often cited early publication, "Evaluating the Quality of Medical Care" (1966) continues to be a foundational work in the study of QA. Although his topic is medical care, the description and discussion of methods apply to other disciplines as well.

During the late 1960s nursing leadership in QA became increasingly evident. Phaneuf developed the nursing audit evaluation method, which focused on the functions of nursing as determined in the retrospective review of client records (Phaneuf, 1972). During the same period the Slater nursing competency scale, which focused on nurse performance, was developed and published (Wandelt & Stewart, 1975). Wandelt and Ager published the Quality Patient Care Scale (QUALPACS), which was a concurrent appraisal of patient care (Wandelt & Ager, 1970). Although these QA approaches were developed some time ago, they remain relevant today.

Since the mid-1960s the ANA has been committed to the development of standards of nursing practice (Chapter 1), which is reflected in various nursing practice specialties. During the 1970s the ANA model for QA was developed with Norma Lang's participation (ANA, 1975). During this decade Hegyvary and associates developed a quality monitoring method to investigate the relationship between the nursing process and patient outcomes. Their findings suggested that there was a need to study process as well as outcome in relationship to other variables (Haussman, Hegyvary, & Newman, 1976).

The state of the art in the 1980s was largely governed by accreditation requirements and/or legislation directed toward cost containment. The rapid rise in the number of home health agencies, as well as the demand for increasingly sophisticated levels of patient care, has resulted in an accompanying concern for quality. The concerns about quality or lack of quality in home care are well summarized in the landmark American Bar Association report to Congress entitled *The "Black Box" of Home Care* (1986). Meisenheimer's 1989 publication, *Quality Assurance for Home Care,* presents the current status of QA in home care (1989). Although there is a sparsity of literature devoted to the subject of QA in community health nursing, Flynn and Ray (1987) summarized the state of the art and suggest the importance of recognizing the interactive components of structure, process, outcome, and environment to measure quality. These authors refer to some of the best-known community health QA programs, such as those of the Colorado and Minnesota departments of health, the Visiting Nurse Association (VNA) of New Haven, Connecticut, the VNA of Omaha, Nebraska, and the Ramsey County Public Health Nursing

Service (Flynn & Ray, 1987). These programs are recognized as models for QA in the community setting. For example, the VNA of Omaha has developed a patient classification system that places a major emphasis on the systematic measurement of quality (Peters, 1988).

Societal Context

The major forces that influence the development of QA are found within the societal context. These influences have been felt even more strongly by health care providers within the last few years with the advent of drastic changes in the health care field. An adaptation of Bull's model (Fig. 8-1) shows the societal forces and the major relationships between them. New technology, consumer demands, government legislation, and methods of financing increasingly demand professional accountability. Some of these influences include implicit or explicit QA mechanisms, such as professional accountability measures and accreditation processes. Each of these social forces will be briefly described.

Finance. The rapid rise in health care costs over the past several years, as well as the continuation of this rise, continues to strongly influence the entire health care system (see Chapter 2). The response to rising health care costs by various groups, such as providers, consumers, and legislators, has been one of intense concern, which sometimes has resulted in preoccupation with cost almost to the exclusion of all else. It would seem that the major issue is one of balance between cost and quality. In 1986 an entire issue of the *Journal of Nursing Quality Assurance* was directed toward the integration of cost and quality. In this issue Beyers proposed that an agency should make a determination of the acceptable standards of care, which then would govern administrative policies and

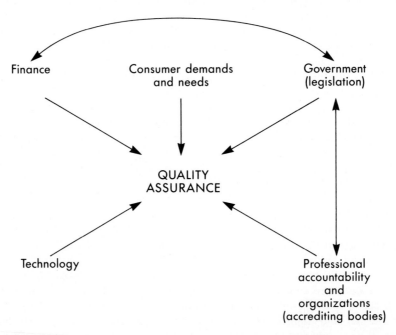

FIG. 8-1 Societal forces influencing quality assurance. *(From "Quality assurance: Its origins, transformation, and prospects" by M. Bull.* In Quality assurance: A complete guide to effective programs *by C. Meisenheimer, Ed., p. 2, 1985, Rockville, MD: Aspen. Copyright 1985 by Aspen Publishers. Adapted by permission.)*

practices. A program integrating both cost and quality could be established if the nursing care required to accomplish the selected standards of care could be made cost effective.

Profit versus nonprofit agencies. The movement toward proprietary (for profit) health care agencies is a concern for many. In a classic article, A. Relman, the editor of the *New England Journal of Medicine,* considered the rise in proprietary health care delivery service as the "single most important health care development of the day" (1980, p. 63). He described this increase in proprietary hospitals, nursing homes, home care, diagnostic laboratories, emergency services, hemodialysis, and many other services as the rise of a medical-industrial complex. The availability of this vast array of profit-making services gives rise to many issues about the quality of care.

Competition. One needs only to examine the availability of competing health care services in one's own community, especially in the urban sectors, to see the rapid rise in competition for the same health care dollar. This competition is not limited to profit versus nonprofit agencies but is rampant among providers of similar services in the same catchment area. There also is debate about whether the majority of health care dollars should be spent on the delivery of expensive acute lifesaving care or on less visible health promotion and disease-prevention activities. In addition, the increased dollars spent for sophisticated marketing of services may cause some to question whether these dollars leave fewer funds for the quality of services. There is little question, however, that the very survival of health care service agencies may be contingent on appropriate marketing. For example, the high level of competition in an oversupplied home care industry has resulted in the closing of many agencies. The ideal, of course, is an agency that is in a sound position to market a high level of quality services.

Consumer demands and needs. Major changes in illness patterns and demographical factors have a great impact on consumer demands and needs. For example, changing patterns of disease, more specifically the identification of the virus in acquired immunodeficiency syndrome (AIDS) in the early 1980s, present major community health concerns. The cost/quality issue in caring for this group of clients continues to create consumer and provider problems that strongly affect the delivery of community health services.

In addition, it is projected that the proportion of elderly persons in the population will continue to increase rapidly until the mid-1990s. According to the Health Care Financing Administration (HCFA), "By 2010 the post-war baby boom will reach retirement age and the rapid growth of the aged population will resume until the peak year birth cohort (about 1970) reaches 65 in 2035" (HFCA, 1987, pp. 14-15).

The rise in consumerism—that is, the public's increasing knowledge about health care matters—is greatly influencing the roles of consumers and providers in the health care system. This trend is reflected in the self-help sections in popular book stores and the rapidly expanding self-care health supply stores. The almost-overwhelming number of self-help books and materials, as well as the increasing media coverage of health matters, offers an insight into the level of sophistication of today's health care consumer. Whether the consumer is prepared and ready to make health care decisions remains an issue. There are those who believe that the majority of consumers are inadequately prepared and perhaps too ill-informed to make health care decisions. The contrasting, perhaps more popular, view is that consumers have not only a right but a responsibility to be actively heard in decisions relating to their health care. These opposing views affect approaches to quality assurance. For example, a community health agency that supports the value that consumers should participate actively in health care matters will review the quality of consumer participation. This review frequently is accomplished by determining the consumer's perceptions, expectations, and/or met and unmet needs. Those agencies that do not value consumer participation will review other aspects of quality instead.

Government. The single most influential economic factor to impinge on American health care and its delivery system has been the legislation leading to the prospective payment system (PPS) (see Chapter 2). In this system, hospitals are paid a predetermined fee for each medical diagnostic category. The PPS legislation also mandated quality review, which led to the creation of professional review organizations (PROs). Hospitals were required to contract with the PROs to determine the quality of care, appropriateness of admission, and appropriateness of care to clients who were "outliers" (persons having unusually extended hospital stays or costs) (Shaffer, 1984). Although original passage of the legislation was related to Medicare patients in hospitals, this system of payment has and will continue to be extended to other populations and third-party payers as well. The impact of the PPS has been felt throughout the health care system. Hospital providers now have a monetary incentive to avoid and/or shorten hospitalization whenever possible. This has resulted in a rapid increase in discharges and referrals to home health care agencies, with increasingly serious concerns about quality.

Professional accountability. The concept of accountability implies being *answerable* to *someone* for *something*. Professional nurses are answerable to the public (their clients) for the safe and professional practice of nursing. The mechanisms that direct the practice of nursing and those that govern accreditation procedures are in themselves basic QA approaches.

Licensure. The State Board Test Pool Examination provides the entrance to practice professional nursing (McCloskey, 1981, p. 336):

> Licensure is a legal process, meant to assure the public of a minimum level of competent care, and controlled in nursing by state laws called nurse practice acts. These laws are interpreted and enforced by an arm of government, the state boards of nursing. The State Board Test Pool Exam is the means by which the state boards (the public) evaluate the applicants' qualifications for practice.

Certification. Common use of the term *certification* implies the recognition of an individual's qualifications in a nursing specialty practice by attesting that the individual possesses the "predetermined skills and knowledge in a specialized field of study" (Jones, 1981, p. 353). Criteria are specified by the certifying agency. Qualifications may include "(a) graduation from an accredited or approved program, (b) acceptable performance on a qualifying examination or series of examinations, and/or (c) completion of a given amount of work experience" (ANA, 1975, p. 5). Although there are other organizations that certify nurses, the ANA is the major certifying agency. According to the ANA, in 1989 there were 61,016 ANA-certified nurses. Of these 2738 were certified in community health nursing. The three specialty areas with the highest number of certified nurses were psychiatry and mental health, medical-surgical, and nursing administration. The newest certification programs are in perinatal nursing and gerontological clinical specialist nursing practice (ANA, 1989). A comparison of the major differences in the processes of licensure and certification is shown in Table 8-1.

Accreditation. Accreditation is a voluntary system in which institutions or organizations are recognized as having met the predetermined standards of an accrediting body. Probably the best known example is the Joint Commission on Accreditation of Healthcare Organizations (Joint Commission). Although accreditation is voluntary, federal funding may be contingent upon it; thus in reality the voluntary nature of the process may be somewhat token. This frequently is the case with Joint Commission–accredited hospitals.

TABLE 8-1 Comparison of licensure and certification

	Licensure	Certification
Regulatory agency	Governmental	Nongovernmental
Action	Mandatory	Voluntary
Level of practice	Entry	Advanced
Area of practice	Basic	Specialized
Purpose	Protection of public	Career advancement
Testing process	State board test pool	Certifying examination

The Joint Commission also affects community health in the form of home health care accreditation. In 1988 the Joint Commission began a new accreditation process for all home health agencies. Before this the Joint Commission had accredited hospital-based home care as part of the hospital accreditation program (Joint Commission, 1988b).

Other accrediting bodies also affect community health. Recently the NLN accreditation process for community health agencies has been revised to reflect the changing health care environment. It now includes the major areas of (1) strategic planning and marketing (formerly community assessment), (2) organization and administration, (3) program, (4) staff, and (5) overall provider evaluation. The focus has moved from structure (resources) and process (activities) to the measurement of outcome (results) (NLN, 1987).

Accrediting agencies have a strong impact on the health care delivery system. Some accrediting bodies have been given the authority to ensure that a health care agency has met the Medicare requirements, thus certifying the agency for Medicare reimbursement. The agency then is recognized to have preferred status, for example, the pending federal legislation to designate either the Joint Commission or the NLN, or both, home health accrediting agencies.

Technology. The rapid advances in technology and the associated use of drugs, equipment, and supplies have strongly influenced the health care delivery system. The availability and use of these "high-tech" treatments often present two major issues: (1) who shall live and (2) who shall pay? According to Shepherd, "Trading off between quality and cost is a difficult decision, and whoever makes that decision—physicians, patients, supplier, payers, or the hospital—needs to evaluate all available data to make informed choice" (1988, p. 3). The use of high technology extends beyond the hospital to the home or community. For example, it is not unusual for home health care givers to plan and deliver care to clients who are dependent on ventilators.

QUALITY

The emphasis on excellence and quality is widespread throughout today's corporate sector. Although the health care arena in general has increasingly emphasized quality matters, the corporate sector appears ahead in many ways. Only recently have health care personnel begun to consider the successful corporate developments in quality management (Gillem, 1988). Some of the best-known corporate ideas that have implications for the future are presented here because of their applicability to the health care field.

Although the image of American industrial products still is one of lack of quality, Knowlton (1988) suggests that the increasing concern for quality is improving American products to the point where they are highly competitive in the world market. The attainment of quality depends on two major principles: (1) the top level administration must have a commitment to quality so that the organization will perceive it as an "ethic" and (2) it is imperative to know and respond to customers' changing needs and expectations (Knowlton, 1988). The applicability of these principles to health care is easily seen.

In the post–World War II era, Japan's recognition of its serious deficiencies in quality and productivity led to the use of a consultant from the United States. Edward Deming, a widely recognized international consultant, is given credit for the current success of Japanese industry. Deming's idea was that improved quality would lead to increased productivity and ultimately to a more highly competitive position in the market (Deming, 1982).

The work of Philip Crosby, who is considered a contemporary guru in the field of quality, might best be summarized in the following quotation (1979, p. 1):

> Quality is free. It's not a gift, but it is free. What costs money are the unquality things—all the actions that involve not doing jobs right the first time.

Crosby is a quality-improvement consultant who insists that the beginning of any quality improvement program must begin with top management.

Peters and Waterman (1982) are well known for their classic work, *In Search of Excellence,* in which 62 companies were studied in an effort to determine the attributes of innovative and excellent companies. Although these attributes are deceptively simple, they are based on principles of excellence that can be applied to health care:

1. It is essential that managers be committed to quality.
2. Consideration of the consumer's perceptions and needs is vital.
3. Employees who are encouraged to be autonomous in their areas of expertise will offer effective solutions to problems.
4. The simply structured organization with well-established missions and values offers an environment that contributes to the quality of the service.

Peter's second work, *A Passion for Excellence* (Peters & Austin, 1985), conveys the idea that it is leadership that makes the difference in the excellence of the organization. P￼h books deal with organizations in a relatively predictable and stable environment. With the advent of rapid societal changes, however, Peter's third book (1987) suggests that organizational survival depends on rapid adaptability, as well as a high level of consumer responsiveness. Even in the health care arena, there is no reason to think otherwise.

QUALITY ASSURANCE IN HEALTH CARE
Concept

Avedis Donabedian is considered one of the best-known experts and most prolific of writers on the subject of quality of health care. He states that "for purposes of assessment the definition of quality must be made precise and operative in the form of specific criteria and standards which respectively specify the desirable attributes and their quantitative measurements" (1978, p. 113). Donabedian is credited with the development of the assessment areas of (1) structure, (2) process, and (3) outcome. *Structure* refers to resources that are used to provide care. Examples of structure are staff (qualifications, number, and mix), space, equipment, and other physical facilities. *Process* means those activities that are performed in the delivery of care. Examples include the nursing process (assessing, planning, implementing, and evaluating) or other activities or tasks that may be performed, such as teaching, counseling, or physical care activities. *Outcome,* which refers to results, often is reflected in the measurement of health status in such areas as functional ability, mortality, mobility, and recidivism (Donabedian, 1978). During the past 20 years, in his numerous writings Donabedian seldom used the words *quality assurance*. Only recently he stated that "the term 'quality assurance,' though firmly ensconced is a misnomer; quality at best can be protected and enhanced but not assured" (1988, p. 184). It is important to recognize the soundness of Donabedian's idea that there really can be no *assurance* of quality. Perhaps a more fitting term would be *quality management*. However, because of its widespread use, the term *quality assurance* will continue to be used throughout this chapter.

Lang, a nurse well-known for her early work in QA, states that "the broadest meaning of quality assurance includes all activities aimed at defining and measuring multiple aspects of quality nursing care and those activities which are planned and implemented as a result of the measurement of care" (ANA and Sutherland Learning Associates, 1982, p. vii). Burgess and Ragland offer a succinct summary statement by indicating that QA "was adopted as the commonly accepted title for programs that assessed, evaluated and improved care given to consumers in the health care system" (1983, p. 442).

According to Donabedian, when the focus of QA is population groups, "the quality of care depends first on access to care, then on the performance of practitioners in case finding, diagnosis, and treatment, and then on the performance of patients and family members through participating in care. Equal access to and enjoyment of the highest level of quality in care may now become the community's ideal" (1988, p. 174).

Donabedian's view is in keeping with ANA statements that direct the practice of community health nursing toward the promotion of the public's health: "The programs, services, and institutions involved in public health emphasize promotion and maintenance of the population's health, the prevention and limitation of disease. Public health activities change with changing technology and social values, but the goals remain the same: to reduce the amount of disease, premature death, discomfort, and disability" (ANA, 1986a, p. 2).

Models of Quality Assurance

A variety of QA models provide the user with an operational framework for implementation. Three representative models are those of the Joint Commission, the program evaluation, and the ANA. Each of these models, as well as several others, have applicability to community health. The ANA model will be discussed in greatest depth because of its generic applicability at all levels of service in community health nursing (individual, family, group, and community).

Joint Commission model. The QA model developed by the Joint Commission can be used as a generic model for community settings. Because the Joint Commission has a home health accreditation program, this model is especially applicable to home health.

The Joint Commission QA model, which is considered a monitoring and evaluation model, provides a step-by-step approach (1988a, p. 6):

1. Assign responsibility.
2. Delineate scope of care.
3. Identify important aspects of care.
4. Identify indicators (criteria).
5. Establish thresholds for evaluation.
6. Collect and organize data.
7. Evaluate care.
8. Take action to solve identified problems.

9. Assess actions, and document improvement.
10. Communicate relevant information to organization-wide QA program.

The following example illustrates how the Joint Commission QA model was used in one specific home health setting. It is not a comprehensive application of the model for a total home health program; rather it includes only representative selected items for each step of the process:

1. *Assign responsibility.* The nursing supervisor for the home health agency was made accountable for the QA program by the agency's administrator. She then formed a QA committee of interested staff nurses.
2. *Delineate scope of care.* The scope of care, which was identified in the agency mission statement, included the delivery of nursing care in the home to medical-surgical, maternity, elderly, and pediatric clients.
3. *Identify important aspects of care.* The QA committee met to determine the diagnostic and therapeutic activities that most affect the quality of care. Based on Joint Commission recommendations (1988a) to include high-risk, high-volume, and problem-prone situations, the following important aspects of care were identified:
   • Ventilatory care, high risk
   • Mobility of the elderly, high volume
   • Catheter care, problem prone
4. *Identify indicators.* Mobility of the elderly population was identified as the aspect of care for study; thus the following indicators (criteria) were developed:
   • Assistive devices will be provided—structure.
   • A functional assessment will be performed by means of the mobility section of the tool (LaLonde, 1986)—process.
   • Clients' mobility will be maintained or improved as shown by functional status—outcome.
5. *Establish threshold for evaluation.* It was predetermined that if more than 20% of the clients had a decline in their mobility level, an in-depth evaluation would be performed.
6. *Collect and organize data.* An audit of the clinical records of 30 patients older than the age of 65 years was performed by QA committee members.
7. *Evaluate care.* Data from the records showed that 40% of the clients declined in mobility level. Because the threshold for evaluation was exceeded, nurses were involved in an in-depth problem-solving session to determine the cause of the diminished mobility. The cause was determined to be the lack of client involvement in the identification and ownership of the goal of maintenance of mobility.
8. *Take action to solve the identified problem.* The selected action recommended by the QA committee was for the nurse to include the patient, or significant other, in mutual goal setting related to mobility.
9. *Assess actions and document improvement.* The nurse made deliberate efforts to include clients in mutual goal setting. Data again were gathered after 3 months and showed that only 11% of the clients now had a decline in mobility level. Because this percentage was now below the threshold for evaluation, no further action was taken. It was then decided that mobility levels would again be monitored in 3 months.
10. *Communicate relevant information to organization-wide QA program.* A sum-

mary report of the findings was sent to the agency administrator in charge of the organization-wide QA program.

The impact of the Joint Commission approach to quality assurance is felt most strongly in the acute care setting. With the advent of Joint Commission accreditation of home health agencies, however, the use of the 10-step model will become more prevalent in community health agencies. It is noteworthy that the model can be considered a generic model and used in any setting to improve the quality of care.

Program evaluation model. A *program* is a systematically designed set of activities that are performed to bring about a certain outcome. *Evaluation* is a cognitive process of placing a value on something. It has been defined as "the attaching of meaning to data. This process is usually based on a series of measurements or a specific set of data that are interpreted on the basis of the professional judgment of the faculty or supervisor" (Litwack, Linc, & Bower, 1985, p. 5). Thus program evaluation can be considered a systematic collection of "information about how the program operates, about the effects it may be having and/or to answer other questions of interest" (Herman, Morris, & Fitz-Gibbon, 1987, p. 8). The three major purposes of program evaluation activities are planning programs, monitoring program implementation, and assessing program utility (Rossi & Freeman 1985; Sandefer, Freeman, & Rossi, 1986).

There are two major types of program evaluations. One is *formative* evaluation, which is the process of making judgments about each phase of the program in an ongoing manner from beginning to end. The other is *summative* evaluation, which is the judgment about whether a program outcome was met. An example of formative evaluation of a community-based support group for unwed mothers is the judgment about whether the group's ground rules are helpful to the group's interaction. Because formative evaluations take place throughout the entire process, there is an opportunity to make needed changes at any stage during the establishment of the program. An example of a summative evaluation is the determination, based on data, of whether the support group met its predetermined outcome objectives.

In some instances neither a formative nor a summative evaluation is indicated; rather a needs assessment related to the specific program area is needed (Herman, Morris, & Fitz-gibbon, 1987). This type of assessment would uncover problem areas or concerns that future programs may address. An example of this is a concern for bereaved parents of children. Thus an assessment would be made of the occurrence of bereavement within a defined geographical area, as well as the community resources available to that area. The needs assessment may indicate that the number of bereaved clients who are not already receiving bereavement counseling is minimal and thus a counseling group is not indicated at this time. It is vital therefore that the sponsor (one who requests the evaluation) clarify the purpose of the evaluation—assessment, formative, or summative, or any combination of these three. In addition, it is imperative for the sponsor and the evaluator to reach consensus about the precise purpose of the evaluation.

The boxes on pp. 168-169 present questions that can be asked during assessment, formative, and summative program evaluations. These questions, which differentiate between needs assessment and formative and summative evaluations, can be used as guidelines to evaluate specific community concerns and/or programs. After the evaluation is completed, it is appropriate to formulate a summary report that will meet the needs of the sponsor.

In summary, the major considerations of program evaluation are as follows:

1. Determine focus (target population and program).
2. Establish purpose.
3. Define appropriate type of evaluation (assessment, summative, or formative).
4. Formulate data-gathering questions.
5. Gather data.
6. Make a data-based judgment.
7. Formulate report.

The role of the staff nurse usually is that of a participant or data gatherer, or both, under the direction of the evaluator. In most cases the evaluator will be someone who has had special training or experience in evaluation.

Program evaluation can be relatively simple or highly sophisticated, depending on the complexity of the program and the purpose of the evaluation. The program evaluation model is particularly relevant for community health programs. For those nurses who become heavily involved with program evaluation, a variety of resources are available. The program evaluation kit consists of nine publications that offer a step-by-step evaluation approach (Herman, Morris, & Fitz-Gibbon, 1987). The nine books have varying degrees of sophistication and can be used singly or as a package. In addition, the classic evaluation research work of Rossi and Freeman (1985) is a well-known approach to evaluating social programs.

The following is an evaluation plan based on the program evaluation model:

1. *Determine focus.* The nutritional program for low-income mothers and children (women, infants, and children [WIC]) will be the focus of the evaluation.
2. *Establish purpose.* The evaluation will be performed to determine the outcome of the WIC program.
3. *Define appropriate type of evaluation.* A summative evaluation to determine the outcome of the program will be completed.
4. *Formulate data-gathering questions.* Guidelines for Summative Evaluation (p. 169) will be used.

GUIDELINES FOR NEEDS ASSESSMENT

Questions on the minds of the sponsors and audiences

What needs attention?
What should our program(s) try to accomplish?
Where are we failing?

Kinds of questions the evaluator might pose

What are the goals of the organization or community?
Is there agreement on the goals from all groups?
To what extent are these goals being met?
What do clients perceive they need? What problems are they experiencing?
What do staff perceive they need? What problems are they experiencing?
How effective is the organization in addressing problems perceived by clients?
What are the areas in which the organization is most seriously failing to achieve goals?
Where does it need to plan special programs or revise old programs?

From *Evaluator's handbook* (p. 16) by J. L. Herman, L. L. Morris, and C. T. Fitz-Gibbon, 1987, Newbury Park, CA: Sage. Copyright 1987 by The Regents of the University of California. Reprinted by permission of Sage Publications, Inc.

GUIDELINES FOR FORMATIVE EVALUATION

Questions on the minds of sponsors and audiences

How can the program be improved?

How can it become more efficient or effective?

Kinds of questions the evaluator might pose

What are the program's goals and objectives?

What are the program's most important characteristics—materials, staffing, activities, administrative arrangements?

How are the program activities supposed to lead to attainment of the objectives?

Are the program's important characteristics being implemented?

Are program components contributing to achievement of the objectives?

Which activities or combination best accomplish each objective?

What adjustments in the program might lead to better attainment of the objectives?

What adjustments in program management and support (staff development, incentives, etc.) are needed?

Is the program or some aspects of it better suited to certain types of participants?

What problems are there and how can they be solved?

What measures and designs could be recommended for use during summative evaluation of the program?

From *Evaluator's handbook* (p. 17) by J. L. Herman, L. L. Morris, and C. T. Fitz-Gibbon, 1987, Newbury Park CA: Sage. Copyright 1987 by The Regents of the University of California. Reprinted by permission of Sage Publications, Inc.

GUIDELINES FOR SUMMATIVE EVALUATION

Questions on the minds of sponsors and audiences

Is Program X worth continuing or expanding?

How effective is it?

What conclusions can be made about the effects of Program X on its various components?

What does Program X look like and accomplish?

Kinds of questions the evaluator might pose

What are the goals and objectives of Program X?

What are Program X's most important characteristics, activities, services, staffing, and administrative arrangements?

Why should these particular activities reach its goals?

Did the planned program occur?

Does the program lead to goal achievement?

What programs are available as alternatives to Program X?

How effective is Program X? In comparison with alternative programs?

Is the program differentially effective with particular types of participants and/or in particular locales?

How costly is the program?

From *Evaluator's handbook* (pp. 16-17) by J. L. Herman, L. L. Morris, and C. T. Fitz-Gibbon, 1987, Newbury Park CA: Sage. Copyright 1987 by The Regents of the University of California. Reprinted by permission of Sage Publications, Inc.

5. *Gather data.* The program head will respond to the questions, using available program reports and client visits.
6. *Make a data-based judgment.* The information obtained will show whether the program is meeting the outcomes objectives.
7. *Formulate report.* A brief summary report is prepared and directed to the administrative head.

American Nurses' Association model. The ANA, with the participation of Lang, has developed and popularized the ANA QA model. This model has widespread applicability in any health care setting and can be used as a guide to implement a QA program in the community. The model was developed in 1974 and modified and adapted to its present form as shown in Fig. 8-2. The model is a circular step-by-step approach that is ongoing and can be entered at any point. However, the identification of values is the logical entry point because values provide the basis for actions that follow. The ANA offers a succinct overview of the model (ANA & Sutherland, 1982, p. 112):

Once values have been identified, structure, process, and outcome criteria can be developed. These criteria are made operational by tools of measurement. When the measurements have been taken, the data can be interpreted. With these interpretations in mind, the nursing staff identifies possible courses of action and chooses the action most likely to resolve the problems. When the action has been taken, the model suggests that continued evaluation and review can

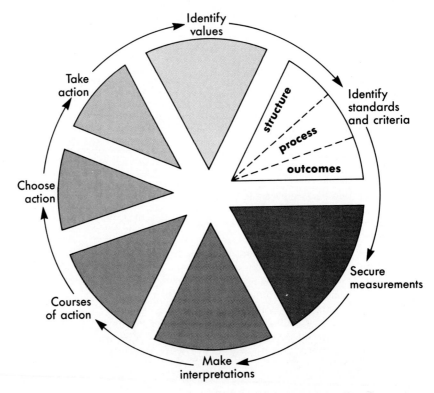

FIG. 8-2 The ANA model for QA in nursing. *(From* Workbook for nursing quality assurance committee members: Community health agencies *by ANA and Sutherland Learning Associates, 1982, Kansas City, MO: ANA. Copyright 1982 by the American Nurses' Association. Reprinted by permission.)*

determine the effectiveness of the action and the progress of health care delivery. Values and criteria are also reevaluated.

The ANA has developed various publications to assist the nurse in using the model. Probably the most well known still is applicable, *A Plan for Implementation of the Standards of Nursing Practice,* published in 1975. This publication presupposes the extremely important, but often neglected, basic idea that standards can be implemented through a QA program. A second, more recent set of three self-contained publications offers step-by-step workbooks to implement the QA model. These workbooks are guides that direct the various roles of persons involved with the QA program: staff nurses, QA committee members, and QA coordinators and administrators. One of the workbooks, written for committee members, is directed specifically to community health agencies (ANA & Sutherland, 1982).

The steps of the ANA model can be summarized as follows:

1. Identify values.
2. Identify structure, process, and outcome standards and criteria.
3. Secure measurements.
4. Make interpretations.
5. Identify courses of action.
6. Choose action.
7. Take action.
8. Reevaluate.

Resource material from the previously mentioned ANA publications will be used to examine the steps of the model in more detail.

Step one: identify values. The importance of reflecting on individual, professional, and agency values cannot be overestimated. Rapid changes in the environment surrounding the delivery of health care strongly influence and impinge on these values, which in turn influence the way health care is delivered, as well as the focus of QA activities. For example, in a given home health agency, if the nursing process is valued as the basis of professional nursing practice, the evaluation of this process will emerge as a vital part of the QA program. In contrast, if in another home health agency, the major value is placed on carrying out physician orders, this action will receive major attention. These values can be determined in various ways: by reading, discussing, and redefining the nursing philosophy or by identifying the key aspects of nursing practice within the agency. It is important to articulate the values that relate to the specific QA focus or program.

Step two: identify structure, process, and outcome standards and criteria

Focus. Initially the focus of the QA activity will need to be defined. The focus may be the staff, the clients, the organization, or all three, or any combination of the three. Another way to look at focusing is to decide which program is to be evaluated. For example, in an agency that values the importance of health promotion in schools, the focus might be on the clients and the staff in a school nursing program.

Standards and criteria. After the focus of the QA activity is decided, standards must be selected or formulated. Standards are defined as an "agreed upon level of practice" (ANA, 1986a, p. 1). (ANA community health nursing standards are discussed in Chapter 1.) These standards generally are broad statements that reflect values and the level of care. There are many sources of standards, such as professional organizations, accrediting bodies, and agency policies and procedures. The ANA practice standards are based on the nursing process and include various specialties that are applicable to community nurse practice. Examples of these community areas are community health, hospice, home care, and schools (1983, 1986a, 1986b, 1987).

Another source of community health standards is the *Model Standards: A Guide for Community Preventive Health Services,* which was developed in 1985 as a collaborative project of several community health organizations. These standards, which relate to the 1990 Objectives for the Nation, deal with various community programs. An example of a standard with a school health focus is that "the school health program will be planned and implemented to ensure that each student and staff person is provided with a healthful environment in which to work and study, together with needed preventive health services and health instruction (American Public Health Association [APHA] et al., 1985, p. 145). If standards that are already written are used, it is desirable to discuss them thoroughly and ratify them with staff members so that ownership of the standards will be established.

After identification of standards the criteria or items by which to measure the accomplishment of the standard will be formulated. To continue the school health example, the following criteria illustrate the three types of assessment measures:

- *Structure:* A problem-oriented health record (POHR) will be maintained for each student.
- *Process:* The nurse will document problem-related data, using the POHR format.
- *Outcome:* The student health record will serve as a comprehensive data source for educational health team conferences.

The number of standards and criteria developed and used depend on professional judgment based on identification of priority standards and criteria. Generally, the development of a small, manageable number of priority standards and criteria that will truly identify the key aspects of care is considered more effective than an all-inclusive agenda.

Step three: secure measurements. "The degree to which actual practice conforms to established criteria provides the information used for making judgments about the strengths and weaknesses of nursing practice" (ANA & Sutherland, 1982, p. 113). Thus the predetermined criteria are formulated into some type of a measuring tool that will be applicable to whatever data collection method is chosen, for example, audit, observation, and client self-report. The methods are discussed in greater detail later in this chapter. To develop the measuring tool an appropriate set of response types is assigned to each item. There is value in selecting simple, easily marked responses such as "yes/ no," "criterion met/criterion not met," or a scale from 1 to 5 that indicates "worst care to best care." A numerical value may be assigned to the total responses, which sums up the final evaluation of attainment of criteria. In addition, it is helpful to specify on the measuring tool what the source of the evidence will be. A simple example is shown in Fig. 8-3.

After the measuring tool is developed or selected, the data then would be gathered from a representative sample of the unit of study by means of the chosen method.

Step four: make interpretations. The degree to which the predetermined criteria are met is the basis for interpretation about the strengths and weaknesses of the program. The rate of compliance is compared against the expected level of criteria accomplishment. The expected level may be determined in various ways, such as a realistic improvement over previous rates. In some instances national norms are available such as the norms presented in the previously discussed model standards. For example, the compliance rate expressed according to these norms might be that "90% of the two-year-old population will have completed primary immunization for the officially designated vaccine-preventable diseases" (APHA et al., 1985, p. 41).

Instructions: Please indicate whether or not each criterion was met.

Criteria

1.   Structure: A Problem Oriented
        Health Record (POHR) will
        be maintained for each
        student. (See student   Not
        health file.)   _____ Met   _____ met

2.   Process: The nurse will
        document problem related
        data using the POHR
        format. (See student   Not
        health file.)   _____ Met   _____ met

3.   Outcome: The student health
        record will serve as a
        comprehensive data
        source for educational
        health team conferences.
        (Observe health team   Not
        conference.)   _____ Met   _____ met

FIG. 8-3   Example of section of measuring tool for school nursing QA audit.

Step five: courses of action. If the compliance level is above the norm or the expected level, there is great value in conveying positive feedback and reinforcement to those delivering the care. On the other hand, if the compliance level is below the expected level, it is essential to improve the situation. A necessary first step is to identify the cause of the deficiency. Then it is important to identify various solutions to the problem.

Step six: choose action. Usually various alternative courses of action are available to remedy a deficiency. Thus it is vital to weigh the pros and cons of each alternative while considering the environmental context and the availability of resources. In the event that more than one cause of the deficiency has been identified, actions may be needed to deal with each contributing cause. For example, the compliance level of immunizations was below the norm of 90% in the example in step four. Causes were identified as (1) parents' lack of awareness about the need for immunizations and (2) the lack of accessibility of the immunization clinic in a certain geographical area. Of the possible solutions an intensive media campaign to raise the awareness level of the clients was chosen, and well-publicized immunization clinics were set up in a shopping center on two consecutive weekends.

Step seven: take action. It is important to firmly establish accountability for the action to be taken. In other words, it is essential to answer the questions of *who* will do *what* by *when?* This step then concludes with the actual implementation of the proposed course(s) of action.

Step eight: reevaluate. The final step of the QA process involves an evaluation of the results of the action. This reassessment is accomplished in the same way as the original assessment and begins the QA cycle again. Careful interpretation is essential to determine whether the course of action improved the deficiency. If the deficiency was remedied, positive reinforcement is offered to those who participated and the decision is made about when to again evaluate this aspect of care. If the deficiency was not remedied, the problem-solving process is repeated.

Application. The following example applies the ANA QA process to a school nurse program. The example is not intended to be complete; only selected items for each step are included for illustrative purposes. Assume that a school nurse task force with an administrative representative has been designated to develop the QA program.

Step one: identify values. On the basis of the ANA standards for school nursing practice the task force identified the key value — that the main purpose of the school nurse program is "to enhance the educational process by the modification or removal of health related barriers to learning and by promotion of an optimal level of wellness" (ANA, 1983, p. 1).

Step two: identify standards and criteria. Various sets of standards, policies, and procedures were reviewed in preparation for the development of standards and criteria. A standard with accompanying criteria was established by the task force for structure, process, and outcome:

- *Standard:* A component of the school health program will be directed toward the prevention of disease.
- *Structure criterion:* An updated immunization record will be maintained for each student.
- *Process criterion:* The nurse will assess the immunization status of students.
- *Outcome criterion:* 100% of the students will have received mandatory immunizations before attending school.

Step three: secure measurements. The method chosen to measure the standards was a record audit. The rating response selected for each criterion was "met/not met." A simple tool was developed by means of the format shown in Fig. 8-3.

Steps four, five, and six: make interpretations, identify courses of action, and choose action. The data gathered from the school files revealed that (1) immunization records were maintained for 100% of the students, (2) the nurse assessed the immunization status of each first grader during the enrollment process, and (3) 90% of the students had received their required immunizations. Data was interpreted as showing that there were no problems in the area of criteria 1 and 2, and positive reinforcement was given to school nurses for the fulfillment of these criteria. However, it was noted that there was a deficiency in the lack of accomplishment of the outcome criteria related to mandatory immunizations (criterion 3). A problem-solving session of the task group explored several possible reasons: parents had not been informed of the necessity of immunizations, immunization records had not been retained by parents, parents were not aware of readily available immunization clinics, and parents had misinformation about the cost of the immunization. It was determined that the cause of the problem was lack of parent accountability for immunization of their children. The short-term solution decided upon was to obtain the vaccines from the health department, secure permission from the parents, and immunize the children on the first day of school. The long-term plan was to prepare a parent information packet dealing with the necessity of the mandatory immunizations. Evidence of immunization was required before any child could be enrolled in the first grade.

Step seven: take action. The school nurse, who carried out both the short- and long-term plan as described in *step 6,* updated the immunization records accordingly. Plans were made to reaudit the immunization criteria on an annual basis thereafter.

Note that the preceding example consisted only of selected aspects of the program. If the entire program were to be evaluated, a similar process would be used for prioritized key aspects of all structure, process, and outcome standards of the school nursing program.

After identifying the key aspects, the task force might then prioritize them according to importance. For example, during the first year, the task force may decide to emphasize the elements of the nursing process (assessment, planning, implementation, and evaluation) and selected outcomes such as immunizations, school attendance, dental health, first aid, and needs of the handicapped. It is considered more effective to evaluate a small number of the high-priority standards and criteria rather than to attempt an all-encompassing evaluation. The ability to prioritize according to the program values is vital to effective completion of the QA process.

QUALITY ASSURANCE METHODS

There are various ways to accomplish quality assessment with a variety of data sources and methods of gathering data. The same criteria can be used or modified for the various data-gathering methods. Some of the most common methods applicable to community health are discussed briefly here.

Audit

Audit is defined as "a review of clinical records used to determine the presence or absence of predetermined criteria. A retrospective audit deals with the clinical record after the discharge from the service, while a concurrent audit is accomplished while the the client or patient is still receiving services" (Schmele, 1989a, p. 73). It is important to recognize that audit is only one of several QA methods; it is, however, one of the most frequently used methods when the individual is the unit of service, such as in the instance of home health care. The audit method receives a great deal of emphasis from evaluators, especially third-party payers, because the quality of care is considered to be reflected in the documentation. Reimbursement for nursing services such as home health is contingent on the documentation that demonstrates the client's specific need of skilled nursing services. Some federally mandated QA processes for home health call for periodic audit of the clinical record. According to two authors, "Examination of the documentation of care in clinical records and minutes of patient care conferences should provide the surveyor with information to measure the agency's adherence to its stated standards in acceptance, continuance of care, and discharge of patients" (Balaka & Smith, 1986, p. 19).

It is likely that the audit method will continue to be widely used inasmuch as it is a part of accreditation and Medicare certification requirements. This is evidenced in the Joint Commission home care standard: "An accurate home care record is maintained to document the home care or service provided to each patient/client" (1988a, p. 15). In addition, the clinical record is a practical source of relatively accessible data that ordinarily can be obtained without a great expenditure of time and money.

Direct Observation

Direct observation is the watching or viewing of the client-nurse interaction, usually by a nonparticipant observer. This method can be used for various levels of service such as that for individuals, families, or groups. Most frequently the observation method involves visual inspection of the process aspect of care. An advantage of the method is that the actual giving of care is observed. A disadvantage is the probability that the presence of an additional person may affect the nurse-client relationship in various ways, such as changing the nurse's behaviors and/or the client's response. A second disadvantage of the method is the additional resource expenditure of the time and cost of the presence of an additional professional person during the care.

Peer Review

Peer review is defined as a QA method in which "a professional of equal standing reviews the quality of care" (Schmele, 1989a, p. 73). An example of peer review is the use of the QA process by nurses who are caring for clients with AIDS as a group; they would define standards and criteria and then use the criteria to evaluate each other's practice. An advantage of peer review is that clinical nurses who have the greatest expertise develop the standards and criteria rather than nurse managers or administrators who may lack clinical expertise. There also is value in using a participative approach to help establish ownership of the QA process and the subsequent investment in the QA program.

Supervisory Evaluation

In supervisory evaluation the performance of the nurse is reviewed by the employee's superior. Performance appraisal, sometimes called employee evaluation, commonly is a management function. In terms of the broad definition of QA, however, supervisory evaluations are directed toward the improvement of practice. Thus it is important that the criteria used in performance evaluations reflect nursing practice standards and criteria.

Self-Evaluation

Sometimes, in addition to supervisory evaluation, individuals may be asked to evaluate their own performances. For example, Knox has developed a system of self-appraisal and goal setting for community health nurses (1985). Her system, which is based on the nursing process, emphasizes nurses' accountability for their own professional performances. This is accomplished by comparing one's own behavior with predetermined criteria of the expected practice behaviors. When combined with goal setting, self-appraisal provides direction to professional development and helps measure progress toward performance goals.

Client Satisfaction

With the rise in consumerism and competition, there is growing interest in assessing the client's level of satisfaction with the care received. This usually is achieved through a survey in which clients are asked to respond to a number of criteria about their care. Although recent literature indicates a lack of consensus about the precise role of consumer satisfaction as a measure of quality, it substantiates patient satisfaction as an essential part of the evaluation of quality of care (Donabedian, 1987; Flynn & Ray, 1987; Schroeder, 1988).

One of the drawbacks of client satisfaction surveys is the likelihood of biased responses. That is, the clients may tell the providers what they think providers want to hear. With the increasing knowledge and sophistication of consumers, client expectations may become more openly expressed in the future. In addition, in the future clients themselves may have an active role on the health care team in determining what the quality of care should be.

Tracers

The tracer method (Kessner, Kalk, & Singer, 1973) requires the selection of a set of specified health problems in a given population. For example, in a given community the selected tracer was the diagnosis of AIDS. "By evaluation of the diagnostic, therapeutic, and follow-up processes of the set of tracers and the outcome of treatment, it is possible to assess the quality of routine care provided in a health care system" (p. 189).

Trajectory

The trajectory method of assessment begins with a "cohort of persons who share a distinguishing characteristic, such as a diagnosis, a laboratory finding, or a set of signs and symptoms. It then follows the path of this company of people through the health care system, noting what happens at important junctures along the way, and what outcomes are achieved by the end of the journey" (Donabedian, 1985, p. 311). An example of this method in the community is the follow-up of prenatal care throughout the pregnancies of a group of women below the poverty level. The final step would be to look at the outcome of the care provided.

Staging

Staging is defined as "the measurement of an adverse outcome and the investigation of its antecedents" (Donabedian, 1985, p. 311). For example, if a client's disease process such as tuberculosis had progressed to an extreme stage, it may indicate that care was inaccessible. This of course would require further retrospective probing into the situation and follow-up problem solving.

Criteria Mapping

Criteria mapping, also known as decision trees or flow diagrams, is a branching framework that is used for discussion-making points to specify a strategy of care (Donabedian, 1985; Wilbert, 1985). The most well-known use of criteria mapping is seen in the process of case management. A case management plan and critical path are used to "map, tract, evaluate, and adjust the patient's course and achievement of outcome" (Zander, 1988, p. 23).

Sentinel

The sentinel approach involves the monitoring of factors that may result in disease, disability, or complications (Donabedian, 1985). An example of this approach is the monitoring of incidences and prevalence of influenza before and after establishment of a comprehensive care program in the community.

RELATED PROGRAMS

The major focus of QA programs is clinical care, whereas risk management and utilization review are administrative programs that relate closely to QA (Gould & Ruane, 1988). An overview of these two programs follows.

Risk Management

Risk management can be defined as a program that is developed for the purpose of eliminating or controlling health care situations that have the potential to injure, endanger, or create risk to clients. The philosophical intent of such a program would be to "do the client no harm," that is, to administer safe care to whichever clients, groups, or populations are being served.

Risk management activities are directed toward the identification, analysis, and evaluation of situations to prevent injury and subsequent financial loss (Culp, Goemaere, & Miller, 1985). This focus contrasts with the goal of QA, which is to improve care; combined, these approaches facilitate problem solving and improved care. For example, all blood donors are screened for human immunodeficiency virus (HIV) before their blood is accepted. This activity is directed toward problem solving by eliminating a possible source of HIV transmission. In addition to protecting transfusion recipients, this procedure provides an opportunity for follow-up assessment and treatment of those persons who show HIV positivity during the screening process.

Within recent years the development of risk management programs has received much attention, especially in the acute care setting. This concern is related to changes that have occurred in the health care environment. Some of the major factors leading to the development of organized risk management programs are the complexity of the health care system, rising costs of health care, increasing litigations, treatments that require the use of high technology, and increased consumer awareness and sophistication. Although the development of risk management programs has occurred mostly in hospitals, it is anticipated that this movement will spread to community agencies as well. Certainly, the philosophy of risk management is already inherent in the community health practice of disease prevention in high-risk groups, for example, the licensure requirements and regulations to ensure safe health practices in day-care centers.

Utilization Review

Utilization review (UR) activities are directed toward the monitoring of health care services for appropriateness. For example, UR programs are developed to control costs through cost-effective use of services. "By providing explicit criteria for admission to the agency, continuation of services, and for discharge, utilization review can contribute significantly to providing only appropriate services as well as to preserving the agency" (Meisenheimer, 1989, pp. 35-38). Federally funded home health agencies that participate in Medicare/Medicaid programs are required to perform a clinical record audit to comply with UR guidelines. According to Meisenheimer, such aspects of care are the appropriateness of admissions and discharge and the use of personnel services. Although the goal of UR is to provide cost-efficient services, there is a need for integration and coordination of UR activities that have concerns in common with QA. For example, a home health UR audit shows that clients with indwelling urinary catheters are requiring prolonged home health coverage because of a high rate of urinary tract infections. This information is valuable to the nurse manager because it raises a red flag that the care of these particular clients needs to be assessed and followed closely. A problem-solving approach may lead to interventions that are directed toward earlier removal of the catheter.

QUALITY ASSURANCE ROLES

Every professional nurse who practices in the community is accountable for both personal nursing practice and maintenance of standards of practice. The ANA's standards that govern community health nursing practice apply to all community health nurses (see Chapter 1). The ANA rationale and criteria for the standard on QA and professional development are presented in the box on p. 179, which outlines QA role expectations for every community health nurse.

In addition, there are various ways in which nurses can actively participate in QA program activities such as problem solving, data collection, development of standards and criteria, interpreting results of QA studies, and implementing corrective action. Some activities are performed on an individual basis and others as peer-group activities. Additional QA roles that community nurses can assume depend on their competence, education, experience, and interest.

In some instances nurses may have opportunities to become QA committee members. Committee membership and responsibility usually are designated by an administrative head. The makeup of the committee may vary from a peer group to a multidisciplinary or interdisciplinary group. Committee functions also may vary from total accountability for a QA program to a specific assignment such as evaluating a particular program. In

---

THE AMERICAN NURSES' ASSOCIATION STANDARD FOR QUALITY ASSURANCE
Standard VII. Quality Assurance and Professional Development
The nurse participates in peer review and other means of evaluation to assure quality of nursing practice. The nurse assumes responsibility for professional development and contributes to the professional growth of others.

Rationale
Scientific, cultural, social, and political changes in society require a commitment from the nurse to the continuing pursuit of knowledge to enhance professional growth. Continuing education and evaluation of nursing practice by peer review and other methods of quality assurance are ways to ensure excellence.

Structure criteria
1. A mechanism for peer review is provided within the practice setting.
2. Nurses are represented on quality assurance teams that evaluate health care outcomes.
3. Policies exist within the practice setting that provide opportunities for continuing education.
4. Opportunities are provided for participation in professional organization activities.
5. Opportunities for self-evaluation and evaluation by communities, families, and individuals are provided in the practice setting.

Process criteria
The nurse:
1. Initiates and participates in the peer review process.
2. Participates in professional development programs, such as in-service sessions, conventions, and formal academic study, to increase knowledge and skills.
3. Assists others in identifying areas of educational needs, and communicates new knowledge to others.
4. Incorporates appropriate changes in his or her own practice suggested by self-evaluation, clients' evaluations, peer review, and professional development activities.
5. Demonstrates professional responsibility by participation in appropriate professional organizations.

Outcome criteria
The nurse:
1. Meets continuing education requirements for relicensure and recertification as appropriate.
2. Incorporates new information and methods into practice.
3. Participates in self-evaluation, the peer review process, and professional development programs.
4. Participates in professional and community organizations.

From *Standards of community health nursing practice* (pp. 13-14), by the American Nurses' Association, 1986, Kansas City, MO: Author. Copyright 1986 by the ANA. Reprinted by permission.

agencies in which a QA coordinator position is in place, that coordinator usually chairs and/or facilitates the work of the committee. In agencies without a QA coordinator position, a committee member usually is designated as chairperson. Ideally, the chairperson of the QA committee is a community nurse specialist with a master's degree or a nurse with a baccalaureate degree who has had additional education and experience in quality management. It is vital that nurses who perform key QA functions and activities have a strong interest in and enthusiasm for QA.

RESEARCH AND QUALITY ASSURANCE

Although the processes of QA and research have certain similarities, such as data gathering and analysis, their purposes are different. The purpose of QA is to improve care, whereas the purpose of research is to generate knowledge. An additional difference is that the sample for QA, as well as the results, usually are agency specific. In contrast, the sample for research generally is obtained from a larger population, which allows the researcher to generalize results.

Although the research process and the QA process are different, it is important to note that the research process frequently is used in studies that relate either explicitly or implicitly to the quality of care. Frequently, research questions relate to structure, process, or outcome variables. Another research area currently receiving attention is the development and testing of valid and reliable instruments to measure the quality of care. I have used the ANA *Standards of Community Health Nursing Practice* (1986a) (see Chapter 1) as a framework for developing and testing instruments to measure the quality of care for a nursing process perspective (Schmele, 1985). Later work focused on the testing and comparison of instruments in home health (Hough & Schmele, 1987; Schmele, 1988 and 1989b).

A current research emphasis is on outcome of care. An example of this type of research is the work of LaLonde (1986), who developed, tested, and refined outcome measures of quality in home health in the following areas: general symptom distress, discharge status, taking prescribed medications, care-giver strain, and functional status. Rinke and Wilson (1988), under the auspices of the NLN, published an anthology that contains selected approaches to the use of outcome measures in home health, and Waltz and Strickland (1988) are the authors of two volumes of research findings related to nursing outcomes. Several of these studies apply either explicitly or implicitly to community health nursing.

An even greater emphasis on research related to quality can be anticipated. Two vitally important research questions as yet remain unanswered: (1) What is the relationship among structure, process, and outcome? (2) What is the relationship between cost and quality? Research in quality measurement in community health nursing holds many challenging opportunities for the future.

THE FUTURE OF QUALITY ASSURANCE

There is little doubt that the rapid changes in the health care system will continue and may even accelerate. The precise direction of these changes, which is yet to be decided, is likely to have profound effects on community health nursing. These changes continue to be a response of the health care system to the impact of such issues as the rapid rise in health care expenditures, the advent of expanding and more sophisticated technology, increasing consumer knowledge, a rapidly aging sector of society, and the AIDS epidemic. Many unanswered questions remain: "Who shall have access?" "Who shall pay?" "What shall be the level of care?" There is increasing widespread concern about the cost-versus-quality issue. In many instances causes for concern coincide with challenging opportunities for improvement and change. The following nonprioritized list presents some of the most pertinent community health issues and concerns that require creative problem-solving responses:

- Continuing debate over cost expenditures for acute care, which requires high technology versus disease prevention and health promotion activities
- Increasing problems of lack of access to health care (currently approximately 37 million persons in the United States are without health care coverage)
- A large segment of the homeless who are increasingly prone to illness
- The high percentage of elderly persons in the population
- Increasing number of persons with AIDS
- Home care involving increasing numbers of acutely ill persons and treatments that require the use of high technology
- Heavy financial, physical, and emotional burdens on family care givers in the home
- The likelihood of prospective payment reimbursement in settings other than acute care
- Increasing complexity of health care problems, with need for interdisciplinary collaboration and case management approaches
- Increasing amounts of data, with need for computerized systems of information management
- High level of competition and marketing of health care services and products
- Continuation of public interest and involvement in self-care and wellness activities
- Increasing consumer and governmental roles in health care
- Growing emphasis on quality of care
- Increasing emphasis on researchable questions related to quality of care

The community health nurse is in a position to take a leadership role in planning the health care system of the future. This system, which may bear only minimal resemblance to the present system, will have many opportunities for client advocacy as well as quality management of care.

SUMMARY

Quality assurance is that systematic process by which client care or service is measured against predetermined standards and criteria, followed by appropriate remedial action. The single goal of QA programs and activities is to improve the quality of care.

The community health nurse has the opportunity and responsibility to be actively involved with quality assurance, whether in the role of a professional nurse accountable for his or her own practice or in the more formal role as part of a QA team. It is clear that in the future, community health nurses will have even greater opportunities and more responsibility to be a part of programs that are directed toward the improvement of the quality of care.

CHAPTER HIGHLIGHTS

- Quality assurance is a systematic, planned approach to improve the quality of client care.
- The development of the Joint Commission on the Accreditation of Hospitals in 1951 had a major impact on the development of QA programs.
- The rapid increase in health care costs over the past several years, increased competition

for health care clients, increased consumer demand for quality services, and the institution of prospective payment systems all increased the need for QA programs.

- Licensure is a legal process designed to assure the public that an individual or institution has met minimum requirements. Certification is a voluntary process designed to indicate that an individual has reached a specified level of expertise in a given area of practice.
- The Joint Commission model of QA is a monitoring and evaluation model that uses a step-by-step approach.
- The program evaluation model may be used to plan programs, monitor program implementation, and assess program utility.
- The ANA model of QA is a cyclical model that includes the steps of identifying values, identifying standards and criteria, securing measurements, making interpretations, identifying courses of action, choosing a specific action, and taking action.
- Methods that may be used within the QA cycle include audit, observation, peer review, patient satisfaction surveys, supervisory evaluations, and self-evaluations. Other more complex and less commonly used methods are termed criteria mapping, staging, sentinel, tracers, and trajectory.
- Risk management and utilization are two programs related to QA programs.
- All professional nurses are held accountable for their own nursing practice. Therefore all nurses must be familiar with the principles of quality assurance.
- The research process frequently is used in studies that relate to the quality of care. A current research emphasis is on outcome of care.
- Quality assurance will become even more important in the future as rapid changes continue to take place within the health care system.

STUDY QUESTIONS

1. How have changes in the health care system affected the development of QA programs?
2. Compare and contrast three models of QA with regard to their applicability to community health nursing.
3. Select a community health setting or agency to which you have recently been assigned. How would you apply the ANA QA process to that setting or agency?
4. How are risk management and utilization review similar to QA? How are they different?

REFERENCES

American Bar Association. (1986). *The "black box" of home care.* (A report presented by the Chairman of the Search Committee of Aging, House of Representatives, Ninety-Ninth Congress, Second Session). Washington, DC: U. S. Government Printing Office.

American Nurses' Association. (1975). *A plan for implementation of the standards of nursing practice.* Kansas City, MO: Author.

American Nurses' Association. (1983). *Standards of school nursing practice* (Publication No. NP-66). Kansas City, MO: Author.

American Nurses' Association. (1986a). *Standards of community health nursing practice* (Publication No. CH-2). Kansas City, MO: Author.

American Nurses' Association. (1986b). *Standards of home health nursing practice* (Publication No. CH-14). Kansas City, MO: Author.

American Nurses' Association. (1987). *Standards and scope of hospice nursing practice* (Publication No. CH-16). Kansas City, MO: Author.

American Nurses' Association. (1989). 61,016 certified by ANA in 19 practice areas. *American Nurse, 21*(3), 33.

American Nurses' Association and Sutherland Learning Associates. (1982). *Workbook for nursing quality assurance committee members: Community health agencies.* Kansas City, MO: Author.

American Public Health Association, Association of State and Territorial Health Officials, National Association of County Health Officials. U. S. Conference of Local Health Officers, and Department of Health and Human Services, Public Health Service Centers for Disease Control. (1985). *Model standards: A guide for community preventive health sources* (2nd ed.). Washington D.C.

Balaha, A. J., & Smith, A. S. (1986). Medicare standards for home health agencies: A basic approach. *Caring, 5*(8), 18-20.

Beyers, M. (1986). Cost and quality: Balancing the issues through management. *Journal of Nursing Quality Assurance, 1*(1), 47-54.

Bull, M. (1985). Quality assurance: Its origins, transformations, and prospects. In C. Meisenheimer (Ed.), *Quality assurance: A complete guide to effective programs* (pp. 1-16). Rockville, MD: Aspen.

Burgess, W., & Ragland, E. C. (1983). *Community health nursing.* Norwalk, CT: Appleton-Century-Crofts.

Christy, T. E. (1971). The first 50 years. *American Journal of Nursing, 71,* 1778-1784.

Codman, E. A. (1914). The products of a hospital. *Surgery, Gynecology, and Obstetrics, 18,* 491-496.

Crosby, P. R. (1979). *Quality is free.* New York: New American Library.

Culp, B., Goemaere, N. D., & Miller, M. E. (1985). Risk management: An integral part of quality assurance. In C. Meisenheimer (Ed.), *Quality assurance: A complete guide to effective programs* (pp. 169-192). Rockville, MD: Aspen.

Deming, W. (1982). *Quality, productivity, and competitive position.* Cambridge, MA: M.I.T. Center for Advanced Engineering Study.

Donabedian, A. (1966). Evaluating the quality of medical care. *Millbank Memorial Fund Quarterly, 44,* 166-204.

Donabedian, A. (1978). The quality of medical care: Methods for assessing and monitoring the quality of care for research and for quality assurance programs. In *Health United States* (DHEW Publication No. [PHS] 78-1232, pp. 111-126). Hyattsville, MD: U. S. Department of Health, Education and Welfare.

Donabedian, A. (1985). *Explorations in quality, assessment and monitoring* (Vol. 3). Ann Arbor, MI: Health Administration Press.

Donabedian, A. (1987). Five essential questions from the management of quality in health care. *Health Management Quarterly, 9*(1), 6-9.

Donabedian, A. (1988). Quality assessment and assurance: Unity of purpose, diversity of means. *Inquiry, 25,* 173-192.

Flynn, B. C., & Ray, D. W. (1987). Current perspectives in quality assurance and community health nursing. *Journal of Community Health Nursing, 4*(4), 187-197.

Gillem, T. (1988). Deming's 14 points and hospital quality: Responding to the consumer's demand for the best value health care. *Journal of Nursing Quality Assurance, 2*(3), 70-78.

Gould, E. J., & Ruane, N. D. (1988). Quality assurance

in home health. In M. Harris (Ed.), *Home health administration* (pp. 393-439). Owing Hills, MD: Rynd Communications.

Haussman, R. K., Hegyvary, S. T., & Newman, J. F. (1976). *Monitoring quality of nursing care, Pt. II* (DHEW Publication No. HRA 76-7). Bethesda, MD: U. S. Department of Health, Education & Welfare.

Health Care Financing Administration, 1987, pp. 14-15.

Herman, J. L., Morris, L. L., & Fitz-Gibbon, C. T. (1987). *Evaluator's handbook.* Newbury Park, CA: Sage..

Hough, B. L., & Schmele, J. A. (1987). The Slater Scale: A viable method for monitoring nursing care quality in home health. *Journal of Nursing Quality Assurance, 1*(3), 28-38.

Joint Commission on Accreditation of Healthcare Organizations. (1988a). *Assuring quality care in nursing services.* Chicago: Author.

Joint Commission on Accreditation of Healthcare Organizations. (1988b). *Standards for the accreditation of home care.* Chicago: Author.

Jonas, S., & Rosenberg, S. N. (1986). Measurement and control of the quality of health care. In S. Jonas (Ed.), *Health care delivery in the United States* (3rd ed., pp. 416-464). New York: Springer.

Jones, F. M. (1981). ANA's certification for specialization. In J. McCloskey & H. Grace (Eds.), *Current issues in nursing* (pp. 353-359). Oxford: Blackwell.

Journal of Nursing Quality Assurance, (1986) 3(3).

Kessner, D. M., Kalk, C. E., & Singer, J. (1973). Assessing health quality—The case for tracers. *New England Journal of Medicine, 288,* 189-194.

Knowlton, C. (1988, March 28). What America makes best. *Fortune,* pp. 40-53.

Knox, L. J. (1985). *The Knox guide to self-appraisal and goal setting for community health nurses.* Ottawa: Canadian Public Health Association.

LaLonde, B. (1986). *Quality assurance manual of the Home Care Association of Washington* (1st ed.). Edmonds, WA: Home Care Association of Washington.

Lee, R. I., & Jones, L. W. (1933). *The fundamentals of good medical care.* Chicago: University of Chicago Press.

Litwack, L., Linc, L., & Bower, D. (1985). *Evaluation in nursing: Principles and practice.* (Publication No. 15-1976). New York: National League for Nursing.

McCloskey, J. C. (1981). The state board test pool exam: Entrance to professional nursing. In J. McCloskey & H. Grace (Eds.), *Current issues in nursing* (pp. 336-347). Oxford: Blackwell.

Meisenheimer, C. G. (Ed.). (1985). *Quality assurance: A complete guide to effective programs.* Rockville, MD: Aspen.

Meisenheimer, C. G. (Ed.). (1989). *Quality assurance for home health care.* Rockville, MD: Aspen.

National League for Nursing. (1987). *Accreditation criteria, standards, and substantiating evidence* (Publication No. 21-1306). New York: Author.

Nightingale, F. (1969). *Notes on nursing* (Dover ed.). New York: Dover.

Peters, D. (1988). Classifying patients using a nursing diagnosis taxonomy. In M. D. Harris (Ed.), *Home health administration* (pp. 311-322). Owing Mills, MD.: National Health Publishing.

Peters, T. J. (1987). *Thriving on chaos.* New York: Knopf.

Peters, T. J., & Austin, N. K. (1985). *A passion for excellence.* New York: Random House.

Peters, T. J., & Waterman, R. H. (1982). *In search of excellence.* New York: Harper & Row.

Phaneuf, M. C. (1972). *The nursing audit: Profile for excellence* (p. 15). New York: Appleton-Century-Crofts.

Relman, A. S. (1980). The new medical-industrial complex. *New England Journal of Medicine, 303,* 963-970.

Rinke, L. T., & Wilson, A. A. (Eds). (1988). *Outcome measures in home health.* (Publication No. 21-2195). New York: National League for Nursing.

Rossi, P. H., & Freeman, H. E. (1985). *Evaluation: A systematic approach* (3rd ed.). Beverly Hills, CA: Sage.

Sandefer, G. D., Freeman, H. E., & Rossi, P. H. (1986). *Workbook for evaluation.* Beverly Hills, CA: Sage.

Schmele, J. A. (1985). A method to evaluate nursing practice in a community setting. *Quality Review Bulletin, 11*(4), 116-122.

Schmele, J. A. (1988). A process approach to measurement of health care in home health [Summary]. *Proceedings of the 15th Midwest Nursing Research Society,* p. 254.

Schmele, J. A. (1989a). Data collection mechanisms. In C. Meisenheimer (Ed.), *Quality assurance for home health care* (pp. 72-80). Rockville, MD: Aspen.

Schmele, J. A. (1989b). A process method for clinical practice evaluation in the home health setting. *Journal of Nursing Quality Assurance, 3*(3), 54-63.

Schroeder, P. (Ed.). (1986). Balancing quality and cost. *Journal of Nursing Quality Assurance, 1*(1).

Schroeder, P. (Ed.). (1988). The consumer's view of quality. *Journal of Nursing Quality Assurance, 2*(3).

Shaffer, F. A. (Ed.). (1984). *DRGs: Changes and challenges* (Publication No. 29-1959). New York: National League for Nursing.

Shepherd, T. (1988, November). Cadillac care: Advances in technology raise cost control questions. *Healthcare Financial Management,* pp. 23-28.

Sledin, D. W. (1984). The medical model: Biomedical science as the basis of medicine. In P. R. Lee, C. L. Estes, & N. B. Ramsey (Eds.), *The Nation's Health* (2nd ed.). pp. 55-762. San Francisco: Boyd & Fraser.

Strickland, O. L., and Waltz, C. F. (Eds.). (1988). *Measurement of nursing outcomes* (Vol. 2). New York: Springer.

Waltz, C. F., & Strickland, O. L. (Eds). (1988). *Measurement of nursing outcomes* (Vol. 1). New York: Springer.

Wandelt, M. A., & Ager, J. (1970). *Quality patient care scale.* Detroit: Wayne State University.

Wandelt, M. A., & Stewart, D. S. (1975). *Slater nursing competencies rating scale.* New York: Appleton-Century-Crofts.

Webb, P. R. (1988). Agency standards. In M. Harris (Ed.), *Home health administration* (pp. 61-132). Owing Hills, MD: Rynd Communications.

Wilbert, C. C. (1985). Selecting topics/methodologies. In C. Meisenheimer (Ed.), *Quality assurance: A complete guide to effective programs* (pp. 103-131). Rockville, MD: Aspen.

Zander, K. (1988). Nursing care management: Strategic management of cost and quality outcomes. *Journal of Nursing Administration, 18*(5), 23-30.

The Individual in the Community

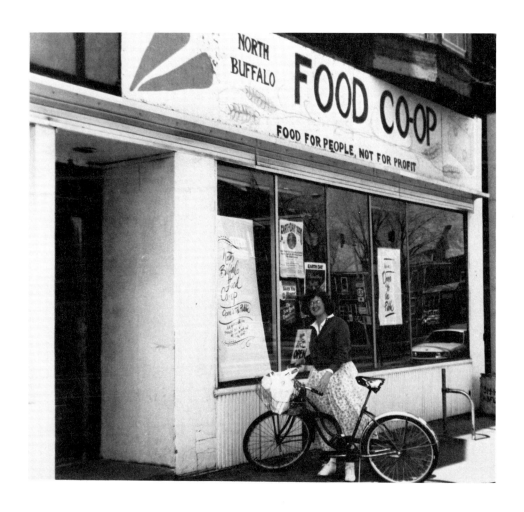

In working to promote health within the family system, the community health nurse often will face a situation in which members of the client family are at different stages of development. Individuals across the life span have varying needs, both psychologically and biologically. In addition, nurses who work with age-specific populations, such as those in child day-care centers or senior citizen centers, must be aware of their clients' specific stages and how those stages influence interactions and plans of care.

Chapter 9 describes concepts that relate to growth and development of infants, toddlers, and preschoolers. Chapter 10 applies this topic to primary and secondary school-age children. The chapter also outlines the role of the school nurse in promoting the health of both age-groups.

Chapters 11 and 12 deal with the individual needs of adults. Young and middle-aged adults, mature adults, and those in late maturity are all experiencing age-specific threats to health and life tasks that relate to their chronological stage of development.

The nurse's role in health promotion is enhanced by a knowledge of the life process experienced by individuals from birth to death. This unit supplies information that will contribute to that knowledge and assist the nurse in planning health interventions at primary, secondary, and tertiary levels across the life span.

CHAPTER 9

The Child from Birth to Five Years

JANET T. IHLENFELD

The child, to learn at all, must play.

EDWARD SPESCHA, Swiss Committee for UNICEF

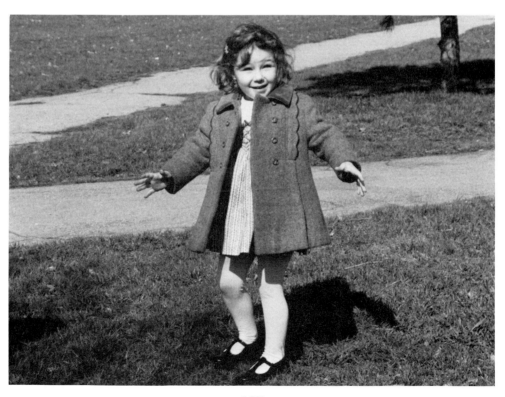

OBJECTIVES

At the conclusion of this chapter the student will be able to:
1. Define the key terms listed
2. Describe concepts of growth and development in infants, toddlers, and preschoolers
3. Describe the play activities of toddlers and preschoolers
4. Identify health problems common to this age-group
5. Describe the roles of the community nurse who cares for infants, toddlers, and preschoolers
6. Describe the use of day-care for infants, toddlers, and preschoolers

KEY TERMS

Autonomy versus shame and doubt	Preoperational phase
Day-care center	Preschool
Family day-care	Preschooler
Infant	Sensorimotor period
Initiative versus guilt	Therapeutic play
Latchkey child	Toddler
Play	Trust versus mistrust

PHYSICAL GROWTH AND DEVELOPMENT

The greatest rate of growth in the human being occurs during the first year of life. Although general rates of growth indicate that the birth weight doubles by 6 months of age (Fig. 9-1) and triples by 1 year of age (Fig. 9-2), growth rates for each individual child are variable. As the infant grows, the degree of gross motor skill increases, as does fine motor skill development. By 13 months the toddler should be able to take approximately 10 unaided steps. Between the age of 8 months to 2 years the teeth begin to appear and the toddler graduates to solid foods. The development of teeth also helps the newly communicating toddler to make specific sounds during acquisition of language. From 2 to 3 years the rate of growth slows; however, the intellectual and neurological capacity continues to grow and develop (Hinson, 1985).

The child from 3 to 5 years of age becomes leaner than the chubby, active toddler. Coordination improves, and the head and face develop more adult proportions than those of the round-headed, large-eyed infant and toddler (Hinson, 1985).

COGNITIVE DEVELOPMENT
The Infant and Toddler

Cognitive development occurs during the rapid growth period of the first few years. According to Piaget (1974, 1978), from birth to 2 years of age is a period of sensorimotor development in which the infant explores the environment through the five senses, especially taste, touch, and sight. Patterns of action called *schemes,* in which ways of doing things are explored and tried out, develop. The concept of object permanence begins during this time period and is fully in place by 2 years of age.

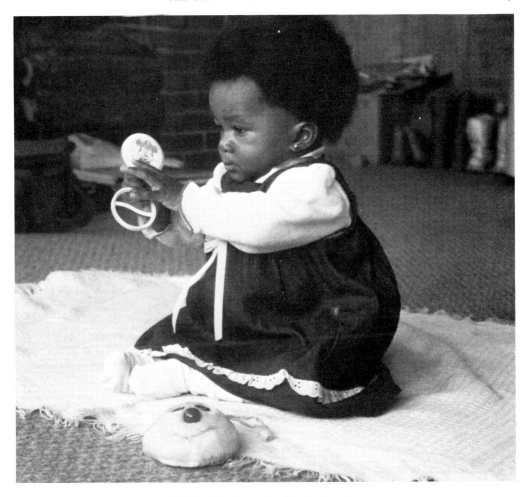

FIG. 9-1 The 6-month-old infant at play.

Erikson (1963) calls the period from birth to 2 years of age in the child's life the time of trust versus mistrust when the infant develops and interacts with parents and learns that the parents care for its needs. Consequently, the infant who lacks a stable caretaker learns mistrust of the world. The next stage of development, according to Erikson, is that of autonomy versus doubt and shame. Here the toddler wishes to gain control of the world but doubts whether it can be attained. It also is the appropriate time for toilet training; the toddler wishes to please the parent but sometimes feels ashamed after toileting accidents.

The Preschooler

The 3 to 4 year old often is called the preschooler because the child is approaching the age for kindergarten and elementary school. According to Piaget (1974, 1978) the preschooler is in the preoperational phase of development. This is a period when representational thought develops and the child learns to solve simple problems. Because language skills become more precise, communication is easier.

According to Erikson (1963) this age-group is dealing with initiative versus guilt in

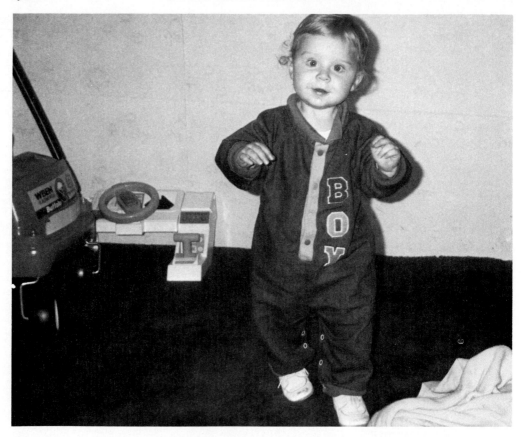

FIG. 9-2 The 1-year-old toddler is starting to walk.

an effort to grow up. This is a time when children begin to spend more time with peers and explore their ability to be independent. This conflict between independence and dependence on the parents is the central part of the initiative-versus-guilt stage. The desire to make decisions is important, and the ability to say "No!" to another's requests provides the child with a source of control. At the same time the potential for guilt arises because the child's search for control also brings conflict when control is exerted by others. This control often is held by the parents or other adults, and the child's reaction reflects a belief that he or she has done something wrong.

These egocentric years (i.e., focus on self) are filled with fantasy and other types of make believe. The preschooler's imagination is very vivid, and the child seems able to play for hours without food or sleep. Eventually, of course, the need for both catch up with the child. The preschool child, continually busy at play, learns at a very fast pace (Meer, 1985).

PLAY

Play is an all-encompassing activity that occupies the child during all waking hours (Leifer, 1982). Some have said that play is a child's work; however, this is not true. Work has a structured objective and defined outcomes. Play can be structured or unstructured and, more important, is fun for its own sake.

Play has several functions. It expresses feelings, teaches and refines developmental skills, provides a way of developing cognitive skills, and helps the child socialize. Developmental trends occur within play; for example, the complexity of play increases as growth and development progress. Each stage becomes more elaborate and is combined into more and more complex events. The child incorporates new life experiences into play as new events and ideas occur. For example, a child playing with blocks or wood may begin by piling them up but later can build walls and still later can create a make-believe fort from those same blocks as the ability to create new ideas grows.

Types of Play

Recreational play can be divided into several categories. *Unoccupied play* occurs when children watch anything of interest. They might wander around, stand, or sit or just do nothing. *Solitary play* occurs when children play by themselves rather than interact with other children. This may be seen when children color or draw or when they play in sandboxes or perform other quiet activities such as riding a tricycle. *Onlooker behavior* is seen when the children observe others playing but do not join in. They see and hear what is going on but resist any urging to join in. Play is occurring, as well as a subtle learning about how to play, because the child is gaining satisfaction from watching others play. Very often onlooker play is the first stage of preschoolers' play (Harris & Liebert, 1984).

Parallel play, also often an early part of the play activity of the preschooler, occurs when the child plays side by side with other children, doing the same activity as the other children—such as threading macaroni onto string—yet there is no interaction among the children. In *associative play* the children are doing the same thing, but there is no group goal in mind nor is there an end product. Although the play lacks visible organization, there is some degree of interaction among the children in that they share materials and ideas and often talk about what they are doing as they do it. *Cooperative play* is an organized activity in which roles are assigned by the children to reach a common goal. An example is playing school, with one child the teacher, another the principal, and the rest are students. Playing games such as "Duck, Duck, Goose" or "Ring-Around-the-Rosey" are cooperative games in that all involved are playing by rules and know their own particular place in the game, whether it is running away from the "goose" or "all falling down." Cooperative play begins during the preschool years and develops during elementary school years. *Fantasy play* is pretending. It begins in the preschool period, usually is spontaneous, and changes as the play goes on to satisfy the child's needs. At this time "dress up" play also occurs (Dickey, 1987).

Structured Play

Structured play is that play in which adults decide on the focus of the play activity or those games that require the players to follow specific rules. Both structured and unstructured play are essential in the play world of the preschool-aged child.

Preschool Toys

It is important to provide the preschooler with toys for both structured and unstructured play. The preschooler likes unstructured materials, or raw materials, for play (Hinson, 1985). Different types of materials, colors, textures, sizes, and shapes are a must (Rubin & Fisher, 1982); suitable materials are crayons, construction paper, nontoxic paste, paint, clay, pencils, and ribbon. The excitement of discovery—children thinking up and creating new things all by themselves—is basic to play. Trial and error, rather than preconceived goals, are used. Blocks allow children to create and then to tear down, an activity of destruction that normally is forbidden to them. This type of fantasy play teaches the concepts of temporary and permanent. It also teaches balance, shape, form, distance, and organization.

Painting is a favorite activity of preschoolers and helps them to create their own viewpoint of the world. Clay also teaches forming skills, helps children interpret ideas, and is fun because, like painting, it permits the child to be messy.

Supervision of Play Activities

To prevent accidents, the play of infants, toddlers, and preschoolers should be supervised by adults. Accidents can range from ingestion of nonedible objects (also called *pica*) such as nontoxic paste to placing small items such as dry macaroni into the mouth to injury from falling objects such as blocks. A child can make a missile out of a stick and hurt someone severely and unintentionally because of absorption with the act of play and lack of understanding of cause and effect.

Special attention should be given to play activities on the playground. Prevention of injuries is paramount here. The adult can guide and structure play by organizing games such as "Duck, Duck, Goose" and "Ring-Around-the-Rosey." Supervised walks around the neighborhood should include instruction on traffic safety precautions.

HEALTH PROBLEMS OF INFANTS, TODDLERS, AND PRESCHOOLERS
Accidents and Accident Prevention

Non—motor vehicle accidents from drowning, fires, burns, falls, or ingestion of foreign objects are the most serious health threats to infants, toddlers, and preschoolers. Fatality rates in the United States in 1982 were 22.4 per 100,000 children under the age of 1 year and 14.5 per 100,000 for those aged 1 to 4 years (Miller, Fine, Adams-Taylor, & Schorr, 1986). At highest risk for accidents are those children in low-income, poorly educated families who live in substandard housing. In addition, the younger the mother the higher the risk of an accident to the child.

The nurse must emphasize safety. The high activity level of infants, toddlers, and preschoolers increases the likelihood that accidents will occur. Falls, burns, poisonings, and other accidents may occur in many settings such as homes, grandparents' homes, and day-care centers, and steps should be taken by all caretakers to prevent their occurrence.

Children are prone to injury while playing. Because they are so absorbed in their play activities or are developmentally unaware of dangers, accidents can occur even when there is adult supervision. Studies have shown that most injuries are due to one of the following events: the child fell from a piece of play equipment, used a toy inappropriately, or was the object of aggressive behavior by another child (Chang, Lugg, & Nebedum, 1989).

Injuries from playground accidents are the most frequently cited injury to children in day-care centers. Severe injuries may be sustained by falls from climbers or jungle gyms, slides, swings, and other climbing apparatus, as well as injuries from running and falling or tripping over objects in the playground (Aronson, 1985, 1986). Nurses who supervise playground activities should make sure that equipment is safe and that sharp edges on wooden or metal structures are shielded. Rules should be developed and enforced regarding use of the equipment. Insurers of day-care centers often recommend that jungle gyms, which trigger many accidents, be removed to reduce liability claims. Shock-absorbing surfaces such as sand or foam may be installed under playground equipment to cushion falls from the apparatus (Chang, Lugg, & Nebedum, 1989).

Although indoor safety is equally important, frequently it is overlooked (Mayer, 1981). Problem areas should be reviewed and frequently checked, for example, nonskid rugs in high-traffic areas, prohibition of running, prohibition of children's access to areas where food is prepared to prevent burns, the use of safety electrical outlets in all areas of the center, quick wipe-ups of spills, and the use of child-proof cupboards and locked cabinets where detergents, pesticides, and other chemicals are stored.

The nurse can assess the home for apparent dangers and teach safety measures as part of health promotion. The nurse also should teach about personal safety and how to deal with strangers. The children should be taught how to call police and fire/rescue departments and also should be able to give their own name, address, and telephone number to appropriate officials. Safety should be stressed as a positive and not as a defensive, frightening aspect of life.

Passenger vehicle safety. It is important for the nurse to stress to preschoolers the need to be safe when they are passengers in a vehicle. This teaching can begin with preschoolers and continue with their parents (Aronson, 1986; Nachem & Bass, 1984).

Most states require that passengers in cars be restrained by vehicle-equipped seat belts and shoulder harnesses. In addition, car seats are required for infants and small children up to 40 pounds or 4 years of age because their body size does not allow for proper restraint by the belts that are installed by automobile manufacturers. These infant or child seats should meet governmental guidelines. Those that do usually note that the product conforms to federal motor vehicle safety standards.

The nurse should emphasize that both children and parents should buckle up every time they are in a car. Parents who usually do not wear seat belts should be encouraged to do so for their own safety, as well as to serve as role models for their children. Seat belt and car seat use also reduces the sometimes exuberant activity of children. The nurse can use this fact to further explain the benefits of belt use to resistant parents.

One aspect of teaching may be difficult for the nurse. The preschoolers may ride a bus, either a large school bus or a van, to a day-care center. Many school buses are not equipped with restraint systems whereas some vans have car seats. Legislation for this safety requirement for buses has not caught up with that for cars, and many state legislatures currently are discussing laws regarding restraints in buses. At this time, however, it would be best for the nurse to emphasize that children in such vehicles always should hang on to the handles on the seats in the buses, remain seated, and face forward. This will help emphasize order and promote use of belts when they are available in buses. The nurse in the community is the logical person to lobby the state for legislation in this area.

Iron Deficiency Anemia

Iron deficiency anemia is the most common nutritional problem in the United States today. Many children do not get enough iron in their diet, which results in susceptibility to infection, poor weight gain, and lower than normal height and weight. These children tend to do poorly in school because of poor oxygenation. The nurse should emphasize proper nutrition and a diet of red meats, fruits, vegetables, grains, and dairy products and should teach parents how to give the prescribed oral iron supplements (Miller et al., 1986).

Dental Problems

Poor dental hygiene also is a health threat to toddlers and preschoolers. Once teeth appear, so does the potential to develop dental caries. Many parents send their child to bed with a bottle of milk or another liquid that contains sugar, which predisposes the toddler to "nursing bottle syndrome." Thus the maxillary anterior teeth are destroyed and the remaining teeth form dental caries because of the milk in the sleeping child's mouth. If the decay is severe, these teeth may require extraction. Parents should be taught to begin brushing the child's teeth gently on a daily basis as soon as the teeth appear. To prevent further cavities and tooth decay they also should be cautioned not to send the child to bed with a bottle (Clemon-Stone, Eigsti, Gerber, & McGuire, 1987). The establishment of good dental hygiene in the early years will help ensure healthy adult teeth and dental hygiene in the future.

Plumbism, or Lead Poisoning

According to the National Center for Health Statistics, 4% of the preschoolers in the United States showed elevated lead levels in 1980. The U.S. Centers for Disease Control defines elevated lead levels as more than or equal to 25 micrograms of lead per deciliter of blood (≥ 25 µg/dl) (Miller, Fine, Adams-Taylor, & Schorr, 1986). Children are exposed to lead in a number of ways. They may eat paint chips from woodwork in their homes, they may inhale automobile emissions in urban areas in which leaded gasoline is still available for purchase, or they may ingest the lead from dietary sources such as from the lead solder in plumbing joints or the solder in the seams of food cans. Those at highest risk for iron deficiency anemia are low-income urban families. Elevated lead levels are difficult to detect; however, any child who shows developmental delay should be evaluated by means of a blood test. If untreated, lead poisoning may result in delayed mental development, severe anemia, and mental retardation. Chelation therapy with calcium disodium edetate ($CaNa_2EDTA$) is the treatment of choice to eliminate lead from the child's system. This treatment, however, will not reverse any preexisting physical or brain damage caused by high lead levels (Whaley & Wong, 1987).

Child Abuse and Neglect

Child abuse constitutes physical or psychological damage inflicted on a child. Neglect is the absence of reasonable care required by a child, such as shelter, food, supervision, or health care. Factors indicating that a child has a potentially high risk for being abused include a history of premature birth, low birth weight, and chronic illness. Factors that place adults at high risk for becoming abusers include alcoholism, substance abuse, the absence of a biological parent in the home, and violence or excessive stress in the family because of such factors as financial difficulties, history of abuse of the parents as children, and immature parents whose expectations of the child are unrealistic (Miller, Fine, Adams-Taylor, & Schorr, 1986). The nurse has a responsibility to be on the lookout for children who may have been abused or for families in which the potential for abuse is suspected. The nurse should intervene by documenting facts and alerting the appropriate authorities; for example, calling the state child-abuse hotline, which is listed in the telephone book, or by informing the local social services or child welfare agency (Dickey, 1987).

HEALTH PROMOTION ACTIVITIES
The Use of Play in Health Promotion

The nurse should use play to help teach the preschooler concepts of health promotion; play facilitates learning because it is applicable to the preschooler's world. For instance, a lesson on brushing the teeth can begin by having preschoolers fashion a crude tooth in clay and then, while the nurse demonstrates, use a stick to "brush" the clay tooth. Children also can help the nurse make up a poem or a song to help them remember to brush and have them recite or sing it before they brush their teeth. Drawing posters is another technique to help children remember. The use of play as a mode to learning is a valuable aid in health promotion for preschoolers.

Therapeutic play. Therapeutic play, or medical play, is used to help children learn about and prepare for health care procedures and activities. Not only is it useful to help hospitalized children deal with their experiences; it also is helpful in preparing children who are well for experiences they may have with the health care system (Meer, 1985).

Preschoolers can use therapeutic play under the supervision of the nurse to dress up as nurses or physicians or use puppets to play out hospital or clinic scenes. Giving injections to dolls and stuffed toys can help children understand why "shots" are necessary. With supervision preschoolers can handle plastic syringes without the needle to work through the immunization process and other instances that require injections. Therapeutic play also helps prepare children for hospitalization and is particularly beneficial to children who will be having tonsillectomies and other surgeries. They can pretend to administer anesthesia to stuffed animals and dolls to prepare for the surgery. The ability of the preschooler to concentrate on make believe and fantasy helps make therapeutic play an important technique to teach children to deal with the health care system.

Parent Education

The nurse is in an excellent position to help teach parents about health promotion activities for infants, toddlers, and preschoolers. The nurse can help parents understand the elements of nutrition, which is particularly important for this age-group, and the need for disease prevention, including the immunizations recommended for all children.

Education in accident prevention, as discussed earlier in this chapter, is paramount. The nurse can make home visits to help assess the home for hazards and to advise parents on how they can "child proof" their homes. Grandparents' or babysitters' homes also can be assessed for these hazards so that they can be made safe before an accident occurs, for example, child-proofing medicine cabinets and removing medications, including vitamins and over-the-counter drugs such as aspirin and acetaminophen, from kitchen counter tops and kitchen tables.

Parents also need to be taught the usual developmental milestones of their young children. Many times, parents expect too much too soon from children, and this lack of understanding of the child's capabilities and resultant frustration tend to place a family at risk for child abuse.

Screening of Preschoolers

Nurses in many health care settings screen children for both health problems and developmental problems. Screening tests do not provide a diagnosis of how far behind his or her peers a child may be; rather screening indicates areas in which further evaluation of the child by other health professionals is needed.

Developmental screening. The Denver Developmental Screening Test (DDST) is the most widely used screening test for young children. Its categories of personal-social, fine motor adaptive, language, and gross motor development serve to indicate general standing on the basis of the average development for children of a certain age (O'Pray, 1980).

Screening tools should reflect sensitivity to cultural and geographical backgrounds. For instance, children who live in urban areas might not know about cows because their frame of reference is city life. The nurse should be aware of the possibility that biased questions may result in lower scores for some children and thus realize that developmental

---

RESEARCH HIGHLIGHT

To assess whether prior parental preparation of preschoolers will affect the process of vision and hearing screening, 389 children between the ages of 2½ and 5 years were assigned to either an experimental or a control group. Parents of 194 preschoolers in the experimental group asked their children to match shapes on flashcards while the child alternately covered each eye. For the hearing test preparation the preschoolers were asked to put a stick in a bowl every time they heard a bell ring. The control group received none of these preparations.

Subsequent professional vision and hearing screening of both groups showed that the average test time was less for those children who were prepared for the screening. It also was shown that the older the child, the less time the screening tests took.

The results of this study indicate that preparation for vision and hearing screening helps the preschooler cope with the screening process and will enable children who have vision or hearing deficiencies to be identified during their preschool years.

Brown, M.S. and Collar, M. (1982). Effects of prior preparation on the preschooler's vision and hearing screening. *MCN: American Journal of Maternal Child Nursing, 7*(5), 323-328.

---

screening tests are used only as a guide rather than a diagnostic tool (O'Pray, 1980).

Health screening. The nurse is in an ideal position to screen children for vision and hearing defects and to keep up with immunization schedules and assessment for child abuse and neglect (Fleming, 1986). The standards of the American Academy of Pediatrics and the standards of maternal and child health nursing practice also serve to guide the nurse in health screening efforts (Rustia & Barr, 1985). (See research highlight.)

Most communities have screening programs to provide low-income families with access to health services. The nurse should be aware of Head Start facilities in the community, which screen for vision, hearing, and anemia (Aronson, 1986). The Early and Periodic Screening, Diagnosis and Treatment Program (EPSDT) provides 14 screenings for each low-income child from birth to 21 years of age (Rustia & Barr, 1985). The program, jointly funded by the federal government and each of the states, is a Medicaid supplemental program created to provide primary health care to Medicaid-eligible children (Harvard Child Health Project Task Force, 1977). These agencies, as well as community health centers, are referral sources for the nurse who conducts health screening.

ROLES OF THE COMMUNITY HEALTH NURSE
The Nurse and Children in the Community

The community health nurse sees children in the community in a variety of settings in which the emphasis is on the health of infants, toddlers, and/or preschoolers. For example, the nurse may be employed in a well-baby clinic where infants are assessed for appropriate growth and development, as well as given immunizations and screened for health problems. Here the nurse can teach parents regarding all aspects of infant and child care (Friedemann, 1983).

The nurse may work in an independent maternal-infant nursing center, employed by parents to assess the mother and newborn after birth and to follow up their care after early discharge from the hospital after birth (Clemen-Stone, Eigsti, & McGuire, 1987). The nurse also may teach prenatal classes to expectant parents.

The community health nurse may be a home visitor from such health care agencies as the Public Health Service or the Visiting Nurse Association. Here the nurse provides primary, secondary, and tertiary care to children and parents who need health assessment and intervention (Clemen-Stone, Eigsti, & McGuire, 1987).

The nurse may be a coordinator of community resources, an advocate for children regarding safety and health promotion matters in governmental agencies, a teacher of health promotion in a clinical agency, or a case finder, that is, identifying and referring high-risk children and families to appropriate health care agencies. Some nurses are active in gathering data about health within a community, carrying out the responsibilities of a nurse epidemiologist (Clemen-Stone, Eigsti, & McGuire, 1987). The nurse may care for children and their families in outpatient or ambulatory clinics, in physicians' offices, in health maintenance organizations (HMOs), in schools, and in day-care settings.

The highest concentration of infants, toddlers, and preschoolers in the community today is in the day-care center. The following section illustrates the application of the Neuman systems model (Neuman, 1989) to nursing in the day-care center. The Neuman model was presented in detail in Chapter 3.

The Nurse in the Day-Care Center

The community health nurse is the professional health care provider most frequently consulted by day-care centers. This nurse has the opportunity to nurse the well child

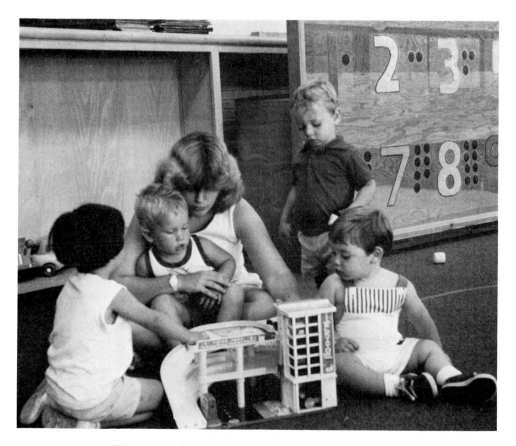

FIG. 9-3 Preschoolers playing together in a day-care center.

from infancy through school age; however, preschoolers are the largest group within this population (Fig. 9-3). This community of well preschoolers gives the nurse the opportunity to use primary prevention and positive reinforcement during interaction with the children and parents concerning self-care.

The nurse may be employed part-time or full-time by the day-care center or may be a paid consultant or a community health nurse who visits the day-care center as part of his or her nursing responsibilities. Because the arrangement depends on state or local community regulations, it may be different in various parts of the country.

Nurses associated with a day-care center help maintain the children's health records, including physical examinations and immunization records, and may assist in keeping track of the children's current health problems. Nurses also perform health surveillance and health screening in areas such as vision and hearing. Their ability to observe and assess allows them to continually look for cues that suggest health problems such as instances of child abuse, child neglect, and infection. They can respond to and give nursing care in emergency situations in the day-care center and thus are excellent providers of accident prevention and injury-control health teaching. Their knowledge of the health care system in the community also facilitates referral of children, families, and staff members to available community agencies. In addition, they can help the staff and board to assess the day-care center in the areas of organization, policy, discipline of children, and noise control (Ferholt, 1980; Fleming, 1986).

Assessing children of all ages for evidence of child abuse should be part of the community health nurse's responsibilities. The nurse also should be mindful that preschoolers may be abused by staff members in day-care centers. Such abuse has been seen in much-publicized instances of sexual abuse of children in day-care centers by the centers' owners. Although such episodes are rare, the nurse should be aware that they can occur (Berkelman, Guinan, & Thacker, 1989; Wilson & Steppe, 1986). Although such a suspicion may cause difficulty if the nurse is an employee of the center, all nurses should be on the lookout for signs of abuse in all settings where they practice. Registered nurses are required in most states to notify appropriate authorities by calling a child-abuse hotline or by going through other official channels (Dickey, 1987).

The nurse in the day-care center is not only a consultant and teacher of children, parents, and staff regarding health issues but also someone children can trust and play with: someone who is an appropriate role model for children as they progress through their preschool years.

The basic structure: infants, toddlers, and preschoolers in day-care. There is a growing need for day-care facilities. It is estimated that 11 million children are in some kind of day-care, and this number grows daily (Wald, Dashefsy, Byers, Guera, & Taylor, 1988). Many children are from single-parent families in which the parent must have someone care for the children during work hours. Other families need the money that two incomes provide, which necessitates the placement of children in day-care. It is estimated that more than half of all children younger than 6 years of age have mothers who work outside the home (Kahn & Kamerman, 1987; Morgan, 1985).

Children of all ages are in day-care: infants, toddlers, preschoolers, and school-aged children. It is of primary concern, however, to ensure that these facilities do not replace the importance of parents in the care of children (Murray & Zentner, 1985). The main responsibility of child care belongs to the parents or legal guardians. These individuals contract for day-care services; at no time do they give up the responsibility of child care, nor should the agency attempt to provide care that is contrary to their wishes. Communication between staff members and parents is essential to keep in perspective the purpose of child care: caring for children at the request of parents, not taking their place (Caldwell, 1986).

Parents send their children to day-care facilities for multiple reasons, ranging from the desire to place the child in contact with other children, to learn new things in an organized setting, or as already discussed, to provide care for the child while the parent is at school or at work. Several types of care are available to families. Some parents choose to have their children supervised by relatives or friends, whereas other parents choose a community facility geared to caring for children (Kahn & Kamerman, 1987). Some parents, even those of preschool children, leave the children alone, with increasing numbers of "latchkey" children as the result. There are estimated to be up to 5 million latchkey children in the United States; approximately half a million of these are preschool children who take care of themselves while parents work (Morgan, 1985). Because this arrangement may be construed as neglect, controversy surrounds this issue. Therefore parents and children conceal the fact that the youngsters are alone at home. Studies indicate, however, that the practice is increasing (Long & Long, 1983).

Lines of resistance: types of day-care centers. Early childhood programs sometimes are generically referred to as day-care centers, nursery schools, preschools, family day-care, or child-care centers. There are, however, subtle differences among these types of facilities.

A day-care center is a state-licensed facility where children ranging from infancy through school age are cared for while parents work or attend school. This type of care provides meals, snacks, and naps, as well as structured and unstructured play activities. Children may arrive at different times of the day, depending on the parent's schedule (Webb, 1984). A nursery school or preschool program is a half-day or full-day program geared to preparing the child for kindergarten and elementary school and often is associated with a school (Blum, 1983; Webb, 1984).

Family day-care is offered in a home setting that provides care for up to six children. Because many of these facilities are in neighborhood or relatives' homes on the basis of informal arrangement, they are largely unregulated by state laws. (Murray, 1984).

Other types of day-care include for-profit centers, nonprofit centers, school- or church-affiliated centers, and day-care within a corporate setting for the children of the employees.

Normal lines of defense: policies and procedures of a day-care center. The community health nurse must begin the assessment of the day-care center by evaluating the facility's policies and procedures. Although all states in the United States require licensing for day-care centers, not all preschools or nursery schools are required to be licensed by all states (Rustia & Barr, 1985). Where they exist, these licensing requirements, which vary from state to state, mandate minimum standards of educational preparation of the director and staff members, health and safety requirements, and financial statements. Other agencies that inspect day-care centers to ensure conformity with licensing requirements are city and county health departments, which regulate such matters as sanitary lavatory facilities, and fire departments, which examine smoke alarms, fire extinguishers, and emergency exits from the building. Regardless of the regulating agency, Kotin, Crabtree, and Aidman (1981) have categorized nine areas in which standards usually are set.

Staff-to-child ratio. Staff-to-child ratio is based on the age of the children in the facility. The younger the children the smaller the ratio, and conversely, the older the children the larger the ratio. Ratios also are based on the numbers of children in the center. In addition, to prevent injury during vigorous play more adults are needed to supervise children while they are engaged in outdoor activities. Conversely, fewer adults are needed to supervise children involved in a quiet activity such as drawing or coloring.

For children between the ages of 3 to 6 years the standard staffing ratio is one staff member for every eight children. Ratio guidelines differ from state to state and from locality to locality. For example, in Massachusetts the recommendation is three infants per caretaker whereas in Florida it is six infants per caretaker (Kahn & Kamerman, 1987).

Group size. The younger the children, the smaller the group in a particular room should be. For example, if the children are between the ages of 3 and 6 years, there might be as many as 16 children in the group.

Staff qualifications. Ideally, the director of a day-care center possesses a Bachelor of Science degree in early childhood education; however, it is not a requirement in all states. Staff members may have associate degrees in various areas, such as early childhood education, but many times they have only on-the-job-training. Salary may be an indicator of the educational level of staff members. The lower the salary the more likely that employees lack formal education for working with preschool children.

Client records. Each day-care center is required to keep written records regarding each child's health, immunization records, name of attending physician or health clinic, emergency telephone numbers to reach the parent or guardian, current medications, list of allergies, and history of illness and surgeries, both the child's and any siblings. All information is confidential and filed separately from other records that include such information as attendance and financial arrangements.

Physical space. Standards that regulate space usually require that a certain number of square feet be allocated per student, especially for play or nap areas.

Equipment. Specifications regulate the construction and safety features of such equipment as slides, swings, and sandboxes and the amount of materials for play, such as crayons, paper, and paste.

Health and safety. The use of separate areas for cooking and handling food and for diapering babies reduces infections, especially diarrheal infections. (These procedures are discussed at greater length later in the chapter). Fire safety includes policies regarding smoke alarms in every room, marked emergency exits, regularly scheduled fire drills, and the presence of fire extinguishers, child-proof electrical outlets, prohibition of extension cords, and the use of electric ranges and ovens (which reduce the risk of fire). Other safety requirements include well-lighted rooms, lighted stairways with banisters on the open side(s), and safety railings to block off stairs from young children. A day-care center that adheres to these safety requirements meets minimum standards.

Nutrition. Most day-care centers provide both snacks and meals. Those that meet standard requirements include selections from each of the major food groups.

Health care and emergency treatment. Of major concern to the community health nurse in a day-care center are the written policies and procedures for health care and emergency treatment, which should be kept in an accessible place and should be familiar to all staff members. Those that relate to emergency procedures and the maintenance of health records are of course mandatory; however, additional policies that regulate such matters as financial arrangements or reporting suspected child abuse or neglect should be considered.

Emergency procedures should include guidelines for staff behavior. Staff members first of all should be trained in first-aid procedures. If the nurse is present during an emergency in the facility, he or she should quickly assess the situation. If further care is needed, a parent or legal guardian should be contacted because that is the only person who can give consent for further care unless there is a life-threatening crisis. There also should be provision for transportation of the ill or injured child. Is there a day-care center bus or staff member's car for emergency use? Does the insurance policy of the center cover the use of the vehicle for emergency transportation? Should the center call 911 or a similar number to reach the fire department, rescue squad, hospital, or ambulance? In addition, a consent form, signed by the parents or legal guardian, although not considered a legal document in all states, should be on file. It should authorize emergency treatment and transportation to a health care facility in the event that the parents cannot be reached. At all times in the development of the written guidelines, the liability of the day-care center must be considered, along with the child's need for care.

Use of medication. The day-care center should be aware of the state's requirements regarding medication and should include these regulations in their policies. Insurance companies also may require that, because of the liability of the day-care center and the nurse or other individual who administers the medication, only certain medications or no medications be given to children.

The nurse in the day-care center should be very careful in dealing with children who take medication. Physician- or clinic-prescribed medication should be given to the center by the parent or guardian in the original container, with written instructions regarding the use of the medication such as dosage and times of doses.

Attendance by ill children. Most day-care centers exclude children who are ill, and these policies need to be established and understood by the parents, the staff, and the community health nurse. The nurse can help the family by recommending alternative arrangements when the child cannot attend the regular day-care center, for example, a "sick child" day-care center if one is available or a baby sitter. (A more detailed discussion is presented later in the chapter.)

Flexible lines of defense: interactions with peers and parents. Infants, toddlers, and preschoolers in day-care settings are exposed to a great number of new experiences during their day-care experiences. The parents' involvement and interest are of paramount importance to the healthy development of their child. Preschoolers in day-care have been found to develop faster socially than their stay-at-home peers. However, they also have been found to become more aggressive and tend to use violence to settle disputes (Kahn & Kamerman, 1987). The involvement of parents in acknowledging that such changes in child behavior exist can help buffer these unintended but seemingly inevitable changes. In this setting the community health nurse can intervene to help identify changes when they occur so that those who are involved can cope with and alter negative behavior.

One study shows that infants are exceptionally vulnerable to the social changes in the day-care setting. Belsky (as cited in Kahn & Kamerman, 1987) found that infants younger than 1 year of age are more likely to have problems bonding with parents after extended day-care experiences. Whether this difficulty was specific only to this study group remains to be seen, especially with the increasing number of infants in day-care. More research is required to ascertain whether these changes persist into older age-groups or whether they are only temporary reactions to the initial experience away from mother and father. With the increasing number of mothers who work full time to support families, this issue will continue to remain a focus of child care research. The community health nurse in the day-care center is the ideal person to collect data and conduct research on this issue. Alternatives such as increasing day-care facilities within the employment setting or close to it so that mothers can see their babies several times during the day, for example, during lunch breaks, may help mitigate these reported effects.

These aspects of the flexible line of defense become problems only when environmental stressors, which are discussed next, conflict with the basic structure, in this case the infants, toddlers, and preschoolers in day-care.

Stressors (in day-care)

Intrapersonal stressors. Intrapersonal stressors are those stressors that impact on the client system, or here, that personally affect the infant, toddler, or preschooler in day-care. These stressors are the growth and development changes that all children undergo, as well as their separation from the home environment.

Interpersonal stressors. Getting along with new people is one aspect of the interpersonal stressors that affect youngsters in day-care. The need to interact with new adults as caretakers and to meet new children are stressors with which the child must cope. It is less of a stressor at the pretoddler stage, before the child begins to engage in parallel play and has to learn to share. Managing these interactions and the occasional conflict that occurs within these relationships is an interpersonal stressor.

Extrapersonal stressors. The totally new environment of the day-care center is an extrapersonal stressor for children. The exposure to new rules and regulations is a stressor, such as sharing a bathroom or learning to wash their hands before meals. Although concern about safety and infection control is also an extrapersonal stressor, children do not recognize it because of their immature stage of development.

Nursing intervention

Primary prevention: prevention of infection in day-care centers. Whether children who attend day-care are sick more frequently than their stay-at-home peers is controversial. What is certain, however, is that they are exposed to *Haemophilus influenzae* (influenza virus type B), cytomegalovirus, hepatitis A, various diarrheal diseases, otitis media, and various respiratory diseases (Berkelman, Guinan, & Thacker, 1989; Henderson, 1985; Rustia & Barr, 1985).

In a prospective study of children at home, in group care, and in day-care, it was found that those in day-care averaged 7.1 illnesses per year whereas those at home averaged 4.7 illnesses per year. Children in day-care also had more sick days per year than those in home care. Because of the close contact of children in day-care, they tended to pass their respiratory and gastrointestinal diseases to their playmates. Those at home have less contact with other children and therefore are less likely to infect or be infected by others (Wald, Dashefsky, Byers, Guera, & Taylor, 1988).

An earlier study (Henderson, 1985) also found that preschool children who attended a day-care center had an average of 6.5 illnesses per year, most of them common colds or respiratory infections with fever. Respiratory diseases again were passed from child to child because of close contact and poor hygiene regarding nasal drainage and coughing.

Gastrointestinal or enteric infections also are seen in day-care and constitute the greatest disease problem seen in day-care today (Hadler, 1985). This is due largely to poor handwashing by children and caretakers in a setting in which food preparation takes place and there are children in diapers and children with poor hygiene habits. Daily cleaning of objects and toys that children place in or near their mouths helps to prevent the spread of enteric diseases, as does the use of disposable towels and soap in a liquid dispenser rather than cake soap.

One common enteric infestation that occurs in day-care centers is that of giardiasis, or infestation by the protozoa *Giardia lamblia.* It is transmitted via the oral-fecal route by swallowing the cyst of protozoa. The incubation period is 5 to 25 days, and explosive diarrhea is its main manifestation. Although a largely self-limiting disease, medication such as quinacrine (Atabrine) or furazolidone (Furoxone) prescribed by a physician may be needed. Good hand washing after toileting or diapering and before food preparation is essential, as well as separating diapering tables from those used for play and food preparation (Bonner & Dale, 1986).

Another infectious disease that has begun to affect children, including those in day-care, is hand, foot, and mouth disease. This coxsackievirus, which causes sores in the mouth and on hands and feet, is self-limiting. Cases were seen in day-care centers and schools in the eastern part of the United States during the summer of 1989. Good hand washing has been shown to minimize cross-infection of the disease (Raeburn, 1989).

The incidence of communicable diseases in day-care may be further decreased by the nurse implementing an educational program for caretakers to teach proper hand washing and use of equipment in the day-care center (Lewis, Gilliss, Pantell, & Holaday, 1989). Research has shown that the use of vinyl gloves and diaper changing pads during diaper changes decreases the cross-infection rates in day-care centers (Butz, Fosarelli, & Larson, 1989).

Secondary prevention: day-care centers for sick children. A real dilemma exists for parents when children who usually attend day-care centers cannot be admitted during acute illness or convalescence from minor surgery. The community health nurse should be sensitive to this concern as working parents try to arrange substitute care. Often the only alternative is that one parent must stay home from work to care for the ill youngster. Because children tend to have several illnesses each year, ranging from the common cold to influenza and chickenpox, the parent faces the loss of work days, which can result in loss of pay or even loss of job. Thus the child who is too ill to attend the day-care center must stay with a grandparent or other willing adult or at a baby-sitting service or, in extreme but by no means rare cases, stay home alone. The nurse would agree of course that the latter choice is unacceptable and, depending on the child's age, may even be illegal, and the former choice may not be feasible.

Choices now exist, in geographically limited areas, that provide a safe, reliable alternative. Special day-care centers are opening in some cities to provide care to children during acute illness. These agencies operate within a hospital or clinic setting, and nursing assistants supervised by registered nurses provide the care. Children usually are grouped by the nature of their illness; provision is made for isolation of children with contagious diseases.

The TLC Center at the Mercy Medical Center in Denver, Colorado, is such a center; it cares for children with minor illnesses in a set of rooms separate from the pediatric inpatient units of the hospital. Registered nurses and licensed practical nurses assess and supervise care of these children. The usual parental consent and emergency policies are in place, and the children receive prescribed medication that the parents have brought from home. The children, usually grouped by symptoms such as those of respiratory illness, are provided with the same aspects of care that they receive in the regular day-care center, such as opportunities for play, meals, naps, and appropriate systems of infection control (Donovan, 1986).

Tuscaloosa, Alabama, is served by a day-care center for ill children at the DCH Regional Medical Center. Similar to the TLC Center, this facility is housed in a unit separate from the pediatric unit of the hospital. It provides care and supervision by nursing assistants in consultation with a registered nurse for children from infancy through 15 years of age who have a minor illness or who have had minor surgery. Isolation facilities are available inasmuch as chickenpox is a common ailment of their clients. As in all centers, recreation is also provided (Harrison, Logan, Townsend, Yeatman, & Williams, 1987).

The community health nurse should become aware of the existence of such facilities in the area and thus be a source of referral for day-care centers and parents. The community health nurse also may serve as a consultant to or initiate the development of a day-care center for ill children. The need for such facilities is great. Given the large number of children of working parents in day-care centers, such facilities would be a welcome addition to any community. This is an excellent way of providing service to the community through nurse entrepreneurship.

Tertiary prevention: day-care for children with special needs. Nurses in the community may have the opportunity to consult with or provide nursing care for day-care centers whose main objective is to serve children with special needs. These children, once termed developmentally or physically handicapped, have the same needs as all children: the need for play, health promotion, and safety. Therefore nurses who serve these children practice the same assessment skills required in regular day-care centers. Some centers also serve as respite centers that care for handicapped children for a set period of time, such as one weekend, to provide parents and other care givers a break from day-to-day care. Thus these day-care centers may have regular clients who attend every day, as well as clients who attend only on certain days as respite clients. The nurse should carefully assess and assist those clients who attend on a one-time or occasional basis to the same degree that they care for the everyday clients.

The nurse should be aware of community agencies that specialize in helping families of children with special needs and be ready to recommend and assist parents in pursuing help from these agencies, for example, local offices of the Association for Retarded Children, Epilepsy Association, Inc., Muscular Dystrophy Association, the United Cerebral Palsy Association, Catholic Charities, and the United Way. To serve clients more fully the nurse should develop some connections with these agencies.

Recommended policies and procedures of the day-care center apply to these special facilities. Of special interest and concern to the nurse are the provision of ramps for wheelchair access to the building, ideally a one-floor plan or service by elevators, lavatories equipped for persons with handicaps, special eating utensils, and fire exits for wheelchairs.

An example of a day-care center for children with special needs is Medi-Kid, Inc. in Jacksonville, Florida. It provides day-care for ill children up to 5 years of age who have a long-term disease and gives convalescence care to children released from the hospital who are younger than 10 years of age. This facility, run by registered nurses with the consultive services of a part-time clinical nurse specialist, provides care for children with tracheostomies, gastrostomies, intravenous therapy, peritoneal dialysis, and other chronic diseases (Special day-care, 1986).

SUMMARY

The first five years of the child's life includes the infant, toddler, and preschool periods. Rapid physical and cognitive growth occurs as the child develops from a helpless infant to an independent person.

The community health nurse can promote the young child's development in a number of ways, including health education, accident and disease prevention, and client advocacy in cases of child abuse or neglect.

The nurse has the opportunity to interact with young children and their families in a variety of settings, including physicians' offices, ambulatory clinics, preschools, and day-care centers. The nurse's responsibilities can include caring for sick and injured children, preventing infection, screening for health problems, providing health and safety education, and helping the facility to comply with state and local licensing requirements. As more mothers of young children continue to be employed, the importance of the nurse's role in the day-care center is likely to increase.

CHAPTER HIGHLIGHTS

- The infant grows quickly in the first year of life, usually doubling birth weight within 6 months and tripling it within 1 year.
- According to Piaget the infant and toddler are in the sensorimotor stage of development and the preschooler is in the preoperational stage.
- According to Erikson, the infant is in the stage of trust versus mistrust and the toddler is in the stage of autonomy versus shame and doubt. The preschooler is in the stage of initiative versus guilt.
- Play is an important activity for children. Its functions include expressing feelings, learning cognitive skills, and socializing with others.
- The various types of play include unoccupied play, solitary play, onlooker behavior, parallel play, associative play, cooperative play, and fantasy play.
- The nurse must emphasize safety and educate children and their parents about the importance of accident prevention, particularly in motor vehicles and during outdoor play.
- Health problems among young children include iron deficiency anemia, dental problems, lead poisoning, and child abuse and neglect.
- The nurse can use play in health promotion with children. Therapeutic play is useful in preparing children for experiences such as hospitalization.
- Health screening of preschoolers includes screening for developmental, hearing, and vision problems.
- The nurse in a day-care center should be familiar with the center's policies and procedures. Procedures cover categories such as staff-to-child ratio, educational requirements of the staff, physical space and materials, safety procedures, nutrition, and health care and emergency treatment.
- In addition to using primary and secondary prevention to care for healthy children, the nurse also may use tertiary prevention to care for children with special needs.

STUDY QUESTIONS

1. On the basis of the stages of Piaget and Erikson, compare and contrast growth and development of infants and toddlers.
2. What are two major health problems facing infants, toddlers, and preschoolers? How can the nurse use primary, secondary, and tertiary prevention to prevent or treat these problems?
3. Give an example of a health-promotion activity that may be carried out with a preschooler and one that may be carried out with the parent of a preschooler.
4. How can the nurse promote the health of children in a day-care center?

REFERENCES

Aronson, S.S. (1985). Health care providers and day-care. In M.C. Sharp & F.W. Henderson (Eds.), *Day-care: Report of the sixteenth Ross roundtable on critical approaches to common pediatric problems* (pp. 71-82.) Columbus, OH: Ross Laboratories.

Aronson, S.S. (1986). Maintaining health in child care settings. In N. Gunzenhauser & B.M. Caldwell (Eds.), *Group care for young children: Considerations for child care and health professionals, public policy makers, and parents, Pediatric round table series, 12,* (pp. 137-146). New Brunswick, NJ: Johnson & Johnson Baby Products Co.

Berkelman, R., Guinan, M., & Thacker, S.B. (1989). What is the health impact of day care attendance on infants and preschoolers? *Public Health Reports, 104(1),* 101-103.

Blum, M. (1983). *The day-care dilemma: Women and children first.* Lexington, MA: Lexington Books.

Bonner, A., & Dale, R. (1986). *Giardia lamblia:* Day care diarrhea. *American Journal of Nursing, 86,* 818-820.

Brown, M.S., & Collar, M. (1982). Effects of prior preparation on the preschooler's vision and hearing screening. *MCN: American Journal of Maternal Child Nursing, 7,* 323-328.

Butz, A., Fosarelli, P., & Larson, E. (1989). Reduction of infectious disease symptoms in day care homes [Abstract]. *Proceedings of the 29th Annual Meeting of the Ambulatory Pediatric Association.* In *American Journal of Diseases of Children, 143,* 426.

Caldwell, B.M. (1986). Professional child care: A supplement to parental care. In N. Gunzenhauser & B.M. Caldwell (Eds.), *Group care for young children: Considerations for child care and health professionals, public policy makers, and parents, Pediatric round table series, 12,* (pp. 3-13). Skillman, NJ: Johnson & Johnson Baby Products Co.

Chang, A., Lugg, M.M., & Nebedum, A. (1989). Injuries among preschool children enrolled in day-care centers. *Pediatrics, 83,* 272-277.

Clemen-Stone, S., Eigsti, D.G., & McGuire, S.L. (1987). *Comprehensive family and community health nursing* (2nd ed.). New York: McGraw-Hill.

Dickey, S.B. (1987). *A guide to the nursing of children.* Baltimore: Williams & Wilkins.

Donovan, D. (1986). Hospital-based day care. *American Journal of Nursing, 86,* 1098.

Erikson, E.H. (1963). *Childhood and society* (2nd ed., rev.). New York: Norton.

Ferholt, J.D.L. (1980). *Clinical assessment of children: A comprehensive approach to primary pediatric care.* Philadelphia: Lippincott.

Fleming, J.M. (1986). Nursing education to meet child care needs. In N. Gunzenhauser & B.M. Caldwell (Eds.), *Group care for young children: Considerations for child care and health professionals, public policy makers, and parents, Pediatric round table series, 12,* (pp. 114-123). Skillman, NJ: Johnson & Johnson Baby Products Co.

Friedemann, M.L. (1983). *Manual for effective community health nursing practice.* Monterey, CA: Wadsworth.

Friedman, A.S., & Friedman, D.B. (1986). Interdisciplinary involvement in child care. I: The resources. In N. Gunzenhauser and B.M. Caldwell (Eds.), *Group care for young children: Considerations for child care and health professionals, public policy makers, and parents, Pediatric round table series, 12,* (pp. 124-131). Skillman, NJ: Johnson & Johnson Baby Products Co.

Gunzenhauser, N., & Caldwell, B.M. (Eds.). (1986). *Group care for young children: Considerations for child care and health professionals, public policy makers, and parents, Pediatric round table series, 12.* Johnson & Johnson Baby Products Co.

Hadler, S.C. (1985). Enteric infections in daycare centers. In M.C. Sharp & F.W. Henderson (Eds.), *Daycare: Report of the sixteenth Ross roundtable on critical approaches to common pediatric problems* (pp. 64-71). Columbus, OH: Ross Laboratories.

Harris, J.R., & Liebert, R.M. (1984). *The Child: Development from birth through adolescence.* Englewood Cliffs, NJ: Prentice-Hall.

Harrison, L., Logan, E., Townsend, J., Yeatman, P., & Williams, G. (1987). Establishing and evaluating a children's sick room program. *MCN: American Journal of Maternal Child Nursing, 12,* 204-206.

Harvard Child Health Project Task Force. (1977). *Developing a better health care system for children (Vol. 3).* Cambridge, MA: Ballinger.

Henderson, F.W. (1985). Respiratory infections and illnesses in daycare. In M.C. Sharp & F.W. Henderson (Eds.), *Daycare: Report of the sixteenth Ross roundtable on critical approaches to common pediatric problems* (pp. 47-52). Columbus, OH: Ross Laboratories.

Hinson, F. (1985). *Handbook of paediatric nursing.* Baltimore: Williams & Wilkins.

Kahn, A.J., & Kamerman, S.B. (1987). *Child care: Facing the hard choices.* Dover, MA: Auburn House.

Kotin, L., Crabtree, R.K., & Aidman, W.F. (1981). *Legal handbook for day care centers* (Administration for Children, Youth and Families, Office of Human Development Services). Washington, DC: U.S. Department of Health and Human Services (Contract No. 105-77-1083).

Leifer, G. (1982). *Principles and techniques in pediatric nursing* (4th ed.). Philadelphia: Saunders.

Lewis, C., Gilliss, C., Pantell, R., & Holaday, B. (1989). Reducing illness in child care centers [Abstract]. *Proceedings of the 29th Annual Meeting of the Ambulatory Pediatric Association.* In *American Journal of Diseases of Children, 143,* 426.

Long, L., & Long, T. (1983). *The handbook for latch-key children and their parents.* New York: Arbor House.

Mayer, G.G. (1981). Choosing daycare. *American Journal of Nursing, 81,* 346-348.

Meer, P.A. (1985). Using play therapy in outpatient settings. *MCN: American Journal of Maternal Child Nursing, 10,* 378-380.

Miller, C.A., Fine, A., Adams-Taylor, S., & Schorr, L.S. (1986). *Monitoring children's health: Key indicators.* Washington, DC: American Public Health Association.

Morgan, G. (1985). Child care options for working parents. In M.C. Sharp & F.W. Henderson (Eds.), *Daycare: Report of the sixteenth Ross roundtable on critical approaches to common pediatric problems* (pp. 4-12). Columbus, OH: Ross Laboratories.

Murray, K.A. (1984). Child care standards and monitoring. In M.C. Sharp & F.W. Henderson (Eds.), *Daycare: Report of the sixteenth Ross roundtable on critical approaches to common pediatric problems* (pp. 23-28). Columbus, OH: Ross Laboratories.

Murray, R.B., & Zentner, J.P. (1985). *Nursing assessment and health promotion through the life span* (3rd ed.). Englewood Cliffs, NJ: Prentice-Hall.

Nachem, B., & Bass, R.A. (1984). Children still aren't being buckled up. *MCN: American Journal of Maternal Child Nursing, 9,* 320-323.

Neuman, B. (1989). The Neuman systems model (2nd ed.). Norwalk, CT: Appleton & Lange.

O'Pray, M. (1980). Developmental screening tools: Using them effectively. *MCN: American Journal of Maternal Child Nursing, 5,* 126-130.

Piaget, J. (1978). *Success and understanding* (A.J. Pomerans. Trans.). Cambridge, MA: Harvard University Press. (Original work published 1974)

Raeburn, P. (1989, August 4). Contagious virus spreads minor childhood ailment. *The Buffalo News,* p. A4.

Rubin, R.R., & Fisher, J.J. III. (1982). *Ages three and four: Your preschooler.* New York: Macmillan.

Rustia, J., & Barr, L. (1985). Wanted: More health services in early-education programs. *MCN: American Journal of Maternal Child Nursing, 10,* 260-264.

Sharp, M.C., & Henderson, F.W. (Eds.). (1985). *Daycare: Report of the sixteenth Ross roundtable on critical approaches to common pediatric problems.* Columbus, OH: Ross Laboratories.

Special day-care. (1986). *Nursing 86, 16*(3), 87.

Wald, E.R., Dashefsky, B., Byers, C., Guera, N., & Taylor, F. (1988). Frequency and severity of infections in day care. *Journal of Pediatrics, 112,* 540-546.

Whaley, L.F., & Wong, D.L. (1987). *Nursing care of infants and children* (3rd ed.). St. Louis: Mosby.

Webb, N.B. (1984). *Preschool children with working parents: An analysis of attachment relationships.* Lanham, MD: University Press of America.

Wilson, C. & Steppe, S.C. (1986). *Investigating sexual abuse in day care.* Washington, DC: Child Welfare League of America.

The Child of Primary and Secondary School Age

JOAN M. COOKFAIR

My heart leaps up when I behold
A rainbow in the sky:
So was it when my life began;
So is it now I am a man

. . . .

The Child is father of the Man.   WILLIAM WORDSWORTH

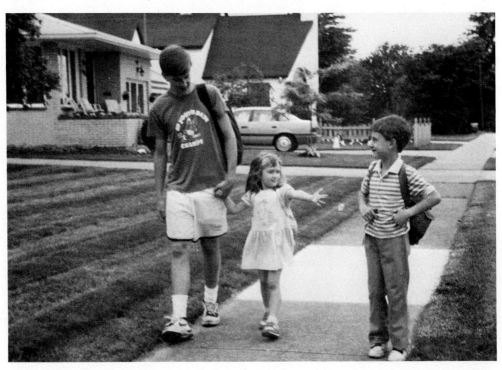

OBJECTIVES

At the conclusion of this chapter the student will be able to:
1. Define the key terms listed
2. Describe the normal growth and development of school-aged children
3. Identify causes of mortality and health problems that face children of primary and secondary school age
4. Discuss the roles of the community health nurse in the schools, historical and current
5. Apply Neuman's model to primary, secondary, and tertiary prevention of illness in school-aged children

KEY TERMS

Adolescence
Asthma
Congenital anomaly
Dental caries
Immunization
Immunoglobulin
Latchkey child
Menarche

Molestation
Morals
Puberty
School nursing
Scoliosis
Spermatogenesis
Tinea capitus
Turner syndrome
Values

The children pictured on the previous page appear to be in excellent health as they walk toward school, and they probably are. Normal growth and development in children, however, do not occur without nurturing and protection against trauma and disease. The openness on the face of the 5 year old, the energy radiating from the 7 year old, and the concern for them reflected on the face of the 15 year old will stay there only if the children remain physically and spiritually healthy.

The school-age years begin when the child is about 5 years old. It is a time when children need peer association and generally enjoy interaction with other children. At this age most healthy children, especially boys, are very active physically. The preadolescent period, between the ages of 9 and 12 years, is characterized by the development of friendships in groups, and/or with one special friend, usually of the same sex. Adolescence, which begins with puberty, is a time when the peer group strongly influences the individual. Puberty generally begins around ages 11 to 14 years for girls and 13 to 18 years for boys. Late adolescence (about 18 to 21 years) marks a time when the need for intimacy with a person of the opposite sex becomes paramount.

PHYSICAL GROWTH AND DEVELOPMENT OF THE PRIMARY-SCHOOL CHILD
Height and Weight

The average schoolchild grows from 2 to 2.5 inches (5 to 6 cm) per year and gains 1 to 2 feet (30 to 60 cm) by age 12 years. The average weight for a 6-year-old boy is 48

TABLE 10-1 Height and weight measurements for boys

Age*	Height by percentiles						Weight by percentiles					
	5		50		95		5		50		95	
	Cm	Inches	Cm	Inches	Cm	Inches	Kg	Lb	Kg	Lb	Kg	Lb
Birth	46.4	18¼	50.5	20	54.4	21½	2.54	5½	3.27	7¼	4.15	9¼
3 months	56.7	22¼	61.1	24	65.4	25¾	4.43	9¾	5.98	13¼	7.37	16¼
6 months	63.4	25	67.8	26¾	72.3	28½	6.20	13¾	7.85	17¼	9.46	20¾
9 months	68.0	26¾	72.3	28½	77.1	30¼	7.52	16½	9.18	20¼	10.93	24
1	71.7	28¼	76.1	30	81.2	32	8.43	18½	10.15	22½	11.99	26½
1½	77.5	30½	82.4	32½	88.1	34¾	9.59	21¼	11.47	25¼	13.44	29½
2†	82.5	32½	86.8	34¼	94.4	37¼	10.49	23¼	12.34	27¼	15.50	34¼
2½†	85.4	33½	90.4	35½	97.8	38½	11.27	24¾	13.52	29¾	16.61	36½
3	89.0	35	94.9	37¼	102.0	40¼	12.05	26½	14.62	32¼	17.77	39¼
3½	92.5	36½	99.1	39	106.1	41¾	12.84	28¼	15.68	34½	18.98	41¾
4	95.8	37¾	102.9	40½	109.9	43¼	13.64	30	16.69	36¾	20.27	44¾
4½	98.9	39	106.6	42	113.5	44¾	14.45	31¾	17.69	39	21.63	47¾
5	102.0	40¼	109.9	43¼	117.0	46	15.27	33¾	18.67	41¼	23.09	51
6	107.7	42½	116.1	45¾	123.5	48½	16.93	37¼	20.69	45½	26.34	58
7	113.0	44½	121.7	48	129.7	51	18.64	41	22.85	50¼	30.12	66½
8	118.1	46½	127.0	50	135.7	53½	20.40	45	25.30	55¾	34.51	76
9	122.9	48½	132.2	52	141.8	55¾	22.25	49	28.13	62	39.58	87¼
10	127.7	50¼	137.5	54¼	148.1	58¼	24.33	53¾	31.44	69¼	45.27	99¾
11	132.6	52¼	143.3	56½	154.9	61	26.80	59	35.30	77¾	51.47	113½
12	137.6	54¼	149.7	59	162.3	64	29.85	65¾	39.78	87¾	58.09	128
13	142.9	56¼	156.5	61½	169.8	66¾	33.64	74¼	44.95	99	65.02	143¼
14	148.8	58½	163.1	64½	176.7	69½	38.22	84¼	50.77	112	72.13	159
15	155.2	61	169.0	66½	181.9	71½	43.11	95	56.71	125	79.12	174½
16	161.1	63½	173.5	68¼	185.4	73	47.74	105¼	62.10	137	85.62	188¾
17	164.9	65	176.2	69¼	187.3	73¾	51.50	113½	66.31	146¼	91.31	201¼
18	165.7	65¼	176.8	69¼	187.6	73¾	53.97	119	68.88	151¾	95.76	211

From *Nursing care of infants and children* (3rd ed.) (p. 1847) by L.F. Whaley and D.L. Wong, 1987, St. Louis: Mosby. Copyright 1987 by The C.V. Mosby Co. Reprinted by permission. Adapted from National Center for Health Statistics (NCHS), Health Resources Administration, Department of Health, Education and Welfare, Hyattsville, MD. Conversion of metric data to approximate inches and pounds by Ross Laboratories.
*Years unless otherwise indicated.
†Height data include some recumbent length measurements, which makes values slightly higher than if all measurements had been of stature (standing height).

TABLE 10-2 Height and weight measurements for girls

	Height by percentiles						Weight by percentiles					
	5		50		95		5		50		95	
Age*	Cm	Inches	Cm	Inches	Cm	Inches	Kg	Lb	Kg	Lb	Kg	Lb
Birth	45.4	17¾	49.9	19¾	52.9	20¾	2.36	5¾	3.23	7	3.81	8½
3 months	55.4	21¾	59.5	23½	63.4	25	4.18	9¼	5.40	12	6.74	14¾
6 months	61.8	24¼	65.9	26	70.2	27¾	5.79	12¾	7.21	16	8.73	19¼
9 months	66.1	26	70.4	27¾	75.0	29½	7.00	15½	8.56	18¼	10.17	22½
1	69.8	27½	74.3	29¼	79.1	31¼	7.84	17¼	9.53	21	11.24	24¾
1½	76.0	30	80.9	31¾	86.1	34	8.92	19¾	10.82	23¾	12.76	28¼
2†	81.6	32¼	86.8	34¼	93.6	36¾	9.95	22	11.80	26	14.15	31¼
2½†	84.6	33¼	90.0	35½	96.6	38	10.80	23¾	13.03	28¾	15.76	34¾
3	88.3	34¾	94.1	37	100.6	39½	11.61	25½	14.10	31	17.22	38
3½	91.7	36	97.9	38½	104.5	41¼	12.37	27¼	15.07	33¼	18.59	41
4	95.0	37½	101.6	40	108.3	42¾	13.11	29	15.96	35¼	19.91	44
4½	98.1	38½	105.0	41¼	112.0	44	13.83	30½	16.81	37	21.24	46¾
5	101.1	39¾	108.4	42¾	115.6	45½	14.55	32	17.66	39	22.62	49¾
6	106.6	42	114.6	45	122.7	48¼	16.05	35½	19.52	43	25.75	56¾
7	111.8	44	120.6	47½	129.5	51	17.71	39	21.84	48¼	29.68	65½
8	116.9	46	126.4	49¾	136.2	53½	19.62	43¼	24.84	54¾	34.71	76½
9	122.1	48	132.2	52	142.9	56¼	21.82	48	28.46	62¾	40.64	89½
10	127.5	50¼	138.3	54½	149.5	58¾	24.36	53¾	32.55	71¾	47.17	104
11	133.5	52¼	144.8	57	156.2	61½	27.24	60	36.95	81½	54.00	119
12	139.8	55	151.5	59¾	162.7	64	30.52	67¼	41.53	91½	60.81	134
13	145.2	57¼	157.1	61¾	168.1	66¼	34.14	75¼	46.10	101¾	67.30	148¼
14	148.7	58½	160.4	63¼	171.3	67½	37.76	83¼	50.28	110¾	73.08	161
15	150.5	59¼	161.8	63¾	172.8	68	40.99	90¼	53.68	118¼	77.78	171½
16	151.6	59¾	162.4	64	173.3	68¼	43.41	95¾	55.89	123¼	80.99	178½
17	152.7	60	163.1	64¼	173.5	68¼	44.74	98¾	56.69	125	82.46	181¾
18	153.6	60½	163.7	64½	173.6	68¼	45.26	99¾	56.62	124¾	82.47	181¾

From *Nursing care of infants and children* (3rd ed.) (p. 1848) by L.F. Whaley and D.L. Wong, 1987, St. Louis: Mosby. Copyright 1987 by The C.V. Mosby Co. Reprinted by permission. Adapted from National Center for Health Statistics (NCHS), Health Resources Administration, Department of Health, Education and Welfare, Hyattsville, MD. Conversion of metric data to approximate inches and pounds by Ross Laboratories.

*Years unless otherwise indicated.

†Height data include some recumbent length measurements, which makes values slightly higher than if all measurements had been of stature (standing height).

pounds (21.5 kg), and the average height is 46 inches (117 cm). By age 12 years the average boy weighs approximately 88 pounds (40 kg) and is 59 inches (150 cm) tall. The average weight for a 6-year-old girl is 43 pounds (19.5 kg), and the average height is 45 inches (114.6 cm) tall. By age 12 the weight is appropriately 91 pounds (43.33 kg), and the height is 59¾ inches (15.5 cm). Statistically there is considerable difference in children of lower socioeconomic classes. They tend to be smaller in weight and height (Diseker, Whaley, & Wong, 1987). Although there is some genetic variation in height and weight, healthy children, by and large, fit somewhere in the normal range of the growth charts depicted in Tables 10-1 and 10-2.

Vital Signs

The normal temperature of a primary schoolchild is 98° to 98.6° F (36.7° to 37° C); the pulse rate typically is 70 to 80 beats per minute; the respiration rate is about 18 to 21 breaths per minute, and the blood pressure is 94 to 112 (systolic) and 56 to 60 (diastolic) mm Hg (Murray & Zentner, 1989).

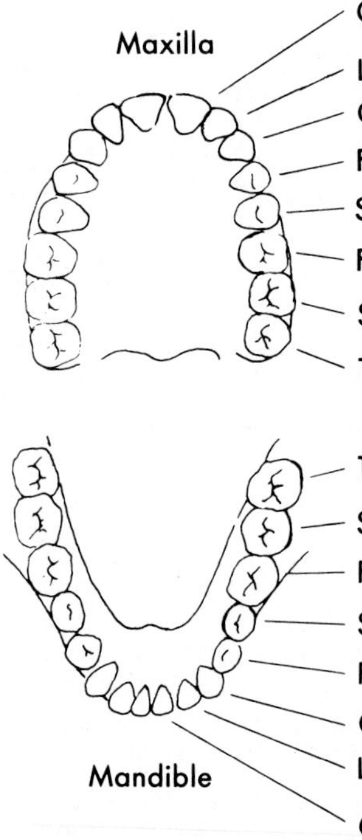

	Average age (months) of eruption of primary teeth	Average age (years) of shedding of primary teeth	Average age (years) of eruption of secondary teeth
Maxilla			
Central incisor	9.6	7.5	7.5
Lateral incisor	12.4	8.0	8.5
Canine	18.3	11.5	11.5
First premolar	15.7	10.5	10.5
Second premolar	26.3	10.5	11.1
First molar			6.3
Second molar			12.4
Third molar			17.0-21.0
Third molar			
Second molar			11.5
First molar			6.0
Second premolar	26.0	11.0	11.2
First premolar	15.1	10.0	10.3
Canine	18.2	9.5	10.1
Lateral incisor	11.5	7.0	7.5
Central incisor	7.8	6.0	6.4
Mandible			

FIG. 10-1 Sequence of eruption of secondary teeth. (*From* Nursing care of infants and children (*3rd ed.*) *by L.F. Whaley and D.L. Wong, 1987, St. Louis, Mosby. Copyright 1987 by the C.V. Mosby Company. Reprinted by permission.*)

Teeth

The young child begins to lose the "baby look" as the permanent teeth erupt. Fig. 10-1 shows the normal tooth formation in a child. During this time the jaw bone extends—more in boys than in girls—and the face assumes a more adult look (Murray & Zentner, 1989).

Other Signs of Physiological Maturation

Maturity of the gastrointestinal system results in fewer stomach upsets. By the time the child is 10 years of age, the kidneys have almost doubled in size. The normal farsightedness of the preschool child converts to 20/20 vision by age 8 years, and peripheral vision is fully developed. The immunoglobulins A and B (IgA and IgB) become functionally mature by preadolescence (around age 12 years). Maturation of the central nervous system results in a continuous improvement in coordination. Children grow less restless after 9 years of age and become more skillful in manual activities (Murray & Zentner, 1989).

Secondary sexual characteristics can become evident in the prepubertal period, with increased growth of body hair, increased perspiration, and active subaceous glands.

PHYSICAL GROWTH AND DEVELOPMENT OF THE SECONDARY-SCHOOL CHILD (ADOLESCENCE)
Height and Weight

During adolescence a growth spurt usually occurs. It begins earlier in girls than it does in boys. During this period girls grow 2.5 to 5 inches (6 to 12.5 cm) and gain 8 to 10 pounds (3.5 to 4.5 kg), whereas boys grow 3 to 6 inches (7.5 to 15 cm) and gain 12 to 14 pounds (5.5 to 6.5 kg). The most significant change during adolescence, however, is the onset of puberty.

Puberty

For girls menarche is the indicator of puberty. The average age of occurrence varies somewhat with population groups. In the United States the average age is 12.6 to 12.9 years; in Sweden, 12.9 years; in Italy, 12.5 years; and in Africa, 13.4 to 14.1 years (Murray & Zentner, 1989). Maturation of secondary sexual characteristics may take 2 to 8 years.

Spermatogenesis (formation of spermatozoa) and seminal emissions signal puberty in boys. Nocturnal emission (loss of seminal fluid during sleep) occurs at about age 14 years (Murray & Zentner, 1989). Around this time secondary sexual characteristics develop, such as increased body hair, enlarged penis and testes, and a deeper voice. Most boys begin to shave sometime during early adolescence.

Skin texture changes in both boys and girls. Sebaceous glands become extremely active . Sweat glands also become more active. Blood pressure increases to a range between 100/50 and 120/70 mm Hg. Pulse rates average 60 to 68 beats per minute, and the respiratory rate is 16 to 20 per minute (Murray & Zentner, 1989).

Boys typically have greater shoulder width than do girls, and their muscle growth continues later in adolescence because of androgen production. Muscle growth in girls is proportionate to the growth of other tissue. Adipose tissue distribution over thighs, buttocks, and breasts is related to estrogen production.

Gradually the physical characteristics of the adult develop in the adolescent. During the high school years rapid growth and hormonal change can predispose adolescents to identity confusion and periods of emotional lability. Certainly it is a time of rapid change in body image and in expectations regarding the place they will occupy in the family and society.

COGNITIVE DEVELOPMENT

Cognitive development is a process that depends on maturation, experience, social interaction, and internal regulation. It is influenced by innate intelligence, environment, and culture.

According to Jean Piaget (1963), primary school–aged children (ages 5 to 12 years) are in the concrete operational phase. They are able to classify objects and think logically. Children between the ages of 12 and 15 years enter the formal operational stage, when they begin to think in terms of concepts and abstractions. Exceptions to this progression are those children who are developmentally delayed or whose innate intelligence does not enable them to think conceptually.

PERSONALITY DEVELOPMENT

According to Erik Erikson (1963), for a child who has acquired self-trust and trust of others and has a sense of autonomy (see Chapter 9), starting school will mark a healthy beginning to the development phase known as initiative versus guilt. The young school-aged child wants to initiate action, be assertive, and stay fairly autonomous. Children who are unable or not allowed to develop initiative will acquire a sense of guilt, defeatism, and anger. A sense of guilt can be instilled by sibling rivalry, lack of opportunity to try things, repressive authoritarian control, or developmental lag (Murray & Zentner, 1989).

The developmental crisis of the older school-aged child revolves around a feeling that he or she can or cannot solve problems. Erikson calls this state industry versus inferiority. Repeated failure can give the individual a sense of inadequacy and defeat.

As the child in secondary school reaches adolescence, the developmental task, according to Erikson, is identity versus diffusion. How well the child accomplishes the development of a sense of identity depends on how well the developmental tasks that preceded it have been completed. Adolescents have the task of discovering who they are, where they are going, and what is the meaning of their lives. Successful accomplishment in these areas depends on earlier gender identity, parents, peers, social class, and prior successful resolution of developmental tasks. Identity diffusion, which results if the adolescent fails to achieve this sense of identity, can lead to alienation, insecurity, and antisocial behavior (Murray & Zentner, 1989).

MORAL AND SPIRITUAL DEVELOPMENT

Lawrence Kohlberg (1978) developed a theory of moral development that parallels Piaget's beliefs about cognitive development. In contrast to Piaget's stages, Kohlberg's stages are hierarchical and overlapping. *The first stage* (toddler to 7 years) is preconventional and based on an obedience versus punishment orientation. The child is good in order to avoid punishment. *Stage two* (preschool and school age) finds the child obeying rules in order to get something in return (reciprocity). *Stage three* (school age through adulthood) is the "good boy" or "nice girl" stage, in which behavior is controlled in an effort to gain acceptance. *Stage four* (also school age through adulthood) is the law-and-order stage wherein the individual focuses on maintaining social order and obeys the rules because they are there. *Stage five* is a more completely developed moral level. Individuals at this stage (middle adulthood) may work to change the law for the good of society. *Stage six,* or the universal-ethical principle of conscience orientation (middle and older adulthood), is the stage in which the individual makes decisions by self-chosen ethical principles (King, 1964). According to Kohlberg (1978), not all persons progress to stage six in moral development even if they achieve Piaget's description of the formal operational level. This degree of maturation depends on personality, education, and environment (King, 1984).

Values, or those ideals that are prized and chosen, are an inherent part of the culture in which a child matures. The family is the culture bearer (see Chapter 14), and values are reflected in the socially acceptable standards of behavior in a particular culture. Many families attend churches, synagogues, and other places of worship, and children are instructed in historical and contemporary spiritual concepts. Schools reflect the accepted norms within a culture. In recent times, television also has been proved to exert a powerful influence on a child's behavior patterns. Physical and emotional violence, shown to children before they develop a strong ego control, can thwart the development of positive values and healthy spirituality. Sexually seductive portrayals on television of instant physical satisfaction may provide an undesirable replacement for the teaching of traditional family values (Murray & Zentner, 1989). Parents should be advised to monitor the programs their children watch so that what the child observes is consistent with the family's value system.

MAJOR CAUSES OF MORTALITY AND ILLNESS

Accidents are the major cause of death in school-aged children. Malignant neoplasms and congenital anomalies rank second and third. Unfortunately, homicide ranks fourth among the 5 to 14 year age-group.

As the child progresses to adolescence and secondary school, accidents remain the major cause of death, with homicide and suicide second and third. Malignant neoplasms are fourth. Table 10-3 describes the latest age-ranked statistics of causes of death in children (National Center for Health Statistics, 1987).

Accidents

Many accidents that injure and kill children can be avoided. Seat belt laws should be enforced, and school instruction should include bicycle and skateboard safety awareness. The National Safety Council in 1987 recorded that 1450 children were killed in home fires between 1985 and 1986. Teaching children what to do in case of fire and emphasizing the use of smoke detectors can help to protect them if a fire should occur. Other accidents that threaten children are falls, drownings, and poisonings. Community health nurses, teachers, and other health professionals can help by promoting safety and increasing public awareness of these hazards to the lives and health of young children.

Chronic Illness and Congenital Anomalies

Chronic illnesses and disabilities in children include asthma, cystic fibrosis, diabetes mellitus, cerebral palsy, blindness, deafness, and cancer. Although some of these conditions remain stable, others may be progressive and even fatal. Many can cause impaired physical or mental functioning or may impede the child's physical or emotional development. In addition, a child's prolonged chronic illness or the anticipation of the loss of a child may significantly affect parents and siblings to the point where the nurse must assist the family, as well as the child, to cope with the disability.

The child with asthma is at added risk for infection, which can result in impaired oxygenation and anxiety. The child who is blind or deaf may be at risk for injury, impaired communication, and social isolation. A young child with diabetes mellitus may be at risk for infection, altered nutrition and in cases of noncompliance, even death. Children with developmental disability sometimes have difficulty as a result of immobility or altered coping.

TABLE 10-3 Deaths and death rates for the 10 leading causes of death in specified age-groups in the United States, 1987

Rank order	Cause of death and age*	No.	Rate
1-4 yr			
—	All causes	7,473	51.6
1	Accidents and adverse effects	2,921	20.2
	Motor vehicle accidents	989	6.8
	All other accidents and adverse effects	1,932	13.3
2	Congenital anomalies	924	6.4
3	Malignant neoplasms, including neoplasms of lymphatic and hematopoietic tissues	548	3.8
4	Homicide and legal intervention	334	2.3
5	Diseases of heart	322	2.2
6	Pneumonia and influenza	199	1.4
7	Meningitis	139	1.0
8	Certain conditions originating in the perinatal period	121	0.8
9	Human immunodeficiency virus infection	104	0.7
10	Septicemia	90	0.6
—	All other causes (residual)	1,771	12.2
5-14 yr			
—	All causes	8,743	25.6
1	Accidents and adverse effects	4.198	12.3
	Motor vehicle accidents	2,397	7.0
	All other accidents and adverse effects	1,801	5.3
2	Malignant neoplasms, including neoplasms of lymphatic and hematopoietic tissues	1,138	3.3
3	Congenital anomalies	448	1.3
4	Homicide	407	1.2
5	Diseases of heart	324	0.9
6	Suicide	251	0.7
7	Chronic obstructive pulmonary diseases and allied conditions	119	0.3
8	Pneumonia and influenza	94	0.3
9	Benign neoplasms, carcinoma in situ, and neoplasms of uncertain behavior and of unspecified nature	81	0.2
10	Cerebrovascular diseases	73	0.2
—	All other causes (residual)	1,610	4.7
15-24 yr			
—	All causes	38,023	99.4
1	Accidents and adverse effects	18,695	48.9
	Motor vehicle accidents	14,447	37.8
	All other accidents and adverse effects	4,248	11.1
2	Homicide and legal intervention	5,354	14.0
3	Suicide	4,924	12.9
4	Malignant neoplasms, including neoplasms of lymphatic and hematopoietic tissues	1,939	5.1

Modified from *Monthly vital statistics report* by the National Center for Health Statistics, 1987, Washington, DC: U.S. Department of Health and Human Services. (Pub. No. PHS 84-1232). Government Printing Office.
International classification of diseases (9th rev.), 1975.

TABLE 10-3 Deaths and death rates for the 10 leading causes of death in specified age-groups in the United States, 1987—cont'd

Rank order	Cause of death and age*	No.	Rate
15-24 yr—cont'd			
5	Diseases of heart	1,062	2.8
6	Congenital anomalies	499	1.3
7	Human immunodeficiency virus infection	492	1.3
8	Pneumonia and influenza	268	0.7
9	Cerebrovascular diseases	244	0.6
10	Chronic obstructive pulmonary diseases and allied conditions	209	0.5
—	All other causes (residual)	4,337	11.3

Cancer, the next leading cause, after accidents, of death in school-aged children can result in altered nutrition, fatigue, pain, feelings of powerlessness, and spiritual distress for the child and family.

Children who are seropositive for human immunodeficiency virus (HIV) may experience social isolation because of the extreme stigma connected with AIDS. Unless the child actually is ill, confidentiality and advocacy are appropriate responses by the nurse who supervises the care of the child.

The box on p. 218 lists numerous nursing diagnoses that can guide the nurse in planning interventions for care of the chronically ill school-aged child.

Homicide

Homicide, according to the National Center for Health Statistics (1983), is increasing in the 15 to 24 year old age-group. It occurs more often in highly stressed and disorganized families than in organized ones, and single-parent families are at high risk (Murray & Zentner, 1989). Physically and mentally handicapped children are at risk when parents become overwhelmed by the child's handicap. Although homicide is a consequence of various forms of violence, hand guns are the weapons most frequently used against older children, sometimes by each other (Murray & Zentner, 1989).

Child Abuse

Physical abuse of children is not a new phenomenon. Unfortunately, situations have always occurred in which child abuse results from actions of adults who themselves have altered coping mechanisms, are stressed, or honestly believe children are better behaved if corporal punishment is used. In 1871 the Society for the Prevention of Cruelty to Children was founded in New York City. Today all states have child protection laws and encourage residents to report suspected child abuse to police or child welfare agencies. Nurses and other health care professionals can be charged with criminal misdemeanor if they do not report known incidents (Creighton, 1986). Presently child abuse and neglect are increasing in the United States. The stresses of modern society and the increasing problems connected with alcohol abuse and drug abuse may be only two of many factors that lead to abuse. Studies have shown that adults who have been abused as children are

SELECTED NURSING DIAGNOSES RELATED TO THE SCHOOL AGE CHILD

Pattern 1: Exchanging

Altered nutrition: more than body requirements
Altered nutrition: less than body requirements
Altered nutrition: potential for more than body requirements
Potential for infection
Potential for injury
Potential for trauma
Potential impaired skin integrity

Pattern 2: Communicating

Impaired verbal communication

Pattern 3: Relating

Impaired social interaction
Social isolation

Pattern 4: Valuing

Spiritual distress

Pattern 5: Choosing

Ineffective individual coping
Impaired adjustment
Health seeking behaviors

Pattern 6: Moving

Impaired physical mobility
Fatigue
Sleep pattern disturbance
Diversional activity deficit
Bathing/hygiene self care deficit
Dressing/grooming self care deficit
Altered growth and development

Pattern 7: Perceiving

Body image disturbance
Self-esteem disturbance
Sensory/perceptual alterations
Hopelessness
Powerlessness

Pattern 8: Knowing

Knowledge deficit

Pattern 9: Feeling

Pain
Dysfunctional grieving
Anticipatory grieving
Anxiety
Fear

From "NANDA approved nursing diagnostic categories," by North American Nursing Diagnosis Association, Summer 1988, *Nursing Diagnosis Newsletter, 15*(1), p. 2. Copyright 1988 by NANDA. Reprinted by permission.

much more likely to be abusive to their children. Also, violence in the media may affect immature adults and older siblings adversely.

In the United States specific definitions of child abuse are established at the state level. Most state definitions are based on federal law, the Child Abuse Prevention and Treatment Act of 1974 (PL 93-247). Section 3 of the act defines abuse and neglect as:

> The physical and mental injury, sexual abuse, negligent treatment or maltreatment of a child under the age of 18 by a person who is responsible for the child's welfare under circumstances which indicate that the child's health and welfare is harmed or threatened thereby (Wissow, 1990, p. 1).

Nurses should be on the alert for sign of abuse such as multiple bruises, burns from immersion in hot water or lighted cigarettes, detached retinas, bruises to the head, and other unexplained injuries. In addition, children who fail to thrive despite absence of organic illness should be thoroughly checked and followed up.

There is no predictable profile for the family of an abused child. Both stress and psychological history are factors. Children left in the care of older siblings sometimes are at risk; at high risk are children in single-parent families, particularly if the parent is young. Surveillance, follow-up, reporting, education, and providing parents with access to support groups can be helpful. Occasionally it is necessary to remove the child from the environment temporarily or permanently.

Sexual Molestation

The use of a powerless child for purposes of adult sexual gratification includes fondling the child's genitals, incest, rape, oral contact, and exhibitionism (Murray & Zentner, 1989). Children frequently do not tell their parents about the sexual abuse of siblings or neighbors because they fear reprisal.

The child or adolescent may not report an incident of pressured sexual activity with an older family member because of feelings of shame. In contemporary society coercion by force and drugs sometimes occurs. The nature of sexual activity, especially with children, is so insidious that on some occasions they are unaware of wrongdoing. Children generally believe adults who tell them that something is "all right to do." Sometimes the sexual offender will make sure the contact is pleasurable so that the child feels wanted and loved. Older children, particularly adolescent girls, in distress because of difficult home situations that sometimes result in their running away often are defenseless and thus severely traumatized when singled out as helpless victims.

Sexual molestation can be avoided or minimized by various means. Education of youngsters as early as possible in the realities of the need for self-protection can be helpful. Support groups for immature parents and follow-up of child molestation cases can protect vulnerable school-aged children to some extent. Well-publicized shelters for troubled teens and outreach school programs for counseling of families can be effective.

Latchkey Children

Of growing concern to health professionals is the latchkey child, that is, the child who has the door key because no one is home when the child returns from school (Murray & Zentner, 1989). This phenomenon appears to result from the growth in the number of single-parent families and two-career households. Teaching children survival skills may decrease the number of accidents, injuries from fire, and sexual molestation by persons who become aware that the child is at home alone.

MENTAL HEALTH

The school-aged child undergoes daily stress and anxiety. Yet the need to experience success, establish a firm identity, and be socially accepted are driving forces in a young child. The attainment of life goals and fulfillment of emotional, moral, and spiritual development are desirable. However, poor health, lack of self-esteem, and other unmet needs may make it difficult for the school-aged child to experience success. In one research study (see box) 500 elementary school staff members identified the following unmet needs of their students: poor decision-making and problem-solving skills, poor self-image, low self-confidence, and inability to solve interpersonal conflicts.

Suicide

Depression may occur in schoolchildren whose scholastic performance or social interaction, or both, do not measure up to their own or their parents' expectations. The result may be a rise of the incidence of suicide in this age-group. Children younger than 5 years of age generally are not afraid of death. If abused, they may have guilt feelings for causing their parents trouble. As they become older, they may form attitudes that reflect a feeling such as "you'll be sorry when I'm gone" (Newton, 1984). Children from unstable or broken homes are at high risk for depression, which can take the form of hostility, delinquency, or dare-devil or self-destructive behavior. The incidence of suicide in adolescents between the ages of 12 and 19 years also is rising. Community health nurses should be alert for danger signals such as the following (Newton, 1984):

1. Writing of notes or poetry with themes related to death
2. Giving away prized possessions
3. Repeated serious trauma (burns or accidents)
4. Family history of suicide.

Health professionals who observe such signals might consider intervention on the child's behalf and referral for counseling and family assistance.

Teen-age Pregnancy

Various theories have been advanced to explain the epidemic-like increase in teen-age pregnancy in the United States. Some blame the media for exposing young people to suggestive sexual material. Rarely are responsible sex, the use of contraceptives, and birth control information discussed. Other factors that influence teen-age pregnancy are the strong sex drive in the teen years, rebellion over authority, lack of responsibility because of identity diffusion, the need to be close to someone, and relief from loneliness (Murray & Zentner, 1989). Pregnant teen-agers frequently have low birth weight babies and are apt to receive a minimum of prenatal care. Consequently, education on responsible birth control and more responsible media programming would be helpful to decrease this maladaptive response to a stressful environment and a culture that is in a period of rapid change.

Alcohol and Drug Abuse

Drug abuse is a common and frightening phenomenon in contemporary America. The romanticizing of the drug culture by segments of the media, the availability of drugs, and the stress on children to excel in our culture appear to contribute to the problem. Media reports indicate that schoolchildren, adolescents, and young adults increasingly are using toxic drugs that result in addiction. Most nurses are familiar with barbiturates and mar-

RESEARCH STUDY

More than 500 elementary school personnel from a large Colorado school district provided perceptions of the unmet needs of their students, the likely causes of the needs and suggestions about solutions or programs to meet the needs. The district's definition of mental health—positive self-image, healthy interrelationships with peers and adults and acquisition of school skills and competencies—guided the questionnaire design. Respondents perceived numerous unmet mental health needs, most involving about 15% of the student population. The most frequently perceived problems were poor decision-making and problem-solving skills, poor self-image, low self-confidence, inability to resolve interpersonal conflicts, depression/unhappiness, low motivation, and various conduct disorders. Further, most respondents believed children's unmet mental needs are increasing, and the causes for most problems are family- and home-related, but most suggested solutions were *school based.* Recommendations include increasing the involvement of school nurses in programs aimed at improving children's mental health.

From "The mental health needs of elementary school children" by L. W. Goodwin and J. Cantrell, 1988, *Journal of School Health, 58,* p. 282. Copyright 1988 by the American School Health Association. Reprinted by permission.

ijuana, but a newer agent, "crack," or "rock," a form of cocaine, is especially dangerous and addictive. It may cause heart or respiratory failure and result in death. One experiment with crack may result in addiction. The box on p. 222 outlines some of the behaviors seen in children and adolescents who are abusing drugs. Schoolchildren often begin to use alcohol as a result of such stresses as peer pressure or lack of self-confidence.

For the young adolescent who is experimenting with drugs or alcohol, a counseling session with the family may be in order. The child with a supportive family may be helped by making a "no use" contract with the parents and being referred for regular family counseling sessions. The nurse should provide emotional support to the child and the family. The child who does not have a supportive family or who is beyond the experimentation stage may need hospitalization for withdrawal, treatment, and intensive counseling.

THE COMMUNITY HEALTH NURSE IN THE SCHOOLS
Historical Perspective

Lillian Wald was instrumental in establishing one of the first school nursing programs. She perceived public health nursing as having a strong educational component and in 1902 appointed Lina Rogers Struthers to serve four New York City schools. Struthers visited sick children in the home and taught parents how to care for them to prevent further illness. In every school she visited, absence because of illness decreased. Shortly thereafter the New York City school board hired 25 more nurses (Wold, 1981).

From the early development of the school nursing role during the 1920s and 1930s (Table 10-4) until the Second World War school nurses continued to develop their role in three areas: medical inspection, medical examination, and health education. The shortage of nurses during the war necessitated the delegation of many school nursing services to volunteers and assistants. Nurses continued to educate families by making home visits and providing in-service training to teachers, but screening tests such as those for vision, hearing, and weight were performed by others.

DRUG-RELATED BEHAVIOR

Primary and general signs of drug abuse in the young person include:

- Decrease in quality of school work without a valid reason. Reasons given may be boredom, not caring about school, not liking the teachers.
- Personality changes, behaving in unexpected ways; becoming more irritable, less attentive, less affectionate, secretive, unpredictable, uncooperative, apathetic, depressed, withdrawn, hostile, sullen, easily provoked, oversensitive.
- Less responsible behavior, not doing chores or school homework, school tardiness or absenteeism, forgetful of family occasions such as birthdays.
- Change in activity, antisocial pattern, no longer participating in family activities, school or church functions, sports, prior hobbies, or organizational activities.
- Change in friends, new friends who are unkempt in appearance or sarcastic in their attitude; the youth is secretive or protective about these friends, not giving any information.
- Change in appearance or dress, in vocabulary, music tastes to match that of new friends, imitating acid rock and roll stars.
- More difficult to communicate with, refuses to discuss friends, activities, drug issues; insists it is all right to experiment with drugs; defends rights of youth, insists adults hassle youth; prefers to talk about bad habits of adults.
- Irrational behavior, frequent explosive episodes, driving recklessly, unexpectedly stupid behavior.
- Loss of money, credit cards, checks, jewelry, household silver, coins, in the home that cannot be accounted for.
- Addition of drugs, clothes, money, albums, tapes, or stereo equipment that are suddenly found in the home.
- Presence of whisky bottles, marijuana seeds or plants, hemostats, rolling papers, drug buttons, and marijuana lead buttons. There may also be unusual belt buckles, pins, bumper stickers, or T-shirts, and the *High Times* magazine in the car, truck, or home.
- Preoccupation with the occult, various pseudo-religious cults, satanism, or witchcraft; and evidence of tattoo writing of 666, drawing of pentagrams on self or elsewhere, or misrepresentation of religious objects.
- Signs of physical change or deterioration; including pale face; dilated pupils; red eyes; chewing heavily scented gum; using heavy perfumes; using eye wash or drops to remove the red; heightened sensitivity to touch, smell or taste; weight loss, even with increased appetite (marijuana smoking causes the "munchies"—extra snacking).
- Signs of mental change or deterioration, including disordered thinking or illogical patterns, decreased ability to remember or in rapid thought processes and responses, severe lack of motivation.

From *Nursing assessment and health promotion strategies through the life span* (4th ed.) (p. 368) by R. Murray and J. Zenter, 1989, Norwalk, CT: Appleton & Lange. Copyright 1989 by Appleton & Lange. Reprinted by permission.

During the 1950s the number of preschool children increased because of the post—World War II baby boom. The complexity of school nursing duties is emphasized by the following definition: "School nursing is a varying combination of what an administrator wants, teachers expect, students need, parents demand, the community is accustomed to, the situation requires, and the nurse believes" (Gair, 1966, p. 401).

Economic circumstances and resultant budget cutbacks in the 1970s compelled school boards to decrease the number of school nurses. Once again, nurses were obliged

TABLE 10-4 The developing role of the school nurse during the 1920s and 1930s

Phase	School health program activity	Goal	School nurse's role
I	Medical inspection	Control of contagion	Assist school physician *or* independently inspect children in classroom Visit home for follow up
II	Medical examination	Identification of physical defects	Assist school physician with examination Disability limitation through correction of defects
III	Medical inspection Medical examination	Same as for phase II	Same as for phase II
	Health education	Student attainment of responsible health behavior	Stage one: develop and implement own health education program Stage two: incorporate health education program into teacher's program
		Student and parental attainment of responsible health behavior	Stage three: mutual planning of health education program by teacher and nurse

From *School nursing: A framework for practice* (p. 8) by S. J. Wold, 1981, St. Louis: Mosby. Copyright 1981 by The C.V. Mosby Co. Reprinted by permission.

to delegate tasks, particularly screening programs. Although this alternative appears to be a desirable cost-saving measure, in reality it denies the nurse access to the student and interferes with the development of rapport and the management of health surveillance by a trained professional. A vision and screening session can be an isolated technical process, or it can be an opportunity for the student to communicate a problem to the nurse or for the nurse to observe the student. The entry of professionals such as social workers began to create overlap and ambiguity in the school nurse's role (Wold, 1981).

Another factor that contributes to the ambiguity of the nursing role is the absence of uniform guidelines regarding the educational preparation of the school nurse. Some school districts require only R.N. licensure to cover minimum legal requirements. Others require certification in health education, guidance and counseling, parenting, vision and screening, and control of communicable disease, in addition to a baccalaureate degree. Still others require certification as a school nurse practitioner (Jarvis, 1985).

Regardless of the complexity or ambiguity of the role, school nursing is a critically important community health nursing specialty that can contribute to the health of schoolchildren in a significant way. If school nurses hope to achieve that goal, they need to establish guidelines, set up protocols, and assertively work with parents and teachers to assist the child in primary and secondary school through a difficult final decade of the century and into the year 2000.

Health Promotion in the Schools

Health promotion in the schools can be planned at primary, secondary, and tertiary levels. Chapter 3 contains an explanation of nursing theorist Betty Neuman's interpretation of

TABLE 10-5 Format for prevention as intervention

Nursing action		
Primary prevention	Secondary prevention	Tertiary prevention
1. Classify stressors that threaten stability of the client/client system. Prevent stressor invasion.	1. Follow stressor invasion, protect basic structure.	1. During reconstitution, attain and maintain maximum level of wellness or stability following treatment.
2. Provide information to retain or strengthen existing client/client system strengths.	2. Mobilize and optimize internal/external resources to attain stability and energy conservation.	2. Educate, reeducate, and/or reorient as needed.
3. Support positive coping and functioning.	3. Facilitate purposeful manipulation of stressors and reaction to stressors.	3. Support client/client system toward appropriate goals.
4. Desensitize existing or possible noxious stressors.	4. Motivate, educate, and involve client/client system in health care goals.	4. Coordinate and integrate health service resources.
5. Motivate toward wellness.	5. Facilitate appropriate treatment and intervention measures.	5. Provide primary and/or secondary preventive intervention as required.
6. Coordinate and integrate interdisciplinary theories and epidemiological input.	6. Support positive factors toward wellness.	
7. Educate or reeducate.	7. Promote advocacy by coordination and integration.	
8. Use stress as a positive intervention strategy.	8. Provide primary preventive intervention as required.	

Copyright © 1980 by Betty Neuman. Revised 1987 by Betty Neuman.

Note: A first priority for nursing action in each of the areas of prevention as intervention is to determine the nature of stressors and their threat to the client/client system. Some general categorical functions for nursing action are initiation, planning, organization, monitoring, coordinating, implementing, integrating, advocating, supporting, and evaluating. An example of a limited classification system for stressors is illustrated by the following four categories: (1) deprivation, (2) excess, (3) change, and (4) intolerance.

these concepts. Primary prevention reduces the possibility of encounters with stressors, thereby strengthening the flexible line of defense. Secondary prevention centers around early case finding and prompt treatment of symptoms, whereas tertiary prevention involves readaptation, reeducation to avoid further occurrences, and maintenance of stability (Neuman, 1989). Table 10-5 further expands the concept of primary, secondary, and tertiary prevention and details methods of implementing the concept.

Primary prevention
Immunizations. Identifying stressors that may threaten the stability of the school-aged child can be accomplished by ongoing assessment. For example protection is available for certain communicable diseases. As children enter school, parents should be interviewed regarding the status of the child's immunizations. If immunizations are not up-to-date, the child will need to begin to receive them. The schedule most often used

TABLE 10-6 Recommended schedule for active immunization of normal infants and children*

Recommended age	Immunization(s)†	Comments
2 mo	DTP, OPV	Can be initiated as early as age 2 wk in areas of high endemicity or during epidemics
4 mo	DTP, OPV	2-mo interval desired for OPV to avoid interference from previous dose
6 mo	DTP	A third dose of OPV is not indicated in the U.S. but is desirable in geographic areas where polio is endemic
15 mo	Measles, mumps, rubella (MMR)	MMR preferred to individual vaccines; tuberculin testing may be done at the same visit
18 mo	DTP,‡§ OPV,‖ PRP-D	See footnotes
4-6 yr	DTP,¶ OPV	At or before school entry
11-12 yr	MMR	Second dose recommended in December, 1989
14-16 yr	Td	Repeat every 10 yr throughout life

Adapted from *Report of the Committee on Infectious Diseases* (21st ed.) by the American Academy of Pediatrics, 1988, Elk Grove Village, IL: AAP. Copyright 1988 by the American Academy of Pediatrics. Reprinted by permission.

*For all products used, consult manufacturer's package insert for instructions for storage, handling, dosage, and administration. Biologics prepared by different manufacturers may vary, and package inserts of the same manufacturer may change from time to time. Therefore, the physician should be aware of the contents of the current package insert.

†DTP = diphtheria and tetanus toxoids with pertussis vaccine; OPV = oral poliovirus vaccine containing attenuated poliovirus types 1, 2, and 3; MMR = live measles, mumps, and rubella viruses in a combined vaccine (see text for discussion of single vaccines versus combination); PRP-D = *Haemophilus* b diphtheria toxoid conjugate vaccine; Td = adult tetanus toxoid (full dose) and diphtheria toxoid (reduced dose) for adult use.

‡Should be given 6 to 12 mo after the third dose.

§May be given simultaneously with MMR at age 15 months.

‖May be given simultaneously with MMR at 15 mo of age or at any time between 12 and 24 mo of age.

¶Up to the seventh birthday.

is that of the American Academy of Pediatrics (Table 10-6). Note that after 6 years of age pertussis immunization no longer is necessary.

Education as to the importance of immunizations may be necessary with some groups, such as refugee families and others for whom English is not a primary language. In addition, some children should not be immunized. For example, a child who is ill and receiving steroid therapy or chemotherapy has depressed immunity and should not receive live attenuated vaccines such as those for measles, mumps, rubella, and poliomyelitis. Adolescent girls should be immunized against rubella only when they are menstruating. In addition, the nurse must explain the necessity for adequate contraception 3 months after immunization because of the danger of the rubella virus or of any attenuated vaccine to the fetus should pregnancy occur (Whaley & Wong, 1987). Immunizations never should be given during a severe febrile illness. A final contraindication to immunization is a history of allergic response to a previous vaccine.

Parents and children of responsible age must be fully informed of the reasons for the immunizations, the importance of their use, the contraindications, and the possible side effects. Verbal explanations reinforced by literature to take home (bilingual, if necessary) contribute to compliance and cooperation to prevent stressor invasion before it can threaten the child's stability (Neuman, 1989).

Accident prevention. Accidents remain the major cause of mortality in children. Thus the provision of educational programs to parents and children is particularly important in reducing the number of preventable incidents.

One "kid safe" program was developed by an advertising agency and marketed across the country. Doctor's Medical Center in Modesta, California, implemented the program with the use of hospital personnel and volunteers. Organized by a group of nurse managers, it was held on four consecutive Saturdays. Featured were health and safety information booths, classes in first aid, fire safety, baby sitting, and personal safety. The sensitive topics of molestation and how to avoid abduction were taught by means of puppet shows. More

---

TABLE 10-7 Social behavior development of the school-aged child and the adolescent

Age (yr)	Typical behaviors
6	Constant activity, enjoys group activities; spontaneously dramatic; indecisive, explosive behavior and rudeness; strict literal conscience; cheating common; behaves differently at school than at home; eager to learn and help out
7	Cautious in play; self-critical; anxious to do things right; talkative, uses expressive language; beginning to understand time and money; assumes responsibility; concerned about what is right and wrong; sensitive to feelings of others; concerned about fairness; aware of sexuality; modest
8	Seeks out and initiates group activity; accepts responsiblity with greater ease; friendships are tenuous but enthusiastic; segregated by sex; begins to collect items; can recognize individual differences; begins self-evaluation; relates to past and present (time concepts); begins to resent authority of parents but needs their support
9	Generally responsible and dependable; more reasonable and independent; period of peer group and conformity, as well as hero worship; begins to see parents more realistically (e.g., they can be wrong); expanding interests; increased ability to plan and to see a project through to completion; self-sufficient and self-critical; strong sense of right and wrong; increased awareness of sexuality and reproduction
10	Cooperative projects and activities dominate; follows and submits to rules; friends of same sex; companions and activities most important; beginning of sexual maturation for girls; girls more socially mature than boys; develops distinct hobbies and interests; continues to appraise parents
11-12	Development of "best friends"; feelings of opposition and dislike for opposite sex; characteristic sexual maturation more apparent, especially for girls; increase in physical and intellectual curiosity; group or clubs popular; secretive, demands privacy yet can be unruly, slovenly, and disrespectful; ambivalent feelings regarding parents and independence versus dependence; may develop annoying overt behaviors, e.g., hair twirling and nail biting
13-18	Vacillation and ambivalence; family relationships supportive but tumultuous; peer relationships intense but unstable; develops skills in individual and group relationships; increasing involvement with opposite sex; developing independence, self-image; becoming more responsible; discovering reality of world

From *Ambulatory pediatrics for nurses* (2nd ed.) (pp. 251,252) by M. S. Brown and M. A. Murphy, 1981, New York: McGraw-Hill. Copyright 1981 by McGraw-Hill Book Co. Modified by permission.

than 995 children and 500 adults attended. This innovative method of health promotion can be adapted for use in the schools and the classroom. Enlisting the aid of parents and teachers might further ensure the success of the program (Moore, Strickland, Melcher, & Walker, 1988).

Mental health. All through the school-aged child's developmental stages, care must be taken to reinforce positive coping and functioning. Parents should be educated as to what constitutes normal behavior in children at different ages. For example, if parents understand that explosive behavior and rudeness are common in a 6-year-old, they may attempt to suppress it less punitively to avoid overstressing the child and triggering hostile feelings. Table 10-7 lists some typical behavior patterns in children from ages 6 through 18 years. Sharing this information with parents, teachers, and social workers might help them support the child's positive coping and functioning rather than overreact to such typical developmental experiences as the 9-year-old's resentment of authority.

Alcohol and drug dependence. The school nurse can institute educational programs about the harmful effects of drugs. Special attention should be paid to adolescents who do not appear to be accepted by any particular group. Helping to form youth groups and school clubs and teaching the importance of keeping the body healthy can make a significant difference in the positive adjustment of school-aged children. The nurse also can educate parents and encourage them to be positive role models for their children, and to work actively to reduce the presence of drugs in the neighborhood.

Wellness motivating. Chapter 4 describes concepts of health and wellness. Nurses can provide instruction on such topics as nutrition counseling and positive coping skills. These sessions require a creative approach and careful planning if they are to hold the students' interest.

Inviting parents to weekly coffee hours to provide orientation and guidance and to answer questions about their children can be an effective way to motivate families toward wellness behavior. In addition, networking with teachers and administrators to form an active advocacy group to serve the developmental needs of the children will clearly establish the nurse's role. Finally, providing information to teachers who have questions about children and being available to listen to their concerns and anxieties will establish rapport and ensure their assistance if it is needed.

Secondary prevention. Secondary prevention involves identification of a stressor (early diagnosis) so that treatment can be prescribed to limit disability. One method is to set up screening programs for populations at risk for specific disease and disability. Those individuals who are identified as having early symptoms or changes in healthy body functioning can be referred for treatment or counseling. Most important, appropriate treatment and intervention methods can be set in motion.

All children should have a thorough physical examination before they begin school. Whether the setting is a school health office, a private practitioner's office, or a well child clinic, the procedure should be well organized and the results carefully recorded for later reference. These data provide a baseline for following a child's development so that any deviation from their norm can be quickly noted.

Height and Weight. Height and weight should be assessed yearly. Young children who are not growing normally according to the growth charts (Tables 10-1 and 10-2) may be experiencing an inadequate intake of calories. Poor muscular development and hypochromic anemia may result. Less than normal weight also may be a symptom of undiagnosed disease. Weight that is below or above normal may be a sign of malnutrition in older children. There also may be some physiological or behavioral disease process occurring such as anorexia nervosa or bulimia in underweight children or overweight.

Any deviation from the norm either in the initial physical examination or as the child develops is a reason for referral for medical evaluation.

Physiological measurements. Temperature, pulse, respiration rate, and blood pressure should be taken yearly. A chronic low-grade fever, for example, may indicate a low-grade chronic infection or other underlying disease. In addition, checking the apical pulse in young children may uncover a congenital defect previously missed. On the other hand, consistent tachycardia may indicate an anxiety state. All children with abnormal vital signs should be referred for medical follow-up.

Blood pressure testing is especially necessary in children; an increase, particularly in diastolic pressure, could be the first indication of renal disease.

The physical examination includes the general appearance of the child, for example, facial expression, skin turgor, hygiene, nutrition, overall body language, clothing, and attitude. Results that may require further investigation should be recorded. The skin is assessed not only for turgor but for rashes, bruises, and texture. At this time it is prudent to question the child about bruises, keeping in mind the facts that child abuse is a frequent problem in the United States and that failure to report it is considered a criminal misdemeanor in most states (Northrop & Kelly, 1987).

The discovery of enlarged lymph nodes during a physical assessment is a reason for

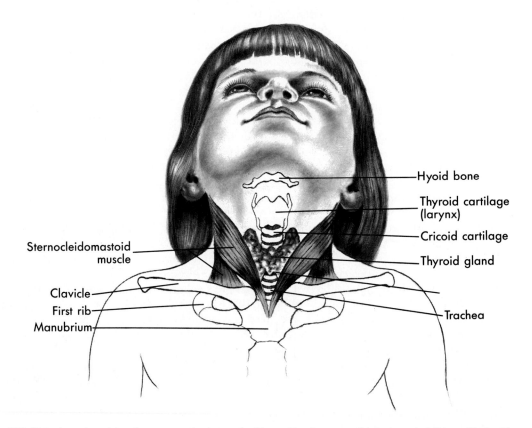

FIG. 10-2 Anterior view of structures in the neck. *(From* Nursing care of infants and children *(3rd ed.) (p. 240) by L.F. Whaley and D.L. Wong, 1987, St. Louis, Mosby. Copyright 1987 by The C.V. Mosby Company. Reprinted by permission.)*

referring a child for a medical examination. This condition may be a symptom of mild infection or of something more severe.

The head is inspected for general shape, symmetry, and range of motion. Limited range of motion may indicate wryneck, or torticollis, as a result of an injury to the sternocleidomastoid muscle. The scalp is examined for head lice (pediculosis), ticks, trauma, and ringworm (tinea capitis).

The nurse also should look for a short webbed neck (Turner's syndrome), edema of the neck, and distended neck veins, which may indicate breathing problems in females.

Checking the teeth for dental caries (decay), the tonsils for chronic infection, and the oral cavity in general should be part of a routine physical examination. The nurse should stress to the parent the need to take proper care of the baby teeth.

Fig. 10-2 illustrates the normal structures of the neck. Deviations from the norm should be referred for medical follow-up.

The chest should be inspected for the normal development of pulmonary function and skeletal formation. Assessment includes such factors as size, shape, movement, and breath sounds (Whaley & Wong, 1987).

Vision testing. Examination of the eyes before the child starts school is of utmost importance. Routine vision testing for binocularity, visual acuity, peripheral vision, and

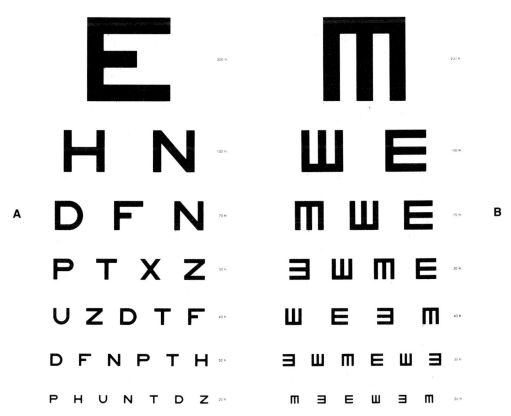

FIG. 10-3 Snellen chart. **A,** Letter (alphabet) chart. **B,** Symbol E chart. *(Courtesy National Society to Prevent Blindness, Shaumberg, IL.)*

color vision can facilitate correction of problems that may cause learning difficulty when the child begins to read.

Binocularity is the ability to fixate on one visual field with both eyes. Nonbinocularity that is uncorrected by the time the child is 4 to 6 years of age can cause amblyopia, vision impairment such as blindness in one eye. Children with this problem should be referred to an ophthalmologist for further testing.

Visual acuity is the ability to see near and far objects clearly. Nurses usually use the Snellen chart (Fig. 10-3) to measure acuity in young children. The chart has nine lines of objects or letters in decreasing size. The child is positioned 20 feet from the chart. Each line is given a value; for example, line eight is 20. If the child can see line eight well, the vision is said to be 20/20, or normal acuity. The youngster who can read only line two, has visual acuity of 20/100. Children with the following test results should be referred or retested to validate the findings:

1. A 4 or 5 year old with a visual acuity of 20/40 or less
2. A child older than 5 years with a visual acuity of 20/30 or less
3. Any child suspected of having strabismus
4. Any child suspected of having cataracts

Children should be tested for acuity on a yearly basis. Older children are tested by means of a Snellen chart that contains letters other than E's.

Strabismus refers to constant misalignment of the two eyes. It seldom affects vision but can cause vision fatigue that inhibits learning. The nurse screens for strabismus by assessing the student's ability to keep both eyes aligned on a small object as it moves medially from about 16 inches away inward to the nose. Referral for misalignment can result in correction of the problem before a reading lag occurs or grades drop (Hall & Wick, 1988).

Hearing. Early intervention for hearing loss can prevent delay, in language development and behavioral problems. Annual testing of children in kindergarten and grades one through three is recommended, and some include annual testing through junior high school. In addition, children with chronic or recurring ear infections should be tested. Auditory screening for hearing loss can be performed by *threshold testing,* which establishes the lowest-volume (intensity) level at which a child can hear tones of a given frequency, and *sweep check testing,* which establishes which frequencies can be heard when the volume remains fixed (Wold, 1981, p. 303). The nurse should suspect a hearing

---

RESEARCH STUDY

In the Victoria, Texas school district 610 high school students were screened for elevated cholesterol levels. Eighteen percent were found to have cholesterol levels above 180 mg/dl. Mean cholesterol values were higher for (1) female than for male students and for (2) black and Hispanic students than for white students. Follow-up questionnaires indicated that students and their parents understood the basic relationship between cholesterol and cardiovascular disease and how to modify the diet to reduce cholesterol intake. Telephone contact with parents of students with elevated cholesterol levels showed that only about 27% had visited a physician before the school-sponsored cholesterol testing.

From "A pilot study on cholesterol screening in the school environment" by A. Weinberg, R. Frost, R. Chamberlain, & C.H. Stroup, 1988. *Journal of School Health, 58 (8),* 62.

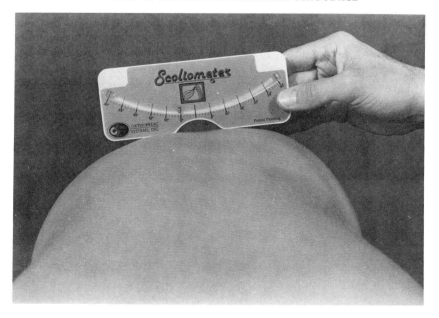

FIG. 10-4 Scoliometer used to document clinical deformity seen in patients with scoliosis. *(From "Nonoperative treatment of spinal deformity: The case for observation" (p. 108) by W.P. Bunnell; in* Instructional course lectures *(Vol. 34) by the American Academy of Orthopaedic surgeons, 1985, St. Louis. Mosby. Copyright 1985 by The C.V. Mosby Company Reprinted by permission.)*

impairment in a child who often asks to have statements repeated, who does not follow directions exactly, and who often is inattentive.

Before the child starts school an otoscopic examination of the ears enables the nurse to assess for excessive wax build-up or any other problems that would indicate a need for further testing.

Cholesterol screening has become a routine part of the physical examination in many schools. (See box for a description of a research study connected with one such program).

Scoliosis. All routine physical examinations should include screening for scoliosis. The term *scoliosis* is used to describe an S-shaped curve of the spine that, if structural, generally is noted at birth. Sometimes, however, scoliosis develops in school-aged children as a result of postural changes. At high risk for idiopathic scoliosis are preadolescent or adolescent girls, although it can be seen at an earlier age. Early intervention with exercise or a simple temporary brace can prevent permanent structural changes. Fig. 10-4 demonstrates how a school nurse can assess a child for scoliosis.

Acne. Most adolescents have some form of skin eruption as a result of hormonal changes during puberty. Mild to severe acne can have a disturbing effect on the self-image of the young person. The nurse's role in helping the adolescent cope with acne is to provide counseling about the importance of getting adequate rest, maintaining proper nutrition and scrupulous cleanliness, and reducing emotional stress. Parental involvement in the management of care also can be helpful. Severe pustular or cystic acne should be referred for medical management.

Tertiary prevention. Tertiary prevention includes coordination and integration of health service resources within the school setting to support the child who is recovering from a major health problem or to enable the child who is chronically ill to remain well as long as possible. Frequent conferences with teachers and parents about the progress of a child with cancer, for example, may enable the child to experience as few disruptions as possible while undergoing treatment. Teachers should be instructed to allow the child to go to the nurse to rest if needed and should be given an explanation as to the unexpected turns, remissions and relapses, bodily changes, and psychological changes that may occur. Special efforts should be made to maintain contact with the family (Wold, 1981).

A very sick child and that child's family can be helped greatly by acknowledging awareness of the stress the disease places on both child and family. In the event that the child dies, classmates and teachers also must be allowed to ventilate their feelings about the death and be offered an opportunity to participate in grief counseling.

Tertiary prevention, with its goal of maintaining the optimum level of wellness for the child who is mentally or physically impaired, can be one of the most challenging roles for the community health nurse in the schools.

SUMMARY

The school-aged population often is pictured as the carefree segment of society. To be carefree the child must be nurtured and protected against trauma and disease, both physically and mentally.

The community health nurse in the schools can institute health promotion at the primary, secondary, and tertiary levels of prevention. Health education should be directed at children, parents, and teachers. Screening and early diagnosis of health problems can prevent many conditions from becoming disabling. School nurses also can be of paramount importance in assisting children, teachers, and parents in coping with chronically ill children and in helping to maintain them at their highest level of wellness for as long as possible.

CHAPTER HIGHLIGHTS

- The school-age years comprise the period from ages 5 to 12 years. Adolescence begins at age 13 years and lasts until approximately age 21 years.
- Puberty begins generally at age 13 years for girls and age 16 years for boys.
- According to Piaget the school-aged child is in the concrete operational stage and the adolescent is entering the formal operational stage.
- According to Erikson the young school-aged child is in the stage of initiative versus guilt and the older school-aged child is in the stage of industry versus inferiority. The adolescent is in the stage of identity versus diffusion.
- The major causes of mortality and illness in school-aged children are accidents, chronic illness, and congenital anomalies. Homicide has become an increasingly common cause of death among adolescents, particularly those in poor neighborhoods and in families that are experiencing stress.
- Child abuse and neglect, particularly sexual abuse, have become greater problems in recent years. The nurse should be alert to signs of abuse or neglect and should report suspected cases to the proper authorities.
- Other problems of children that have increased in prevalence in recent years include depression, suicide, teenage pregnancy, and alcohol and drug abuse.
- The role of the community health nurse in the schools is somewhat ambiguous because uniform guidelines do not exist regarding education, licensing, and certification.

STUDY QUESTIONS

1. Construct a tool that would enable you to perform a complete physical assessment on a well 8-year-old child.
2. Identify the major causes of mortality in primary and secondary school-aged children.
3. Write a nursing care plan within the Neuman framework of primary, secondary, and tertiary prevention that would enable you to assist a chronically ill child in the school setting.

REFERENCES

American Academy of Pediatrics. (1988). *Report of the Committee on Infectious Diseases.* (21st ed.). Elk Grove Village, IL.

American Academy of Pediatrics Committee on Infectious Diseases (1989). Measles: Reassessment of the Current Immunization Policy. *Pediatrics, 84* (6):1110-1113.

Berkow, R. (1982). The *Merck manual of diagnosis and therapy* (14th ed.). Rahway, NJ: Merck.

Brown, M.S. & Murphy, M.A. (1981). *Ambulatory pediatrics for children* (2nd ed.). New York: McGraw Hill.

Creighton, H. (1986). *Law every nurse should know* (5th ed.). Philadelphia: Saunders.

Diseker, R. et al. (1982). A comparison of height, weight, and triceps skinfold thickness of children ages 5-12 in Michigan (1978) Forsyth County, North Carolina (1978), and Hanes, Part I (1971-1974). *American Journal of Public Health, 72,* 730-733.

Erikson, E. (1963) *Childhood and society.* New York: Norton.

Gair, C. (1966). What is school nursing? *Journal of School Health, 36,* 401-402.

Goodwin, L.D., Goodwin, W.L., & Cantrell J. (1988). The mental health needs of elementary school children. *Journal of School Health, 58, (7),* 282-287.

Hall, P., & Wick, B. (1988). Simple procedures for comprehensive vision screening. *Journal of School Health, 58, (2),* 58-61.

Jarvis, L. (1985). *Community health nursing: Keeping the public healthy.* Philadelphia: Davis.

King, E. (1984). *Affective education in nursing: A guide to teaching and assessment.* Rockville, MD: Aspen Pub. Inc.

Kohlberg, L. (1978). The cognitive developmental approach to moral education. P. Scharf (Ed.), *Readings in moral education,* Minneapolis: Winston Press.

Lester, D. (1988). One theory of teen-aged suicides. *Journal of School Health, 58,* 193, 194.

Moore, E., Strickland, R., Melcher, M., & Walker, J.

(1988). Protecting our children through Kid Safe. *Pediatric Nursing, 14(1),* 32-35.

Murray, R. & Zentner, J. (1989). *Nursing assessment and health promotion strategies through the life span.* (4th ed.) Norwalk, CT: Appleton-Lange.

North American Nursing Diagnosis Association. (1988). Approved nursing diagnosis categories. *Nursing Diagnosis Newsletter, 15 (1),* 1-3.

National Center for Health Statistics. (1987). *Health— United States* (DHHS Publication No. PHS 84-1232). Washington, DC: U.S. Government Printing Office.

Neuman, B. N. (1989). The Neuman Systems model (2nd ed.). Norwalk, CT: Appleton & Lange.

Newton, J. (1984). *School health handbook.* Englewood Cliffs, NJ: Prentice-Hall.

Northrop, C., & Kelly, M. (1987). *Legal issues in nursing.* St. Louis: Mosby.

Oberbeck, T. (1988). Vision screening of preschool and school aged children, Bethesda, Maryland. *Journal of Ophthalmic Nursing & Technology, 7 (3),* 96-99.

Piaget, J. (1963). The *origins of intelligence in children.* New York: Norton.

The plague among us. (1966, June 16). *Newsweek,* p. 16.

Robinson, P., & Greene, J. (1988). The adolescent alcohol and drug problem: A practical approach. *Pediatric Nursing, 14 (4),* 305-309.

Spradley, B. (1985). *Community health nursing concepts and practice* (2nd ed.). Boston: Little, Brown & Co.

Stanhope M, & Lancaster, J. (1988). *Community health nursing* (2nd ed.). St. Louis: CV Mosby.

Whaley, L.F., & Wong, D.L. (1987). *Nursing care of infants and children* (3rd ed.). St. Louis: Mosby.

Wissow, L. (1990). *Child advocacy for the clinician: an approach to child abuse and neglect.* Baltimore, MD: Williams and Wilkins.

Wold, S. (1981). *School nursing: A framework for practice,* St. Louis: CV Mosby.

The Young and Middle-Aged Adult

JOAN M. COOKFAIR

Well-being is a state characterized by experiences of contentment, pleasure, and kinds of happiness; by spiritual experiences; by movement toward fulfillment of one's self-ideal; and by continuing personalization.

DOROTHEA OREM

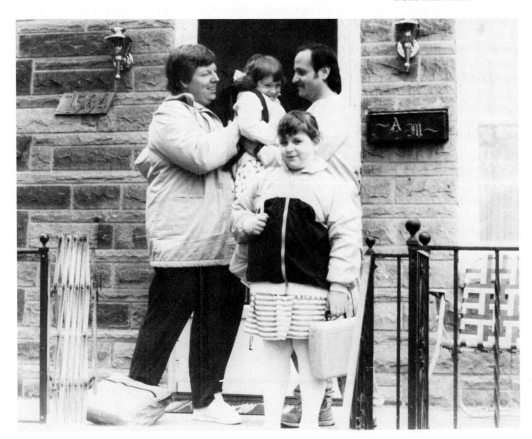

OBJECTIVES

At the conclusion of this chapter the student will be able to:

1. Define the key terms listed
2. Discuss the "death of permanence" that affects the health needs of young and middle-aged adults in the community
3. Describe selected theories of the developmental stages and tasks of young and middle-aged adults
4. Identify causes of mortality and health problems experienced by young and middle-aged adults
5. Describe the use of Neuman's assessment tool in assisting the nurse in planning health care needs at primary, secondary, and tertiary levels
6. Discuss possible resolutions of spiritual dilemmas experienced by middle-aged adults

KEY TERMS

Accelerating change	Logotherapy
Death of permanence	Menopause
Dissonance	Midlife crisis
Generativity versus stagnation	Sandwich generation
Glaucoma	Spiritual development
Hiatal hernia	Stress factors
Intimacy versus isolation	

Much has been written about the school-aged child and the adult in late maturity. In contrast, very little can be found in the literature about the young and the middle-aged adults who, supposedly, are the individuals responsible for the well-being of the other two groups.

This group, in the middle of the age spectrum between school age and retirement, is experiencing stressors and health hazards that are unique in human history. The individuals in this group must learn to live in an environment increasingly polluted by waste, noise, and the products of modern technology. Their world has never been free of the threat of nuclear holocaust. Space travel has enabled them to touch a piece of the old romantic moon; the reality is a cold hard piece of rock. The media constantly reinforce an economic paradise of fast cars, hot tubs, and eternal youth. The reality is an economy that finds many of this group living at a poverty level. The truth is that their bodies age in a predictable way, and eternal youth becomes a mockery. The nature of world politics changes daily. The "cold war" and the KGB now seem irrelevant. Acquired immunodeficiency syndrome (AIDS) looms as a threat to this group and to its children.

The pace of change has accelerated. There is a *death of permanence* (Toffler, 1970), both in relationships and material possessions. Our culture has released a totally new societal force—a stream of change so accelerated that it influences the tempo of daily life and affects the way we feel (Toffler, 1970).

No other group in history has had to adjust to such rapid internal and external dissonance. Surrounded by an unpredictable world, a kaleidoscope of societal change, the individuals in this group still must accomplish certain developmental tasks to be healthy. They live through a predictable span of years in bodies that age and have needs and with personalities that grow and develop in a predictable way.

An awareness of the stressors that affect those in this middle group enables the community health nurse to plan preventive interventions at primary, secondary, and tertiary levels. An understanding of the developmental tasks they must accomplish will equip the nurse with the insight to guide them toward a fulfillment of their self-ideal and ultimate personalization (Orem, 1985).

THE YOUNG ADULT
Developmental Tasks

In contemporary society, young adults are considered those persons between 18 and 35 years of age. With physical growth completed, they are considered to be functioning at the peak of their physical potential. Several theorists have stated that the healthy young adult will process through certain developmental tasks.

Erik Erikson's theory (1968) maintains that after adolescence, there is a crisis of intimacy. Sexual intimacy is only a part of it. Developing a true and mutual psychosocial intimacy with another person, be it in friendship, erotic encounters, or joint inspiration, is important at this stage to the attainment of a healthy personality. Without such an experience the individual may settle for a highly stereotyped interpersonal relationship and retain a deep sense of isolation (Erikson, pp. 135, 136).

Robert Havighurst (1972) suggests that selecting a mate, beginning a family, and assuming civic responsibilities are part of a young adult's developmental tasks.

Gail Sheehy (1976) discusses hallmarks of well-being. According to her theory, young adults have the tasks of making an occupational choice and negotiating a successful transition from childhood to a clear sense of adult role identity. They also must become minimally sensitive to criticism, conquer major fears, and establish sincere friendships. Sheehy links developmental stages in young adulthood to Erikson's developmental stages.

Gallagher (1987, p. 348) maintains that leaving the family home and establishing physical, financial, and psychological distance are part of normal young adult development.

Table 11-1 compares several models of developmental theories. Most of the theorists emphasize that an important task for the healthy young adult is to establish a firm identity as a person by leaving the family home. Because of the state of the economy in the 1990s, this task is difficult for some young people. Some may remain at home for extended periods to acquire education beyond high school in the hope that it will lead to job security (Fig. 11-1). Some put off marriage and childbearing until they can attain financial stability. Others marry and move home to establish what becomes an extended family network in one household.

Prolonged periods of transition into economic independence can delay the achievement of developmental tasks for both young adults and their middle-aged parents. There may be a subtle stressor inherent in the fact that parents who grew up in the 1950s and 1960s, when jobs were plentiful, may have difficulty understanding the obstacles facing their offspring.

Major causes of Mortality

Table 11-2 shows the death rates for the 15 leading causes of death in young adults. Motor vehicle accidents lead the list as the major cause of death. The rate per 100,000 in 1987,

TABLE 11-1 Comparison of developmental tasks of young adulthood

Erickson's stages (1950)	Havighurst's developmental tasks for adulthood (1952)	Levinson's stages (1977)	Gould's stages (1972)	Sheehy's stages (1976)
Identity vs. confusion	*Early adulthood*	*Separating from family (16-24)*	*Ages 18-22*	*Pulling up roots (18-22)*
Commencing adult tasks	Mate selection	Leaving family home and establishing physical, financial, and psychologic distance	Peer group support in separating from family	Becoming part of a peer group
Focusing on an occupation	Learning to live with a partner in marriage		Moving away from family with anxiety	Adopting a sex role
Reviewing of ideals and idols	Beginning a family	*Moving into adult world (20-27/29)*	Receptive to new ideas	Selecting an occupation
Preserving sense of continuity during psychologic turmoil	Raising children	Exploring adult roles in interpersonal occupational areas; making provisional commitments and beginning to develop a life structure	*Ages 22-28*	Developing a world view/ideology
	Managing a home		Feelings of autonomy and self-reliance	Leaving home physically
Imposing a moratorium period if feasible	Starting an occupation		Resolution of separating from family	Beginning emotional distancing
Intimacy vs. isolation	Assuming civic responsibility	*Age 30 transition*	Opportunity for expansiveness, (i.e., living, growing and building)	Deidealizing parental figures
Undertaking specific affiliations	Selecting a social group	Reevaluating and changing commitments	*Ages 29-34*	*Trying twenties (22-28)*
Developing sexual relationships and achieving orgasm		*Settling down (28-32)*	Feelings of doubt, questioning of activities	Clearer definition of major goals
		Making deeper commitments	Weariness about established status	Selecting a mentor
		Achieving occupational fulfillment	Reawakening of strivings	Testing occupational and interpersonal relationships
			Stressful marriage	*Age 30*
				Coping with restless feelings
				Reviewing relationships
				Becoming more introspective
				Searching for identity
				Increased awareness of mortality related to signs of biological aging
				Rooting and extending (early thirties—mid-thirties)
				Renewed moderation
				Committing and investing oneself

From *Maximizing human potential throughout the life cycle* by L. Gallagher and M. Kreidler, 1987, Norwalk, CT: Appleton and Lange, p.348. Modified from *Continuations: Adult development and aging* by L. Troll, 1982, Monterey, CA: Brooks-Cole and *Psychosocial caring throughout the life span* by I. M. Burnside, 1979, New York: McGraw-Hill.

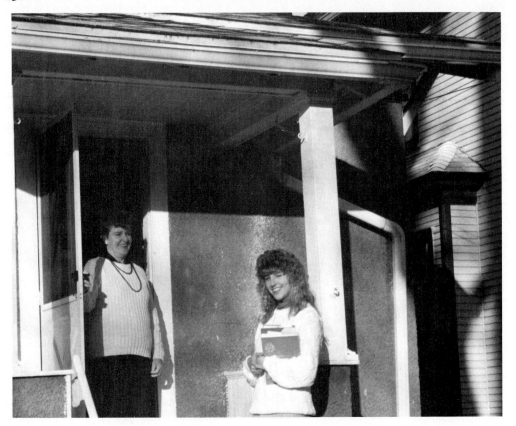

FIG. 11-1 Young adult remaining at home to complete school.

according to the National Center for Health Statistics, was 37.8 per 100,000 for persons between the ages of 15 and 24 years and 24.2 per 100,000 for those between the ages of 25 and 34 years. Fatalities from motor vehicle accidents can be decreased by the use of seat belts. Driver education should be emphasized, and strict penalties for drunken driving should be enforced. Between 50% and 60% of all fatal accidents are caused by drunken drivers (Gallagher & Kreidler, 1987). Industrial accidents and drowning also rank high as major causes of accidental death (Murray & Zentner, 1989). Occupational health nurses can address occupational hazards by initiating safety programs in the workplace. In addition, young adults should be reminded of the safety rules associated with athletic activities such as swimming.

Homicide, 15.1 per 100,000, and suicide, 15.4 per 100,000, are the next leading causes of death in the young adult population. Drug abuse and alcohol frequently are involved in cases of homicide and suicide. Table 11-3 shows the increase in deaths from drug-related causes in the United States from 1979 to 1987. Health education for the prevention of the use of addictive drugs should begin in the elementary schools, and school nurses should be assertive in the planning and implementation of such programs.

Malignant neoplasms continue to cause mortality at the rate of 3.6 per 100,000 in the young adult population. Young men and women should have yearly complete blood counts to detect any sign of neoplasms of hematopoietic tissues.

TABLE 11-2 Age-specific and age-adjusted death rates for the 15 leading causes in 1987 and selected components: United States, 1979, 1986, and 1987

Cause of death†	Year	Age-group (yr)				
		15-24	25-34	35-44	45-54	55-64
All causes	1987	99.4	133.2	214.1	498.0	1,241.3
	1986	102.3	132.1	212.9	504.8	1,255.1
	1979	114.8	133.0	229.8	589.7	1,338.0
Diseases of heart	1987	2.8	8.4	35.6	140.5	408.8
	1986	2.8	8.6	37.5	144.6	424.2
	1979	2.6	8.4	45.3	184.6	499.0
Rheumatic fever and rheumatic heart disease	1987	0.1	0.4	0.7	1.9	4.7
	1986	0.1	0.3	0.7	2.1	5.0
	1979	0.2	0.4	1.4	3.9	8.0
Hypertensive heart disease	1987	0.0	0.3	1.6	5.9	14.2
	1986	0.0	0.3	1.6	5.9	13.8
	1979	0.0	0.4	1.9	7.0	16.2
Hypertensive heart and renal disease	1987	0.0	0.0	0.2	0.3	1.0
	1986	0.0	0.1	0.1	0.3	1.0
	1979	0.0	0.0	0.2	0.4	1.4
Ischemic heart disease	1987	0.3	2.8	20.8	92.0	278.6
	1986	0.3	3.0	22.4	95.9	292.5
	1979	0.3	3.6	30.1	136.1	381.0
Acute myocardial infarction	1987	0.2	1.6	12.3	56.6	165.2
	1986	0.2	1.8	13.5	59.6	176.0
	1979	0.2	2.4	21.1	94.6	258.9
Other acute and subacute forms of ischemic heart disease	1987	0.0	0.1	0.3	1.3	2.9
	1986	0.0	0.1	0.4	1.4	3.4
	1979	0.0	0.1	0.5	2.0	4.8
Angina pectoris	1987	—	0.0	0.0	0.1	0.5
	1986	0.0	0.0	0.1	0.1	0.5
	1979	0.0	0.0	0.1	0.1	0.3
Old myocardial infarction and other forms of chronic ischemic heart disease	1987	0.1	1.1	8.2	34.0	110.1
	1986	0.1	1.1	8.4	34.8	112.6
	1979	0.1	1.0	8.4	39.3	117.0
Other diseases of endocardium	1987	0.1	0.3	0.7	1.6	4.2
	1986	0.1	0.3	0.6	1.4	4.2
	1979	0.1	0.2	0.6	1.5	4.3
All other forms of heart disease	1987	2.2	4.7	11.8	38.9	106.1
	1986	2.2	4.7	12.1	38.9	107.6
	1979	1.9	3.7	11.0	35.7	88.1
Malignant neoplasms, including neoplasms of lymphatic and hematopoietic tissues	1987	5.1	12.4	43.5	164.3	447.0
	1986	5.4	13.1	45.3	165.7	444.4
	1979	6.1	13.3	48.3	181.4	429.4
Malignant neoplasms of lip, oral cavity, and pharynx	1987	0.1	0.1	0.8	4.0	9.9
	1986	0.1	0.2	0.9	4.2	10.3
	1979	0.1	0.2	1.1	5.6	11.8

Continued.

Modified from *Monthly vital statistics report* by the National Center for Health Statistics (DHHS *38 (5)*, September 26, 1989, Washington, DC: U.S. Government Printing Office.
*Rates per 100,000 population in specific group.
†Ninth revision, *International classification of diseases*, 1975.

TABLE 11-2 Age-specific and age-adjusted death rates for the 15 leading causes in 1987 and selected components: United States, 1979, 1986, and 1987—cont'd

Cause of death†	Year	Age-group (yr)				
		15-24	25-34	35-44	45-54	55-64
Malignant neoplasms of digestive organs and peritoneum	1987	0.3	1.6	7.4	32.0	97.9
	1986	0.3	1.5	7.3	32.5	98.0
	1979	0.3	1.8	8.2	36.3	103.9
Malignant neoplasms of respiratory and intrathoracic organs	1987	0.1	0.8	7.7	51.6	160.4
	1986	0.1	0.7	7.9	51.7	157.8
	1979	0.1	0.8	9.8	56.0	140.9
Malignant neoplasm of breast	1987	0.0	1.6	8.9	23.4	43.1
	1986	0.0	1.5	9.3	23.4	43.1
	1979	0.0	1.6	9.1	25.3	41.3
Malignant neoplasms of genital organs	1987	0.3	1.5	3.7	11.5	32.8
	1986	0.3	1.4	4.0	11.8	34.3
	1979	0.5	1.6	4.7	14.5	35.6
Malignant neoplasms of urinary organs	1987	0.1	0.2	1.0	5.2	15.3
	1986	0.1	0.2	1.0	5.2	15.1
	1979	0.1	0.2	1.1	5.7	15.1
Malignant neoplasms of all other and unspecified sites	1987	1.9	3.6	8.6	23.5	56.1
	1986	2.0	4.1	9.2	23.6	54.4
	1979	2.3	3.7	8.6	24.0	49.8
Leukemia	1987	1.3	1.5	2.4	4.8	11.2
	1986	1.5	1.6	2.4	4.8	11.4
	1979	1.3	1.5	2.5	5.0	11.7
Other malignant neoplasms of lymphatic and hemato-poietic tissues	1987	0.9	1.7	3.0	8.2	20.5
	1986	1.0	1.9	3.4	8.3	20.0
	1979	0.9	1.8	3.0	8.6	19.5
Cerebrovascular diseases	1987	0.6	2.2	7.0	20.1	52.2
	1986	0.7	2.2	7.1	20.4	53.0
	1979	0.9	2.6	9.1	26.4	68.1
Accidents and adverse effects	1987	48.9	38.4	31.7	30.0	35.5
	1986	51.2	39.5	31.1	30.7	34.8
	1979	62.6	45.7	38.4	39.4	43.5
Motor vehicle accidents	1987	37.8	24.2	17.3	15.4	15.6
	1986	39.0	24.2	16.6	15.1	15.1
	1979	45.6	28.8	21.0	18.6	18.2
All other accidents and adverse effects	1987	11.1	14.2	14.4	14.6	19.9
	1986	12.2	15.3	14.5	15.6	19.7
	1979	17.0	16.9	17.4	20.8	25.2
Chronic obstructive pulmonary disease and allied condition	1987	0.5	0.6	1.8	9.2	47.4
	1986	0.5	0.6	1.6	9.8	47.2
	1979	0.3	0.5	1.7	9.3	40.2
Pneumonia and influenza	1987	0.7	1.8	3.4	7.0	17.6
	1986	0.7	1.7	3.6	7.0	18.6
	1979	0.8	1.5	3.2	7.1	16.4
Diabetes mellitus	1987	0.3	1.4	3.5	9.7	26.9
	1986	0.4	1.5	3.6	9.5	26.0
	1979	0.4	1.4	3.6	9.0	25.8

TABLE 11-2 Age-specific and age-adjusted death rates for the 15 leading causes in 1987 and selected components: United States, 1979, 1986, and 1987—cont'd

Cause of death†	Year	Age-group (yr)				
		15-24	25-34	35-44	45-54	55-64
Suicide	1987	12.9	15.4	15.0	15.9	16.6
	1986	13.1	15.7	15.2	16.4	17.0
	1979	12.4	16.3	15.4	16.5	16.6
Chronic liver disease and cirrhosis	1987	0.2	2.6	10.0	19.8	32.1
	1986	0.2	2.8	9.6	20.3	32.2
	1979	0.2	3.4	13.9	31.0	40.9
Atherosclerosis	1987	0.0	0.0	0.1	0.7	4.0
	1986	0.0	0.0	0.1	0.8	4.0
	1979	0.0	0.0	0.1	0.9	4.8
Nephritis, nephrotic syndrome, and nephrosis	1987	0.2	0.6	1.2	3.3	9.2
	1986	0.2	0.6	1.3	3.2	9.5
	1979	0.3	0.7	1.5	3.7	8.5
Homicide and legal intervention	1987	14.0	15.1	10.8	7.7	5.5
	1986	14.2	16.1	11.4	8.3	5.4
	1979	14.5	18.2	14.3	10.8	7.0
Septicemia	1987	0.3	0.7	1.4	3.2	9.1
	1986	0.2	0.6	1.4	3.3	8.9
	1979	0.2	0.4	0.8	2.2	4.9
Certain conditions originating in the perinatal period	1987	0.0	0.0	0.0	—	0.0
	1986	0.0	0.0	0.0	0.0	—
	1979	0.0	0.0	0.0	0.0	0.0
Human immunodeficiency virus infection	1987	1.3	11.6	14.0	7.9	3.5
	1986	—	—	—	—	—
	1979	—	—	—	—	—

TABLE 11-3 Deaths from drug-related causes, by sex: United States, 1979 to 1987*

	All races		
Year	Both sexes	Male	Female
1987	9796	6146	3650
1986	9976	6284	3692
1985	8663	5342	3321
1984	7892	4640	3252
1983	7492	4145	3347
1982	7310	4130	3180
1981	7160	3835	3271
1980	6900	3771	3129
1979	7101	3656	3445

Data from *International classification of diseases* (9th rev. ed.) by National Center for Health Statistics, 1989, Washington, DC: U.S. Government Printing Office.

*Rates per 100,000 population in specified group.

Common Causes of Illness

Viruses that cause upper respiratory infections, fever, and malaise are common health problems for young adults, particularly for those who do not get enough rest or whose nutrition is inadequate.

Hepatitis B is increasingly prevalent among users of intravenous drugs. The disease also can be transmitted sexually. In addition, health professionals who work with high-risk populations may be at risk. Health promotion, including distribution of information about methods of prevention and modes of transmission, may be effective in lessening the transmission of the disease.

Skin cancer, which results from excessive exposure to ultraviolet rays during extended time periods in the sun, is a potential threat to young adults, as is lung cancer. The lungs are affected by primary and secondary smoking. Young adults need to be given information about the harmful effects of smoking and its relationship to lung cancer and other life-threatening diseases.

Periodontal disease is chronic infection of the gums. This condition leads to tooth decay and loss of teeth, but it can be prevented by scheduled visits to the dentist and by proper brushing.

Obesity is a major problem for young adults in the 1990s. According to studies published by the Metropolitan Life Insurance Company, excess weight even by 10 pounds increases the possibility of illness. Table 11-4 shows a height and weight chart that can assist the nurse in an assessment of obesity. Discouraging the consumption of junk foods and providing instruction in following a healthy diet may prevent the problem.

TABLE 11-4   Height and weight chart

Men					Women				
Height		Small frame	Medium frame	Large frame	Height		Small frame	Medium frame	Large frame
Feet	Inches				Feet	Inches			
5	2	128-134	131-141	138-150	4	10	102-111	109-121	118-131
5	3	130-136	133-143	140-153	4	11	103-113	111-123	120-134
5	4	132-138	135-145	142-156	5	0	104-115	113-126	122-137
5	5	134-140	137-148	144-160	5	1	106-118	115-129	125-140
5	6	136-142	139-151	146-164	5	2	108-121	118-132	128-143
5	7	138-145	142-154	149-168	5	3	111-124	121-135	131-147
5	8	140-148	145-157	152-172	5	4	114-127	124-138	134-151
5	9	142-151	148-160	155-176	5	5	117-130	127-141	137-155
5	10	144-154	151-163	158-180	5	6	120-133	130-144	140-159
5	11	146-157	154-166	161-184	5	7	123-136	133-147	143-163
6	0	149-160	157-170	164-188	5	8	126-139	136-150	146-167
6	1	152-164	160-174	168-192	5	9	129-142	139-153	149-170
6	2	155-168	164-178	172-197	5	10	132-145	142-156	152-173
6	3	158-172	167-182	176-202	5	11	135-148	145-159	155-176
6	4	162-176	171-187	181-207	6	0	138-151	148-162	158-179

From Metropolitan Life Insurance Company. Source of basic data: *1979 build study* by the Society of Actuaries and Association of Life Insurance Medical Directors of America, 1980, NY: Author. Source of table: *Maximizing human potential throughout the life cycle* by L. Gallagher and M. Kreidler, 1987, Norwalk, CT: Appleton and Lange, p. 335. Weights at age 25-59 based on lowest mortality; clothing weights: 5 lb for men; 3 lb for women; shoes: 1-inch heel.

PRIMARY PREVENTION	SECONDARY PREVENTION	TERTIARY PREVENTION
Stressor* Covert or potential	**Stressors*** Overt, actual or known	**Stressors*** Overt, or residual—possible covert
Reaction Hypothetical or possible based on available knowledge	**Reaction** Identified symptoms or known stress factors	**Reaction** Hypothetical or known—residual symptoms or known stress factors
Assessment† Based on client assess-, ment, experience, and theory Risk or possible hazard based on client/nurse perception Meaning of experience to client Lifestyle factors Coping patterns (past, present, possible) Individual differences identified	**Assessment†** Determined by nature and degree of reaction Determine internal/external available resources to resist the reaction Rationale for goals—collaborative goal setting with client **Intervention as treatment** Wellness variance—overt symptoms-nursing diagnosis Need priority and related goals Client strengths and weaknesses related to the five client variables Shift of need priorities as client responds to treatment (primary prevention needs and tertiary prevention may occur simultaneously with treatment or secondary prevention) Intervention in maladaptive processes Optimal use of internal/external resources such as energy conservation, noise reduction, and financial aid	**Assessment†** Determined by degree of stability following treatment and further potential reconstitution for possible regression factors **Intervention as reconstitution following treatment** Motivation Education-reeducation Behavior modification Reality orientation Progressive goal setting Optimal use of available internal/external resources Maintenance of client optimal functional level
Intervention Strengthen client flexible line of defense Client education Desensitization to stressor avoidance Strengthen individual resistance factors		

*Environmental stressors include intra-, inter-, and extrapersonal factors.
†Assessment/intervention, based on the Neuman Systems Model, ideally would consider simultaneously the interrelationship of the five interacting and interdependent client variables: physiological, psychological, sociocultural, developmental, and spiritual.

FIG. 11-2 An assessment/intervention tool development guide. *(From* The Neuman Systems Model *[2nd ed.] p. 21, by B. Neuman, 1989, Norwalk, CT: Appleton & Lange.)*

Health Promotion Activities

The young adult, supposedly at the height of physical potential, still has a need for health care at primary, secondary, and tertiary levels. Fig. 11-2 shows an assessment and intervention tool designed by nursing theorist Betty Neuman to assist the nurse in the assessment phase of health care and in planning prevention at all three levels.

Primary prevention. Strengthening the client's flexible line of defense by desensitization and client education are examples of primary prevention.

Immunizations are available for influenza, hepatitis B, rubella, rubeola, tetanus, poliomyelitis, and other infectious diseases. Administration of these vaccines is not recommended for individuals whose immune systems are compromised. In addition, immunization for rubella is contraindicated because of possible teratological effects if pregnancy is a possibility. Judicious use of immunizations in healthy young adults can desensitize them to some of the stressors that cause infectious disease.

Intervention such as client education is an example of primary prevention that may strengthen the flexible line of defense. Nurses are in a position to counsel clients about such problems as the hazards of drinking while driving and the risk of lung cancer to the individual who smokes.

Secondary prevention. Intervention through treatment occurs if a client shows symptoms that indicate the presence of stress factors. A woman who has found a lump in her breast should be referred immediately for treatment. A client with a chronic cough from smoking or one who shows signs of becoming significantly overweight may be helped by counseling to encourage changes in life-style to correct maladaptive processes.

Tertiary prevention. Assessment of the client's degree of stability and potential reconstitution after a life-threatening disability may prevent further disability and regression. The following case study is an example of nursing intervention at this level.

 CASE STUDY

Assessment

Charles T, age 28 years, and Rose T, 23 years, have been married for 5 years and have one child, Eric, age 2 years. Charles had been discharged from the Army 1 year previously and went to work in the family construction business. Adjustment to civilian life and working in the family business were difficult for him, and he began drinking heavily. One evening after work he stopped with friends for some drinks at a bar. After leaving the bar, he attempted to drive his truck home but, instead, was critically injured in a one-vehicle accident.

The extent of his injuries included permanent paraplegia and partial paralysis of both arms as a result of a fracture at the level of the fourth thoracic vertebrae. He remained in an intensive care unit for 5 weeks. After 6 weeks of hospitalization Charles was discharged home. Referral to the community health nurse for follow-up care included planning and coordinating extensive rehabilitation. Notation was made that Charles was deeply depressed.

The community health nurse visited the home the day Charles was discharged. The client reported abdominal discomfort and indicated that he did not think his catheter was functioning properly. The nurse found impaction, administered a suppository, and irrigated the catheter. Both procedures gave Charles relief. The nurse spent some time with Rose, gave her a list of soft foods that Charles would be able to digest, and instructed her about what to do for Charles during the night. Rose confided that Charles did not want to get well. He felt "she would be better without him." The nurse listened empathically and

CASE STUDY—cont'd

assured Rose that they would talk more about the problem when she returned the following day. She asked Rose not to encourage Charles to talk a lot yet, just to be there and meet his needs as he made them known.

On the following day the nurse began an in-depth assessment. Rose and Charles both admitted they were in financial difficulty. Rose wished to bring their son, who was staying with grandparents, home. She did not, however, feel that she could care for both Charles and their son. As the nurse attended to Charles's physical care, she encouraged him to talk about his injuries. His response was primarily one of anger. He stated he really was not interested in further treatment and simply wanted to be left alone. The nurse accepted his remarks without comment but told him they would talk more about his wishes on the next nursing visit.

On the third day after his release from the hospital, the nurse found Charles in a more relaxed state of mind. As they talked the nurse asked him to name the three things he wanted most. He responded that he wished (1) to be a father to his son, (2) to be able to walk, and (3) to be able to love his wife as a man. Rose, when asked the same question, hesitantly, looking at Charles: (1) to have Charles believe she needed him, (2) to have him help with their son, and (3) to regain financial stability. The following morning the nurse found Rose and Charles were talking to each other, and there was less tension between them.

The nursing care plan was based on the following nursing diagnosis:

Nursing diagnosis

1. Ineffective family coping, disabling
2. Spiritual distress related to altered health state
3. Altered nutrition, less than body requirements related to altered health state
4. Potential for urinary infection related to indwelling catheter
5. Potential for impaired skin integrity related to immobility
6. Body image disturbance related to altered health state
7. Altered sexuality patterns related to altered health state
8. Potential for muscle atrophy related to immobility

Nursing goals

Nursing goals were established as follows:
1. Arranging for father and son to be reunited
2. Referral for counseling by an accepted professional
3. Planning small, frequent meals, with emphasis on soft foods; assisting with bowel training
4. Irrigating catheter daily and changing it as needed
5. Arranging for daily visits by a home health aide to bathe Charles and change his position frequently
6. Arranging for daily visits by a physiotherapist
7. Arranging for social services to assist with plans for rehabilitation
8. Counseling Charles and Rose about realistic plans for the future.

Nursing outcomes

During the time Charles remained at home (1 month) the nurse visited twice weekly. Charles remained free of infection and began to gain weight. Eric returned home, and Charles was able to reestablish a relationship with him. Continued rehabilitation was planned at a veteran's hospital because of Charles's prior military service. The social service worker was able to obtain some financial help for the family. Extended family members continued to be supportive. Although Charles remained depressed, he was cooperative and seemed less angry.

Continued.

For a while after Charles was admitted to the veteran's hospital, Rose maintained contact with the community health nurse. She wrote that Charles seemed better able to accept his wheelchair existence after meeting other young men who had suffered severe disabilities. The family was planning for Charles to reenter the business with the use of a home computer. They felt he would ultimately be able to take charge of billing and possibly could provide an answering service from his home. Rose felt that, although things would never be the same, they were going to make it together.

This near-fatal family crisis, which allowed stressors to invade the solid line of defense of the family structure, was precipitated by Charles's altered coping after his Army discharge. In addition to the serious threat to the basic family structure, an actual threat to Charles's life existed.

To reestablish the client's family stability, an overall assessment of the family as a system was conducted. Nursing care was planned by means of the Neuman format of nursing diagnosis, nursing goals, and nursing outcomes. Available resources were coordinated to assist in the client family's recovery.

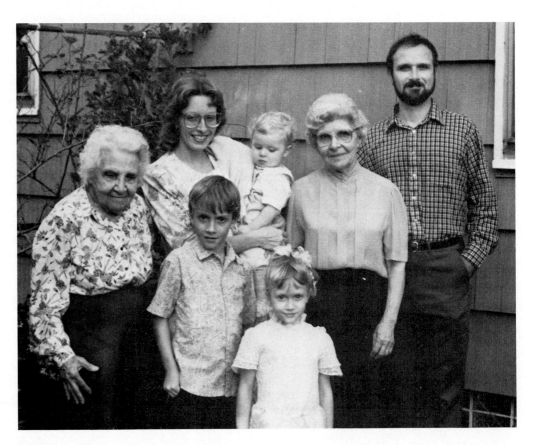

FIG. 11-3 Middle-aged couple responsible for children and older family members at the same time.

THE MIDDLE-AGED ADULT

Middle-aged adults are in a central position in the life cycle. They also are in a central position in terms of responsibility to society. While attempting to complete developmental tasks and fulfill their own needs, this "sandwich generation" is busy raising children and assisting aging parents (Fig. 11-3). In assessing the needs of this particular population, the stress caused by its life position cannot be ignored. A minor illness such as a respiratory infection can be a major catastrophe to a young mother who works and monitors the well-being of a parent living alone. A minor back strain can be a major threat to a construction worker who has small children and extended family members depending on him, particularly if he is not eligible for disability or compensation.

Middle-aged adults who are able to remain healthy physically and emotionally with a sense of well-being are in a position to contribute positively to their nuclear family, their family of origin, the community in which they live, and ultimately to their culture. Those who are unable to do so may weaken the fabric of their family, their community, and their culture.

Middle age is considered that period between the ages of 36 and 65 years. Even the well adult in this central group begins to experience some effects of aging. Body fat, for example, begins to redistribute, centering around the waist, abdomen, and hips. In men the hairline may begin to recede. Both sexes notice some gray in their hair. Skin becomes drier and wrinkles appear, particularly in the face. A subtle, progressive loss of muscle strength begins around the age of 45 years. There may be minor changes in visual acuity and some hearing loss.

During the middle years women experience menopause (cessation of menses). Although it is a normal part of the aging process, it can be a difficult adjustment for some.

Developmental Tasks

Community health nurses can assist their clients to make healthy transitions from youth to middle age if they are aware of the stressors that threaten them and the developmental tasks they are trying to accomplish.

Erikson (1968) maintains that the middle-aged adult (36 to 64 years of age) who does not achieve productivity and a sense of fulfillment in life may become overly concerned with physical and psychological decline and risk excessive inward focusing (generativity versus stagnation). At this stage the attainment of wisdom is a more important value than is the retention of physical powers. Persons who do not move toward perceived life goals may begin to experience a sense of boredom and stagnation. As they begin to lose the physical powers of youth, they may demonstrate an excessive concern for their health and become detrimentally self-preoccupied.

Havighurst (1972) suggests that the following undertakings are part of the middle-aged adult's challenge in society: a satisfying occupation with a specific economic standard in mind, establishing a good relationship with one's spouse, being active in the community, developing meaningful leisure activities, and guiding children, as well as aging parents, through developmental tasks.

According to Peck (1968), the specific developmental tasks that characterize middle age are (1) valuing wisdom versus physical power, (2) socializing versus "sexualizing," (3) cathetic flexibility versus inflexibility, and (4) mental flexibility versus mental rigidity.

People who age well, Peck says, learn to convert their values from their hands to their heads. They add a new dimension to the sexual relationship, which may result in increased loving and intimacy. They are able to shift emotional investments from one person to another and from one activity to another. The successful adult in midlife remains flexible and is able to use life experiences as guidelines on encountering new situations (Gallagher & Kreidler, 1987).

Gould (1980) maintains that midlife is a time of transformation, a period when individuals begin to define themselves in terms of a definite identity. An individual personality emerges, separate from the family of origin, one that is able to risk growth and an acceptance of realities. A period of disenchantment may occur with the realization that the family is not immune to external dangers and that children develop minds of their own.

Major Causes of Mortality

Cardiovascular disease. According to the National Center for Health Statistics, (Table 11-2), cardiovascular disease is the major cause of death among middle-aged adults. Health promotion is important, and the general public should be informed about the major risk factors for cardiovascular disease, for example, cigarette smoking, high serum cholesterol levels and diabetes. Low- or high-density lipoproteins may indicate intracellular abnormalities in lipid or carbohydrate metabolisms. An abnormality in lipoproteins is a reason for further screening and/or diagnostic testing (Harrison, 1977). Lesser risk factors include emotional stress, overweight, sedentary life-style, a family history of heart disease before age 65 years, and aggressive personality (Gallagher & Kreidler, 1987). Primary prevention techniques by community health nurses can help prevent cardiovascular disease.

Malignant neoplasms. Malignant neoplasms are the second highest cause of mortality in middle-aged adults. Clients should be taught the seven warning signs of cancer that, according to the American Cancer Society, should alert them to seek medical care:

1. Change in bowel or bladder habits
2. Any sore that does not heal
3. Unusual bleeding or discharge
4. Thickening or lump in breast or elsewhere
5. Indigestion or difficulty in swallowing
6. Obvious change in wart or mole
7. Nagging hoarseness or cough

Women should be encouraged to have scheduled Papanicolaou's (Pap) smears and mammograms. Men should be encouraged to perform self-examination of the testicles.

Accidents, suicide, and homicide. Motor vehicle accidents, suicide, and homicide are the third, fourth, and fifth causes of death in middle-aged adults. Health education about the advisability of not drinking while driving might cut down on motor vehicle accidents. Addictive drugs often are a factor in suicides and homicides (Table 11-3), and clients should be advised of this added risk.

Common causes of illness

Infectious disease. Upper respiratory infection caused by viruses or bacteria are common in this age-group. Encouraging a regimen of proper diet, rest, and exercise can help to prevent these infectious diseases.

Injury and accidents. Because some adults do not accommodate for physical changes, back and muscle strains are common. Also a concern are serious accidents, both in the home and in the workplace. Occupational health nurses and school nurses can be instrumental in establishing safety programs. In addition, safety consciousness should be encouraged in the home as well as in the workplace.

Hiatal hernia. Hiatal hernia, or herniation of the stomach through the esophagus, can cause pain that mimics a myocardial infarction. Persons with this disability should be encouraged to maintain ideal weight, to avoid tight clothing around the abdomen, and to eat frequently in small amounts and not before bedtime. In addition, elevating the head of the bed and taking antacids help to minimize pain (Murray & Zentner, 1989).

Diabetes. Diabetes mellitus (type II, which is non-insulin-dependent) may occur in middle-aged adults, particularly in the presence of a family history of the disease. Diet regulations, skin and foot care, regular eye checkups, and drug therapy can control the effects of diabetes (Murray & Zentner, 1989).

PRIMARY PREVENTION	SECONDARY PREVENTION	TERITARY PREVENTION
Nursing Action* to: 1. Classify stresssorst as to client/client system threat to stability. Prevent stressor invasion. 2. Provide information to maintain or strengthen existing client/client system strengths. 3. Support positive coping and functioning. 4. Desensitize existing or possible noxious stressors. 5. Motivate toward wellness. 6. Coordinate/integrate interdisciplinary theories and epidemiologic input. 7. Educate/reeducate. 8. Use stress as a positive intervention strategy.	Nursing Action to: 1. Following stressor invasion, protect basic structure. 2. Mobilize and optimize internal/external resources toward stability and energy conservation. 3. Facilitate purposeful manipulation of stressors and reactions to stressors. 4. Motivate, educate, and involve client and client system in health care goals. 5. Facilitate appropriate treatment/intervention measures. 6. Support positive factors toward wellness. 7. Promote advocacy by coordination/integration. 8. Provide primary prevention/intervention as required.	Nursing Action to: 1. During reconstitution, attain/maintain maximum level of wellness and stability following treatment. 2. Educate, reeducate, and/or reorient as needed. 3. Support client/client system toward appropriate goal directedness. 4. Coordinate and integrate health service resources. 5. Provide primary and/or secondary prevention/intervention as needed.

*At first priority for nursing action, in each of the areas of prevention as intervention, is to determine the nature of stressors and their threat to the client/client system.
Some general categorical functions for nursing action are initiation, planning, organization, monitoring, coordinating, implementing, integrating, advocating, supporting and evaluating. An example of a limited classification system for stressors is illustrated by the following four categories: 1) deprivation, 2) excess, 3) change, and 4) intolerance.

FIG. 11-4 Format for prevention as intervention. *(Copyright 1980 by Betty Neuman. Reprinted by permission.)*

Glaucoma. Glaucoma, which is characterized by increased intraocular pressure, can cause progressive loss of sight. A simple test by an ophthalmologist, nurse practitioner, or physician can predict the presence of increased pressure and should be performed every 2 years after the age of 40 years. Administration of pilocarpine eye drops or some comparable medication on a regular basis can decrease the intraocular pressure and prevent blindness or loss of acuity (Berkow, 1982).

Sexual dysfunction. Sexual dysfunction may result from alcoholism, obesity, mental or physical fatigue, or stress. Chronic illness such as diabetes can cause autonomic neuropathy in men in the sacral area and result in impotence. The threat of an attack of angina also can limit an individual's sexual activity. Whatever the reason, listening empathically and referral to an appropriate counselor can assist the client with this problem.

•   •   •

Additional health problems include pulmonary disease, alcoholism, obesity, and other chronic illnesses such as multiple sclerosis. Middle-aged adults should be encouraged to have yearly physical examinations. Many of the illnesses that affect them can be prevented at a primary level or screened at a secondary level and treated before disability occurs. Treatment at a tertiary level also can be important to prevent or limit permanent disability (Fig. 11-4).

Midlife Crisis

Some adults experience a time of dissonance during their forties called a midlife crisis. An individual who has not resolved the identity crisis of adolescence or achieved mature intimacy in adulthood may perceive midlife as a disaster (Murray & Zentner, 1989). In addition, as children leave home and parents become ill or die, thoughts of their own mortality may create periods of emotional distress in middle-aged adults. Such persons may seek counseling or may become highly introspective for a time to attempt to find balance in their lives. This period can be unsettling to those in this age-group and to their families. Nursing intervention can include listening, validation, clarifying, and, if deemed necessary, referral for professional counseling.

Spiritual Development

Doubts and quandries during the forties and fifties can provoke a search for a gestalt structure to answer spiritual needs. Midlife questioning, brought about by a sense of urgency to fulfill life goals, may encompass a search for the meaning and purpose of life. Any family crisis—the illness or death of a member, disappointment in adult children, or divorce—may precipitate questions such as "Why am I doing all this?" "What do I really believe in?" A spiritual dilemma may manifest itself in a number of insidious ways, and unless intervention occurs, a deep sense of depression and despair may lead to clinical depression. One technique, developed by a psychiatrist, Viktor Frankl (1969), is logotherapy.

Frankl developed his theory of logotherapy while he was a prisoner at Auschwitz. One night when the prisoners in his unit were at their lowest ebb from starvation, deprivation, and prolonged illness, he was asked how they could avoid giving up hope. He began by saying that while their bones were still intact, there was hope of regaining health, family, happiness, professional ability, fortune, and position in society. He quoted from Nietzche, "That which does not kill me, makes me stronger." Then he spoke of the future and the small things that might make life easier for them, for example, being attached to a special group with exceptionally good working conditions (small goals). He tried to motivate them to think of the good things that had happened to them in the past and encouraged them to think about those things daily (imaging). He encouraged his fellow prisoners to think of a reason to survive. For one it was a son in another country who needed him. For another it was a scientific work begun, which no one else could have completed (future goals).

Frankl's therapy is anchored in the belief that no matter the circumstances, an individual has choices that affect spiritual freedom. The choices that emphasize personalization and fulfillment of life goals make life meaningful and give it purpose. The choices that lead toward a hopeless, helpless position doom the individual to a kind of spiritual void. Frankl stresses that each person must set daily goals and tasks to give life meaning, that an individual who has a "why" to live can bear the "how." He maintains that individuals in crisis are helped by a process called *self-transcendence* or focusing on others to find a meaning for existence. Middle-aged adults suffering from the loss of valued life experiences (e.g., loss of spouse) might be helped by making a commitment to assist a relative in need or by spending time with children and grandchildren.

Frankl indicates that health is not simply the attainment of physiological and psychological well-being but also must include a component that relates to healthy spirituality. Spirituality is defined as that component of health that relates to core existence—that is, the belief system of the individual—and reflects sensitivity or attachment to religious values.

A nurse who, by observing affect and attitude, perceives a spiritual void or emotional stagnation in a client should remain open and willing to discuss the client's spiritual concerns. Helping the client set daily short-term goals that give life meaning may alleviate some of the spiritual distress. In addition, assisting in the formulation of some long-term goals might motivate the client to move beyond emotional stagnation.

SUMMARY

Young and middle-aged adults in contemporary society are experiencing health stressors and hazards that are unique in the history of human beings. While trying to fulfill developmental tasks, finish school, start an occupation, and begin to raise a family, the young adult may be battling an increasingly competitive job market in a changing society. Middle-aged adults may be attempting to raise children and monitor the well-being of aging parents.

Inability to complete developmental tasks, acute or chronic illness, and excessive stress may lead to a spiritual void in middle-aged adults and predispose them to clinical depression. Helping distressed clients to set daily short-term goals that give life meaning can alleviate some spiritual distress. Assisting them to focus on long-term goals can result in renewed emotional health.

CHAPTER HIGHLIGHTS

- Young and middle-aged adults experience many stresses as a result of increasing changes in the environment. They often are referred to as the "sandwich generation" because they are raising their children at the same time that they are caring for their aging parents.
- According to Erikson the young adult is in the developmental stage of intimacy versus isolation. The middle-aged adult is in the stage of generativity versus stagnation.

- Other theorists who have dealt with the developmental stages of adulthood are Havighurst, Sheehy, Levin, Peck, and Gould.
- The major causes of death in young and middle-aged adults are motor vehicle accidents and other accidents, homicide, suicide, cardiovascular disease, and cancer.
- Diseases that commonly affect young adults include viruses, hepatitis B, skin cancer, lung cancer, periodontal disease, and obesity.
- Diseases and disabilities that commonly affect middle-aged adults include infectious diseases, occupational injury, hiatal hernia, diabetes, glaucoma, and sexual dysfunction.
- Community health nurses can use primary, secondary, and tertiary prevention techniques to prevent or limit the effects of diseases, particularly those that can be predicted.
- Logotherapy was developed to help individuals find meaning and purpose in life. Community health nurses can use principles of logotherapy to help clients fill a spiritual void and avoid emotional stagnation.

STUDY QUESTIONS

1. Describe Erikson's developmental stages for the young and the middle-aged adult.
2. Discuss the stressors placed on young and middle-aged adults today that did not exist in previous generations.
3. Identify the major causes of mortality and morbidity in young and middle-aged adults.
4. Develop a teaching plan that will have as an outcome lowering the incidence of motor vehicle accidents involving young and middle-aged adults.

REFERENCES

Berkow, R. (1982). *The Merck manual of diagnosis and therapy*, (14th ed.). Rahway, NJ: Merck.

Erikson, E. (1963). *Childhood and society*. New York: Norton.

Erikson, E. (1968). *Identity: Youth and crisis*. New York: Norton.

Frankl, V. (1969). *Man's search for meaning*. New York: The World Publishing Co.

Gallagher, L.P., & Kreidler, M. (1987). *Nursing and health: Maximizing human potential throughout the life cycle*. East Norwalk, CT: Appleton & Lange.

Gould, R. (1980). Transformation during early and middle adult years. In N. Smelser & E. Erikson (Eds.), *Themes of work and love in adulthood*. Cambridge: Harvard University Press.

Harrison, T.R. (1977). Principles of Internal Medicine, (8th ed.). New York: McGraw Hill, a Blackiston Publication.

Havighurst, R.J. (1972). *Developmental tasks and education* (3rd ed.). New York: David McKay.

Kimmel, D. (1973). *Adulthood and aging*. New York: Wiley.

Murray, R., & Zentner, J. (1989). *Nursing assessment and health promotion strategies through the life span*. East Norwalk, CT: Appleton & Lange.

National Center for Health Statistics. (1989, September 26). *Monthly vital statistics report* (DHHS 38 (5). Washington, DC: U.S. Government Printing Office.

Neuman, B. (1989). *The Newman systems model* (2nd ed.). Norwalk, CT: Appleton & Lange.

Orem, D. (1985). *Nursing: Concepts of practice* (3rd ed.). New York: McGraw-Hill.

Peck, R. (1968). Psychological developments in the second half of life. In B. Neugarten (Ed.), *Middle age and aging*. Chicago: University of Chicago Press.

Sheehy, G. (1976). *Passages: Predictable crises of adult life*. New York: Dutton.

Toffler, A. (1970). *Future shock*. New York: Random House.

The Adult in Later Maturity

JOAN M. COOKFAIR and PATRICIA A. ANDERSON

To everything there is a season,
and a time to every purpose under heaven.

ECCLESIASTES III:1

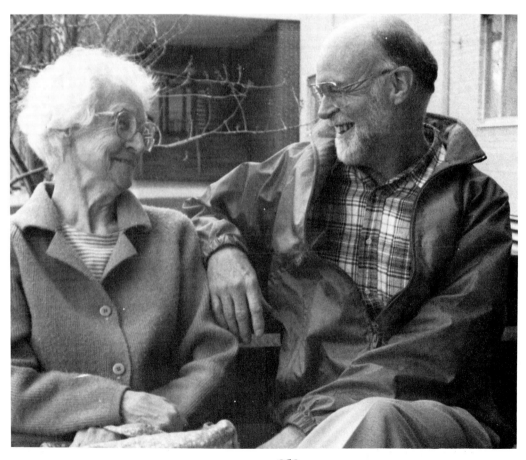

OBJECTIVES

At the conclusion of this chapter the student will be able to:

1. Define the key terms listed
2. Describe the characteristics of the elderly population
3. Describe normal physical and cognitive changes that occur with the aging process
4. Discuss primary, secondary, and tertiary interventions to prevent physical disabilities that may occur as a result of the aging process
5. Describe selected theories of the developmental tasks of aging
6. Describe and compare selected psychosocial theories of aging
7. Describe some health problems that are common to the aging population
8. Describe the role of the nurse in the senior center
9. Identify community resources available to the aging population
10. Discuss the role of the nurse with the fragile elderly population
11. Discuss spiritual nursing

KEY TERMS

Activity theory
Adult day-care
Aging
American Association of Retired Persons
Continuity theory
Disengagement theory
Examination stage

Fragile elderly
Integrity versus anxiety and despair
Later maturity
Presbycusis
Presbyopia
Reality orientation
Spiritual nursing

The photo on the previous page depicts a mother and son who are both in stages of later maturity. The son, aged 62 years, is health conscious, exercises daily, and maintains an active professional career. He does not think of himself as an aging person. His mother, aged 87 years, lives in a senior citizens' apartment building, enjoys good health, and sees her son regularly. Some societal myths about the older population are dispelled by this pair. A few of these myths are as follows (Murray & Zentner, 1989):

1. Most older persons are institutionalized. In reality, approximately 5% of older Americans are institutionalized.
2. Old age brings senility. Approximately 10% of older adults have memory loss.
3. Older persons cannot learn. This is not true. Memorization may take longer, but learning ability remains the same.
4. Old people are all alike. Older people are as different in personality, personal style, and economic status as any other age-group.

Later maturity is a phase of life that begins at about age 65 years and continues to death. Typically it includes the retirement years and may include a period of infirmity and dependence. More people are living to later maturity in this decade than in decades past. This is due, in part, to improved sanitation, better nutrition, fewer deaths from infectious disease, and improved technology. Fig. 12-1 illustrates the increase in the older

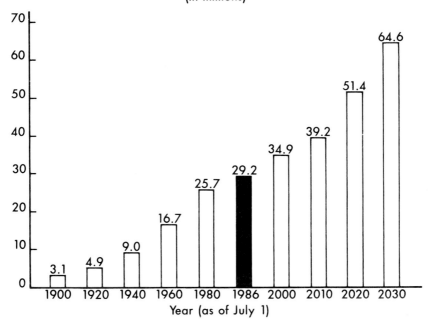

Number of persons 65+: 1900 to 2030
(in millions)

Note: Increments in years on horizontal scale are uneven.

FIG. 12-1 Number of persons aged 65 years and older: 1900 to 2030. *(Based on data from U.S. Bureau of the Census [DHEW Publication No. 79-55071], 1979, Washington, DC: U.S. Government Printing Office.)*

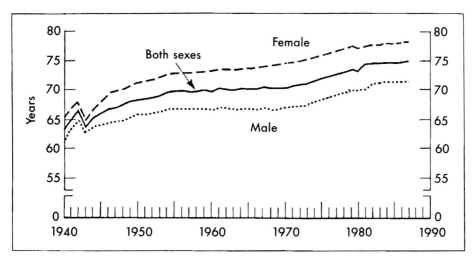

FIG. 12-2 Life expectancy in the United States by sex: 1940 to 1990. *(From Monthly vital statistics report by the National Center for Health Statistics [DHHS Vol. 38, No. 5. Suppl.], September 26, 1989, Washington, DC: U.S. Government Printing Office.)*

population since 1900 and the projected increase through July 1, 2030. The older population is expected to increase most rapidly between the years 2010 and 2030 when the children of the baby boom (those born between 1946 and 1964) reach 65 years of age.

In 1860, 2.7% of the population of the United States reached later maturity. It is predicted that by the year 2030, 21% of the population will be 65 years of age or older.

Fig. 12-2 shows the average life expectancy for persons born in the years between 1940 and 1987 in the United States. The life expectancy for female infants born in 1987 was 78.4 years, compared with 71.4 years for male infants born that year. There is also an ethnic difference in life expectancy. The average life expectancy for the white population between 1986 and 1987 was 75.6 years, whereas the average life expectancy for the black population was 69.4 years. Among the four race-sex groups, white female infants continue to have highest life expectancy (78.9 years), followed by black female infants (73.6 years), white male infants (72.2 years), and black male infants (65.2 years).

THE AGING PROCESS

Despite the research efforts of physical and social scientists, the aging process remains, to a great extent, a mystery. The outward manifestations of aging—the obvious effects of wear and tear and the physiological changes that occur—are observable and even measurable. The causative factors, however, remain unclear. Advances in medical science, improved nutrition, emphasis on health education, and an increase in social awareness have made it possible for many more persons to live to later maturity. On the other hand, there is no evidence that the maximum length of human life has increased. Although more people are living to an older age, there is no research to support the expectation of an increase in the life expectancy of those who survive to 80 years of age.

As persons age, they become more susceptible to specific chronic diseases that impair their functioning and ultimately may cause death. The elderly person may experience physiological changes as a result of the simultaneous effects of disease and the aging process. For a proper understanding of the effects of the aging process, those effects should be considered separately from the effects that can be attributed to disease.

Normal Physical Changes

The older adult gradually experiences normal physical changes. Skin turgor decreases because the sebaceous glands, which normally lubricate the skin with oil, become less active. The skin becomes drier. Irregular areas of dark pigmentation, commonly called age spots, appear on the skin (Murray & Zentner, 1989).

The appearance of the face changes. Wrinkles appear, which are caused by the repeated stress of smiling or frowning.

There are changes in the mouth that may require attention. Periodontal disease in older adults may predispose them to loss of teeth. Dentures can subtly alter the person's appearance. Ill-fitting dentures can be very uncomfortable and interfere with adequate nutrition and speech (Murray & Zentner, 1989).

There is a gradual loss of hair and hair color. Melanin production in the hair follicle diminishes (Murray & Zentner, 1989).

Older adults experience an increasing loss of muscle strength and endurance. Muscle cells atrophy, and lean muscle mass is lost. Planned physical activity and proper nutrition can slow the process.

Nervous system changes accompany the aging process. Older adults, particularly those older than 80 years of age, may have altered sensory response so that nerve transmission is delayed and sensory thresholds increase. The older adult may be slower to make decisions and may be less responsive to pain than is a younger person. The older adult may have decreased equilibrium and coordination (Hogstel, 1981).

There are some visual changes that occur with aging; lacrimal glands produce fewer tears; the lens thickens and there is an impaired ability of the lens to change shape for near vision (presbyopia).

Hearing loss may occur because of changes in the organ of Corti. Approximately 13% of the adult population older than 65 years of age experience progressive loss of hearing (presbycusis) (Murray & Zentner, 1989).

The cardiovascular system changes; vessel membranes thicken and cardiac output decreases. The older adult must learn to adapt to less strenuous exercise; for example, brisk walking may be more appropriate than jogging.

Changes in the respiratory system that result from aging affect both internal and external breathing. There is a gradual decline in the structure and function of the respiratory muscles (Murray & Zentner, 1989).

There is a loss of nephron units in the kidneys, which causes a decrease in the filtration rate. Excretion of toxic substances occurs more slowly than it does in a younger adult. There also is a slowing of peristalsis in the intestinal tract because of fewer stimuli from the autonomic nervous system. The older adult should be encouraged to increase fluid intake and to exercise daily to stimulate filtration. High-fiber foods and exercise can stimulate peristalsis.

The aging man continues to produce testosterone. There is, however, a gradual decline in sexual vigor, muscle strength, and sperm production. The ability of women to continue pleasurable sexual activity remains, although there is a thinning of the vaginal wall that may make penetration difficult and less satisfying to both partners.

Aging depresses immunity in a general way. Older adults who learn to adapt well to the normal changes of aging stay healthy and lead productive lives. Proper nutrition (see Chapter 24), adequate rest and sleep, planned exercise and activity, and lack of emotional stress assist the older adult to remain well. For individuals who are at high risk for infection, immunization against influenza and pneumococcal pneumonia are recommended (Schuster & Ashburn, 1986).

Normal Cognitive Changes

Cognitive changes depend on many factors; however, the innate mental acuity of the individual does not change. An intelligent 7 year old will remain an intelligent person at the age of 70 years if illness does not intervene. Sociocultural influences, life role, adaptability, and motivation all come into play. Wisdom and experience unite in the healthy elderly person so that some may demonstrate crystalized cognition and the ability to perceive relationships, engage in formal abstraction, and understand the ramifications of intellectual and cultural complexities. There may be difficulty in immediate recall of new learning because of delayed sensory input, but the accumulated learning of a lifetime may compensate (Murray & Zentner, 1989).

Table 12-1 describes methods of disability prevention at primary, secondary and tertiary levels relative to the natural aging process.

DEVELOPMENTAL TASKS OF AGING

Erik Erikson (1959) indicates that the crucial task in later adulthood is to evaluate one's life and accomplishments and affirm that the life has been a positive one, that it has not been wasted nor is it meaningless. This conclusion reinforces integrity of the personality in contrast to anxiety and despair. Erikson maintains that to accomplish this developmental

TABLE 12-1	Prevention of disability in the older adult		
Physical disabilities associated with the natural aging process	**Primary prevention**	**Secondary prevention**	**Tertiary prevention**
Hearing			
Presbycusis: loss of auditory acuity associated with age	Encourage avoidance of excessive noise.	Recommend auditory check if speech discrimination skills decrease or if the individual seems inattentive or is giving inappropriate responses to verbal cues.	Encourage examination by otologist to identify possible medical reasons for hearing loss, then to an audiologist for evaluation. Counsel patient and family in communication techniques, for example, to speak slowly and clearly, not louder; face the person to facilitate lip reading; use nonverbal cues when possible (e.g., smiles and waves), write messages and avoid fatigue and environmental distractions; encourage use of hearing aid if helpful.
Taste and smell			
Loss of ability to enjoy food because of decrease in threshhold for taste and smell	Encourage a well-balanced diet and pleasant surroundings during mealtimes.	Recommend listing foods eaten during 24-hour period to determine balanced nutrition.	Encourage vitamin and food supplements if well-balanced diet not adhered to; suggest condiments other than salt to enhance taste of food; Recommend homemaker or family assistance for older adult eating poorly.
Touch			
Decrease in tactile sensation	Encourage avoidance of sudden unexpected changes in body position in space.	Encourage use of cane for extra balance if necessary.	Encourage the individual to allow time before changing position, (e.g., sitting to standing); incorporate sensory stimulation in all aspects of rehabilitation program.
Vision			
Presbyopia (old sight): associated with aging; lens loses ability to accommodate to near and far vision	Encourage regular eye checkups, general check using Snellen eye chart for acuity, general check for peripheral vision; refer for eye examination if necessary.	Recommend wearing bifocals as needed to prevent accidents and mistakes; recommend strong reading glasses to prevent fatigue and disengagement.	Recommend cessation of driving if vision level less than 20/40; recommend magnifying glasses for reading, adequate glare-reduction lighting, use of large print, magnifying glasses and more auditory cues.
Possibility of glaucoma: caused by high intraocular pressure; insidious onset	Encourage regular eye checkups that include screening for glaucoma.	Refer for treatment if glaucoma is detected.	Encourage use of prescribed eye drops, (e.g., pilocarpine and epinephrine); assist with activities of daily living, transportation, and recreation if blindness occurs.

TABLE 12-1 Prevention of disability in the older adult—cont'd

Physical disabilities associated with the natural aging process	Primary prevention	Secondary prevention	Tertiary prevention
Vision—cont'd			
Cataracts: caused by a degenerative opacity of lens of eye, which results in obstruction of light rays to retina	Encourage regular eye checkups.	Recommend surgical intervention if needed.	Encourage cataract lenses, possibly contact lenses; educate to adapt to difficulty in focusing and aphakia (lack of focusing ability) and to compensate for lack of depth perception.
Musculoskeletal			
Decreased skeletal bone mass because of decreased intestinal absorption of calcium; more common in women than in men	Encourage supplemental calcium for postmenopausal women; recommend at least two glasses of milk/day in diet.	Recommend oral daily supplement of vitamin D and calcium (600 mg 4-6 times/day); refer to physician for follow-up calcium levels; counsel to avoid falls and excessive weight bearing.	Recommend hyperextension exercises to strengthen flabby muscles and avoid heavy lifting or accidental falls if osteoporosis is present; counsel in use of orthopedic support walkers, analgesics, heat and massage.
Muscles: progressive loss of muscular strength because of changes in collagen fibers, less flexibility	Encourage daily exercise, walking, rotating hips, straightening legs, and rotating arms and shoulders.	Provide slow, prolonged stretching exercises.	Recommend continuing exercises in a home care program to encourage functional motion; assist with activities of daily living if function is lost or limited.
Joints: decrease in cartilage so that bone makes direct contact with bone and can result in degenerative arthritis	Encourage adherence to moderate exercise program to prevent stiffening of joints; ensure adequate rest, and avoid extreme cold.	Encourage rest of affected joint, analgesics as ordered; recommend adherence to prescribed exercise; encourage weight reduction if appropriate.	Encourage warm soaks, analgesics if necessary, rest, and medical assistance; instruct in the use of canes and walkers; rehabilitate after hip replacement if necessary.
Skin, hair, and toes: wrinkling of skin and graying of hair because the cell layers of the epidermis are thinning Graying of hair because of a reduction in melanin	Encourage staying out of the sun because the sun speeds up the aging process; use sun screen.	Encourage use of moisturizing cream if psoriatic patches begin to appear.	Avoid trauma that may result in senile purpura and lead to skin infection; apply dressings and antiseptics as needed.
Rate of nail growth decreases and causes thickening nails	Encourage soaking before cutting nails to prevent injury.	Refer to podiatrist.	

Continued.

TABLE 12-1 Prevention of disability in the older adult—cont'd			
Physical disabilities associated with the natural aging process	**Primary prevention**	**Secondary prevention**	**Tertiary prevention**
Immunity			
Antibody response to antigen decreased because of fewer cytotoxic T lymphocytes	Encourage annual influenza and pneumonia vaccines and avoidance of stress, cold, and chills; maintain prudent nutrition (see Chapter 25), wear appropriate clothing and avoid exposure to viral infection.	Monitor changes in health status; refer for early medical treatment.	Encourage adherence to prescribed regime; assist in client recovery or adaption to chronic illness.
Nervous system			
Loss of neurons in frontal lobe; decreased availability of neurotransmitters	Encourage stress management, adequate rest, structured environment.	Monitor changes in mental status.	Refer for medical checkup if changes occur; assist with activities of daily living and medical regimen.
Sexuality			
Men, penile erection takes longer; women, loss of vaginal lubrication	Encourage patience; recommend vaginal creams.	Counsel if necessary.	Refer for assistance if chronic illnes interferes with adaptation; counsel as to comfort positions.

task, the individual first must successfully complete other developmental tasks in the life cycle.

Robert Havighurst (1975) calls later maturity the *examination stage* and maintains that the elderly adult must accomplish the following tasks:

1. Decide where and how to live out remaining years.
2. Continue supportive, close relationships with spouse or significant others (including sexual activity).
3. Find a satisfactory and safe living space.
4. Adjust living standards.
5. Maintain maximum level of health.
6. Maintain contact with children, grandchildren, and other relatives.
7. Maintain interest in people and in events, such as civic affairs.
8. Pursue new interests and maintain earlier ones.
9. Find meaning in life after retirement.
10. Work out a philosophy.
11. Adjust to death of spouse and other loved ones.

Carl Jung says about aging, "We cannot live the afternoon of life according to life's morning; for what was great in the morning will be little at evening and what in the morning was true will at evening have become a lie" (1971, p. 17). Jung reports that although many persons reach old age with unsatisfied life goals, it is unwise to look back. It is essential to find a goal for the future. He suggests that in the later years of life individuals need to spend time in reflection to find a meaning and purpose in life that makes it possible to accept approaching death: "An old man who cannot bid farewell to life appears as sickly and feeble as the young man who cannot embrace it" (p. 20).

PSYCHOSOCIAL THEORIES OF AGING

The disengagement theory proposes that older adults and society inevitably undergo a mutual withdrawal that is an essential part of the aging process and that is beneficial to society. In direct opposition to the disengagement theory is the *activity theory,* which maintains that development of a high level of physical, mental, and social activity is needed by the individual past middle age and that if societal roles are given up, new roles must replace them (Burnside, 1984).

The *continuity theory* states that the maturing adult maintains a continuity of personality and that individuals do not drastically change as they age. They simply become more of what they were. Older adults who were healthy emotionally in their earlier life tend to remain so. Healthy older persons have an open attitude, adapt to physical changes, and maintain independence if they stay physically well (Burnside, 1984).

The *activity theory* includes the suggestion that most adults maintain a high level of activity and involvement and that the amount of activity is more influenced by previous life-styles and by socioeconomic forces than by internal or inevitable processes (Burnside, 1988).

COMMON HEALTH PROBLEMS OF LATER MATURITY

Common health problems that face elderly persons are, in part, due to the normal aging process. Some health problems can be prevented at primary, secondary, and tertiary levels as described in Table 12-1. A community health nurse who is performing a physical assessment of an older client may find it helpful to use a systems approach as described in the following section and summarized in Table 12-2.

Constitutional

Any excessive weight gain or weight loss can be a reason to refer a client to a physician for a complete physical examination. Low-grade fever, repeated infections, and fatigue may be symptoms of insidious underlying disease process.

Psychological

Dreams or nightmares, crying, insomnia, and depression are reasons for a complete physical and psychological examination. Depression in persons of later maturity is not uncommon; in rare instances it may be a precursor to dementia.

One life task that may precipitate depression is retirement. Although anticipation of retirement can be stressful, successful transition can be assisted by preretirement planning. Some retired persons find pleasure in doing volunteer work; they remain useful and feel needed but do not have to maintain an exhausting schedule (Fig. 12-3).

Persons in the advanced elderly age-group, especially 75 to 80 years of age and older, sometimes suffer from chronic depression as a result of cumulative losses. Siblings and

TABLE 12-2 Review of systems: physical assessment and health history

Constitutional	Health overall; weight gain or loss; fever; fatigue; repeated infections; ability to carry out activities
Psychological	Dreams or nightmares; crying; depression; anxiety; insomnia; diagnosed mental illness
Integument	General skin condition and care. Any changes; rash; itch; nail deformity; hair loss; moles; open areas
Head, ears, eyes, nose, throat, teeth	Head: aches; evidence of trauma or bumps; hair loss
	Eyes: eye care; poor eyesight; double or blurred vision; use of corrective lenses or medications
	Ears: hearing acuity; reaction to noise level; tinnitus (ringing in ears); presence of infection or pain
	Nose and throat: upper respiratory infections; hoarseness; sore throat; sinusitis; epistaxis (nose bleeds); dysphagia (difficulty swallowing)
	Teeth: dentures or dental work; caries. Pattern of brushing and use of dental floss. Fluoride application
Respiratory	History of respiratory infections; self-treatment of colds
	Cough and its duration; last chest x-ray; tuberculin skin test and results; dyspnea (difficulty breathing) and when (night-time, with exertion); wheezing; asthma or bronchitis; hemoptysis (coughing or spitting up blood)
Cardiovascular	Exercise pattern to maintain cardiovascular health. Edema; varicose veins; heart sounds, including murmur; chest pains; palpitations; hypertension (high blood pressure); electrocardiogram (EKG)
Gastrointestinal	Dietary pattern; amount of fiber in diet. Heartburn; epigastric pain; abdominal pain; nausea and vomiting; food intolerance; flatulence; diarrhea; constipation; clay-colored, tarry, or bright red stools; hemorrhoids; history of ulcers
Genitourinary	Nocturia; dysuria; incontinence; resistance; sexual difficulty; venereal disease; history of stones. Men: slow stream; penile discharge; contraceptive use; self-testicular examination (technique and frequency). Women: breast lumps, breast self-examination and how often; menarche; menopause; intermenstrual bleeding; last menstrual period; contraceptive use; last Pap smear
Musculoskeletal	Exercise pattern. Neck pain or stiffness; joint pain or swelling; incapacitating back pain; paralysis; deformities
Neurological	Syncope; stroke; seizures; paresthesia
Lymphatic and hematological	Enlarged, tender nodes; easy bruising; anemia; bleeding
Endocrine	Polydipsia; polyphagia; polyuria; intolerance of heat or cold; weight gain or loss; changes in skin, hair, or nail texture
Immunological	Immunization record; what diseases and dates

From *Nursing assessment and health promotion through the life span*, (4th ed.) 1989 by R. Murray and J. Zentner, 1989, Norwalk, CT: Appleton & Lange, p. 633. Copyright 1989 by Appleton & Lange. Reprinted by permission.

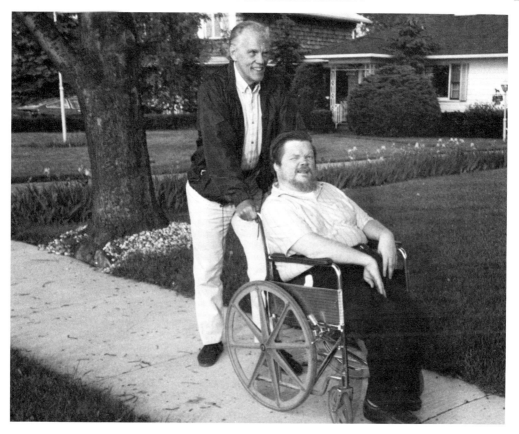

FIG. 12-3 The older adult doing volunteer work.

friends begin to die, they have diminished energy, and some even experience loss of children. Community health nurses should watch for prolonged sadness, withdrawal, irritability, agitation, and excessive fatigue.

Integument

General skin condition should be observed. Aging skin tends to be dry, and sometimes annoying itching can occur. The older client should be advised to lubricate the skin after bathing. The use of bath oil and mild soap may be helpful.

Head, Ears, Eyes

Prevention of disabilities related to ears and eyes is described in Table 12-1. If, however, a client experiences severe visual impairment, both client and family should be instructed to keep the environment free of hazards: no scatter rugs on the floor, well-lighted rooms, no furniture with sharp edges, and few changes in arrangement of the furniture.

Severe impairment in hearing acuity can create a secondary condition. Inability to hear may result in a withdrawal because of communication difficulty. The following techniques are helpful in speaking to a person who is hard of hearing: speaking in a good light to facilitate any lipreading, facing the person, and using a light touch to attract the individual's attention. Facial expression is especially important because open, friendly

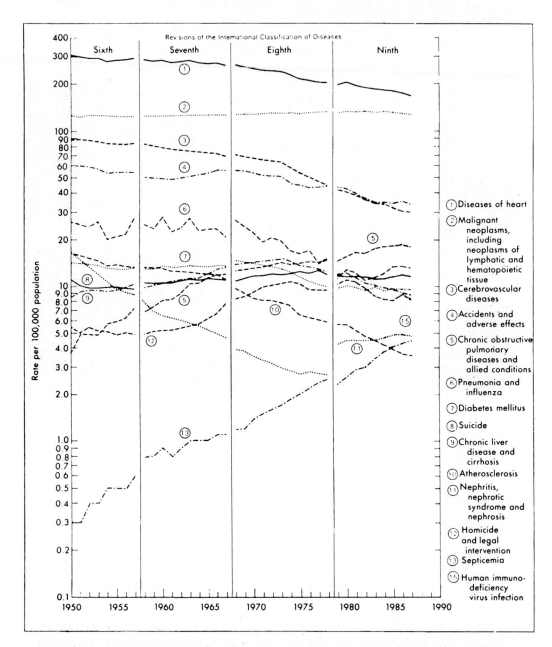

FIG. 12-4 Age-adjusted death rates for 14 of the 15 leading causes of death: United States, 1950 to 1990. *(From* Monthly vital statistics report *by the National Center for Health Statistics [DHHS 38 (5)], September 26, 1989, Washington, DC: U.S. Government Printing Office.)*

communication may be established by what the person can see rather than hear. If possible, important messages should be written as well as verbalized.

Respiratory System

Some form of chronic lung disease, for example, chronic obstructive pulmonary disease (COPD) from emphysema, bronchoconstriction, or bronchitis, may be present in the elderly adult. There also is the possibility, especially in persons older than 80 years of age, that arrested tuberculosis will become active as a result of depressed immunity connected with the aging process. Upper respiratory infections are particularly serious for this group. Any elderly adult who suffers from chronic lung disease should be encouraged to have yearly influenza and pneumococcal vaccine as indicated (Murray & Zentner, 1989).

Cardiovascular System

Cardiovascular disease is the leading cause of death in persons older than 60 years of age (Fig. 12-4). Often arteriosclerosis and hypertension are precursors. Congestive heart failure may be present if the individual complains of ankle swelling, if neck veins are distended, or if rales are heard in the lungs. A low-sodium diet can be recommended to improve renal excretion. Medication can be prescribed for hypertension and digitalis for strengthening the heart beat. Persons with congestive heart failure should be assessed on a regular basis to prevent their condition from becoming life threatening.

Chronic occlusive arterial disease of the extremities may occur because of partial or complete occlusion of one or more of the peripheral blood vessels. Elderly persons who complain of a cramping pain in the muscles, which is relieved by rest, should be assessed for decreased peripheral pulses. If this condition is clinically verified and is accompanied by shiny skin and loss of normal skin hair, the person should be instructed in good skin care and should avoid excessive heat and cold. Smoking and caffeine ingestion also should be avoided.

Stasis ulcers of the lower extremities may result from chronic venous stasis and consequent poor circulation. Although peripheral pulses may be present, pitting edema occurs because of compromised venous circulation. Elevation of the extremities and cleansing with an antiseptic may assist in healing (Murray & Zentner, 1989).

Gastrointestinal System

Because neoplasms are the second highest cause of death in elderly persons (see Fig. 12-4), periodic assessment of the gastrointestinal tract should be conducted.

Genitourinary System

Aging men frequently experience a condition called benign prostatic hypertrophy. This enlargement of the prostate gland is easily corrected by surgical intervention. (Murray & Zentner, 1989).

Musculoskeletal System

Osteoporosis, a decrease in bone tissue mass, is found in one fourth of all white women in the United States who are past menopause. Men older than 80 years of age also are at risk for this problem, which predisposes the person to bone fractures in the affected areas. Some research has shown that taking calcium in the younger years may prevent this condition (Murray & Zentner, 1989).

Neurological System

A number of neurological diseases may cause disability in later maturity. Herpes zoster results in a unilateral vesicular eruption and occurs in persons with altered immune responses. Parkinson's disease is a progressive degenerative disorder that can be highly debilitating and that requires careful monitoring. Alzheimer's disease, also a progressive degenerative disorder, requires not only in-depth monitoring but extensive family therapy to help family members deal with resultant multiple problems (Murray & Zentner, 1989).

Lymphatic and Hematological Systems

Pernicious anemia, which occurs because of a lack of intrinsic factor essential for the absorption of vitamin B_{12}, may require supplemental B_{12} injections on a routine basis. Lymphatic leukemia, which is a neoplasm of blood-forming tissues, is a severe health hazard that may occur in late maturity.

Endocrine System

Diabetes mellitus should be suspected if the older client complains of polydipsia or polyurea, frequent infections, or numbness and tingling of the extremities. This condition is the most common metabolic disorder of the endocrine system in elderly persons (Murray & Zentner, 1989).

The box on p. 267 lists selected nursing diagnoses approved by the North American Nursing Diagnosis Association (NANDA), which relate to persons in later maturity. More detailed explanations of health problems that may affect the individual in late maturity may be found in any medical/surgical textbook.

HEALTH PROMOTION IN THE SENIOR CITIZEN CENTER

The older retired adult who remains healthy may function as well as ever and may enjoy the freedom to pursue interests and hobbies rather than full-time employment. The person who becomes less mobile can benefit from community support services such as Meals on Wheels, transportation, shopping aides, and telephone reassurance programs. Senior citizen centers may provide social outlets, warm meals, and referral services to all citizens who seek them. A useful service to those who need assistance is the adult day-care center, which can uniquely meet the needs of the older age-group in the community in a number of ways. It is primarily a social center that plans events and activities organized to capture the interest of the senior citizen and to stimulate social interaction. In addition, programs for health promotion can be facilitated.

Ideally, the senior citizen centers and adult day-care centers include a nurse and a social worker to assist participants with health problems as well as social and personal problems. Students from various professionally oriented career programs often find the center a place for clinical assignments and projects. The center is a good setting for students because it furnishes them with an opportunity to interact with and to study and understand the unique needs of older citizens in the community. This interaction is beneficial both to students and to clients.

Psychosocial Needs

After a person is retired, social interaction and activity can be reduced severely or ended entirely to the point where the person becomes socially deprived. Interaction and activity can be facilitated at the adult day-care center to overcome potential social deprivation. Interaction on a daily basis with others of the same generation can replace former work companions and social friends. There often is a card game or just a coffee and discussion

SELECTED NURSING DIAGNOSES RELATED TO PERSON IN LATER MATURITY*

Pattern 1: Exchanging

Altered nutrition: more than body requirements
Altered nutrition: less than body requirements
Hypothermia
Hyperthermia
Stress incontinence
Potential for injury
Potential for trauma
Potential for disuse syndrome
Potential impaired skin integrity

Pattern 2: Communicating

Impaired verbal communication

Pattern 3: Relating

Impaired social interaction
Social isolation
Altered role performance
Sexual dysfunction
Altered family processes
Altered sexuality patterns

Pattern 4: Valuing

Spiritual distress

Pattern 5: Choosing

Ineffective individual coping
Impaired adjustment
Defensive coping
Ineffective denial
Ineffective family coping: disabling
Ineffective family coping: compromised
Family coping: potential for growth
Decisional conflict
Health seeking behaviors

Pattern 6: Moving

Impaired physical mobility
Fatigue
Potential activity intolerance
Sleep pattern disturbance
Diversional activity deficit
Impaired home maintenance management
Altered health maintenance
Bathing/hygiene self care deficit
Dressing/grooming self care deficit

Pattern 7: Perceiving

Body image disturbance
Self esteem disturbance
Chronic low self esteem
Situational low self esteem
Sensory/perceptual alterations
Unilateral neglect
Hopelessness
Powerlessness

Pattern 8: Knowing

Knowledge deficit
Altered thought processes

Pattern 9: Feeling

Pain
Chronic pain
Dysfunctional grieving
Anticipatory grieving
Post-trauma response
Anxiety
Fear

*Other of the NANDA diagnoses related to physiological phenomena are applicable to the ill individual in this group.

session in progress. The members of the center become friends and confidants who can partially meet each other's social needs (Fig. 12-5). Other needs can be met and problems solved through the efforts of social workers and counselors, who can help the senior manage many problems that may seem overwhelming at the time. For example, family problems can be discussed discreetly with a staff member, and the client can be supported to cope effectively, or appropriate community referrals can be made. This kind of assistance will reduce the senior's anxiety level and consequently contribute to improved overall health.

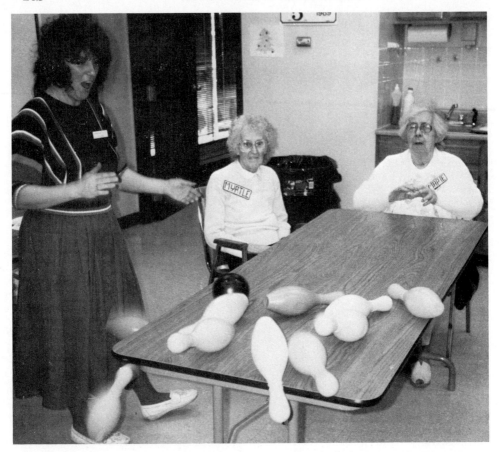

FIG. 12-5 Older adults can enjoy the social activities offered by an adult day-care center.

Physical Needs

The adult day-care center and the senior citizen center can assist the older adult in the community setting in meeting physical and social needs. A community health nurse, on site or on call, can monitor and guide the health care of the clients at the centers. Regularly scheduled blood pressure clinics and physical assessment clinics can be arranged to gather baseline information and to screen for potential or actual health problems. The nurse can answer questions regarding medical diagnoses and medications ordered by physicians that may alarm, confuse, and cause anxiety for the older adult. In addition, information concerning current news items such as cholesterol and diet management can be made available. Subtle changes in the overall health status of the senior citizen can be detected and proper action taken when signs of a potential problem appear. In this case the nurse can make referrals to appropriate health professionals and community resources.

State funding in the form of grants has been made available in some areas to support these centers. This financial aid attests to the invaluable services in the areas of social interaction and health promotion the centers offer mature adults in the community.

Similar services may be provided by various community services and agencies such as the local YMCA or Jewish Community Center. Nurses should become familiar with the available resources in their area and refer clients as appropriate.

OTHER COMMUNITY RESOURCES

Other community resources that are available to the older adult include the following (Murray & Zentner, 1989):

1. The American Association of Retired Persons (AARP), an organization for persons older than 50 years of age. Members are provided with information of interest to retired and preretired persons, such as lobbying activity on behalf of their age-group, and access to discount drug purchases, health and automobile insurance, and other benefits.
2. Respite care, which provides relief for family care givers over a weekend or holiday. This may be provided in the client's home or in another setting, such as a nursing home or senior citizen complex.
3. Adult congregate living facilities (ACLF), which provide room, board, and personal services but no nursing or medical services.
4. Adult day-care for frail or fragile elderly who need care through the day either because they live alone or because family members are absent during certain time periods.

CASE STUDY

The Reverend C was admitted to a skilled nursing facility with a diagnosis of organic brain syndrome. He was 78 years of age and a widower with four adult children. His wife had died 1 year earlier. Until 6 months before admission he had been the pastor of a local church with a large congregation. He frequently had visited members of this church at the facility where he was now living. He had a history of infrequent transient ischemic attacks accompanied by vertigo and confusion and had fallen several times, sustaining minor injuries. His son and daughter reported that his confusion had begun shortly after their mother's death, which they believed had strongly affected him. At about the same time the church secretary had retired. Both women had organized his life for years. His children indicated that the reason for admission was his inability to accept retirement or his wife's death. He returned to the church whenever possible and repeatedly asked where his wife was. On a number of occasions, when he had driven to make calls on church members, he became lost and confused and had difficulty getting home. His son, with whom he had been living, stated that he and his family could not keep their father at home because he would not stay there and became agitated if they attempted to force him to do so. The admitting nurse observed that the Reverend C was agitated the day of admission and then seemed to withdraw. He stopped coming to meals and spoke very little. The nursing care plan for the Reverend C is shown in Table 12-3.

One month after his reality orientation program began, the Reverend C was attending and taking part in group meetings. He regularly visited his clients and interacted appropriately with them. His autobiography was extensive but related only to his early life. He never acknowledged his wife's death by talking or writing about it. He also did not remember the death of one of his children, although his surviving children visited often and he remembered them. He accepted the use of the cane, walked regularly, and went to the dining room for meals. It was found, however, that unless the reality orientation program of one-on-one for 15 minutes daily was continued, the Reverend C once more became depressed and withdrawn.

TABLE 12-3 Nursing care plan for the Reverend C

Nursing diagnosis	Plan	Intervention	Evaluation
1. Alteration in thought process related to loss of short-term memory	1. Rev. C will tolerate 15 minutes of reality orientation daily.	1. Nurse will spend time daily talking with Rev. C, allowing him to express his feelings and answering questions. The room will be equipped with a calendar and clock. Rev. C will be walked to group meetings, recreational programs, and worship services.	1. Rev. C will express understanding of where he is and why; agitation and confusion will decrease within 1 month. He will be able to attend meetings by himself; he will not get lost.
2. Disturbance in self-concept related to altered role performance, self-esteem	2. Arrange to have Rev. C visit and talk to bedridden patients; encourage him to lead group discussions and meetings.	2. Rev. C was given three patients on his floor to visit.	2. Rev. C will speak appropriately with clients, and they will enjoy his visit.
3. Ineffective individual coping related to change in life-style	3. Arrange for writing of past experiences; looking back on things, reminiscing.	3. Rev. C was supplied with a typewriter, paper, and desk.	3. Rev. C will begin writing his autobiography.
4. Potential for injury related to transient ischemic attacks	4. Teach Rev. C to use a cane.	4. Rev. C was instructed to use his cane.	4. Rev. C will use his cane.

THE FRAGILE ELDERLY PERSON

The fragile elderly who require long-term extended care facilities comprise approximately 5% of the older population. Of these, not all are permanent nursing home residents. Some will recover and go back to residences in the community (Spradley, 1985). Those who must remain institutionalized because of chronic illness or cognitive impairment will still benefit from attempts to improve the quality of life within the institutional setting. Encouraging as much autonomy as possible and allowing residents to make decisions and preserve their uniqueness will help keep them functioning at their highest level of wellness for as long as possible.

The older adult who, because of arteriosclerosis, depression, anxiety, or other chronic disease process, is cognitively impaired may be helped by a process called *reality orientation*, programs that focus them on present events. The case study on p. 269 describes one such nursing intervention.

SPIRITUAL NURSING CARE

It should be remembered that adults in later maturity are coping with the knowledge that they are moving toward the part of the life cycle that is a mystery. To some this is viewed as an end to *being* and to others as a peaceful journey. To all it is unknown.

Spiritual nursing care includes listening to concerns, providing an opportunity to talk about death, and assisting in summing up or reminiscing about their life, if they care to do so. An individual with a strongly developed religious life may enjoy quoting familiar Bible passages and praying. It may be even more urgent for persons who regard death as an end to being to discuss anxieties and concerns either about themselves or others at this point in their lives. Anxieties of a practical nature are easier to deal with than are anxieties concerning approaching death. These concerns are best handled with compassion, a nonjudgmental approach, patience, and an honest interest in the client's welfare, thoughts, feelings, and opinions (Carroll, 1985).

SUMMARY

The elderly population is growing at a faster rate today than at any time in the past. This increase is expected to continue; the projection is that approximately 21% of the population of the United States will be 65 years of age or older by the year 2030. Advances in medical science, improved sanitation, improved nutrition, and a greater emphasis on health education have made it possible for people to live longer and remain healthy.

As people live longer, they are affected by normal physiological and cognitive changes of aging. They also become more susceptible to chronic disease. The combination of the two may significantly impair functioning.

Community health nurses can use primary, secondary, and tertiary prevention techniques to promote health and minimize the disabling effects of disease. They must therefore be familiar with the normal effects of aging on all body systems. Settings for practice include outpatient clinics, senior citizen apartment buildings, and senior citizen and adult day-care centers in the community.

CHAPTER HIGHLIGHTS

- The adult in later maturity can enjoy good health and an active life. Approximately 95% of older Americans live independently in the community.
- Physical and cognitive changes are normal with aging. Prevention at primary, secondary and tertiary levels can help prevent disability as these changes occur.
- According to Erikson, developmental tasks of aging include developing a feeling that one's life has not been meaningless. Havighurst calls later maturity the examination stage, and Jung recommends that older people spend time in reflection.
- Psychosocial theories of aging include the disengagement theory, the activity theory, and the continuity theory.
- Mature adults face common health problems. Periodic physical assessment can identify some developing problems before they become disabling.
- Of the several community resources for adults in later maturity, some of the most pleasurable are the senior center and the adult day-care center.
- The fragile, or frail, elderly persons who must be institutionalized can still be helped through nursing intervention to improve their quality of life.

STUDY QUESTIONS

1. Describe three normal physical changes associated with aging.
2. Discuss the nurse's role in the prevention of disability as a result of these physical changes.

3. Discuss and compare the disengagement theory and the activity theory of aging.
4. Identify three health promotion activities the nurse can perform in an adult day-care center.
5. Discuss spiritual nursing care. Why is it particularly helpful with older adults?

REFERENCES

Burnside, I. (1988). *Nursing and the aged: a self-care approach* (3rd ed.). New York: McGraw Hill.

Burnside, I. (1984). *Working with the elderly: Group process and techniques*. Monterey, CA: Wadsworth.

Carroll, D. (1985). *Living with dying*. New York: McGraw-Hill.

Erikson, E. (1959). *Identity and the life cycle*. Selected papers, New York: International University Press.

Havighurst, R. (1975). A social psychological perspective on aging. In W. S. Sze (Ed.), *Human life cycle*. New York: Aronson.

Hochschild, A. R. (1975). Disengagement theory: A critique and proposal. *American Sociological Review, 40,* 553-569.

Hogstel, M. (1981). *Nursing care of the older adult*. New York: Wiley.

Jung, C. (1971). The stages of life. In J. Campbell (Ed.), *The portable Jung*. New York: Viking.

Kimmel, D. (1974). *Adulthood and aging*. New York: Wiley.

Linden, M. & Courtney, D. (1953). The human life cycle and its interruptions: A psychological hypothesis: Studies in gerontological human relations. *American Journal of Psychiatry, 109,* pp. 906-916.

Murray, R., & Zentner, J. (1989). Nursing assessment and health promotion strategies through the life span (4th ed.), Norwalk, CT: Appleton & Lange.

National Center for Health Statistics. (1989, September 26). *Monthly vital statistics report* (DHHS *38* [5]) Washington, DC: U.S. Government Printing Office.

Neugarten, B., & Havighurst, R. (1973). Extending the human life span: social policy and social ethics. Unpublished manuscript, University of Chicago, Committee on Human Development.

Schuster, C., & Ashburn, S. (1986). *The process of human development: A holistic life span approach* (2nd ed.). Boston: Little, Brown & Co.

Spradley, B. (1985). *Community health nursing: Concepts and practices*. Boston: Little, Brown & Co.

The Family in the Community

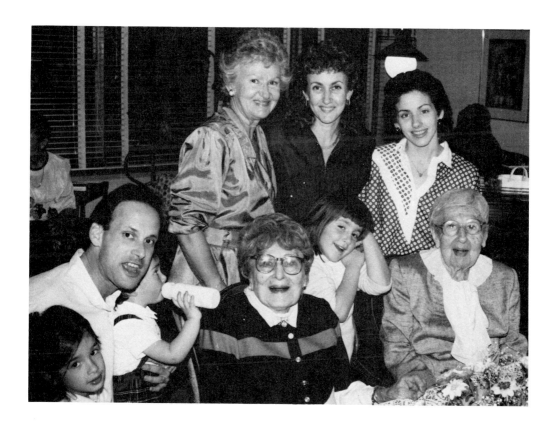

A nurse who practices within a family unit frequently must involve the entire family in a plan of care to promote the wellness of one family member. Most families function as a system, and anything that impairs one part of the system affects the entire system.

Chapter 13 describes various types of families and focuses on the functional family. A functional family develops adaptive coping mechanisms and operates at a level of wellness. This is not to say that stressors do not occur. They simply are dealt with in a way that contributes to the health of the family members and attempts to maintain equilibrium within the family system. The chapter also points out some of the changes that are occurring within the family structure as we approach the year 2000. More women in the work force, increased use of modern technology, and an aging population are subtly influencing the modern family. In this chapter several conceptual frameworks are outlined which nurses can use in the study of family life. Assessment tools for planning care for families also are provided.

To practice effectively in our increasingly diverse cultural population, nurses frequently need a knowledge of the ethnic differences among various groups. Chapter 14 describes several cultural groups and encourages the student to develop an awareness of their cultural patterns, as well as an understanding of the nurse's own ethnicity.

Chapter 15 describes the characteristics of families who are at risk for, or have developed, dysfunctional behavior. The role of the nurse in enabling members of dysfunctional families to move toward wellness behavior is complex. This chapter identifies numerous variables and stressors that can cause or result in dysfunctional behavior and outlines nursing actions for intervention at primary, secondary, and tertiary levels.

Just as the wellness of an individual affects a family, the wellness of a family can affect an entire community. Thus nurses who practice in the community can raise the level of wellness in the community by raising the level of wellness in even one family.

The Family as a Unit of Service

SANDRA L. TERMINI

The family of the future may neither vanish nor enter upon a new golden age. It may break up and shatter, only to come together again in weird and novel ways.

ALVIN TOFFLER

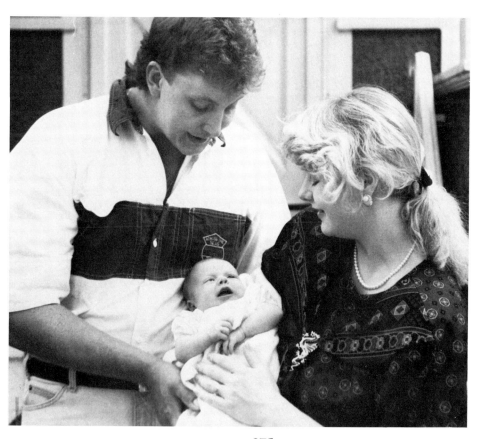

OBJECTIVES

At the conclusion of this chapter the student will be able to:
1. Define the key terms listed
2. Identify five types of families
3. Describe evolving family structures
4. Describe role behavior within the family unit
5. Explain communication theory
6. Describe crisis theory
7. Define the functional family
8. Describe adaptive family coping patterns
9. Discuss three conceptual frameworks that can be used in understanding the family
10. Use a systems framework to identify the interactive aspect of the individual's and the family's level of wellness
11. Use the nursing process to raise the level of wellness in a family
12. Use a systems framework to identify the interaction between the family's and the community's level of wellness

KEY TERMS

Blended family	Genogram
Communication	Kin network family
Crisis theory	Maturational crisis
Ecomap	Metacommunication
Extended family	Nuclear family
Family	Nuclear family dyad
Family developmental tasks	Single-parent family
Family life cycle	Situational crisis

A thorough understanding of the family is essential to the practice of professional nursing. Historically, community health nurses have utilized a family-oriented focus by including all family members in their assessment and involving them in care and counseling. Providing care in the client's home rather than a hospital or a clinic gives the nurse a totally different perspective and presents a more accurate picture of the individual as part of a family and a community system. Home nursing care takes place in the client's territory, and health care planning responsibilities are shared equally by the health care provider and the client/family system.

In this chapter the definition of *family* in contemporary society is reviewed, various types of families are described, several conceptual frameworks for studying the family are discussed, and the process of providing nursing care for the family as a unit is examined.

Knowledge of theory provides only part of a nurse's preparation in planning family care. Nurses also must consider their own personal family experiences and background inasmuch as these experiences form the perceptual field through which they view other families. Understanding one's own culture and values helps a nurse both to respect and to be more objective in evaluating families with differing life-styles.

WHAT IS A FAMILY?

Various disciplines have developed their own definitions of family. Each is based on the particular emphasis of that field. Biological definitions of family describe mating, reproduction, and descent and do not emphasize psychosocial aspects of partnering or parenting. Sociologists view the family as a social group usually related by blood or contract. Legal definitions of family consider the phenomena of marriage, divorce or separation, and adoption, which create nonbiological family configurations. These are only a few examples of the differing focuses of various disciplines.

Common to all definitions of family are that families comprise more than one person, with at least one adult, and that these persons are related to one another by blood or social contract.

It is very important to remember that the structure and form of the family are dynamic and everchanging. Anthropologists acknowledge that some form of family is found in every culture. Historical reference to family forms are found in folklore and in ancient written manuscripts such as the Old Testament of the Bible. Scientists are not in agreement regarding a clear path of evolution from primitive human life forms to the contemporary family. The significant fact is that the concept of family has existed in some form since the beginning of time and has survived centuries of change, disruption, and technological growth.

TYPES OF FAMILIES

Typical family structures vary from culture to culture. Even within one culture the family structure constantly is changing and evolving into new forms. The more common types of families are described here (Friedman, 1981; Hymovich, 1980; Sussman, 1971).

The *nuclear family* consists of husband and wife with one child or more. Although this family type is the idealized or perceived "typical" family, it represented only 38% of American families in 1985 (National Data Bank, 1986).

The *nuclear family dyad* is the term applied to the increasing number of adult couples who choose to remain childless or to "empty nesters" whose children have grown and left home.

The *single-parent* family consists of only one parent with one or more children, an arrangement resulting from divorce, separation, abandonment, death, or a never-married parent.

The *single adult living alone* does not fit the strict definition of a family (comprised of more than one person) but may be viewed as part of a family modified as a result of divorce, abandonment, death, or the choice to live alone. This person still may function as a part of his or her original birth family, also known as the *family of orientation.*

The *three-generation or extended family* can encompass any combination of the nuclear, dyad, single parent, or single adult. At one time it was common for several generations of a family to share a home. With the advent of modern technology, communication networks, and transportation systems, nuclear families are more likely to be geographically mobile. Relatively frequent career-related moves around the state or country have contributed to the separation and fragmentation of the extended family system.

The *kin network family* includes nuclear families or unmarried members living in close proximity and working together in a reciprocal system of exchange of goods and services. This family form probably has arisen to provide the support network once found in extended families.

THE EVOLVING FAMILY STRUCTURE

Life in the United States has changed dramatically in the last several decades. As Americans struggle to keep up with technological developments that alter virtually every aspect of daily life, new family structures emerge to meet the needs of a new day. Economic changes have contributed to an increasing number of women in the work force. In 1960 27.7% of married women between the ages of 25 and 34 years were in the work force. In 1987 67% of married women in the same age-group worked outside the home. In 1960 18% of working women had children under the age of 6 years. This number increased to 56.8% in 1987 (U.S. Department of Commerce, 1988).

Concurrent with these changes were the advent and development of effective methods of family planning. The ability to exert some control over women's reproductive functions has resulted in smaller families and has allowed families greater capability to make a dual-career choice. As more women have developed and continued careers, family members gradually have had to adapt and change their definitions of sharing household responsibilities (Lewis, 1984). Modern-day pursuits of a comfortable life-style, coupled with the expectation that the small nuclear family should meet all the needs of its members for nurturance, affection, and survival, place the family under extraordinary pressure.

Various evolving family structures have resulted from these social changes (Hymovich & Bernard, 1973; Sussman, 1971).

The *unmarried parent/child family* consists of an unmarried adult and children who are biologically produced or adopted by an unmarried adult.

The *unmarried couple/child family* is one in which the adult couple shares emotional bonds without the legal sanction of marriage. The couple may abide by some form of social contract and may or may not have children.

Same sex families consist of two men or two women living together, usually bound by some form of social contract. The couple may or may not have children by adoption or by previous or alternative reproductive arrangements. Their relationship may or may not include a sexual relationship.

The *cohabiting retired couple* is an unmarried retired couple living together without legal sanctions. Often this is due to economic necessity; that is, retirement or Social Security benefits can be lost or negatively affected by marriage.

The *blended family or stepfamily* has evolved as a family form concurrent with the rising divorce rate. This family group results when one or both adults who have been part of a previous family join together to form a new family, which may include children by these previous families or relationships. The new family also may produce offspring of its own. The media commonly refers to this newly evolved family form as "yours, mine, and ours" (Visher & Visher, 1979).

ROLES WITHIN THE FAMILY

Within any social group persons assume responsibilities for various tasks that are defined in terms of a certain role, for example, parent, breadwinner, student, and son or daughter. An individual's understanding of a given role or role expectations governs how he or she expects to interact with others regarding certain issues or tasks. For example, a parental role expectation can include control of a child's bedtime and the child's compliance with the designated time. Obviously expectations are not always met within daily living.

Roles are learned primarily during childhood by examples set by adults, authorities at school, and the media. When two individuals from separate family systems merge to begin their own family, each brings along personal role expectations based on previous experiences. A young woman who was brought up in a traditional home may expect her role to be that of housewife and mother, as was her mother's. If her husband is the product of a two-career family, he may expect his wife to assume a career role, as his mother did. As the two learn more about each other, ideally they develop a new set of roles, based not totally on previous family experiences but established according to the particular needs of their new relationship.

Each change or crisis in the couple's (family's) life and movement through each developmental stage require the family to adapt and perhaps renegotiate various roles to maintain its equilibrium. The career woman who returned to work after the birth of her first child may find that having her second or third child necessitates stepping out of the career role at least temporarily to assume a full-time mothering role. Her partner may be willing to assume some of the caretaking responsibilities associated with child-bearing and homemaking, as well as maintaining the "breadwinner" role. Some families negotiate ways for both parents to share both roles equally. Others decide to maintain the woman as breadwinner and have her partner assume the homemaker/primary parent roles.

The more flexibility individuals can attain in their role expectations, the better able they are to adapt in times of crisis. The ability to adapt and adjust family roles and responsibilities is what ensures that each member's needs are met. For example, when a family member becomes ill or disabled, a void may be created in the usual functioning of the family. In a functional family other family members are able to adapt and change their roles and expectations so that they can assume the responsibilities that belonged to the disabled member. This shifting and sharing of responsibilities enable necessary family processes to continue.

THE FUNCTIONAL FAMILY

Each family is a dynamic, constantly changing system whose individual members interact with one another and form a unit capable of interacting with the community. In the well-adjusted or functional family, each member interacts with others in a positive facilitative manner that provides nurturance and support not obtained from the wider world. Ideally each family member is a better person for having been part of that family. Experts in family studies have identified the following attributes as common to most well-adjusted functional families (Otto, 1963):

- Open effective communication patterns
- Provision for basic physical, emotional, and spiritual needs
- Provision for security, support, and nurturance
- Responsiveness to individual family member's needs
- Equitable division of tasks and responsibilities, with flexibility in assigned roles
- Commitment to family unity
- Regular interaction among members
- Involvement in the community
- Competence in problem solving and crisis management

When assessing a family's state of health, the nurse determines how many of these attributes are manifested in the family's normal daily activities. It is of crucial importance to recognize that these functions and traits describe the ideal family and that only a small percentage of families are "ideal." Although very few families possess all the characteristics noted here, the more that are present, the more functional the family will be.

Each family also must be assessed with the understanding that what normally is described as healthy family behavior actually may be unhealthy for some families. Conversely, behavior patterns that are identified as maladaptive in most families may serve a particular function in maintaining one family's health. For example, it might be considered healthy in a two-career family for all family members to share equal responsibility for household tasks rather than expect the woman to have a full-time career outside the home and also to assume complete responsibility for the household. In some families, however, the attitudes and beliefs regarding the importance of the man's role as "breadwinner" is strong, and household tasks may be perceived as "woman's work." This family may be better able to maintain its equilibrium or well-being by adhering to the traditional sex role—defined areas of responsibility and adjusting the wife's workload in some other way.

Family unity is another important trait of functional families. For the average family this unity may mean spending time together and sharing common interests, hobbies, and goals, as well as a common place of residence. Some families, however, seem to function well on building "space" into their family system by having separate activities, recreation, or vacations. Sometimes career needs conflict, and couples actually may spend time working and living in different cities. At face value this "commuting" life-style may appear dysfunctional, but for some families it may in fact be satisfying and even essential to its survival. Just as individual persons are different from one another, so each family has its own patterns of interaction with one another and with the community. The nurse needs to see each family in its own light, using the criteria of healthy family functioning only as a yardstick and allowing for individuality and the complex diversities that are common in today's society.

ADAPTIVE FAMILY COPING PATTERNS
Crisis Theory

As families develop and grow across the life cycle, they are faced with normal periods of transition or biological growth that require them to undergo new sets of behaviors and psychological growth. These transitional periods are known as *maturational crises*. One example is forming a couple relationship, during which intimacy skills must be mastered. The birth of the first child, which requires parents to adapt to and accommodate the dependency of the new baby through parent-infant bonding and caretaking behaviors, is another maturational crisis.

Other crises that may threaten the family's physical, psychological, and social integrity and that may cause some disequilibrium in the family system are known as *situational crises*. Some examples are the death of a loved one, loss of a job, accidental injuries, and even positive events such as buying a new house or winning the lottery. Crisis theory, which is based on the works of theorists and researchers (Caplan, 1964; Erikson, 1950; Lindeyman, 1944) focuses on the concept of offering preventive mental and emotional health care.

As these examples suggest, a crisis is defined as an "upset in a steady state," when an individual or a family experiences tension that results from a problem the members cannot solve. Some results of the crisis are anxiety, inability to function, and emotional upset (Caplan, 1964). Occasionally the family's customary coping methods are ineffective in resolving the problem and a period of disorganization occurs. Thus a positive focus during a crisis is important, and it should be considered that the crisis is both a problem and an opportunity because it opens the family to becoming receptive to therapeutic care.

Not all families are equally able to cope with crises. These critical periods require the family to be adaptable and flexible and to have strong coping skills. As the crises are weathered in a positive, constructive manner, the family's cohesiveness will improve. The community health nurse is in an excellent position to intervene to restore family equilibrium and prevent ill health. After identifying that the family is in actual or potential crisis, the nurse can take the following steps:

1. Help the family identify the problem leading to the crisis.
2. Help the family to identify its resources to assist in dealing with the problem.
3. Collaborate with the family to formulate and implement an action plan to alleviate the problem.

The family that has flexible role definitions copes much more readily with changes than does the family that rigidly defines what its members can or cannot do. Concern for an individual family member ensures that all are responsive to the one in need and that efforts will be directed toward care for that person while maintaining the needs of other family members.

Communication Theory

One of the most important elements of coping is the ability to communicate openly and clearly regarding problems. Good communication and problem-solving skills then become a means to identify potential solutions. Communication can be described as the giving or receiving of information or messages. This exchange of information involves a complex process, which results in varying degrees of clarity. When a communication is clear, the receiver understands the message sent and communication is said to be functional. When the receiver does not understand the message being sent, that communication is described as dysfunctional (Hall & Weaver, 1985).

There are two levels of communication. One is the denotative or literal message content. The other is the metacommunication portion, that is, the verbal or nonverbal information about the message sent. For example, body language such as positioning, facial expressions, patterns of movement, and tone of voice give the receiver much information about what is being said.

Sometimes our body language does not match the literal message. This is another type of dysfunctional communication pattern, which leaves the receiver uncertain as to the content of the message. An example is the wife who verbally states that it would be acceptable for her husband to spend the holiday weekend hunting with his friends but makes the statement through clenched teeth, with a tense facial expression. She may be intending to be cooperative, but her own feelings of discomfort or resentment are relayed clearly in her body language, or through metacommunication.

Another communication problem that can occur is the assumption a person may make about something someone said without checking it out. In the cited example, the husband simply may decide not to go hunting because he senses his wife's displeasure without asking her what her feelings are. This can be a dangerous and harmful process, and clarification should be encouraged whenever uncertainty exists.

Some families have been culturally conditioned not to share emotions and feelings. This omission can be a major communication block that closes off many possibilities for sharing. The public health nurse who works with such a family can facilitate communication by evaluating the patterns of information exchange and assisting with clarification or sharing of feelings when appropriate.

CONCEPTUAL FRAMEWORKS FOR STUDYING THE FAMILY

Assessing and evaluating family health are extremely complex tasks. One method of systematic study of the family is through the use of various conceptual frameworks that have been developed for the purpose of scientific investigation by various disciplines. A conceptual framework can be defined as a tool or model to organize and interpret data or research and to develop an effective plan for action. Some commonly used concepts for the study of the family are the developmental framework, the structural-functional framework, the symbolic-interactional framework, and the systems theory framework.

Developmental framework. The *developmental framework* is one that is particularly suited to application in many different fields of investigation. This framework was developed in 1948 by Evelyn Duvall and Reuben Hill for use at the First White House Conference on Family Life. It provided a method for social scientists to systematically study the family and to describe and share their findings. It continues to serve as a valuable and reliable method for predicting or anticipating a family's need for assistance or anticipatory guidance during various stages of the life cycle. It incorporates general systems theory in describing family changes or adaptations.

The family developmental framework is based on the predictability of family life experiences, which have been observed to follow a universal sequence across the family's life cycle (Duvall, 1977). To fully comprehend any individual or family one must consider both the uniqueness of the person and the blend of the family members. Two main concepts are important: (1) *family life cycle,* which is that period beginning with the formation of the family and ending with the dissolution of the family through the death, separation, divorce, or physical relocation of its members and (2) *family developmental tasks,* which are defined as responsibilities connected with each particular stage of family life. Developmental tasks need to be accomplished successfully for the family to continue to move successfully through the life cycle. According to Duvall, there are eight developmental stages (see Table 13-1).

Table 13-1 lists the developmental tasks associated with each stage of the family life cycle. The nurse who is planning care can assess the family to determine its developmental stage, evaluate the family's attainment of the appropriate developmental tasks, and then assist the family in possible ways to fulfill the appropriate tasks for that particular stage. Although this theory is extremely valuable in family assessment, it should be noted that Duvall considers the middle-class nuclear family to be the "normal" type. Her framework may be considered less relevant for application to the care of families that are not within the "middle" socioeconomic class definition or for single-parent or blended families.

Structural-functional framework. This approach was developed by sociologists and anthropologists and focuses on the relationships between family systems and other social systems such as school, workplace, or the health care delivery system. Attention also is paid to the interrelationships of family members. Although this framework provides a strong reference for studying the relationships between family members and outside social organizations, it is inadequate in incorporating the processes and dynamics of social change.

Symbolic-interactional framework. This concept was developed within the fields of sociology and social psychology. It focuses on the interactions of family members as described by roles, decision-making processes, communication patterns, and conflict res-

TABLE 13-1 Family life cycle

Family life cycle stages	Family development tasks
Marriage phase	Establishment of: relationship boundaries; roles; financial plans; home; relationships with friends, family members; parenthood plans
Childbearing family	Redefinition of marital relationship; taking on the role of parents; reevaluation of home space arrangements, career plans, financial plans
Preschool-child family	Providing for safety, security, and nurturance needs of child; coping with fatigue and lack of privacy; beginning socialization of child
School-aged-child family	Adjustment to separation from family; development of peer relationships by child; establishing educational goals; entering parent/child/teacher community
Teenager-family	Fostering autonomy while maintaining structure in adolescence; dealing with midlife career and personal issues; beginning concern with providing for grandparents
Launching phase	Assisting young-adult aged children in establishing independent identities; redefinition of marital relationship as children leave home.
Middle-aged family	Rebuilding couple identity; incorporation of new family members—spouses and grandchildren; caretaking of older generation
Elderly family	Adaptation to retirement; financial realignment; bereavement issues; dealing with loneliness; coping with health problems

Adapted from *Marriage and family development* (5th ed.) (p. 144) by E. Duvall 1977, Philadelphia: Lippincott.

olution. Although it provides a thorough view of the interior structure of the family, it does not include or consider the family's interactions with outside social systems.

Systems theory framework. This concept, which initially was developed by biologist Ludwig von Bertalanffy (1968), is used by many disciplines. It extends beyond the theory that the whole is made up of the sum of its parts, which are interdependent and interrelated, and that if change occurs in any one part of the system, the other parts are affected and must regain balance (Brill, 1978). Systems theory, on the other hand, defines the whole as more than the sum of its parts. A system may receive input from outside and may put energy out into its environment, which is known as *output.* These energy exchanges create a change in the system and thus require adjustment of the system.

Although this theory has broad applications, it can be applied to the family in the following manner. The family is a living system whose parts are its individual members. The family is defined as a system because its members are interrelated and interdependent. The patterns of interaction among its members affect each person. The family interacts with a larger system, the community, which also affects its well-being. Systems theory has been used (Ackerman, 1984) to describe how families adapt and change over time through information exchange and feedback processes among themselves and with the community.

As described in Chapter 3, Betty Neuman's systems model for planning nursing care conceptualizes a structural framework that can be used to implement the assessment and intervention portions of the nursing process. Systems theory provides a rationale to explain that the whole of the family is affected by the interaction of its members and by the family's interaction with the community, as discussed later in this chapter.

FAMILY HEALTH

As a system a family is more than its collective parts. Evaluation of a family's level of health cannot occur without a working knowledge of each member's health status. Conversely, evaluation of an individual's health status cannot take place without exploring the dynamics of the family's health. Good planning includes both aspects.

Family health may be described and evaluated by means of the Neuman systems model. The family is considered a system composed of individual members who are interrelated in such a fashion that a change in any one part sets off a series of changes in the other parts. When one member becomes ill, other family members are expected to give assistance. The illness may alter work patterns and require restriction of previous plans. A long-term chronic illness may deplete the family financially and emotionally. If a breadwinner becomes disabled, his or her career may be jeopardized and there will be a loss of earnings. In most instances this change requires the rest of the family members to adapt or alter some aspect of their own life-styles.

On the other hand, when one family member or more subscribe to a healthy life-style, the example each sets by valuing the principles of health maintenance and health promotion can positively affect the family's health. If this person is one of the adult members who shares family caretaking, he or she may foster healthy nutrition, encourage exercise programs, set a good example for stress management, and arrange for preventive medical or dental care.

NURSING CARE OF THE FAMILY

As early as the early 1900s, community health nurses recognized the importance of planning care for the family. Even in instances in which one person had a health problem, the entire family was involved in setting priorities and planning and giving care. Nurses have long recognized that the family's health values, beliefs, and practices influence the health status of its individual members. For example, wellness is more commonly experienced in families in which nutrition and exercise are valued and preventive medicine is practiced. Individuals who are members of families that do not value healthy life-style behaviors may not do so themselves. The opposite effect can be observed when one member of a family that does not value health adopts a wellness consciousness. It is not uncommon for one family member or several members to be impressed enough by the outcome of a healthier life-style that they gradually alter their own attitudes and adopt healthier habits.

Providing high-quality nursing care to the family involves the application of the same principles as are involved in caring for an individual client. The nursing process is the prescribed method because it is based on a scientific approach that involves the collection of data to make appropriate clinical judgments and to plan the care and identify interventions. Evaluation and reassessment are used to determine the effectiveness of the interventions and make necessary revisions or modification in care.

Assessment

Assessment of the family involves the use of the five senses to compile appropriate information that allows for the identification of actual or potential health problems and the development of a plan to improve the level of wellness of the family. A thorough nursing assessment includes family history, family health assessment, and physical assessment.

A variety of tools are available for recording the history, health, and physical assessments. The ideal tool must be easy to use, should take a minimal amount of time to

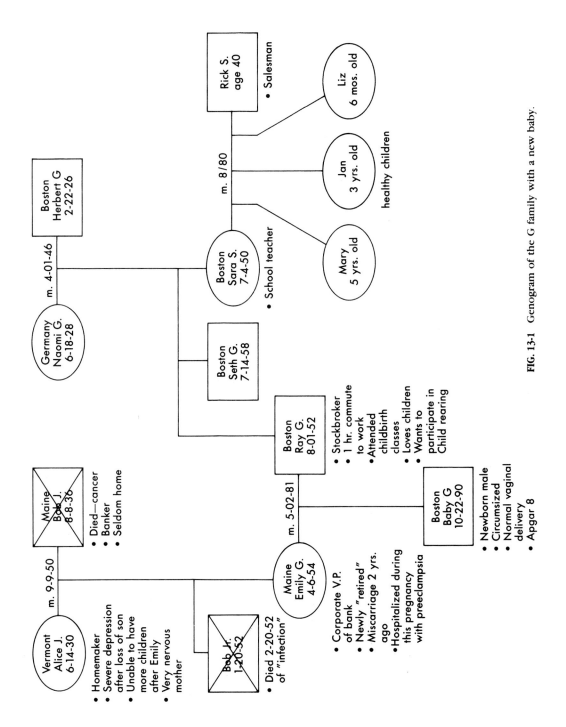

FIG. 13-1 Genogram of the G family with a new baby.

complete, and, when completed, provide a composite picture of that family's strengths and problems or needs. To use an assessment tool in planning care the nurse must be familiar with such concepts as family types, role theory, crisis theory, communication theory, and stages of development, which were discussed earlier in this chapter.

Genogram. One example of an assessment tool is the genogram. It has been used by therapists to gain a retrospective perception of a family system as it has developed over time (Fig. 13-1). This tool is based on generalized information about the evolution of the family over one or more generations and can clearly depict the family structure. The format used for the genogram is a simple family-tree structure. The data elicited by careful interviewing provide information on child-rearing practices, health-valuing beliefs and attitudes, social information, and traditions that can affect the family's health or well-being.

The genogram in Fig. 13-1 shows a family the day after their first baby's birth. A few of the important data include the fact that Emily and Ray, now 34 and 36 years old, have been married 7 years and that Emily had a spontaneous abortion 3 years earlier. Ray is interested in participating in the childbearing/child-rearing experience but is limited by his long hours of work and commuting. Emily is making the transition from a career in corporate management to that of homemaker for a few years while she raises her children.

The genogram also shows that Emily's mother, who Emily describes as nervous and overprotective, has been a widow for many years. She has a history of severe depression following the loss of her first-born in early infancy. It is possible that Emily's mother was not able to provide a strong role model for mothering; this could interfere with Emily's self-confidence and ability to adapt to the mothering role. Ray comes from a larger family, and although his mother is described as "not too affectionate," his father loves children. These facts may enable Ray to feel comfortable in the parenting role. Baby boy G, delivered by a normal vaginal birth, is strong and healthy. Nothing in the genogram indicates any potential health problems.

The completed genogram provided the nurse with a quick and easy way to obtain a family history. The development of the genogram helped Emily and Ray understand that Emily, on the basis of her own family history, may take some time to adapt to the mothering role. The couple also was able to identify a family strength in Ray's comfort with the role of fatherhood.

The genogram may be used in conjunction with one or more other tools described in the following sections to develop a complete assessment.

Ecomap. An ecomap (Fig. 13-2) can be used to provide additional information regarding the family as a system and its interactions with other systems such as work, health care, school, extended family, friends, or recreation. This tool borrows from the science of ecology, which studies the delicate balance that exists in nature between living things and their environment. It looks at the ways in which this balance may be maintained for the good of all (Hartman, 1978). The completed ecomap clearly illustrates all the important interaction patterns between the family and other systems, as well as the nature of the relationship and the direction of the energy flow, or resources.

The completed ecomap (Fig. 13-3) enables both the nurse and the couple shown in the genogram (Fig. 13-1), Emily and Ray, to identify areas in which they may seek help, for example, through friends, Lamaze class members, church, family, and neighbors. They were able to anticipate that Emily's temporary loss of career might become a problem and that Ray might attempt to limit his work hours while the family goes through the parent-adaptation process. Both decided to try to keep in closer contact with Ray's siblings in an effort to strengthen the bond and develop a resource. The lack of any potential

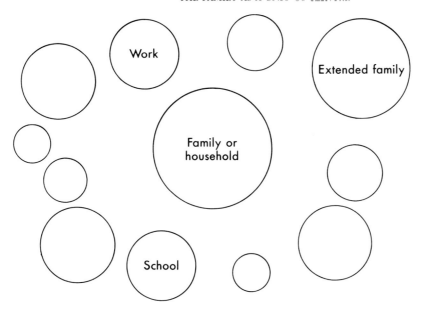

FIG. 13-2 Ecomap. *(From "Diagrammatic assessment of family relationships" by A. Hartman, 1978, Social Casework, 59, 469. Copyright 1978 by Family Service Association of America. Reprinted by permission.)*

child-care persons was clearly evident and was identified as an important priority.

Other assessment tools. Many community health care providers develop their own assessment tools to be used alone or in conjunction with other standardized forms. Fig. 13-4 depicts a family assessment tool that is comprehensive in nature. This tool includes items related to the family structure and resources, the physical and social environments, and family health, health practices, and life-style. These basic demographical and factual data give the nurse an overview of the family system.

Fig. 13-5 provides an example of a modification of a comprehensive family assessment tool that was developed by one home care agency to use with childbearing families. This form is more concise than that of Fig. 13-4 because it is used in conjunction with detailed maternal and newborn assessment tools.

The tool used for physical assessment can follow any problem-oriented format developed for client history and physical examination. In collecting the family's health history, the nurse looks for indicators of factors that might place family members at risk for health problems. For example, Sally B's father, grandfather, brother, and two paternal aunts suffered from alcoholism. Because this family history predisposes Sally herself to alcoholism, this possibility should be carefully investigated.

Another example is that of John S, aged 42 years, whose father and brother both died of myocardial infarctions in their early 50s. The nurse certainly would include in John's physical assessment screening for signs of impending cardiovascular problems. A teaching plan for John would include an evaluation of John's dietary and nutritional habits and a plan for healthy eating developed collaboratively with John and his wife. John, the nurse, and the physician would begin developing a safe plan for exercise, stress management, and realistic dietary strategies. *Text continued on p. 292.*

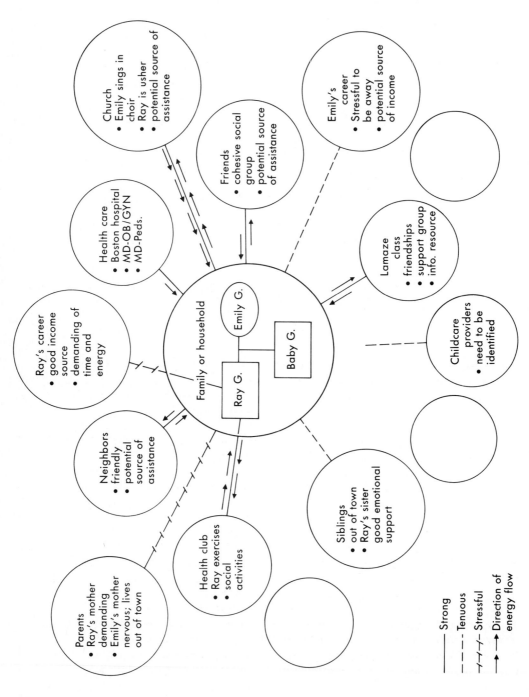

FIG. 13-3 Ecomap showing the G family's systems of support. (*Adapted from "Diagrammatic assessment of family relationships" by A. Hartman, 1978, Social Casework, 59, 469. Copyright 1978 by Family Service Association of America. Reprinted by permission.*)

Client name:	Case no.:
Clients address:	Phone no.:

Reason for admission:

Family constellation:

    Name   Relationship   Age

_____

_____

_____

_____

_____

Social history:

    Name   Ethnicity   Occupation   Income

_____

_____

_____

_____

Neighborhood data: Affluent _____ Moderate _____ Poverty _____

Adequate utilities: Yes _____ No _____

Neighbors: Freindly _____ Noncommittal _____ Hostile _____

Transportation: Convenient _____ Accessible _____ Not available _____

Health care facilities accessible: Yes _____ No _____

Family health care data:

Present family illnesses (list) _____

_____

Past action taken when family member ill _____

_____

_____

_____

Family dynamics:

Role of each member _____

_____

Leadership: Patriarchal _____ Matriarchal _____ Egalitarian _____ Democratic _____

Communication style: Open _____ Closed _____ Direct _____ Indirect _____

Values system: Family ____ Religion ____ Materialism ____ Ethnic beliefs ____ Health ____

Health belidfs: Myths _____ Old wives' tales _____ Cultural beliefs _____ Fact _____

Family priorities _____

FIG. 13-4 Comprehensive family assessment tool and care plan.   *Continued.*

Family coping skills:

	Adequate skills	Needs assistance
Communication patterns: Express thoughts and feelings with one another		
Emotional support: Encourage and care about one another		
Community interaction: Involved in community activities, maintain friendships		
Accepting help: Able to tap resources when needed		
Flexibility of roles: Able to adjust responsibilities in change or crisis		
Crisis management: Draws family together, viewed as a growth experience		

Family wellness behaviors:

	Acceptable habits	Needs Improvement
Nutritional status		
Exercise program		
Alcohol consuption		
Drug habits		
Smoking		
Sleep patterns		
Stress management		
Practices preventative health care		

Risk factors identified: _____
_____
_____

Notes _____
_____
_____
_____

Signature _____
Home Care Nurse

FIG. 13-4, cont'd   Comprehensive family assessment tool and care plan.

Client family:		Case no.:
EDC:	Delivery date:	Date of visit:	Time:

Family constellation:

Name	Relationship	Age

Support persons:

Name	Availability

Home safety plan: Adequate utlities _____
Hazard modification:_____

Neighborhood safety problems:_____
Other:_____

Role behaviors and responsibilities (occupations, household, child care):
Mother: _____

Father: _____

Other: _____

Adaptations: _____

Knowledge of newborn:

	Aware of infant cues	Responsive to cues	Infant care skills
Mother:			
Father:			
Siblings:			

Sibling adjustment: Good _____   Fair _____   Poor_____

Sibling adaptation: Physiologic _____   Psychologic _____   Family planning _____

Coping skills: Good situational adaptation _____   Needs to mobilize resources _____
Needs to reorganize life _____   Needs further information _____
Needs to identify problem _____

Notes: _____
_____

Signature _____
Visiting Nurse

FIG. 13-5 Childbearing family assessment guide. *(Courtesy Birthtrends, Buffalo, NY.)*

Finally, Mary W is a 45-year-old woman with a history of gestational diabetes during her previous two pregnancies. Although Mary presently does not display any overt symptoms of diabetes, it is known that adult-onset diabetes often develops later in life in women who had gestational diabetes. Therefore screening for diabetes will be an important component of Mary's physical assessment. Family teaching will include alerting Mary and her family to the importance of watching for signs of diabetes such as unexplained weight loss, excessive thirst, extreme hunger, and frequent urination. Mary will be encouraged to contact her physician at the earliest sign of any of these symptoms.

In addition to physical assessment of the individual members, assessment of a family's level of health also includes identification of life-style behaviors such as nutritional and exercise patterns, preventive health care, stress management, and identification of risk factors. It may be possible to focus on one member of a family who has an altered health state, or it may be necessary to develop a plan of care that includes all family members because in some way the illness of one member affects each of them.

Nursing Diagnosis

After completing the assessment phase of family care, the nurse will be able to determine the existence of any actual or potential health problems in the family and also to identify family strengths. These factors will be developed into statements called *nursing diagnoses.* In a review of Sally B's assessment the following nursing diagnosis might be formulated: "need for health teaching regarding potential for alcohol dependency." Another example of a nursing diagnosis, this time for Larry M, 245 pounds and 5 feet 9 inches tall, with poor eating habits and an inadequate knowledge of nutrition, might be "obesity related to poor eating habits and knowledge deficit about nutritional requirements."

Planning

The nurse and family work together collaboratively to develop a list of goals, strategies, and expected outcomes. The family prioritizes its identified needs, and a plan of care begins with the formulation of interventions or actions.

Implementation

Once goals and actual or potential problems are identified and then prioritized by the family, the nurse and family define appropriate measures or actions to rectify the problems. These are known as *interventions.* Implementation of the interventions involves the actual execution of the nursing care or client self-care regimen. Interventions may involve administering a prescribed medical treatment or medication, providing comfort measures, giving physical care, or providing health teaching or counseling.

Both Sally B and Larry M in our previous examples are prime candidates for interventions based on health teaching and counseling. Another example of an intervention is the use of positioning to enhance the comfort level of a new mother after childbirth.

Evaluation and Reassessment

To determine the effectiveness of the nursing interventions in alleviating or preventing any given client problem, a regular system of patient observation, interview, and reassessment must be undertaken. This process identifies the problem as remedied, improved, unchanged from previous findings, or worsened. Problems that are remedied are removed from the problem list. Problems that show improvement may warrant continuation of the interventions. Problems unimproved or worsened may require a modification in the problems and may allow for discharging the particular client/family from care.

CASE STUDY

Emily G, aged 34 years, and Ray G, aged 36 years, have just had their first child, a healthy boy, weighing 7 pounds 8 ounces. Emily's pregnancy was normal, she attended childbirth preparation classes with Ray, and she had an uncomplicated labor and vaginal delivery. Emily, a breast-feeding mother, and baby G were discharged to go home after a stable 24-hour recovery period. Because the G's had requested a 24-hour discharge during their pregnancy, a home care nurse visited them during the antepartal period during which time a family history had been completed (see genogram, Fig. 13-2). A health history of the mother, which included a thorough obstetrical history, also was recorded. Nurse S then worked collaboratively with the G's to plan for the birth. During the preparation phase the processes of patient teaching, health counseling, and anticipatory guidance were used. Home visits then were scheduled for post-partum days 1 and 3 to provide for continuity of care after hospital discharge.

Nurse S arrived at the home on day 1 to find the baby frantically crying and Emily close to tears herself. She reported the baby had been crying most of the day, did not eat well, and had wet through his diapers, soaking his sleepers several times.

Nurse S reassured Emily that crying was normal (both for baby and herself!) and that they would review various methods of comforting the baby. Emily's first priority was to quiet the baby. Recognizing that Emily herself needed some comfort measures, Nurse S helped her find a comfortable position and then positioned the baby next to her. Emily requested some assistance with diapering, and together they reviewed how the diaper could be folded to make it fit snugly and prevent leakage. Nurse S then explained and demonstrated the concept of wrapping the baby swaddling style in a blanket because it provides comfort to many newborns.

Emily decided to offer the baby part of his feeding to quiet his crying and to complete the feeding after his bath. She requested assistance in putting the baby to breast. Nurse S helped her to recall the importance of comfortable positioning and relaxation in stimulating the milk "let down" reflex. It was suggested that before breast-feeding

Emily burp the baby to expel any air he had swallowed while crying.

Emily recalled that she had learned to express a drop of breast milk before beginning the feeding both to help stimulate the "let down" reflex and to encourage the baby to take the nipple with the taste of the sweet breast milk. The nurse offered positive feedback and encouragement during the feeding, along with other constructive suggestions for making the feeding time easier. She observed that Emily was not burping the baby correctly and demonstrated a few easy techniques for doing so. Ray came in just as the feeding was ending. He requested the opportunity to help with the feeding, and Nurse S instructed him to wash his hands and encouraged him to complete the burping.

Because baby G was sleeping at the end of the feeding and Emily felt more relaxed, Nurse S believed it was an appropriate time to update the health history by adding data related to the labor, delivery, and early postpartum recovery. A physical assessment indicated that Emily appeared to be recovering well except for sore, edematous hemorrhoids. Nurse S asked Emily to explain the principles of asepsis and perineal care she had learned and reviewed the treatments that her physician had ordered. Comfortable positioning also was discussed.

Emily was concerned that she had not had a bowel movement in the day since her delivery. Because her hemorrhoids were so painful, she was worried that this would be a painful event. Nurse S discussed the restoration of bowel function with a focus on preventing constipation and promoting soft stool. Together, the nurse and the family planned some nutritional approaches that were appealing to Emily and easy for Ray to prepare. They also reviewed the importance of adequate water intake and the gradual increase of physical activity to promote the restoration of normal bowel function. Nurse S emphasized the importance of good hemorrhoidal care to promote comfort and healing. These measures would all be important components of restoring Emily's bowel function.

Nurse S included Emily and Ray in the physical assessment of baby G, explaining the findings. As baby G was awakening, the nurse explained some normal newborn behaviors, neurological reflexes, and other normal deviations of the newborn such as erythema toxicum and breast engorgement. The G's began to prepare for the baby's bath as they had learned in class. Emily assisted Ray while he gave the baby a sponge bath. Nurse S included instruction in caring for the umbilical cord and demonstrated proper care for the circumcision. Once baby G was bathed, dressed, and wrapped, Emily offered the second breast. Nurse S encouraged Emily to share with her husband her recall of the skills she had just acquired regarding feeding techniques and burping the baby.

Once baby G was settled, Nurse S used her health counseling and patient teaching skills to discuss the early postpartum period with both parents. Recognizing postpartum as a period of great adaptation that may create disequilibrium in the family system, Nurse S encouraged the G's to discuss their progress. The G's felt it was important to identify one or two persons who would be available to watch the baby a few times a week. This relief would enable Emily to rest and restore her energy during the first postpartum week. Later these persons could enable Emily to get out of the house for some time alone with Ray, with other friends, or by herself. The nurse then helped them plan for mobilizing these resources for assistance.

Nurse S reassured the G's that it is normal to feel a little overwhelmed when a first baby is brought home. The G's stated that they were both very tired because they had not slept well the week before the delivery and Emily had been in labor all night. Together they reviewed their plan to enable Emily to obtain the needed restorative rest. The G's decided to use one of their resource persons to help with the housework and perhaps even stay with the baby for a few hours each afternoon so Emily could sleep. Ray was encouraged to assume responsibility for meal planning and preparation for the first week. Together they planned a few simple, nutritious meals.

At the completion of the visit, Nurse S and the G family developed the following list of family strengths and nursing diagnoses:

Strengths

1. The G's are well-educated and prepared to care for the infant.
2. The G's are well-motivated to provide for this early period of adjustment.
3. Ray is willing to adapt his role to assist with many household tasks.
4. The G's have good support systems.

Nursing Diagnoses

1. Altered comfort level of Emily related to episiotomy and edematous hemorrhoids.
2. Potential altered bowel functions of Emily related to restoration process and perineal pain.
3. Knowledge deficit in parenting skills of both parents related to inexperience.
4. Altered comfort level of newborn related to parental inexperience.
5. Altered comfort level of both parents related to fatigue.
6. Potential stress of both parents related to postpartum family adjustment.

Fig. 13-6 shows an example of another type of family care plan that might have been used by Nurse S and the G family.

THE FAMILY/COMMUNITY SYSTEM

The interrelationship of the health of the family and the health of the community was recognized by the American Public Health Association (APHA) in 1980 when it described the role of public health nurses in terms of working with families toward the goal of improving the health of the community (APHA, 1980).

Levels of wellness of individuals, families, and communities are directly or indirectly interrelated. The family serves as a moderator between the wellness of its individual members and the wellness of the community (Dunn, 1967). The healthy or functional family contributes to the community by preparing its members to function productively in societal roles in the workplace, in school, or in their own families. Communities with

Assessment	Nursing Diagnosis	Plan/Intervention	Evaluation
Physical findings	Altered comfort level related to edemotous episiotomy and hemorrhoids	Evaluate mother's knowledge of perineal care Reinforce use of perineal treatments Instruct mother in additional comfort measures: positioning, firm seated chair, back rub	Instruction provided
	Potential altered bowel function related to restoration process and perineal pain	Evaluate and encourage increased fluid intake Encourage adequate activities and ambulation Evaluate dietary intake and Instruct regarding high fiber foods	12 oz. juice taken during visit Instruction provided Fiber intake adequate
Behavioral patterns	Altered comfort level of newborn related to possible hypertonic disposition and parental knowledge deficit	Observe and evaluate degree of responsiveness to environmental stimuli	
Knowledge of parenting skills	Knowledge deficit in parenting skills related to being new parents	Demonstrate techniques for diapering, wrapping Demonstrate process for bathing Observe and provide feedback re: feeding technique with emphasis on burping	Demonstration returned by parents Instructed to burp more often
Family interactions	Anxiety of mother related to inexperience and excessive crying of infant	Reinforce instruction of parenting skills Allow mother to ventilate by expressing her feelings Reassure mother of her competence and the normalcy of her feelings	Mother feels frightened Reassurance provided
	Parental fatique related to childbirth experience and disrupted sleep patterns	Encourage frequent rest periods for mother, daily nap for father Identify resource persons to do household tasks and prepare meals Instruct parents that mother should only care for herself and baby during first week	Daily nap period planned Will arrange for assistance

FIG. 13-6 Family nursing care plan.

many unhealthy families will suffer ill effects because these families are less able to fulfill societal roles and they place demands on the community's health care delivery systems (Stanhope & Lancaster, 1988).

The systems theory can be used to describe this relationship between the family and the community. The family is described as a dynamic system made up of smaller parts, which are its individual members. The family system also is conceptualized as a subsystem of a larger system, the community.

Betty Neuman's systems model can be applied to define the family as an open system, that is, a system that exchanges energy with its environment. The family performs certain functions that result in the output of energy into the community. For example, the reproduction and socialization of new family members contribute new persons to the community (Hymovich & Chamberlin, 1980).

Any contributions a family makes to community function can be considered outputs of energy into the community system. Volunteer work performed for community organizations and the contribution of valuable skills in the workplace serve as positive examples. Sometimes the family's output is negative in nature, such as a situation in which a family member's actions result in crime or personal injury to other community members.

Services provided by the community act as energy input into the family system. The adequacy of community functions or services such as security (fire and police protection), the availability of health care providers (hospitals, clinics, and doctors' offices), transportation systems, and educational institutions may determine the level of health or wellness of its families. In a community in which health care facilities are too few or inaccessible because of distance from public transportation, families may be unable to secure adequate primary or tertiary health care. The lack of preventive care and adequate rehabilitation services to segments of the community population impedes the family's ability to attain optimum wellness.

When large segments of a community's families experience impaired health, the community as a whole may suffer. Nursing care provided to the family to enhance its health status serves to increase the level of wellness of the entire community.

SUMMARY

Community health nurses use a family-oriented focus by caring for all family members as part of a system. A change in the health of one family member affects the health of other family members. Similarly, the health of individual families influences the health of the community.

Although the nuclear family, consisting of two parents and one or more children, is considered the ideal "typical" family, it accounts for a minority of families today. Social changes in the recent past have led to an increase in the number of single-parent families and to other evolving family structures.

The use of various conceptual frameworks and the nursing process allows the community health nurse to plan care for the family as a unit, to help the family cope with crises and solve its problems, and to increase the wellness level of all family members.

CHAPTER HIGHLIGHTS

- Although there are many definitions of a family, all include the following characteristics: families are composed of more than one person, they include at least one adult, and the persons are related to each other by blood or formal or informal social contract.
- Family structures are constantly changing. The nuclear family is perceived as the "typical" family but actually represents fewer than half of all American families.
- Members of families learn to assume various roles as children on the basis of examples set by parents, school authorities, and the media. Individuals from different family systems may have different and conflicting expectations of role behavior.
- Characteristics common to functional families include effective communication patterns, provisions for members' physical and emotional needs, flexibility within roles, commitment to family unity, involvement in the community, and ability to solve problems.
- Community health nurses can use their knowledge of crisis theory to help families cope with both maturational and situational crises.

- An understanding of communication theory is important in assessing a family's ability to communicate openly and to solve problems.
- Conceptual frameworks useful for studying the family include the developmental framework, structural-functional approach, and the systems theory approach.
- The health of one family member affects the health of other family members.
- The community health nurse can use the nursing process to provide nursing care to the family unit.
- The genogram and ecomap are assessment tools that allow the nurse to gather information and assess family strengths and weaknesses.
- Healthy families contribute to the health of the community whereas unhealthy families place demands on community resources and lower the community's overall health.

STUDY QUESTIONS

1. Formulate your own definition of a family. How well does this definition fit your own family?
2. Select (a) nuclear family, (b) a single-parent family, and (c) a blended family from those you have seen in your clinical practice. What are the strengths and weaknesses of each? What adaptive coping mechanisms does each use? Are they effective?
3. A family consists of father, mother, and three children. The father is the breadwinner; the mother has never worked outside the home. The ages of the children are 24, 22, and 16 years. Both parents have contributed to several community groups. The father has just received a diagnosis of chronic heart disease. How might this diagnosis affect the other family members? The community?

REFERENCES

Ackerman, N.J. (1984). *A theory of family systems.* New York and London: Gardiner Press Inc.

American Public Health Association. (1980). *The definition and role of public health nursing in the delivery of health care.* Washington, DC: Author.

Aguilera, D. C., and Messick, J. M. (1990). *Crisis intervention theory and methodology* (6th ed.). St. Louis: CV Mosby.

Bell, R. R. (1983). *Marriage and family interaction.* Homewood, IL: Dorsey.

Bertalanffy, L. V. (1968). *Organismic psychology and systems theory.* Worcester, MA: Clark University Press.

Bohannan, P. (1985). *All the happy families: Exploring the varieties of family life.* New York: McGraw-Hill.

Brill, N. K. (1978). *Working with people: The helping process.* Philadelphia: Lippincott.

Caplan, G. (1964). *Principles of prevention psychiatry.* New York and London: Basic Books, Inc.

Carpenito, L. J. (1985). *Nursing diagnosis: Application to clinical practice.* New York: Harper & Row.

Clemen-Stone, S., Eigsti, D. G., and McGuire, S. L. (1987). *Comprehensive family and community health nursing* (2nd ed.). New York: McGraw-Hill.

Clements, I., and Roberto, F. (1983). *Family health: A theoretical approach to nursing care.* New York: Wiley.

Dunn, H. L. (1967). *High level wellness.* (7th ed.). Arlington, VA: Beatty.

Duvall, E. M. (1977). *Marriage and family development* (5th ed.). New York: Lippincott.

Duvall, E. M., and Miller, B. C. (1985). *Marriage and family development* (6th ed.). New York: Harper & Row.

Erikson, E.H. (1950). *Childhood and society.* New York: W.W. Norton & Co.

Friedman, M. M. (1981). *Family nursing theory and assessment.* New York: Appleton-Century-Crofts.

Glick, P. C. (1984). American household structure in transition, *Family Planning Prospective, 16*(5), 204-211.

Hall, J. E., and Weaver, B. R. (1985). *A systems approach to community health* (2nd ed.). Philadelphia: Lippincott.

Hartman, A. (1978). Diagrammatic assessment of family relationships. *Social Casework, 59,* 465-479.

Hymovich, D. P., and Bernard, M. U. (1973). *Family health care.* New York: McGraw-Hill.

Hymovich, D. P., and Chamberlin, R. (1980). *Child and family development.* New York: McGraw-Hill.

Lewis, G. L. (1984). Changes in women's role participation. In I. Frieze, et al. (Eds.), *Women and sex roles: social psychological perspective.* New York: Norton.

Lindemann, E. (1944). Symptomatology and management of acute grief. *American Journal of Psychiatry, 141,* 148.

Miller, J. R., and Janosik, E. H. (1980). *Family-focused care.* New York: McGraw-Hill.

Minuchin, S. (1974). *Families and family therapy.* Cambridge, MA: Harvard University Press.

National Data Bank and Guide to Sources. (1986). *Statistical abstract of the United States* (107th ed.). Washington, DC: U. S. Department of Commerce, Bureau of the Census.

Neuman, B. (1989). *The Neuman systems model* (2nd Ed.). East Norwalk, CT: Appleton and Lange.

Nye, F. I., and Berardo, F. M. (Eds.) (1981). *Emerging conceptual frameworks in family analyses.* New York: Praeger.

Otto, H. E. (1963). Criteria for assessing family strength. *2*(2):329-333, Baltimore, MD: Waverly Press.

Pendagast, B. S., and Sherman, C. O. (1977). A guide to the genogram family systems training. *The family 5,* 3-14.

Queen, S. A., and Haberstein, R. W. (1974). *The family in various cultures.* New York: Lippincott.

Reinhardt, A. M., and Quinn, M. D. (Eds.). (1973). *Family-centered community nursing: A sociocultural framework.* St. Louis: Mosby.

Rodgers, R. H. (1964). Towards a theory of family development, *Journal of Marriage and the Family, 26,* 262-270.

Stanhope, M., and Lancaster, J. (1988). *Community health nursing: Process and practice for promoting health,* (2nd ed.). St. Louis: Mosby.

Sussman, M. (1971). Family systems in the 1970s: Analysis, policies, programs. *Annals of the American Academy of Political and Social Science, 396,* 5-19.

Thorne, B., and Yalom, M. (1982). *Rethinking the family: Some feminist questions.* New York: Longman.

Tinkham, C. W., Voorhees, E. F., and McCarthy, N. C. (1984). *Community health nursing: evolution and process in the family and community.* Norwalk, CT: Appleton-Century-Crofts.

Toffler, A. (1970). *Future shock.* New York: Bantam.

Turner, R. H. (1966). *Family interaction.* New York: Wiley.

U.S. Department of Commerce, Bureau of the Census. (1988). *Statistical abstract of the United States.* Washington, DC: Bureau of the Census.

U.S. Department of Commerce, National Data Bank and Guide to the Sources. (1986). *Statistical abstract of the U.S.,* (107th ed.). Washington, DC: Bureau of the Census.

Visher, E., and Visher, J. (1979). *Step families: A guide to working with stepparents and stepchildren.* New York: Brunner/Mazel.

Walsh, F. (Ed.). (1982). *Normal family processes.* New York: Guilford.

Wright, L. M., and Leahy, M. (1984). *Nurses and families: A guide to family assessment and intervention.* Philadelphia: Davis.

The Family as a Bearer of Culture

DIANA M. STULC

*To seek, to know, and to understand designated
cultures—with their values, beliefs, and daily living
patterns—is probably one of the greatest challenges for
students of human behavior.*

MADELEINE LEININGER

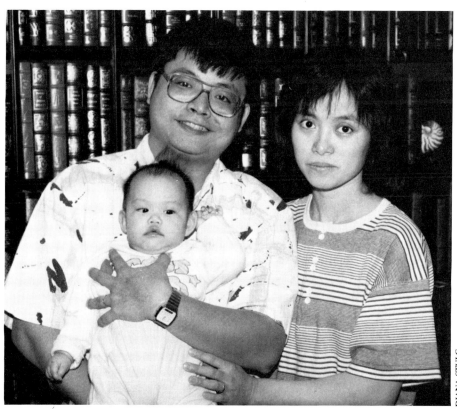

DIANA STULC

OBJECTIVES

At the conclusion of this chapter the student will be able to:
1. Define the key terms listed
2. Differentiate among culture, ethnicity, and race
3. Discuss the role families play in establishing the cultural identity of their children
4. List and discuss aspects of a cultural assessment
5. Compare and contrast the characteristics of four minority ethnic groups
6. Apply the nursing process to families with diverse cultural backgrounds

KEY TERMS

Beliefs   Folk healers
Cultural assessment   Melting-pot approach
Cultural diversity   Parenting
Culture   Race
Culture-bound   Religion
Enculturation   Socialization
Ethnicity   Stereotypes
Ethnocentrism   Values

Each person is born into a family unique in its cultural characteristics, which serve to shape behavioral development. The family unit is the first to teach the child about the culture in which he or she lives. All aspects of the culture are instilled through the primary care givers as part of the socialization process of the child.

North America is rich in its numbers of culturally diverse families. In fact, the United States is facing its largest influx of immigrants since the nineteenth century (Mattson, 1987). Despite this diversity of ethnic groups, American society has been seen predominantly in terms of white, middle-class, Anglo-Saxon values and beliefs. Members of this dominant cultural group were primarily descendants of immigrants of European ancestors who valued self-control, hard work, individuality, physical cleanliness, democracy, time, achievement, and doing (Fig. 14-1). In reviewing these values the student is reminded that nursing has been and continues to be taught with the premise that all clients are members of this dominant cultural group. Therefore nursing as a profession has been "culture-bound," or imprisoned in viewing its approach to health and illness as the only way, with the expectation that clients conform to this view.

Nurses must deal with their ethnocentrism, or the tendency to judge other cultures on the basis of their own group's beliefs and values, and strive to avoid viewing their way as the best and the standard for all judgments. If nurses are not open to the validity of the beliefs of other cultural groups, they may misjudge the impact of their views on their health care behavior. Development of sensitivity and acceptance of cultural diversity are essential requirements of community health nursing in which the client must take responsibility for health practices. It is the client, after all, who decides whether to keep a clinic appointment or to allow a nurse to enter the home. The box on p. 301 lists some of the ways that nurses may develop cultural sensitivity.

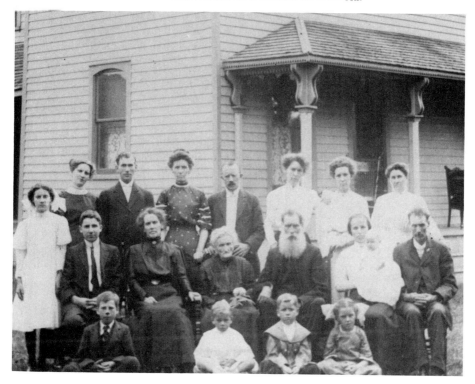

FIG. 14-1 Parents of first generation Americans valued self-control, hard work, physical cleanliness, democracy, time, achievement, and doing.

WAYS TO DEVELOP CULTURAL SENSITIVITY
1. Recognize that cultural diversity exists.
2. Demonstrate respect for people as unique individuals, with culture as one factor that contributes to their uniqueness.
3. Respect the unfamiliar.
4. Identify and examine your own cultural beliefs.
5. Recognize that some cultural groups have definitions of health and illness as well as practices that attempt to promote health and cure illness, which may differ from the nurse's own.
6. Be willing to modify health care delivery in keeping with the client's cultural background.
7. Do not expect all members of one cultural group to behave in exactly the same way.
8. Appreciate that each person's cultural values are ingrained and therefore very difficult to change.

This chapter explores the meaning of culture, the role that families play in their children's cultural development, and the importance of an individualized cultural assessment that is free of stereotypical judgment. Basic components of a cultural assessment are outlined and used as a basis for comparing the dominant cultural group and four minority ethnic groups. Application of the nursing process to families whose cultural background differs from that of the nurse is only one aspect of care. The identification of one's own values and possible biases toward those who are "culturally different" is just as important. Recognition of these feelings and the willingness to accept differences in others are the first steps in the provision of sensitive and effective nursing care.

CULTURE AND FAMILIES

Culture is a term that has various definitions in the literature, each reflecting different theoretical concepts. In its simplest form it is a distinctive way of life that characterizes a given community (Logan & Semmes, 1986). Within the community are families with shared practices, beliefs, values, and customs that are passed down from generation to generation.

Rules that govern behavior also are shared within a culture, although perhaps not on a conscious level. No one is born with knowledge of these rules; rather they are learned through verbal and nonverbal interaction within the family and community. What a family decides is acceptable or not varies. These rules are implied from the behavior and when they are broken, usually cause feelings of discomfort. For example, a Laotian refugee reported his feelings of discomfort when he was greeted with handshakes and physical embraces on entering this country as a refugee. Southeast Asians generally do not touch one another in public, and it is considered an insult for a man to touch a woman in the presence of others.

Children born into diverse cultures appear to enter the world with similiar endowments; yet cultural forces impact their development and lead to increasing differences in the kinds of behaviors adults expect of them. The process of enculturation, also known as socialization, is an anthropological term for parenting or child rearing: "the raising of children within a family to conform to the requirements of the social group in which they were born" (Brink, 1982, p. 67). Parents within the family unit teach their children rules that govern certain behaviors, along with important beliefs and values in life. Thus, child-rearing practices are culturally defined, with each culture providing its own way of socialization so that the child can become an accepted and functioning member of the society. For example, cultural scripts in many communities set boys and girls on different courses by giving them different responsibilities, thus affecting their sex-role development.

Whereas culture refers to learned patterns of behavior, ethnicity can be defined as affiliation with a value system and with those people who share that system. This affiliation provides members with a comfortable sense of security, belonging, and understanding. The development of an ethnic identity also is a function of socialization. Piaget and Weil suggest that by the age of 10 years, children have an awareness of their own nationality, as well as developed attitudes about others (Bonaparte, 1979). Therefore early experiences within the immediate environment of the family establish basic predispositions toward one's own group and toward others that stay with each person throughout life.

North America often has been called the melting pot of the world. As families from various countries and cultures move into communities in this country, they assimilate aspects of the dominant culture in a process called *acculturation.*

The more similarities the family has with the dominant culture, the more readily the process will occur. The melting-pot approach, however, implies that cultural diversity is expected to recede as each group adopts traits from the dominant culture and gradually loses its own distinctiveness. Eventually a new, uniform culture group is expected to appear. This approach, however, is severely limited because it devalues cultural diversity and places a high value on the assumption of the dominant culture's traits.

Historically, families that immigrated to America during the late 1800s and the turn of the century strove to assimilate into the dominant culture as quickly as possible, consciously attempting to submerge their differences. This attitude was challenged in the mid-1960s when the civil-rights movement helped bring about an increased sense of pride in ethnic differences. Families that have immigrated to America since then have been more resistant to assimilation and are maintaining their individuality through the retention of diverse languages, life-styles, and values, for example, the increase in the number of bilingual education programs within the public school system.

The melting-pot approach, because it stresses uniformity, discourages nurses from delivering culturally sensitive care. Thus nurses should seek to intervene in ways that are culturally acceptable to their clients. The overall goal—that of demonstrating respect for cultural differences—supports the client's sense of ethnic identity and power.

CULTURAL ASSESSMENT

A systematic appraisal of a client's cultural beliefs, values, and customs is an essential aspect of the health assessment. According to Leininger (1978) a cultural assessment is as important as a physical or psychological assessment. The information obtained can help the nurse work more effectively and comfortably with persons of different cultural backgrounds. Cultural assessments also can promote understanding of behavior that might otherwise be misjudged in a negative manner. For example, a group of Mexican-Americans believes that a spell will be cast on a newborn infant who is bathed in the first 3 days of life. Most nurses, as members of the dominant American cultural group that values cleanliness and the importance of good hygiene, might find this practice offensive and might tend to label the group as lazy and poor caretakers unless the reason for the practice is understood.

It is important for nurses to remain sensitive to individual variations within cultural groups while performing a cultural assessment inasmuch as families and individuals may not always reflect the "typical" cultural pattern. When nurses assume that clients will conform to a cultural pattern just because they belong to a specific group, stereotyping occurs. A problem arises when one applies a negative component to the stereotype or when the nurse fails to recognize important differences among members of the same cultural group. For example, the expectation that all Indians are alcoholics is based on frequent news reports that alcoholism is prevalent in this group. A biased image is further promoted by the dominant culture's negative attitude toward lack of will power and loss of control, which erroneously are perceived by many as causes of alcoholism. This attitude fails to take into consideration the possibility that biological differences in alcohol metabolism, along with differences in cultural attitudes about alcohol use and drinking behavior, are possible explanations for the higher alcoholism rates. Subsequent failure to recognize individual differences within the group further limits the nurse's accurate perception and understanding of the client and may seriously jeopardize the nurse-client relationship.

An accurate understanding of another culture is a complex process that takes even a trained anthropologist years of study. Nurses should be warned against developing a false sense of knowledge of a culture by learning specific aspects of the culture, such as the use of herbs in healing, beliefs of disease causation, and religious practices. Nevertheless, community health nurses need to spend time learning about a culture before effective interventions can be made. This understanding can be acquired initially by reviewing the literature and interviewing colleagues who are members of the specific cultural group.

Methods of performing a cultural assessment center around observation and interview. The nurse's most important tool is the ability to project a nonjudgmental interest in the client, with careful attention to interpretation of both verbal and nonverbal cues in response to questions. The home visit, as opposed to a clinic or hospital visit, is the ideal setting for a cultural assessment because it is a more natural and comfortable environment for the client. Before the interview begins, it is helpful to identify specific social amenities practiced within the group, such as taking off one's shoes before entering the room or addressing the client by his or her proper name. Spending time in socializing through friendly conversation generally is more beneficial in obtaining information and understanding of a client's lifestyle than is systematically going through a questionnaire. Observing the client's daily living routine and interaction with family members in the home also is an excellent means of assessment. In asking questions it is important to word them in a positive manner without implying a value judgment. For example, asking a pregnant Filipino mother, "Do you really think that eating dark foods will bring you a dark-complexioned baby?" probably will discourage any further discussion of diet. A more positive approach is "Tell me about some of the foods that you feel are important to include in your diet during your pregnancy."

A variety of assessment tools or guides are available (Tripp-Reimer, Brink, & Saunders, 1984). The assessment should include information about the following aspects of the client's background:

1. Ethnic group affiliation and racial background
2. Major values and beliefs
3. Health beliefs and practices
4. Religious influences or special rituals
5. Language barriers and communication styles
6. Parenting styles and role of family
7. Dietary practices

Ethnic Group Affiliation and Racial Background

It is important to identify the specific ethnic group with which the client identifies. Racial background refers to specific physical and structural characteristics such as skin pigmentation, stature, facial features, texture of body hair, and head form. These characteristics, which are trasmitted genetically, distinguish one human type from another. Some diseases are more prevalent in certain racial or ethnic groups because of genetic factors and environmental differences, such as sickle cell anemia among black persons and Tay-Sachs disease among Jews. However, just as there may be predispositions toward certain diseases, there also are ethnic variations in natural resistance toward disease. For example, black Americans have a low incidence of skin cancer and central nervous system malformations.

Minority ethnic groups comprise a large number of the lower socioeconomic class in American society (Bloch, 1983). This unfortunate fact makes it difficult to distinguish cultural characteristics from those of poverty unless the nurse is sensitive to the differences. Both poverty and minority status are subject to discrimination and prejudice, especially within the health care system. Increased vulnerability to disease because of such factors as poor nutrition, overcrowded living arrangements, and decreased personnel and staff members with sensitivity and knowledge of variations in cultural background, all contribute to this situation.

Major Values and Beliefs

Values, which are present in all cultures, describe an orientation or view concerning how members should think, act, and behave. For example, many Americans value punctuality

TABLE 14-1 Comparison of value orientations among eastern Asians, Hispanics, native Americans, blacks, and the dominant American culture	
Value orientation	**Cultural group**
Time orientation	
Present oriented: accepts each day as it comes; little regard for the past; future upredictable	Hispanic, black, native American
Past oriented: maintains traditions that were meaningful in the past; worships ancestors	Eastern Asian
Future oriented: anticipates "bigger and better" future; high value on change	Dominant American
Activity orientation	
"Doing" orientation: emphasizes accomplishments that are measurable by external standards	Dominant American
"Being" orientation: spontaneous expression of self	Hispanic, black, native American
"Being-in-becoming": emphasizes self-development of all aspects of self as an integrated whole	Eastern Asian
Human nature orientation	
Human being basically evil but with perfectable nature; constant self-control and discipline necessary	Dominant Amercian, Hispanic, black
Human being as neutral, neither good nor evil	Eastern Asian, native American
Human-nature orientation	
Human being subject to enviroment with very little control over own destiny	Hispanic, black
Human being in harmony with nature	Eastern Asian, native American
Human being master over nature	Dominant American
Relational orientation	
Individualistic: encourages individualism: impersonal relationships occur more with outsiders and less with family	Dominant American
Lineal: group goals dominant over individual goals; ordered positional succession (father to son)	Eastern Asian
Collateral: group goals dominant over individual goals: more emphasis on relationship with others on one's own level	Hispanic, black, native American

Adapted from "Dominant and variant value orientation" (p. 63-80) by F. Kluckhohn; *Transcultural nursing: A book of readings* by P. Brink (Ed.), 1976, Englewood, Cliffs, NJ: Copyright 1976 by Prentice-Hall. Modified by permission.

and place a high priority on adhering to a strict time schedule. Many black and Hispanic persons have a more flexible orientation of time. Needs of friends and family may take precedence over being on time for an appointment.

Variation in value orientation is believed to be one of the most important differences among cultures; therefore it is an important difference for nurses to recognize (Kluckhohn, 1976). Because the majority of nurses who practice in North America are from the dominant culture, it is vitally important for their practice to demonstrate not only an awareness of their value orientation but also how it may contrast with those from different cultural groups. Table 14-1 outlines five major value orientations and implications for health care practice.

Health Beliefs and Practices

Ethnic groups vary in the way they view illness and health and how healing takes place. The definition of illness by the dominant American culture is based on Western scientific thought, which views illness as a breakdown in a body part because of invasion by an organism. The roots of this belief can be traced to Galileo, Newton, and sixteenth century Pythagoreans who dealt with the universe in terms of the parts that make up the whole. Thus, instead of treating the whole person, Western medicine treats a diseased organ. In contrast, other cultural groups such as native Americans view illness and disease as a lack of harmony with nature. Health care not only treats the whole person but includes active participation of the family, neighbors, and community. It is interesting to note in recent years the attempt by Western society to develop a holistic approach to health care whereas native Americans and other older cultures have used this approach for centuries.

Perhaps one of the difficulties encountered in implementing this concept has been that nursing and medical personnel, as members of the dominant culture, are culture-bound by their heritage to view health and illness traditionally. It takes extreme effort and special diligence to force oneself to see things from a different point of view—an important fact to keep in mind in working with clients and families whose cultures define illness in their own way. Open communication and active participation in developing a plan of care with the client and family are essential for successful interventions and improved health. Lack of effective communication also may affect patient safety. For example, many Laotians believe in the use of various herbs and roots for cures of certain illnesses. The concurrent use with Western drug therapy may have hazardous effects. Thus the assessment process is vital to reveal information that affects the client's well-being.

In many cultures folk healers or other individuals are consulted for advice and treatment of illness. It is important for the community health nurse to work with such members of the client's group and respect their status within the community. Folk healers can be an important source of information because they usually live in the client's community and are sensitive to the individual's cultural needs.

Ethnic groups tend to vary in their beliefs about the cause of pain and suffering and how it should be managed. In Zborowski's classic study (1952), various ethnic groups reacted differently to pain. It was discovered that health providers from the dominant American culture valued stoicism and limited, nonemotional expressions of pain. They found it difficult to help clients who were complaining of pain through screams, moaning, and verbal complaining. Thus, it becomes clear that nurses who develop awareness of their own value orientation toward pain and its expression can more effectively assist clients with appropriate supportive measures for their pain.

Religious Influences or Special Rituals

In many cultures religion has a strong impact on beliefs concerning health and illness, views on death and chronic illness, and adherence to nursing or medical practices. Religious beliefs, sacred rituals, and the use of talismans may play an important role in the treatment of disease. For example, certain types of medical procedures may be forbidden because of religious beliefs and practices, as in the case of those who belong to Jehovah's Witnesses.

It is important to assess the role of significant religious persons during health and illness. For example, the American Indian medicine man also is a priest and a highly respected tribal leader. For nursing interventions to be successful it is essential to involve these significant individuals in planning the client's care.

Approaches to various life-cycle events such as death and dying differ from one culture to another. Nurses with a Christian background may be comforted by the belief of an afterlife. Many native Americans, however, do not believe in an afterlife and view death as a natural part of life that is celebrated with feasting and gift giving. In some Eastern Asian families it is important for the ill member to die at home surrounded by other family members.

Language Barriers and Communication Styles

The nurse should determine which language is spoken in the home. Many times, non-English-speaking clients have learned some English words as a part of the acculturation process and begin to use them when speaking with professionals. Their skills in English, however, may not be developed to the point that they are adept at cognitive expression. Therefore an interpreter is essential in explaining potentially complex topics such as those involved in health education. In addition, assessing whether the client can read or write in English is important because this ability determines whether the nurse can use written materials in client teaching.

Certain nonverbal expressions may have different meanings or social significance. Nodding the head often is perceived by nurses as a sign of comprehension by the client. Many Eastern Asian Americans, however, may nod during a conversation to indicate respect and deference, not necessarily an understanding of the information being presented. In some cultures direct eye contact is considered a sign of disrespect and thus is avoided. Nurses who view eye contact with the client as a valued communication tool and are unaware of this cultural difference may erroneously perceive this behavior as a sign of disinterest.

Many resources are available to nurses to help break language barriers. The nurse can assess whether other family members or close friends are proficient in English. In addition, interpreters may be available at larger institutions such as universities, health departments, and welfare agencies. More and more communities are developing organizations that provide trained cultural informants who can assist not only in translating language but in providing insight into the cultural beliefs of individuals as well.

If resources are unavailable, the nurse should make every effort to communicate with the client through the use of alternative methods such as diagrams, drawings, and pointing. Behaviors such as talking loudly or showing frustration and anger can lead to alienation and the client's withdrawal from the interaction. Sometimes learning and using some key words from the client's native language can greatly enhance the communication process because it minimizes the perceived superiority of the English language and demonstrates the nurse's interest and respect for the client.

Parenting Styles and Role of Family

Since the late 1920s social and cultural anthropologists in various cultures throughout the world have studied child-rearing practices. The predominant finding has been that these practices vary from culture to culture and need to be viewed within the context of the client's culture; that is, "parenting is neither good nor bad in any culture, simply different" (Brink, 1982, p. 81).

Child-rearing or parenting is dysfunctional only when it fails to provide the child with the tools for surviving in a particular society. Yet anyone who walks into a bookstore in this country sees countless books and magazine articles on how to be a "good parent," all of which contribute to the erroneous idea that there are right and wrong ways of parenting. Probably no other area of nursing practice is fraught with more ethnocentrism than nursing concepts about parenting. Just the assumption alone that nurses can teach others to be better parents and that they have all the answers concerning parenting is culturally biased. The dominant cultural group places a high value on self-expression and independence in children and discourages physical punishment in children who misbehave. Yet another culture may value submissiveness and strict discipline of its children. Who can say what the best approach is as long as it is functional for that parent-child interaction system and instills within that child a sense of belonging and the ability to function within the community?

Nurses who work with parents of diverse cultural backgrounds should assess what parents believe is good or bad behavior in a child; at what age the child is expected to achieve certain types of learning (for example, toilet training); what kinds of supports are given to children as they are developing; methods of discipline; roles played by parents, siblings, and extended family members; and what values are important to instill in their children. Other assessment factors include determining if the family is nuclear or extended and whether relatives are available for support.

Attitudes toward family members also vary from culture to culture. Many groups identify grandparents or elders as leaders and persons to respect and to seek for advice. Developing a positive relationship with these members can be crucial for an effective plan of nursing care because at times decisions will not be made without their advice. The culture also affects the value placed on children, as well as the child's role within the family structure and differences in treatment on the basis of sex.

Dietary Practices

Diet is an integral part of a person's culture. In addition to influencing food preferences and dislikes, culture influences style of food preparation and consumption, frequency and time of eating, and types of eating utensils. This is not to say that Hispanics eat only Mexican food. Certain foods, however, are more apt to be a major part of a client's diet because of his or her ethnic group.

As part of the cultural assessment, it is important for nurses to explore the kinds of foods the client eats, as well as general eating patterns; for example, particular foods the client is encouraged to eat or expected to avoid. This knowledge is essential if the nurse is to effectively assist the client to implement a prescribed diet. Diet recommendations should reflect as little variation as possible from the client's food choices and method of food preparation. The nurse may find this approach difficult because nursing programs traditionally have taught in terms of the nutritive values of the dominant middle-class culture's typical diet. Consultation with a nutritionist, cultural informant, or colleagues of various ethnic backgrounds can be helpful. When foods that are part of the client's usual diet are included in the treatment plan, adherence to that diet is more likely. After all, it is the client who determines what he or she will eat.

CULTURALLY DIVERSE FAMILIES

This section concerns some characteristics of four large cultural groups in the United States and Canada. It is important to note that certain generalizations may or may not be true for individual members of those groups. There is a tendency for nurses to assume that all members of similiar cultural backgrounds share a common religion, language, and world view (Thierderman, 1988). For example, the Eastern Asian group includes Japanese, Chinese, Koreans, Vietnamese, Laotians, and Cambodians. Each group has a different language, a different religion, and varying practices. Making assumptions about them would be similiar to making assumptions about families whose European ancestry includes such diverse ethnic groups as Italians, Germans, and Swedes. The information presented here should assist, not substitute for, a careful cultural assessment by the nurse.

Families of Eastern Asian Origin

Ethnic group affiliation and racial background. The Eastern Asian group comprises families of ethnic groups from the continent of Asia and from the Pacific Islands and includes Japanese, Chinese, Filipino, Korean, and most recently, refugees from Vietnam, Cambodia, and Laos. These are widely diverse ethnic groups with important differences in language, religion, dietary practices, and various other cultural customs. Racial and anatomical characteristics vary as well and include brown skin tone for the Filipinos and Vietnamese and yellow skin tone for the Chinese and Japanese. The presence of inner eye folds contributes to their characteristic almond-shaped eyes. Dark hair and short stature also are typical; however, with the increase in interracial marriages among persons of Eastern Asian ancestry who were born in America, the distinctiveness of these characteristics has begun to diminish. Other characteristics include Mongolian spots or irregular areas of deep-blue pigmentation, commonly seen in the sacral and gluteal regions of babies. Lactase deficiency, common among many Eastern Asians, is believed to have a genetic link (Chen-Louie, 1983). Sensitivity to alcoholic beverages, characterized by flushing and other biological symptoms such as hypotension, tachycardia, and bronchial constriction, is common among the Japanese; it too is thought to reflect genetic involvement (Hashizume & Takano, 1983).

Major values and beliefs. A common value among many Eastern Asian families is harmony in social relationships. Any direct expression of conflict is suppressed to maintain dignity or to "save face." Many believe that emotions should be controlled to think logically and make objective judgments. This contrasts with the dominant American culture, which values assertiveness and open verbal expression of both positive and negative feelings. Many Eastern Asians value self-sufficiency; therefore dependency on a person outside the family, such as a visiting nurse, may cause embarrassment. The tendency to keep problems to themselves may prevent some families from using community resources (Hashizume & Takano, 1983).

Health beliefs and practices. The ethnic groups of Eastern Asia have various health beliefs and practices. A common theme, however, is one that portrays disease as caused by an imbalance of forces, with healing aimed at restoring the balance. Health requires a balance between the opposing forces of yin and yang, also known as the "hot" and "cold" concept, which includes the five elements of the body: metal, wood, water, fire, and earth. Disharmony as a result of improper care of the body or unhappiness with oneself or society can result in disease. For example, poor diet, lack of sleep, lack of exercise, or problems with interpersonal relationships can cause illness as a result of a physiological imbalance. Therefore preventive health measures to preserve health and avoid illness generally are well received and followed by these families. Because balance of the body fluids is disrupted by such practices as having blood drawn for laboratory tests, some Eastern Asians may be reluctant to allow this procedure.

Eastern Asian families may seek treatment from both physicians and cultural healers (Chen-Louie, 1983). Cultural healers are believed to have supreme power that is passed from elderly healers to the new generation. A potential problem can arise when herbal medicines recommended by a cultural healer are taken along with medications prescribed by a physician. Because effects of this combination are unknown, clients should be warned of the risk that one medication might potentiate or weaken the other.

Religious influences. It is no more accurate to discuss one Asian American religion than it is to discuss one European religion. Great diversity of religion exists among and within the various countries. Families of Eastern Asian origin may practice Buddhism, Confucianism, Taoism, or "Western" religions such as Judaism or Christianity. Confucian principles stress the importance of duty toward others instead of individual rights. Taoism, which teaches self-realization through the achievement of harmony, influences its followers to avoid conflict. Thus the nurse may mistake a cultural characteristic for passivity. Many practicing Buddists believe that their present lives predetermine their own future lives and those of their dependents. Ancestors are respected, and great importance is placed on visiting and caring for the tombs or memorials of deceased relatives. Newly arrived immigrants may find separation from their homeland difficult because of their inability to visit the graves of their ancestors. Death is accepted as a natural part of the life cycle, and many prefer to die in the comfort of their own homes. This custom stems from the belief that a person who dies outside the home will become a wandering soul with no place to rest.

Language barriers and communication styles. Eastern Asians have distinct communication practices. Verbal expression is more restrained because of the value placed on harmony in interpersonal relationships. They may smile or laugh to mask emotions or nod "yes" even when they disagree. To question perceived authority figures and to look directly into the eyes of another person are considered signs of disrespect. Eastern Asians may wait silently rather than ask a question because they may believe that the health provider knows best and will meet their needs without being asked.

During home visits the nurse should be aware of some practices that involve social etiquette. Use of touch through hand shaking is uncomfortable for many Eastern Asians and should be avoided unless the client offers a hand first. Because many believe that the head is the most sacred part of the body, the nurse should obtain permission before touching the client's head. The foot is considered the lowliest part of the body; thus it may be considered disrespectful to point a toe in someone's direction or show the bottom of one's shoe. Therefore nurses should refrain from crossing their legs to show the bottom parts of their shoes while talking to clients. Within the home setting many Eastern Asian families show hospitality by offering food or drink. Consequently, it would be impolite to refuse such offers. In partaking of any food or drink, it is important to wait until the client has eaten or drunk first. Appreciation for nursing services may be demonstrated by gift giving, and the client might feel slighted if the gift is refused.

Parenting styles and role of family. The traditional kinship system is the extended family, with as many as three generations living under one roof. Today's families of Eastern Asian origin tend to be more nuclear, although close ties still are maintained, with many relatives outside the immediate family (Suzuki, 1980). In more traditional families the father is viewed as the authority figure. Grandparents and elders are respected for their wisdom, and their advice is sought on important family matters.

Child-rearing practices during the early years are characterized by parental permissiveness. Infants seldom are allowed to cry for prolonged periods before the mother picks them up. They usually are fed on demand rather than by scheduling. On the average, weaning takes place later than for Anglo-American infants. Parents may allow the young child to sleep with them, occasionally tolerating such behavior until the child reaches the age of 5 or 6 years. At that age parents adopt a sterner form of discipline in which obedience is stressed. Nonphysical disciplinary techniques are employed, usually through scolding or instilling shame. Aggression, especially fighting, is strongly disapproved of and quickly admonished. The mother is the primary disciplinarian and plays the major role in child-rearing (Suzuki, 1980).

Dietary practices. Typical meals and patterns of eating vary from one region to another. Rice is the main starch, although in some regions the use of wheat products in the form of noodles is prevalent. Either may be taken with many vegetables and smaller amounts of meat or fish, depending on availability. Chopsticks or fingers may be used as eating utensils, and it is the custom for some to hold their bowls of rice or soup under their chins.

Milk is not readily consumed because a taste for it has not been acquired and, as mentioned previously, there may be a possible lactose intolerance. Calcium is acquired through a diet rich in soybean products, small bony fish, sesame seeds, and tofu. Although Eastern Asian diets tend to be low in cholesterol, they are high in sodium. The frequent use of soy sauce and monosodium glutamate makes adjustment difficult for those who require low-sodium diets. Many food stores now offer low-sodium soy sauce and other condiments in response to the present emphasis on a diet of decreased sodium.

Families of Hispanic Origin

Ethnic group affiliation and racial background. The term *Hispanic American* is used to categorize those people of Puerto Rican, Cuban, Mexican, and Central and South American backgrounds. Their ancestry can be traced to several Indian tribes such as the Aztecs and Mayans, the Spanish, and the African black people. A recent cultural movement among this population has encouraged the use of the term *La Raza* to recognize the many Indian tribes and ancestors of this group. La Raza is the word for race, and although this population is not officially recognized as a race separate from the white population, the increased use of this term demonstrates increased pride in cultural diversity. Physical appearance may vary from light hair, blue eyes and fair complexion to dark hair, eyes, and skin tone. Although many families pride themselves in their "mixed" descent, some do not. Consequently, the nurse who works with the population always should assess the particular ethnic group with which the client identifies, such as Puerto Rican or Mexican.

Major values and beliefs. Many Hispanic persons value their diverse culture and take pride in maintaining their language. Loyalty to family is considered more important than meeting individual needs. This attitude contrasts with that of the dominant American society, which values individualism. Religion plays an important role in the lives of many Hispanic persons and influences their daily lives and attitudes toward health. They believe that human beings have very little control over their future and stress the "will of God."

Health beliefs and practices. For many Hispanic persons health is considered a gift from God and illness is believed to be a punishment for wrongdoing. Cure is sought from the *curanderos* (folk healers) who use prayers, rituals, and laying on of hands in their treatment. Less common disorders are believed to be the will of God and part of one's destiny—something that must be endured. Thus treatment and preventive measures may have a low priority. A Hispanic description of some common clinical conditions is presented in Table 14-2.

Health is considered a balance among the four humors of the body (blood, phlegm, black bile, and yellow bile). This belief is derived from ancient times and was used by Hippocrates. Each humor possesses different characteristics in terms of temperature and moisture. Blood is hot and wet, yellow bile is hot and dry, phlegm is cold and wet, and black bile is cold and dry. "Hot" diseases such as rashes, fever, and ulcers require treatment with "cold" medications and diet. Penicillin is considered a "hot" medication, and if the

TABLE 14-2 Common clinical conditions described by Hispanic Americans

Syndrome	Cause	Symptom	Treatment
Mal de ojo ("evil eye")	Individuals with this power gaze enviously at child or pregnant woman without touching them	Illness and misfortune	That person must touch or pat the child or woman when admiring them; if person not found, an egg is cracked and placed in a bowl at the head of the bed
Calda de la Mollera ("fallen fontanel")	Arises from the nipple being removed too quickly from the infant's mouth; bouncing or dropping infant	Diarrhea, restlessness, fever, inability to suck	Prayers, pushing up the palate from inside infant's mouth, holding child by feet over pan of tepid water, applying eggs or warm salted olive oil to scalp
Empacho ("blocked intestine")	Arises from bolus of food becoming stuck to abdominal lining	Abdominal pain, vomiting, decreased appetite, crying; common in infants, children, and immediate postpartum period	Massage, herbal cathartics
Susto ("fright sickness")	Results from frightening or upsetting experience	May have anorexia, listlessness, languor	Curandero rubs body with special herbs; herbal teas and sugar water; prayers

client who adheres to these beliefs has a fever as a result of an infection, noncompliance with the treatment plan may result if it includes this drug. Nurses who are aware of these beliefs can advise the client to take the penicillin with fruit juice or any other "cold" substance to neutralize its "hot" properties.

Religious influences. Religion plays an important role in the lives of many Hispanic persons and influences their attitude toward life, health, illness, and death. Approximately 85% to 90% are Catholic (Monrroy, 1983) and follow the religious practices of this religion. The priest often plays an important role as spiritual leader and adviser in many family matters.

Language barriers and communication styles. Spanish is the predominant language of Hispanic Americans, although it may be spoken with many different accents, depending on the country of their ancestor's origin. A large number speak only Spanish, which has implications for nurses who speak only English. Translators must be carefully picked to avoid the use of Hispanic translators who recently have risen from the lower ranks into a white-collar job and may be "disdainful of the plight of their uneducated countrymen" (Murillo-Rhode, 1981, p. 235). Translators also should be the same sex as the client inasmuch as modesty is valued in this group and a translator of the opposite sex might result in reluctance to discuss sexual matters. Touch is an acceptable form of expression and may be used in greetings among friends and family through hugging, kissing, and holding hands.

Parenting styles and role of family. There is a strong sense of family among Hispanic persons, and many live in extended families. Men, who historically assume a paternalistic role, must be consulted for all decisions. However, they tend to be minimally involved in child care, which is believed to be the mother's responsibility. Children are highly valued and receive much physical affection and cuddling from both parents. Relatives such as godparents and the parents, brothers and sisters assume many child care responsibilities. Boys are encouraged to be independent whereas girls are protected. Discipline of children involves teaching them to respect authority figures, although there is less emphasis on rigid rules and harsh punishments. Respect for authority figures may cause adults to feign agreement and understanding of the treatment plan so as not to offend the nurse. The nurse may be viewed as a health official. Consequently, it may not be productive to ask if the client understands the information presented. Instead the nurse might more accurately evalute the client's understanding by an open-ended question such as "What would you do if . . . . " The attitude that family problems should remain within the family is common, and care should be taken to avoid asking too many questions about family matters, which may be viewed as an invasion of privacy.

Dietary practices. As is true for many cultures, food is a symbol of hospitality and friendship in the Hispanic culture. Although Latin American countries vary in diet, the basic staples usually include rice and beans, along with corn and such vegetables and fruits as green bananas *(plantanos verdos),* chilis, and *cassavas* (from the yucca plant and used in making tapioca, bread, and starch). The diet tends to be high in vegetable protein and carbohydrates and contains smaller amounts of animal protein and calcium (Monrroy, 1983). Hispanic persons value fat babies as a sign of health, and infant feeding practices may include the addition of cereal to the baby's bottle.

Foods that are considered "hot" and "cold" should be taken into account when diet is part of the treatment plan for Hispanic Americans. "Cold" foods include most fresh vegetables and tropical fruits, dairy products, poultry, and fish. "Hot" foods include chili peppers, cereal grains, kidney beans, alcoholic beverages, evaporated milk, beef, and lamb. It is believed that "hot" foods are more easily digested than "cold" (Currier, 1978).

Families of Native American Origin

Ethnic group affiliation and racial background. The term *native American* encompasses more than 400 Indian tribes in the United States and Canada alone and there are approximately 280 reservations (Miller, 1982). It is important to realize that there is no one language or style of dress among this group, which is contrary to the pervasive stereotype of buckskin, beaded headband, and feathers. Despite these differences, the ethnicity of native Americans is delineated by many values, beliefs, and customs. Many have characteristic features such as a long, narrow nose and dark skin tone.

Major values and beliefs. Some of the values and beliefs shared among many native Americans are respect for harmony between human beings and nature, generosity and sharing of possessions, personal integrity and bravery, brotherhood, and compassion for others. Competitive behavior generally is discouraged because of the value placed on generosity and compassion.

Health beliefs and practices. Health is defined as a state of harmony between the human being and nature as well as with the universe. Illness most often is believed to be caused by (1) witchcraft, (2) violation of a taboo, (3) becoming possessed by spirits, (4) loss of soul, and (5) disease or object intrusion into the body (Vogel, 1981). Loss of soul typically occurs during a dream, and if it is not recovered, the person is believed in danger of dying. Spirit intrusion occurs when the body is possessed by the spirits of human beings and animals. Disease or object intrusion refers to the lodgement inside the body of some type of animal, worm, or insect.

Preventive health practices may involve wearing a talisman or carrying a special sac that contains herbs or objects with special curative powers. Healing ceremonies often consist of prayers and songs that offer spiritual renewal and are carried out by a medicine man or family members.

Religious influences. Religion is an integral part of life in native American culture. The mountains, rivers, and all geographical features are considered sacred and must not be abused or treated disrespectfully. Religion and health beliefs are closely interwoven with the power of the medicine man who functions both as priest and as healer of sickness. Types of medicine men vary from tribe to tribe, but most are believed to possess supernatural powers and are responsible for the care of the soul.

Language barriers and communication styles. Many different languages are spoken among the various tribes. In addition, many tribes value nonverbal communication and periods of silence as a means of becoming more sensitive to the environment and as a way to help the individual formulate thoughts for greater impact while speaking. Therefore they do not value individuals who hurry conversation, interrupt, and interject. Many are sensitive to nervous or hurried mannerisms and other forms of body language. They appreciate a handshake and eye contact during an interview, but unwavering eye gaze should be avoided because it is viewed as insulting and is likened to controlling one's spirit.

Parenting styles and role of family. The kinship structure is extended. In many tribes there is a matriarchal dominance and clan membership is inherited through the mother's family. Clan refers to a much wider group than the immediate family and consists of aunts, uncles, cousins, and grandparents. Elders are respected, and grandparents play a special role as teacher and counselor of their grandchildren in such topics as the human being and nature. Family membership is highly valued: "to be poor in the Indian world is to be without relatives" (Henderson & Primeaux, 1981).

Parents highly value their children and may engage only in those social activities that include children. Children seldom are disciplined by raising the voice or using physical force. Parents instill respect not only of elders but of worthy objects within nature. Competitiveness is discouraged, especially if it involves hurting another person.

Dietary practices. Food plays an important role beyond that of nutritional value in native American culture. Foods may be used in ceremonies to help ward off an illness or to help regain health. For example, before a person enters a home, cornmeal may be sprinkled on the shoulders to ward off bringing in illness. Because the concept of sharing and generosity is important, eating serves an important social function. Food restrictions are observed by many as part of religious ceremonies, and other customs may vary from tribe to tribe. The Delaware Indians actually prohibit the consumption of meat during febrile illness. Some restrictions, such as not drinking undiluted cow's milk, may be based on biological conditions inasmuch as lactose intolerance is prevalent (Wilson, 1983). Corn, squash, and beans are typical staple foods of the native American diet.

Black American Families

Ethnic group affiliation and racial background. Black American families historically have been the most oppressed minority group in the United States and Canada, culturally distinctive because of appearance, origins, and experience with slavery. Although black Americans are a heterogeneous group, the majority are descendents of the people of the West African countries of Ghana and Cote D'Ivoire (formerly called the Ivory Coast). Their ancestors were forcibly separated from highly developed civilizations in which the concept of family was well-defined and served important economic and political functions.

With the organization of slave trade more than 300 years ago, this family life was disrupted as members were separated and forced to tend to the needs of plantation owners before the needs of their families.

The black race is distinguished from other races primarily by darker skin tones and hair texture. Because of intermixture with other races, variations of these features exist. Sickle cell anemia is a common genetic disease among black persons, along with another hematological problem, glucose-6-phosphate dehydrogenase (G6PD) deficiency, in which anemia results after certain drug therapies or stress conditions.

Major values and beliefs. Several cultural values vary in their occurrence and degree among black American families, for example, orientation to the present rather than to the future, which has implications for preventive health teaching. In addition, orientation to time is flexible in terms of meeting schedules or appointments so that needs of family or friends, which are valued above punctuality, can be met.

Health beliefs and practices. The health beliefs of black Americans have evolved over the years from those brought over by African slaves. Snow (1974) described the health beliefs of low-income black Americans from the southwest as a blend of elements from Africa, folk medicine of a century ago, and selected beliefs of modern scientific medicine, interwoven with aspects of Christianity, voodoo, and magic. As in other cultures there is an underlying belief that health is a state of harmony within oneself and with the environment. Illness is defined as a sense of physical, emotional, or spiritual disharmony.

In many southern communities of the United States the use of roots, herb potions, oils, powders, tokens, rituals, and ceremonies continues. These customs are observed primarily by elderly black persons when scientific medical approaches have been employed without success. The practice of self-treatment of illness evolved as a result of inaccessibility to health care because of prohibitive cost and racism. Prayer as a method of treatment for illness also has been used because of the belief that illness is a punishment for failure to abide by God's rules.

Religious influences. Religion served as an escape from the harsh realities of the slaves' daily life. After the American Civil War the church provided a supportive environment for those caught in the struggle with poverty, unemployment, and overcrowded living. Through the church black Americans were able to assume leadership roles as ministers and other church administrators. Ministers always have played an important role in the black American culture as community leaders who provide significant support to families during times of stress. Thus the nurse should include black ministers as part of the health team because they often help bridge the gap between the health care providers and the client by serving as a cultural informant.

Language barriers and communication styles. Despite the fact that black American families speak English, many health care providers from the dominant white culture inevitably create barriers that prevent effective communication. For example, attempts to imitate the highly stereotyped and stylized "black English" may be perceived as mockery and should be avoided. The demonstration of respect for the client as a unique individual influenced by his or her culture is essential for any effective interaction.

Parenting styles and role of family. The black American family survived through the harsh realities of slavery and racism with a strong sense of kinship among its members. The kinship structure frequently is extended, with a close-knit circle of relatives and friends—aunts, uncles, grandparents, brothers, sisters, boyfriends, ministers, and friends— all participating in aspects of child rearing. This family structure is seen as a "buffer against the stress of living" (Thomas, 1981, p. 212). Thus nurses should involve not only the client but the key members of the family in planning nursing care.

Socialization of black children has been described in the literature as posing special challenges (Billingsley, 1968; Williams, 1988). Parents must teach their children how to be black in a white society, that is, to realize that the dominant white culture may judge black persons as inferior while at the same time learning to move beyond those factors by developing self-confidence and pride in their cultural background: "to raise a black child without any notion that he is viewed differently because of his race would be disastrous" (Williams, 1988, p. 50).

Individuality of the child is highly valued from infancy because "each grasp, movement, burp, or cry is interpreted as expressive of the child's own unique personality" (Leigh & Green, 1982, p. 116). First-born children tend to receive more mothering and stimulation in early infancy, with emphasis on instilling assertiveness and leadership qualities in the child. As children reach adolescence, however, girls are encouraged to take on adult responsibilities whereas boys are permitted more freedom.

Dietary practices. Salt pork as a seasoning is a key ingredient in many dishes, especially with greens such as collard and mustard greens, chard, and kale. Other ingredients such as vinegar and hot pepper sauce are added as condiments. Chicken and pork are commonly served meats, along with their less desirable parts, which are included in gumbos, hash, and pot pies. Boiling and frying tend to be the main methods of meat preparation. Some foods, such as black-eyed peas, served on New Year's day for good luck, may have spiritual overlays.

Hypertension and strokes cause the highest mortality among black Americans, with men 15.5 times more affected than their white counterparts (Thompson, 1980). Obesity and consumption of a diet that is high in sodium and fats are believed to be precipitating factors, along with a genetic tendency for cardiovascular disease.

USING THE NURSING PROCESS TO PROVIDE CULTURALLY APPROPRIATE CARE
Assessment

This chapter has focused primarily on factors that should be assessed in working with culturally diverse families. The box on p. 317 provides an assessment guide that can be used to assist the nurse in understanding the client's cultural framework. It is important to develop awareness of one's own behaviors, feelings, and value system in the areas listed in the guideline before working with clients from different cultures. Self-awareness and recognition of personal biases or prejudice enable the nurse to develop a nonjudgmental approach.

The home setting is an ideal place to learn about culturally diverse families. Flexibility in scheduling home visits, such as during evening hours when more family members are present, enables the nurse to consider the whole extended family. A series of on-going visits, as opposed to a single visit, assists not only in the development of accurate assessments but also demonstrates genuine interest. Whenever possible, it is helpful if the nurse avoids advocating any health measures until sufficient time has been spent listening to clients' perspectives of their health problems.

Nursing Diagnosis

The North American Nursing Diagnosis Association (NANDA) does not include nursing diagnoses that refer specifically to cultural problems or situations. However, factors related to problems encountered with culturally diverse clients may be noted, for example, nursing diagnoses such as "impaired verbal communication related to use of Vietnamese as the primary language" and "anxiety related to disregard of cultural practice observed to prevent illness."

CULTURAL ASSESSMENT GUIDE

Health beliefs and practices

How does the client define health and illness?

Are there particular methods used to help maintain health, such as hygiene and self-care practices?

Are there particular methods being used by the client for treatment of illness?

What is the attitude toward preventive health measures such as immunizations?

Are there health topics that the client may be particularly sensitive to or that are considered taboo?

What are the attitudes toward mental illness, pain, handicapping conditions, chronic disease, death, and dying?

Is there a person in the family responsible for various health-related decisions, such as where to go, whom to see, and what advice to follow?

Religious influences and special rituals

Is there a religion that the client adheres to?

Is there a significant person that the client looks to for guidance and support?

Are there any special religious practices or beliefs that may affect health care when the client is ill or dying?

What events, rituals, and ceremonies are considered important within the life cycle, such as birth, baptism, puberty, marriage, and death?

Language and communication

What language is spoken in the home?

How well does the client understand English, both spoken or written?

Are there special signs of demonstrating respect or disrespect?

Is touch involved in communication?

Are there culturally appropriate ways to enter and leave situations, including greetings, farewells, and convenient times to make a home visit?

Parenting styles and role of family

Who makes the decisions in the family?

What is the composition of the family, how many generations are considered to be a single family, and which relatives comprise the family unit?

When the marriage custom is practiced, what is the attitude about separation and divorce?

What is the role of and attitude toward children in the family?

When do children need to be disciplined or punished, and how is this done (if physical means are used, in what way)?

Do the parents demonstrate physical affection toward their children and each other?

What major events are important to the family, and how are they celebrated?

Are there special beliefs and practices surrounding conception, pregnancy, childbirth, lactation, and child rearing?

Dietary practices

What does the family like to eat, and does everyone in the family have similar tastes in food?

Who is responsible for food preparation?

Are any foods forbidden by the culture, or are some foods a cultural requirement in observance of a rite or ceremony?

How is food prepared and consumed?

Are there specific beliefs or preferences concerning food, such as those believed to cause or to cure an illness?

Planning

Collaboration between the client and the nurse for the development of goals is essential, inasmuch as the client and nurse may define health and illness differently and therefore disagree on the plan of care. The nurse should not attempt to change the client's values but work with and involve the client in determining the plan of care. Consideration must be given to include cultural healers, religious leaders, and significant family members in the planning process when appropriate. Areas of conflict between the nurse and client need to be identified and mediated. For example, should a woman with diabetes believe that the development of ketoacidosis is the will of God, the nurse who is sensitive to the client's belief could respond that it is the will of God that she was sent to her to instruct her on what to do should it occur.

Implementation

Whenever possible it is helpful to use visual aids to demonstrate health practices, especially when English is not the client's native language. In cultures in which ritual acts are important, it may be helpful to break down the separate components of a procedure. For example, the nurse can teach the steps involved in cleaning a wound by means of a technique, equipment, and sequence of activities to help establish a ritual practice.

Evaluation

Nurses must avoid the tendency to label the client as "difficult" or "uncooperative" when the health plan does not work out in the anticipated way. Noncompliance often reflects the failure to recognize and understand conflicts in health value orientations when the nurse and client have different cultural perspectives. Client involvement throughout the planning process helps prevent noncompliance as a result of these cultural differences. Effective modifications in health practices are much more likely to occur if the nurse acknowledges and understands cultural factors.

SUMMARY

Community health nurses who work with culturally diverse families first must assess their personal values and beliefs if they are to provide nonjudgmental and culturally sensitive care. These values are taught by each family from the moment of birth through the process of enculturation.

In the past, nurses have failed to recognize the significance of cultural orientation and its influence on their clients' behavior, especially in health-related behaviors. Through careful cultural assessments, community health nurses can develop understanding of their clients' behavior, which enables more effective interventions to occur. Familiarization with typical characteristics of their clients' ethnic group can provide an initial data base and thus assist nurses involved in the process of cultural assessment. However, nurses must recognize that each person is unique and that many important differences exist among members of the same cultural group. Collaboration with the client enables the establishment of mutually determined goals, which results in culturally sensitive nursing care.

CHAPTER HIGHLIGHTS

- A person's culture includes values, beliefs, and customs that are learned within the family and that govern most aspects of behavior.

- Nurses who care for individuals and families from cultural backgrounds that are different from their own must become sensitive to and accepting of the client's cultural practices.
- In the nineteenth century, immigrants to the United States strove to assimilate as quickly as possible into the dominant culture. More recent immigrants have attempted to retain their individuality and cultural practices.
- A cultural assessment should include information about the client's ethnic affiliation and racial background, values and beliefs, health beliefs and practices, religious beliefs, language barriers and communication style, parenting style and role of family, and dietary practices.
- Members of certain racial and ethnic groups may be genetically predisposed toward certain diseases and naturally resistant to others.
- Value orientations that have implications for health care include attitudes toward time, activity, human nature, the individual's relationship with nature, and individual and group relationships.
- If a client believes in the use of folk healers or other nontraditional methods of treatment, the nurse should incorporate these methods into the care plan whenever possible.
- Communication includes both spoken language and nonverbal expressions.
- Child-rearing practices vary from culture to culture and are dysfunctional only when the child is not provided with the tools needed to survive in society.
- To encourage compliance with dietary regimens the nurse should allow the client to retain as many elements as possible from his or her traditional diet.
- Cultural groups in the United States and Canada include East Asians, Hispanic persons, black Americans, and native Americans.
- The community health nurse can use the five steps of the nursing process to assist in delivering culturally appropriate nursing care.

STUDY QUESTIONS

1. Describe, in a one-page narrative, the meaning of culture, ethnicity, and race and the differences among the three.
2. Compare and contrast the characteristics of families of the following origins with respect to religious beliefs, health beliefs and practices, and parenting style: (a) Eastern Asian, (b) Hispanic, (c) native American, and (d) black American.
3. Discuss the role that culture plays in parenting.

REFERENCES

Billingsley, A. (1968). *Black families in white America.* Englewood Cliffs, NJ: Prentice-Hall.

Bloch, B. (1983). Bloch's assessment guide for ethnic/cultural variations. In M. Orque, B. Bloch, and L. Monrroy, (Eds.), *Ethnic nursing care: A multicultural approach.* St. Louis: Mosby.

Bonaparte, B. (1979). Ego defensiveness, open-closed mindedness, and nurses' attitude toward culturally different patients. *Nursing Research, 28,* 166-167.

Brink, P. (1976). *Transcultural nursing: A book of readings.* Englewood Cliffs, NJ: Prentice-Hall.

Brink, P. (1982). An anthropological perspective on parenting. In J. Horowitz, C. Hughes, and B. Perdue,

(Eds.), *Parenting reassessed: A nursing perspective.* Englewood Cliffs, NJ: Prentice-Hall.

Chen-Louie, T. (1983). Nursing care of Chinese American patients. In M. Orque, B. Bloch, and L. Monrroy, (Eds.), *Ethnic nursing care: A multicultural approach.* St. Louis: Mosby.

Currier, R. (1978). The hot-cold syndrome and symbolic balance in Mexican and Spanish folk medicine. In R. Martinez (Ed.), *Hispanic culture and health care: Fact, fiction, and folklore.* St. Louis: Mosby.

Hashizume, S., and Takano, J. (1983). Nursing care of the Japanese American patient. In M. Orque, B. Bloch, and L. Monrroy (Eds.), *Ethnic nursing care: A multicultural approach.* St. Louis: Mosby.

Henderson, G., and Primeaux, M. (1981). *Transcultural health care.* Menlo Park, CA: Addison-Wesley.

Kluckhohn, F. (1976). Dominant and variant value orientation. In P. Brink, (Ed.) *Transcultural nursing: A book of readings.* Englewood Cliffs, NJ: Prentice-Hall.

Leininger, M. (1978) *Transcultural nursing: Concepts, theories, and practices.* New York: Wiley.

Logan, B., and Semmes, C. (1986). Culture and ethnicity. In B. Logan and C. Dawkin, (Eds.), *Family-centered nursing in the community.* Menlo Park, CA: Addison-Wesley.

Mattson, S. (1987). The need for cultural concepts in nursing curriculum. *Journal of Nursing Education, 26,* 206-208.

Miller, N. (1982). Social work services to urban Indians. In J. Green, (Ed.), *Cultural awareness in the human services.* Englewood Cliffs, NJ: Prentice-Hall.

Monrroy, D., Bloch, B., & Orque, M.S. (1983). *Ethnic nursing care: A multicultural approach.* St. Louis: Mosby.

Snow, L. (1974). Folk medical beliefs and their implications for care of patients. *Annals of Internal Medicine, 81,* 82-96.

Suzuki, B. (1980). The Asian American family. In M.

Fantini and R. Cardenas, (Eds.), *Parenting in a multicultural society.* New York: Longman.

Theirderman, S. (1988). Workshops in cross-cultural health care: The challenge of "ethnographic dynamite." *Journal of Continuing Education in Nursing, 19* (1), 25-27.

Thomas, D. (1981). Black American patient care. In Henderson, G., Primeaux, M. (Eds), *Transcultural health care.* Lopec, CA: Addison-Wesley.

Thompson, D. (1980). Hypertension: Implications of comparisions among blacks and whites. *Urban Health, 9,* 31-33.

Tripp-Reimer, T., Brink, P., and Saunders, J. (1984). Cultural assessment: Content and process. *Nursing Outlook, 32*(2), 78-82.

Vogel, V. (1981). American Indian medicine. In G. Henderson and M. Primeaux, (Eds.), *Transcultural health care.* Menlo Park, CA: Addison-Wesley.

Williams, J. (1988). The color of their skin. *Parenting, 3,* 48-53.

Wilson, U. (1983). Nursing care of American Indian patients. In M. Orque, B. Bloch, and L. Monrroy, (Eds.), *Ethnic nursing care: A multicultural approach.* St. Louis: Mosby.

Zborowski, M. (1952). Cultural components in response to pain. *Journal of Social Issues, 8,* 16-30.

The Dysfunctional Family

JANICE COOKE FEIGENBAUM

Just as the individual consists of internal factors, so the family can be similarly viewed as one singular internal environment or system where each individual within helps define it by their interactions as they become a composite of total family relationship characteristics.

BETTY NEUMAN

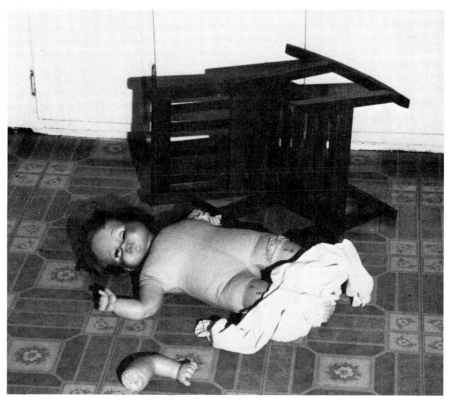

OBJECTIVES

At the conclusion of this chapter the student will be able to:
1. Define the key terms listed
2. List behaviors associated with dysfunctional family interactions
3. Describe the impact of dysfunction on the integrity of family units and on the health and development of family members
4. Describe the impact of a large number of dysfunctional families in a community
5. Use the nursing process to implement and evaluate nursing care provided to dysfunctional families

KEY TERMS

Disengagement	Ineffective family coping
Dysfunctional family	Interfamily stressors
Enabling	Intrafamily stressors
Enmeshment	Regression
Extrafamily stressors	Scapegoating
Family violence	Substance abuse
Hopelessness	

CHARACTERISTICS

The dysfunctional family can demonstrate a wide range of behaviors. In effect many of these behaviors are almost the opposite of those observed in healthy or functional families (see Chapter 13). Maribelle Leavitt (1982) distinguished dysfunctional families from healthy ones by explaining that the former tend to experience severe levels of anxiety and respond to a crisis by perceiving it as an "overwhelming burden" and "annihilating" problem, whereas the latter view the stressor as a challenge. The expression of a need to escape from a situation also is an important cue of dysfunction. Further, "there are intergenerational patterns of unresolved grief, loss, violence, and major psychopathology" (Weitzman, 1985, p. 475).

Family Structure

The family structure influences the course of illness in family members in a number of ways. According to Murray Bowen, (Friedman, 1985) it can even account for the reason that the health status of one family member changes and that of the others in a family does not. A family member can have all the physical prerequisites for a disease, including the promoting agent (e.g., bacterium, virus, or carcinogen), but the symptoms may not occur until some of the emotional conditions (prerequisites) in that family were satisfied. Conversely, a person who assumes particular family roles, on being subjected to certain triggering emotional, contextual, or physical factors, would be particularly at risk for "picking up" a disease, "catching it," or "getting sick." All this does not mean that "correct" or "positive" thinking can prevent illness. It does, however, strongly suggest that the way persons think about themselves and their family relationships can minimize the risk of becoming sick and, if illness occurs, can maximize the possibility of recovery (Friedman, 1985).

The boundaries of dysfunctional families tend to be rigid and impermeable. These closed systems are suspicious of persons, objects, and knowledge outside their own boundaries, which means that the family may view the nurse with suspicion. Further, "the closed family system is rigid in its authoritarianism; it needs children who conform and comply with the family rules" (Amundson, 1989, p. 288).

Dysfunctional families further tend to encourage dependency and learned helplessness instead of motivating each member to develop autonomy and individuality. If a member within the system attempts to develop these characteristics, the family usually responds negatively.

Severe chronic health problems, such as substance abuse (especially alcoholism), mental illness, incest, and violence, frequently occur in dysfunctional families. Jack Weitzman described these families as ones in which "the most obvious defining characteristic is the presence of a serious symptom, often multiple symptoms, of long duration and high intensity" (Weitzman, 1985, p. 474). He further noted that "these are families greatly at risk for symptom production and further disintegration. They are highly volatile entities in which the basic building blocks of family life are badly damaged. . . . The ideas of members actually enjoying one another's presence, sharing in activities, and having fun is rare indeed" (p. 475).

Susan Meister (1984) suggested that a poor fit between the family's resources and the demands for them leads to dysfunction. She explained as follows (p. 67):

> When the family does well in achieving resource/demand fit, then it has a greater capacity to contribute to the members—who are also juggling personal resources and demands. Similarly, members achieving functional degrees of fit have greater capacity to contribute to family-level resource.
>
> If the family is not able to "fit" resources to demands, then the family is less able to contribute to the efforts of its members as they face the individual requirements to "fit" resources and demands. Over time, members who are struggling to meet demands become less able to contribute to the family's processes or coping with demands. . . . It is the **dysfunctional fit of resources and demands** that bears directly upon family violence.

The North American Nursing Diagnosis Association (NANDA) classified dysfunctional families under "ineffective family coping: disabling" and defined it as "the state in which a family demonstrates destructive behavior in response to an inability to manage internal or external stressors due to inadequate resources (physical, psychological, cognitive, and/ or behavioral)" (Carpenito, 1989, p. 260).

To formulate this nursing diagnosis for a family, the nurse must identify the presence of at least one of the following major defining characteristics: "neglectful care of the client; decisions/actions which are detrimental to economic and/or social well-being; neglectful relationships with other family members" (Carpenito, 1989, p. 260).

It is difficult to estimate the percentage of families that are dysfunctional because many of their problems and attempts to resolve them are hidden from health-care and legal professionals. It is, however, possible to infer this number by considering statistics related to one problem frequently exhibited by dysfunctional families, namely alcoholism.

It is estimated one in every 10 Americans is an alcohol abuser, and these individuals create serious problems for others: "on the average, (for) some four to six other persons, including mates, children, friends, employers, and even total strangers" (Carson, Butcher, & Coleman, 1988, p. 368). In the United States the effects of alcoholism include more than 50% of deaths and major injuries caused by automobile accidents, 50% of murders, 40% of assaults, 35% of rapes, and 30% of suicides. Further, "the financial drain imposed on the economy by alcoholism is estimated to be over $25 billion a year, in large part comprised of losses to industry from absenteeism, lowered work efficiency, and accidents" (Carson et al., p. 369).

The incidence of another dysfunctional family behavior, violence (including sexual abuse), is more difficult to confirm. It is estimated that annually 3.8% (1.5 to 2 million) of American children between 3 and 17 years of age, who live in homes with two parents, and 3.8% (1.8 million) of married women are victims of abuse within families; in addition, *wife abuse occurs more often than rape by a stranger and child abuse is more prevalent than chickenpox* (Humphreys & Campbell, 1984). It is also estimated that *"about 1 woman in 12 in prenatal clinics may be in an abusive relationship"* (Tilden, 1989, p. 311). This abuse occurs more commonly during pregnancy than does placenta previa or diabetes (Campbell, 1984).

These statistics show how the presence of large numbers of dysfunctional families within the community may create problems for all members of the society. The community health nurse, who frequently encounters dysfunctional families, is in an ideal position to care for them, to act as their advocate, and in effect, to improve the health of the community at large.

Careful consideration of the criteria for dysfunction is mandatory. It is important for the nurse to recognize that a family should be diagnosed as dysfunctional only when it demonstrates behaviors related to this nursing diagnosis and not because the family does not fit the nurse's idea of a healthy family. That is, homosexual family units, single-parent units, childless couples, dual-career families, blended families, and families receiving welfare are not dysfunctional just because they exhibit characteristics different from the ideal image of a middle-class family of mother, father, and two or three children. In effect, a nuclear family, just as any of the others mentioned, may be a dysfunctional one if it demonstrates behaviors associated with the nursing diagnosis of ineffective family coping.

Nursing Concerns

It is important that nurses who work with dysfunctional families develop an awareness of their personal thoughts and feelings regarding each family's situations. Because dysfunctional families are prone to experiencing hopelessness, worthlessness, powerlessness, and high levels of anxiety, the nurse also may begin to feel these emotions. In addition, the family may be suspicious of anyone who is not a member of its system and thus may respond to the nurse as a threat to its existence. This reaction frequently leads the family to reject the nurse's overtures of help. Thus the nurse may be prone to experiencing frustration, rejection, and uselessness.

The potential for violence among dysfunctional families may cause concern for personal safety, particularly among community health nurses as they make home visits, working in these environments alone and with minimal access to support in time of danger. If safety is a concern in a specific situation, two nurses can be assigned to work together with the family.

The nurse also needs to develop an awareness of the strengths and liabilities of his or her own present family system and family of origin. Knowledge of personal desires for change is important to prevent nurses from reacting to client family members as if they belonged to their own family system. Judith Nelsen highlighted this tendency as follows (1983, p. 56):

> Practitioners having fantasies that they will tell off parents they see, tell children to shape up, coerce couples on the verge of divorce into reconciling, or otherwise do something likely to meet their own needs rather than clients' are not ready to see families. Such negative motivations need not persist if they are recognized and discussed, perhaps with a supervisor.

The nurse needs to acknowledge that negative feelings, as well as caring, concern, love, and a desire to help, are part of therapeutic relationships with individuals and families. Thus the occurrence of these emotions should not threaten the nurse's feeling of competence. Instead the nurse should recognize that identification of these reactions is the initial step in being able to set them aside so that they do not interfere with the caring implementation of the nursing process. It is helpful before each visit to a potentially dysfunctional family, or to one already diagnosed as such, for the nurse to ask the following questions:

- How do I feel about caring for this family today?
- What do I think about caring for this family today?
- How might these feelings and thoughts influence my abilities to care for this family today?
- How may I set aside these feelings and thoughts so I may effectively care for this family today?

ASSESSMENT

After dealing with personal assessment, the nurse begins to care for the family by implementing the nursing process: gathering data about the family by observing how members relate with each other, with the nurse, and with the home setting (Table 15-1). Both verbal and nonverbal behaviors provide information. The assessment process also involves identifying the family's strengths as well as its problems.

Physiological Variables

The nurse assesses the family for signs of physical health problems. Within these families, these problems may result from neglect, malnutrition, physical abuse, hyperactive behaviors, lack of attention to symptoms of illness, and noncompliance with health care regimens (Shealy, 1988). Betty Neuman suggested that the presence of a "suboptimal energy level" within family members indicates family instability inasmuch as the system's energy is "consumed by immediate interpersonal conflicts, emergencies, and basic survival" (Neuman, 1983, p. 244).

Substance abuse. The use of alcohol and other chemical substances such as marijuana and cocaine should be investigated. Some family members coping with alcoholism or drug dependency or both, may view this problem as the major stressor confronting the family. Other families may use these substances as they attempt to cope with other stressors in their lives.

Both situations create grave problems for the family because of the properties of these chemical substances and the results of their use as they relate to physical and psychological dependency and to tolerance and cross tolerance. **Physical dependency** develops when physiological symptoms such as tremors, nausea, diaphoresis, and abdominal cramps occur unless the individual ingests the substance. **Psychological dependence** refers to a compulsion and craving for the effects of the substance to create a feeling of self-esteem and well being. When either one or both develop, the individual needs the effects of the chemical substance to experience a sense of normalcy. At this point the substance controls the individual's life and that of the family instead of vice versa.

This situation is further complicated when chemical substances have tolerance and cross-tolerance properties. **Tolerance** refers to the need for increasing amounts of the substance to achieve the effect previously gained from smaller amounts. **Cross-tolerance**

TABLE 15-1 Characteristics of dysfunctional families

Stressors	Variables				
	Physiological	Psychological	Sociocultural	Developmental	Spiritual
Intrafamily	Physical neglect Malnutrition Physical/sexual abuse Hyperactivity Low energy level Lack of attention to symptoms Noncompliance with health-care regimens Physical dependence on drugs	Lack of warmth Anger/hostility Depression Dysfunctional grief Hopelessness Helplessness Powerlessness Worthlessness Frustration Avoidance of feelings View of stressors as burden Desire to escape Guilt Dependence on drugs	Perpetuation of family myths Distortion of reality Rigid rules Lack of empathic communication Ineffective role patterns Lack of interdependence Scapegoating/enabling Lack of fit between resources and demands	Insufficient knowledge of phases Unrealistic expectations Regression Learned helplessness	Rigid spiritual beliefs Religious conflicts Overdependence on supreme being
Interfamily	Avoidance of contact	Avoidance of contact	Suspicion of others Belief that no one can help Belief that no one cares Bitterness toward others	Lack of interdependence Fear of asking for help	Belief that situations will only get worse Cynicism regarding motives of others
Extrafamily	Limited housing resources Lack of mobility	Fear of accepting help from agencies Fear of loss of control View of schools/governmental agencies as interfering	Lack of money Unemployment	Avoidance of interdependence	Belief that helpers have failed Belief that nothing can help Rejection of support groups Withdrawal from religious groups Lack of faith in the system

TABLE 15-2	**Types of family violence**
Type	**Characteristics**
Physical	"Malnutrition and injuries such as bruises, welts, sprains, dislocation of extremities, lacerations"*
Psychological	"Verbal assault, threat, fear, or isolation"*
Material	"Theft or misuse of money or property"*
Medical	"Withholding of required medication or aids (e.g., false teeth, glasses, hearing aids)*
Sexual	"Any sexual activity between a child and an adult (or any individual significantly older than the child), whether by force or what may appear to be consent (Kelley, 1985, p. 234)
Family	"At least one member is using physical force against another, resulting in physical and/or emotional destructive injury" (Campbell, 1984, p. 217)
Incest	"Sexual relations between blood relatives or members of the same socialization unit other than husband and wife" (Wilson & Kneisl, 1988, p. 1169)
Violence	"Behavior by an individual that threatens or actually does harm or injury to people or property" (Wilson and Kneisl, 1988, p. 1176)

*Fulmer and Cahill, 1984, pp. 17-18.

is the extension of the tolerance effect to other drugs in the same classification that have similar pharmacological properties. When drug (including alcohol) tolerance and dependencies develop, the person requires larger amounts to prevent withdrawal symptoms and to feel "normal."

The individual also is at risk for problems associated with substance abuse, such as violence, employment difficulties, financial drain, and physical complications. These problems frequently confront dysfunctional families again and again as a result of substance abuse. (Substance abuse is discussed in greater detail in Chapter 26.)

Family violence. Cues of abuse and violence within the family must be assessed. Within a family system, violence may be directed at any member by another and can include sexual acts, as well as other forms of physical aggression.

Family violence is a profound event that will affect each member of the system. A violent family is one in which all members are in pain. All are capable of hurting each other, all are learning that violence is an acceptable form of behavior, and all are at increased risk of resorting to the use of violence (Campbell, 1984). This reality means the cycle of violence will be perpetuated for another generation.

The problem of violence is difficult to define and approach. Table 15-2 lists the types of abuse found in dysfunctional families. The fact that only physical, sexual, and incestuous abuse are beginning to be studied must be highlighted. Nevertheless other forms of family abuse are important and should be considered as the nurse cares for a family.

Some theories that concern causative factors of family violence include a low level of frustration tolerance, a family's beliefs that crises should be resolved with aggression, and the lowering of inhibitions against violence caused by the use of alcohol and other central nervous system depressants (Campbell, 1984). In fact, family violence may result from the interactions of many of these factors.

Table 15-3 outlines the results of many research studies regarding the profiles of violent families. The nurse, on initiating a relationship with a family, considers these factors.

TABLE 15-3 Profile of the violent family

Identifying data	Child physical abuse		Child sexual abuse	
	Abuser	Victim	Abuser	Victim
Age	Mother, average age = 26; father average age = 30; all ages	Most under 2 years; average age = 4 years; all ages	All ages; 21 to 30 years old most often; 11 to 20 years old next often	All ages; 6 to 9 years old at onset; 12 years old when disclosed; mean age = 7.9 years
Sex	Male and female; father more often than mother, but mother more violent	Not a factor	Male; accomplice sometimes female	Male and female; most reported cases are female (7 females to 1 male); in females, 63% are younger than 12 years old; in males, 64% are older than 12 years old
Relationship	Father or stepfather; not a stranger most often (e.g., babysitter or guardian)	Acquainted or known; oldest/youngest daughter or only child most often	Father more often than mother	Son/daughter or stepchild
Marital status	Married and living with spouse	Single	Married and living with spouse	Single
History of childhood physical/sexual abuse	60% of cases	Repeated multiple victimization or neglect	70% of cases	Repeated multiple victimization
Socioeconomic status (SES)	Evident at all SES levels; rate twice as high in reported cases of families under the poverty line ($5999) as in families of $20,000+ income		Evident in all SES levels; found cases most often lower SES	
Occupation	Reported cases most often skilled or semiskilled	Student	Found cases most often professional, skilled, or semiskilled	Student

From "Nursing intervention in family abuse and violence" by T. Foley and B. Grimes (pp. 930-933) in *Principles and practice of psychiatric nursing* (3rd ed.) (1987) by G. W. Stuart and S. J. Sundeen (Eds.), St. Louis: Mosby. Copyright 1987 by The C.V. Mosby Co. Reprinted by permission.

Spouse abuse		Sibling abuse		Elder abuse	
Male	**Female**	**Abuser**	**Victim**	**Abuser**	**Victim**
Often 17 to 30 years old at disclosure; all ages; seen in abuse of elders		All ages; most reported cases are 17 years old or less; rate decreases as age increases		40 to 60 years old	60 years old and older
Male and female; most reported cases have female victims		Male most often; higher incidence in all male–sibling families	Male most often; higher incidence in all male–sibling families	Female	Not a factor; more elder are female
Spouse or partner		Brother to brother as victim most often; brother to sister as victim next often		Son/daughter, relative, or caretaker	Parent of abuser most often
Married most often; living together next often		Single	Single	Married	Widowed
Most were subject to repeated victimization as children		Live in abusive/violent home; often victims of parent/guardian as well		Data not widely available; positive history in some cases	Positive history in some cases; repeated victimization
Evident at all SES levels; five times more common in families at or below poverty line than in families over $20,000 income in reported cases		Evident at all SES levels		Not a factor; evident at all SES levels; founded cases mostly lower to middle class and found through health care systems	
Reported cases skilled or semiskilled most often		Childhood (or history of delinquency)		Professional or semiskilled	Not employed

Continued.

TABLE 15-3 Profile of the violent family—cont'd

Identifying data	Child physical abuse		Child sexual abuse	
	Abuser	Victim	Abuser	Victim
Employment status	Unemployment not disproportionately prevalent; abuse twice as high if father is employed part time	Not employed	Employed; higher rate if part time or unemployed	Not employed
Race	Blacks and minorities inaccurately represented; all races	Same as abuser	Not a factor	
Religion	Highest, one or more parents of minority religion; lowest, Jewish	Mixed religious background	Highest, highly religious family, rigid inflexible belief system; lowest, realistic balance of religion in family belief system	
Education	Most violent, high school diploma for both men and women; least violent, grammar school dropout or some college education	Mostly preschool; if in school, performance may be poor (stress symptom)	Inaccurately presented	
			Often high school and some college	Grammar and high school student; performance may be poor (stress symptom)
Residence	Large city most often Evenly distributed in United States		Evenly distributed in United States	

The nurse who suspects abusive behaviors should meet individually with each member of the family. This subject is a difficult one to discuss, yet it must be explored to prevent further abuse and to break the cycle of intergenerational violence. It is especially necessary that the nurse pursue comments by individuals that appear to suggest that they are the victims of abuse or are concerned about becoming violent toward a family member. John Flynn's (1977) research revealed that "almost all" of his sample of abused wives had sought help from a variety of sources, including police, marriage counselors, or clergy. Frequently these pleas for help were not taken seriously. Instead the person from whom help was sought continued to attempt to keep it hidden.

Spouse abuse		Sibling abuse		Elder abuse	
Male	Female	Abuser	Victim	Abuser	Victim
Violence two or three times higher if man is unemployed or has part-time employment		Not employed		Least violence in homes of retired men; victim often physically/mentally impaired	
All races; reported most by minorities; black more than whites (2:1)		Highest, racial minorities; lowest, blacks		Highest, American Indians, orientals, minorities; blacks = 12%, whites = 88%, also reported as no difference	
Highest, minority religions and Jewish women; lowest, Protestants and Jewish men		Highest minority religions (excluding Jewish, Catholic, or Protestant)		Protestant	
Victim more often without high school diploma and less often with college education		Most violent if father/male highly educated and mother/female high school diploma or some college education		High school diploma or some college	
Most violent husbands, high school diploma; least violent, grammar school dropout or some college	Most violent, wives without high school diploma				
Evenly distributed in United States	Abused by male in large city or rural area; rate decreased by half in suburbs	Higher rates in rural area and large cities Not Southern phenomena		Limited data, evenly distributed with more reports in large cities Not Southern phenomena	

Barbara Limandri suggested the "most critical element in helping abused women is the nurse's response to the women's disclosure" (1987, p. 10). The box on p. 332 lists the facilitative and inhibitive helper responses identified in Limandri's research. The nurse uses the first set of responses to help women discuss the reality that they are victims of abuse.

Psychological Variables

As the nurse explores the psychological variables of the family system, cues such as a lack of warmth within the family; avoidance of the expression of feelings; intense levels

RESPONSES TO ABUSED WOMEN

Facilitative helper responses

- Helper asking woman if abuse is occurring
- Helper identifying described behavior as abusive
- Helper acknowledging seriousness of abuse
- Helper expressing belief in woman's description of abuse
- Helper acknowledging that woman does not deserve the abuse
- Helper being directive in exploring resources
- Helper telling the man to stop the abuse
- Helper aiding woman consider full range of available options
- Helper avoiding telling woman what to do
- Helper aiding woman to assess her internal strengths
- Helper suggesting tangible resources (e.g., shelters, financial aid)
- Helper offering support groups with other abused women
- Helper active in listening and empathizing

Inhibitive helper responses

- Helper demonstrating irritation/anger with woman
- Helper blaming woman
- Helper advising woman to accept abuse as better than nothing
- Helper refusing to help until woman left abuser
- Helper aligning with abuser
- Helper disbelieving woman
- Helper not responding to abuse disclosure
- Helper advising woman to leave abuser

From "The therapeutic relationship with abused women" by B. Limandri, 1987, *Journal of Psychosocial Nursing,* 25 (2) p. 11. Copyright 1987 by Charles B. Slack. Reprinted by permission.

of anger, hostility, and aggression; depression; expressions of guilt, hopelessness, worthlessness, powerlessness, cynicism, and bitterness; and dysfunctional grieving are considered important in identifying a dysfunctional system. Feelings of hopelessness usually can be identified by one or more of the following cues:

- Inability to set goals
- Perception of unachieved outcomes as personal failure
- Emphasis is on failure in light of accomplishments while healthy
- Rigid adherence to the possibility of achieving goals only when healthy
- Making no effort to consider alternatives
- Increasing agitation over accomplishing nothing
- Verbalization of self-doubt, therapy, and life
- Verbalization of giving up as the only solution
- Giving up

During the assessment of psychological variables the nurse observes how the family perceives itself and its health problems. Dysfunctional families tend to distort reality, frequently by means of unconscious denial, projection, and/or fantasty formation. The result is rationalization by means of blaming, scapegoating, and wishful thinking as the family tries to solve its problems (Leavitt, 1982). The reliance on these coping mechanisms leads to the perpetuation of family myths. Cues that reflect rigid family rules, such as "We are a strong family so none of us cry" or "We'd be okay if everybody like you would leave us alone" may indicate a dysfunctional family.

Spiritual Variables

As highlighted in Table 15-1, cues of extremely rigid spiritual beliefs, opposing religious loyalties, and an overdependence on supreme powers frequently are observed among families prone to violence. In addition, the families "may not participate in therapy because of their belief that a supreme being will solve the problems, if it is His will" (Shealy, 1988, p. 555).

Sociocultural Variables

Sociocultural variables can be the most difficult to assess in a caring and empathic manner because of the wide differences of cultural orientations among families encountered by community health nurses. When the nurse and the family members have different cultural backgrounds, misunderstandings frequently arise. Toni Tripp-Reimer and Sonja Lively aptly illustrated this phenomenon with the following case study (1988, p. 185):

> A case of reported child abuse was reported recently to the staff of a county mental health facility. The case involved a Vietnamese refugee family newly arrived in the United States. The referral was made by a school nurse who, while conducting routine physical assessments, identified long bruised areas on the chest and back of a girl in the second grade. However, rather than being caused by incidents of child abuse, the marks were the results of the lay practice or dermabrasion (*cao gio*), a standard home treatment for the symptoms of fever, chills, and headaches that accompany "wind illness." This practice consists of applying oil to the back and chest of the child with cotton swabs. The skin is massaged until warm and then rubbed with the edge of a copper coin until marks (bruises) appear. Thus the parents had not been abusing the child but rather were following a culturally prescribed and sanctioned mode of folk therapy.

To avoid misunderstandings such as this, the nurse must be aware of the cultural orientation of the family. (Chapter 14 presents detailed information regarding cultural issues.)

As sociocultural variables are reviewed, behaviors that indicate dysfunction may be observed by the way members communicate with each other. Depending on the family's cultural orientation, the avoidance of eye contact, excessive agreement or disagreement, and individuals' interrupting each other, changing the topic, silencing some members, and being sarcastic may indicate a dysfunctional family. Conversations often are dominated by vague, confusing, unempathic, negative, critical, and mixed messages.

The family's method of role allocation and handling of role relationships are considered under the sociocultural dimension, as well as the family's cultural norms. Cues of dysfunction include parent-child role reversals, role deficiencies, disengagement, enmeshment, and rigid role assignments. These behaviors are demonstrated by inappropriate role expectations; that is, they do not correspond to the individual's age, developmental phase, and capabilities.

Enmeshment and disengagement are two extremes of the range of family interaction patterns. *Enmeshment* refers to a pattern in which the sharing among the members of the system is extreme and intense. Individuality and independence are viewed negatively. An example of enmeshment occurred in a family that reacted to the 14-year-old daughter's request to see a movie with two friends in school by telling her what a "bad girl" she was for wanting to do something away from the family and then punishing her by giving her extra housework to do. At the other extreme is *disengagement*. In this pattern, rigid, impermeable boundaries separate the members of the system. Thus interactions among the individuals within the family seem to lack response and connection. A sense of abandonment pervades the system as communication among the members is discouraged. An example of disengagement is the case of a 10-year-old who brings home a report card that none of the family members review.

Neither pattern promotes interdependence: "the close relationships of people that involve the willingness and ability to love, respect, and value others, and to accept and respond to love, respect, and value given by others" (Hanson, 1984, p. 306).

Two specific role patterns frequently observed in dysfunctional families are scapegoating and enabling, both of which develop unconsciously within the system.

Scapegoating occurs when one member bears the blame for the problems confronting the family. Frequently, a child or a member with a chronic health problem falls into this role. This person then unconsciously acts out the family's conflict by developing a problem or symptoms of a physical, psychological, or social nature. The other members of the system unite to focus on the scapegoat's situation. They further express their frustration and anger toward this person for causing the family problems.

According to Murray Bowen (Friedman, 1985), scapegoating can even account for the reason that the health status of one family member changes and that of the others in a family does not. A family member can have all the physical prerequisites for a disease, including the promoting agent (e.g., bacterium, virus, or carcinogen), but the symptoms may not occur until some of the emotional conditions (prerequisites) in that family were satisfied. Conversely, a person who assumes particular family roles, on being subjected to certain triggering emotional, contextual, or physical factors, would be particularly at risk for illness. All this strongly suggests that the way persons think about themselves and their family relationships can minimize the risk of becoming sick and, if illness occurs, can maximize the possibility of recovery.

Enabling is defined as any conscious or unconscious behavior that encourages an individual to continue acting in a specific manner primarily by shielding the person from the consequences of the behavior. An example of enabling is the wife who calls her husband's boss to explain that her husband is too ill to work when in reality he has a hangover. In effect, the wife is saving her husband from the consequences of his behavior, rewarding him, and thus encouraging him to continue the pattern.

Developmental Variables

In assessing developmental variables, the nurse observes the family for its knowledge of both individual and family developmental tasks (see Chapter 13). Among the variables that cause dysfunctional behaviors within a family is insufficient knowledge of the different phases of growth and development. Frequently, this causes parents to have unrealistic expectations of their children, for example, a mother who believes her 13-month-old daughter should be toilet trained.

In dysfunctional families the nurse may observe high levels of regression in individual members and in the system itself. Frequently, this behavior occurs because those involved are so overwhelmed by a stressor that they believe they cannot resolve the situation.

Stressors

According to Betty Neuman (1983) the family system faces many stressors throughout its life. Stressors are forces that produce a reaction from the system, which tends to create instability within it. Stressors can affect an organism either negatively or positively. Neuman emphasizes that the manner in which the family reacts to the stressor depends on its subjective perception of the problem. Further, the family's potential for change as it reacts to stressors is contingent on its previous coping patterns, especially the rigid use of defensive patterns such as the denial or the rejection of help from others. However, the reality is that a family who can cope with a stressor shows adaptive facility, that is, the ability to change.

Neuman identifies three types of stressors: intrafamily, interfamily, and extrafamily. Intrafamily (that is, within the unit itself) stressors include the allocation of roles and conflict among the members. An important intrafamily reaction occurs because "family stressors usually require some changes in role function. The change process itself may become a stressor" (Neuman, 1983, p. 247).

Interfamily stressors develop as the family interacts with other systems in the environment that directly influence the family, such as schools, health-care agencies, or the workplace. The nurse, in initiating a relationship with a family, also becomes an interfamily stressor.

Extrafamily stressors occur as the family is influenced indirectly by political, social, and cultural issues. This type of stressor includes limited housing resources, political decisions that restrict the minimum wage and cut back health-care funding, and cultural stigmas that perpetuate the myths of hopefulness and helplessness of individuals who experience problems related to alcoholism or mental illness. The nurse needs to be aware that all these forces may be at work and that the effects of these stressors require continual assessment as the nurse cares for the family.

Influence of lines of defense and lines of resistance. All these previously described behaviors and cues result in a weakening of the family's flexible and normal lines of defense and flexible line of resistance (see Chapter 3 for a review of these terms). Thus the flexible line of defense is unable to change as needed to respond to the everyday stressors of life. In effect, it will no longer provide a buffer zone to screen out the pressures from these problems.

Because the flexible line of defense is not functioning effectively, the family's normal line of defense is under constant pressure to help it address the immediate pressures of daily existence. The result is that the family's normal level of adaptation, or state of wellness, becomes relatively low.

Finally, the flexible line of resistance is under constant attack as it tries to protect the family's basic energy resources. As demonstrated by the variables already described, this line becomes rigid. Thus the sense of interdependence within the family is limited as members are unable to rely on one another.

The weaknesses of these protective lines result in the family's increased susceptibility to the threat of stressors. The thrust and penetration ability of even weaker stressors becomes relatively strong as the family's resistance level and its ability to change are lowered. At this point "death of the family is imminent" (Reed, 1982, pp. 192-193) as it attempts to prevent the stressors from destroying its limited energy resources and integrity as a unit.

NURSING DIAGNOSIS

After assessing the family system, the nurse formulates the nursing diagnoses that provide the focus for planning and evaluating care. If a family system is determined to be dysfunctional, the nurse identifies the stressors—intrapersonal, interpersonal, and/or extrapersonal—that are confronting the unit and creating the dysfunction. Possible nursing diagnoses include the following:

- Ineffective family coping related to substance abuse
- Ineffective family coping related to family violence
- Ineffective family coping related to hopelessness

PLANNING AND INTERVENTION

After formulating the nursing diagnoses the nurse and family establish the goals for intervention and the plan of intervention. The nurse attempts to capitalize on the strengths of the system that were identified during the assessment.

Engaging the family in care. In planning care for dysfunctional families within Neuman's theoretical framework, the nurse primarily uses the secondary and tertiary prevention/intervention strategies. Thus the overall goals of nursing intervention will be to "attain/maintain [a] maximum wellness level" (Neuman, 1983, p. 249). This is accomplished by supporting the internal and external resources of the system to strengthen the family's flexible and normal lines of defense and line of resistance. The result is strengthening the family's abilities to withstand the threats of stressors in the future in an adaptive manner.

The nurse, however, does not employ these terms when meeting with the members to establish the goals. Instead, the nurse uses nontechnical language to emphasize the family's ability to confront its problems so that it may experience a healthier future.

Capitalizing on strengths of the family system. The nurse continues to encourage the family to capitalize on its strengths. Frequently the family is so overwhelmed by the stressors it is facing that it is unable to recognize any assets or even the potential for change. It is important that the nurse emphasize the family's ability to attempt to carry on despite difficult circumstances (Fleishman, Home, & Arthur 1983).

Weitzman (1985) stressed the deep level of loyalty that tends to exist within families. Consequently, the nurse should move slowly, at the family's pace, and not expect to accomplish major changes quickly. The nurse must especially be sensitive to the fact that "unlike the stable family, the severely disturbed family is heavily invested in its own stabilization, often resorting to old dysfunctional patterns with increased vigor, especially when threatened by imminent breakdown. It can tolerate a challenge to its rules only slowly and with thought-out consequences for the family" (Weitzman, 1985, p. 476).

The nurse must acknowledge that these families are interested primarily in regaining a sense of stability by returning to their previous level of wellness.

Empathizing with the family's predicament. The nurse initially empathizes with the family's difficulties, acknowledges past efforts to gain help, and attempts to reduce the level of conflict among family members. The nurse must maintain a balance between accurately recognizing the gravity of the problems that confront the family and maintaining the belief that there is hope and help for the system.

To accomplish these objectives the nurse initially can assume an authority position within the unit, taking the role of a warm and concerned, yet controlling, person who can meet the adults' needs for support and direction (Hallowitz, 1980).

Encouragement of realistic goal setting. In establishing goals the nurse should discuss with family members how each would like the situation within the family to be different (McKinney, 1976). The nurse should encourage the members to be realistic but also to identify some solutions to their problems.

It is imperative that the nurse focus the discussion on current, here-and-now problems so that the family does not become overwhelmed by past problems and interpersonal conflicts. The nurse also encourages members to express the anger, hostility, and frustration they are feeling while avoiding the ventilation of numerous grievances against each other, such as constant complaints by parents about their children. These accusations lead only to increased tension in the family and may cause it to reject the nurse's help because of the resultant discomfort. Instead the nurse should listen to the complaints one time, elicit the individual's feelings regarding them, and then focus the family's attention on what can be done to improve the situation, at least minimally (Fleishman et al., 1983).

Encouragement of the acceptance of three primary rules. In meeting with the family the nurse should encourage the acceptance of three primary rules. First, everyone present has an opportunity to speak and to participate. Second, only one individual speaks at a time. Thus, while one is speaking, all others should be listening and focusing their attention on what is being said (Fleishman et al., 1983). Third, individuals will not be "permitted to attack one another (verbally or otherwise), be overly critical, disruptive or punitive" (Weitzman, 1985, p. 480).

Relabeling all members of the system as victims. Being part of a dysfunctional family means that an individual experiences intense anger and a feeling of hurt. Frequently one member is blamed for the family's problems and failures. It is important that the nurse avoid perpetuating this belief. To counteract this phenonmenon the nurse attempts to redefine the problem as one that affects the whole family and every person within it. "This is best done by focusing on how each person is, in fact a 'victim' of the problem" (Fleishman et al., 1983, p. 27).

IMPLEMENTATION

Considering the principles already presented, the nurse then works with the family to develop realistic plans of care related to the family's priority nursing diagnoses. Three suggested plans are offered here.

Ineffective Family Coping Related to Substance Abuse

When the nursing diagnosis of ineffective family coping related to substance abuse has been formulated, the nurse and the family members work toward achieving the goals of avoiding substance abuse and developing more adaptive coping mechanisms. The plan of care might include some of the following nurse-centered interventions (Neuman, 1988).

Primary prevention

1. Recognize the reality that substance abuse may be a threat to the stability of the family and plan how the family may attempt to prevent the invasion of this stressor.
2. Use stress as a positive intervention strategy by encouraging the family to view stress as a challenge it can meet. Empathize with how difficult this may be in light of the family's other stressors.
3. Educate members regarding the effects of various substances such as alcohol, diazepam (Valium), cocaine, and marijuana. Discuss terms such as *physical* and *psychological dependencies,* as well as *tolerance* and *cross-tolerance*.
4. Support the efforts of members toward positive coping and functioning.

Secondary prevention

1. Recognize the extent of invasion of the family system by substance abuse, especially the phenomena of psychological and physical dependencies.
2. Mobilize and optimize the family's resources and energy by focusing on the reality that substance abuse is a problem that can be overcome.
3. Encourage the family members to observe within themselves the signs of enabling,

denying, and minimizing. Encourage the family to confront the reality of this stressor (substance abuse) directly, and emphasize that avoidance will compound the severity of its impact.

4. Motivate the family to seek treatment for this problem with education regarding the fact that substance abuse affects every member of the family and that the sooner treatment is sought, the weaker these effects will be.

5. Facilitate the seeking of appropriate treatment. If physical dependence is present, the individual should be referred to a detoxification unit. Once withdrawal from the physical effects of the drug and/or alcohol has occurred, participation in a rehabilitation program is helpful. This program should include educational sessions, along with individual, group, and family psychotherapy. During the rehabilitation program the persons who have been abusing the substances should begin attending self-help support groups such as Alcoholics Anonymous, Narcotics Anonymous, or Women for Sobriety. After discharge from the program, active and frequent participation in the therapeutic work of these support groups is necessary to maintain sobriety. Attending meetings daily during the first year of sobriety is recommended. Family members also should attend similar meetings of groups such as Al-Anon, Al-Ateen, and Adult Children of Alcoholics.

6. Support the family's efforts toward health by empathizing with the difficulty of recovery and the need for a day-by-day commitment. Help the members focus on the here and now instead of the future.

Tertiary prevention

1. Coordinate the family's efforts to seek and follow through on treatment for substance abuse as already explained.

2. Support the family's efforts to cope with family members' relapses as they try to maintain sobriety.

3. Educate family members regarding adaptive coping mechanisms, such as sublimation, to deal with stressors that attempt to invade the flexible line of defense of both the individual and the family system.

4. Educate regarding the effects of substance abuse.

Ineffective Family Coping Related to Family Violence

When the nursing diagnosis of ineffective family coping related to family violence has been selected, the nurse and family members work toward achieving the goals of avoiding violence as a means of coping with stressors and developing more adaptive coping mechanisms. The plan of care might include some of the following interventions (Neuman, 1988).

Primary prevention

1. Classify violence as a stressor that may threaten a family's stability.

2. Educate the family regarding the dynamics of anger, frustration, aggression, hostility, and violence. Empathize with members' feelings that "it's difficult to cope when you reach your breaking point."

3. Support the members' efforts to develop adaptive methods of coping with anger and frustration, especially sublimation.

4. Provide information to the parents on how to discipline their children in nonviolent ways, such as the withdrawal of privileges or time-out periods.

5. Educate the parents regarding the stages of child development so that they become

PRIMARY PREVENTION OF FAMILY VIOLENCE THROUGH POLICY CHANGES

1. Eliminate the norms that legitimize and glorify violence in the society and family. The elimination of spanking as a child rearing technique, gun control to get deadly weapons out of the home, elimination of corporal punishment in school and the death penalty, and an elimination of media violence which glorifies and legitimizes violence are all necessary steps. In short, we need to cancel the hitting license in society.
2. Reduce violence-provoking stress created by society. Reducing poverty, inequality, unemployment and providing for adequate housing, feeding, medical and dental care, and educational opportunities are steps which could reduce stress in families.
3. Integrate families into a network of kin and community. Reducing social isolation would be a significant step that would help reduce stress and increase the abilities of families to manage stress.
4. Change the sexist character of society. Sexual inequality, perhaps more than economic inequality, makes violence possible in homes. The elimination of men's work and women's work would be a major step toward equality in and out of the home.
5. Break the cycle of violence in the family. This step repeats the message of step 1— violence cannot be prevented as long as we are taught that it is appropriate to hit the people we love. Physical punishment of children is perhaps the most effective means of teaching violence, and eliminating it would be an important step in violence prevention.

From *Intimate violence in families* (p. 144) by R. Gelles and C. Cornell, 1983, Beverly Hills, CA Sage. Copyright 1983 by Sage Publications. Reprinted by permission.

aware of the normal characteristics of a maturing individual. Teach the use of reinforcement of positive behaviors as a parenting technique.

6. Educate the parents regarding the importance of their having time alone together, without the children or older family members, so that their relationship may be sustained.
7. Support each member's attempts to build a positive sense of self-esteem. Emphasize each person's ability to continue trying to cope, despite overwhelming stressors.
8. Encourage the family to build support systems through interactions with other families and significant others.
9. In addition to working with families, the nurse should become politically active to bring about social changes to reduce violence (see box).

Secondary prevention

1. After the invasion of the family by the stressor of violence, protect the system's basic structure by recognizing the existence of family violence as early as possible.
2. Use the theories and skills of crisis intervention to help the family members confront the reality of the abusive situation.
3. Depending on the legal implications of the nature of the violence, if warranted report the incidence of abuse to the proper authorities. Each state requires that nurses report suspected child abuse or neglect: physical abuse, emotional abuse, some forms of physical neglect, and sexual abuse. Failure to report results in specific penalties (Munro, 1984).

The nurse should include the following information in a report to the authorities (Rhodes, 1987):

- Name and address of child

- Name and address of parent or caretaker
- Age and present location of child
- Nature and extent of injuries
- Any evidence of previous injuries such as scars or healing bruises
- Name, age, and condition of other children in the home
- Parent's or caretaker's description of injury
- Person responsible for injury (if known) or name of person caring for the child at the time of the injury
- Statement summarizing why child abuse is suspected
- Any other information that may be helpful in establishing the cause of the injury or that will provide assistance to the child

Currently nurses are mandated by law to report only incidences of suspected child abuse. Situations that involve the abuse of adults, such as spouse or elder abuse, are not covered under these laws. Wide variations exist concerning how the legal system addresses these episodes of adult violence.

The health care and legal systems view family violence from two widely different philosophies, control versus compassion (Gelles & Cornell, 1985). The compassionate view is that the abusive parents are also victims themselves. Thus intervention involves the support of both abuser and family by providing homemaker services, health and child care, and other supports. The opposite view, that of control, involves aggressive intervention, including the punishment of violent behaviors. The abuser is considered fully responsible, and consequences include removal of the child from the home, separation of the abused wife from her violent spouse, and full criminal prosecution of the offender.

Problems are inherent in each approach. One recommendation combines both: the use of control in assessment and compassion in treatment (Gelles & Cornell, 1985).

This dilemma confronts the nurse who suspects family violence. It is imperative, however, that the nurse first follow the mandates of the state and then work to coordinate the treatment plan that is established for the family.

4. If the abuse involves adults, support the victim's efforts to deal with the situation.
5. Facilitate appropriate intervention for all family members. The abuser especially will benefit from individual and group psychotherapy to learn adaptive methods of handling frustration and to develop a higher level of self-esteem (Swift, 1986). Refer victims to group-support programs that will help them to realize that they did not deserve the abuse and also to increase their levels of self-esteem. Encourage other family members to attend meetings of self-help support groups to help them recognize how they have been affected by the violence within their homes.
6. Refer the family members to Parents Anonymous. One study (Hunka, O'Toole, & O'Toole, 1985) analyzed the functioning of one of these support groups to identify how the group process effected change. The authors concluded that

> the group becomes a surrogate family through the process of identification and emotional bonding. Veteran members resocialize a new member ... to learn new ways of coping with their psychological problems, their feelings toward the child, and means to handle the crisis. At the same time, they learn to identify and relinquish old, maladaptive behavior. ... Emotional bonding in PA also tends to increase the abusive parent's self-esteem (p. 29).

Tertiary prevention

1. During reconstruction of the family's stability and health, acknowledge the need to break the vicious cycle of intergenerational family violence.

2. Support the members' efforts to deal with stressors in nonviolent manners.
3. Acknowledge the reality that relapses may occur and should be discussed immediately.
4. Encourage the members to continue to participate in the activities of self-help support groups such as Parents Anonymous.
5. If the violence has led to the break-up of the family, support the members' efforts to start a new life.

Ineffective Family Coping Related to Hopelessness

When the nursing diagnosis of ineffective family coping related to hopelessness has been selected, the nurse and family members work toward fulfilling the goals of gaining a sense of hope for the future and developing more adaptive coping mechanisms. The plan of care might include some of the following nurse-centered interventions (Neuman, 1988).

Primary prevention

1. Classify hopelessness as a stressor that may be a threat to the family's stability, and prevent the invasion of this stressor. NANDA defined hopelessness as a "subjective state in which an individual sees limited or no alternatives or personal choices available and is unable to mobilize energy on own behalf" (Bruss, 1988, p. 28).
2. Provide information to the family regarding its existing strengths as a basis for facing problems that seem overwhelming.
3. Emphasize the positive value of stress as a challenge rather than a threat.

Secondary prevention

1. Protect the basic structure of the family by recognizing hopelessness as an invader as soon as possible (Bruss, 1988). Verbal cues of hopelessness are considered to be most significant.
2. Optimize the resources of the family toward stability and energy conservation by encouraging it to find "clues which substantiate hope, [feel it] has something to anticipate, and [discover] a sustaining supernatural love" (Miller, 1983, p. 297).
3. Educate the family members to develop the coping skill of maximizing experiences, that is, to appreciate to the fullest extent even the smallest positive event (Miller, 1983). The box below lists activities the nurse can suggest to help clients achieve a state of hopefulness.

ACTIVITIES OF DAILY LIVING THAT MAY HELP MAXIMIZE HOPEFUL EXPERIENCES

- Savor the richness of coffee in the morning.
- Note the crystal-clear blue sky.
- Feel the warmth of a sunbeam.
- Watch activities of animals in a tree outside a window.
- Share children's experiences.
- Note loving characteristics of a significant other.
- Appreciate expressions of caring concern.
- Build highlights into each day, such as meals, visits, inspirational reading.
- Study a favorite photograph or painting.
- Listen to a favorite song or symphony on the radio.

From *Coping with chronic illness* (p. 293) by J. Miller, 1983, Philadelphia: Davis. Copyright 1983 by F. A. Davis Co. Modified by permission.

---

4. Empathize with the client's frustration and fatigue in feeling that everything appears hopeless and how difficult it is to attempt to change this feeling.

Tertiary prevention

1. Support the family's efforts to sustain a sense of hope while recognizing that relapses will occur.
2. Acknowledge the difficulty of sustaining hope, and educate the family in coping with the difficulties.

EVALUATION

The nurse evaluates the effectiveness of nursing intervention for dysfunctional families by analyzing whether changes have occurred within the system. Positive outcomes are reflected in the strengthening of the unit's flexible line of defense, which enables it to respond in a more adaptive manner to the everyday stressors of life. In effect, these families then have a more effective buffer from stressors. In terms of the nursing diagnoses discussed in the previous section, family members might maintain sobriety, react adaptively to feelings of anger and frustration, or maintain a sense of hope even in the face of problems.

Cues of the reactions of the family's normal line of defense also are evaluated. Although realistically this line would be strengthened by the nursing intervention, it probably will be functioning at a relatively low level because of the overwhelming odds facing the dysfunctional family compared with a healthy family.

The system's flexible line of resistance also will be strengthened by the intervention, which will allow the family greater interdependence and an increased ability to adapt to change.

In evaluating the effectiveness of the nursing intervention, the nurse should observe for small markers of progress and recognize that they are positive signs of the family's advancement toward health.

The following case study highlights some of the important components of the nursing process applied to a dysfunctional family.

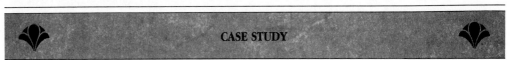

CASE STUDY

Margaret T is a married, 32-year-old mother of three. She has been discharged from the hospital against medical advice after a 3-day stay with a medical diagnosis of diabetes mellitus and a compound fracture of the left proximal humerus (upper portion of the arm). She had initially gone to the emergency room of the hospital for treatment of her "broken arm" after a "fall down the basement stairs." During her examination the physician determined that she also was experiencing symptoms of diabetes mellitus. She was admitted to the hospital for further tests that confirmed that diagnosis. Her left arm has been immobilized in a sling, and she has been referred for physical therapy twice a week.

During her stay the nurse who specialized in diabetes education taught Margaret how to administer insulin injections and modify her diet. The nurse observed that Margaret appeared depressed and sullen, avoided eye contact, and answered all questions with one or two words. The nurse also noted that Margaret had not had any visitors during her stay. The nurse decided that home care follow-up was indicated because Margaret seemed vague and insecure about her condition even though she verbalized a complete understanding of her diet and was able to administer her injections safely. The visit was planned for the day after discharge.

During the first home visit the nurse found that Margaret had given herself the injection but had not eaten because "there was no food in the house." She explained, "My husband didn't have time to shop while I was in the hospital." The nurse also observed that the house appeared cluttered but was relatively clean. A case of empty beer bottles was sitting on the counter.

Margaret appeared very tense and agitated. She told the nurse, "Let's get this over with fast before my husband wakes up. He'll be upset if he sees a stranger here. I wish you'd just leave me alone. I'll be fine. As soon as my 8-year-old daughter gets home from school, she'll go shopping for me."

The nurse empathized with Margaret's feelings and then emphasized the importance of eating scheduled meals and following the prescribed menu. Margaret then began crying and said, "I can't believe this has happened to me. I've never been sick before. How am I going to handle my kids? They're driving me crazy. Besides, I have to get back to work because my husband isn't working now."

The nurse asked Margaret if she could look for something she could make her for breakfast. Margaret hesitantly agreed. While the nurse prepared oatmeal, she encouraged Margaret to talk about her family.

Margaret smiled as she mentioned her 8-year-old daughter and said, "She's my biggest help. She cleans the house when I don't have the time and looks after my other two kids." Her other children are a 6-year-old son and a 5-year-old daughter. Margaret sounded angry when she mentioned her son, saying, "He never listens to me." She added, "I don't know how much more of him I can take. Even spanking him with the belt doesn't make him behave."

The nurse noted that Margaret never mentioned her husband. So she said, "Tell me about your husband." Margaret averted her eyes and looked fearful. She whispered, "He's asleep now. He had a very bad night."

The nurse followed up by focusing on the husband's use of alcohol and specifically asked if her husband was the cause of her arm injury. Margaret answered that he had thrown her down the stairs when he was drunk. She added, "I know he didn't mean it. He's a wonderful husband and father when he isn't drunk. We just have to act better so he'll love us enough to stop drinking."

The nurse explained that his alcohol abuse was not due to the behavior of Margaret and her children. She also emphasized that Margaret was going to have to have help if she was going to regain her physical health. She gave Margaret the name of a local priest whose parish supplied groceries to families in need. The nurse also gave Margaret the number of Parents Anonymous, adding, "If you feel like talking to someone when you feel like exploding at your son, call this number any time, day or night." The nurse encouraged Margaret to consider attending Al-Anon meetings as soon as she felt better. The nurse also arranged for home visits three times a week for 2 weeks to help Margaret adapt to her new diet and medication regimen. Margaret tentatively agreed.

At the completion of the first visit, the nurse completed a family assessment guide (see Chapter 13) and formulated the following list of priority nursing diagnoses:

- Lack of knowledge and financial resources related to following regimen for diabetes
- Ineffective family coping related to alcohol abuse
- Potential ineffective family coping related to wife and child abuse

When the nurse visited again the next morning, Margaret appeared calmer and more rested. She had given herself an injection and had eaten breakfast made with food donated by the local parish. Margaret explained that her husband had become very angry when the food had been delivered, had left the house, and had not returned. The nurse empathized with the difficulty of Margaret's situation and then emphasized that help was available. The nurse then began to formulate a plan of care for Margaret and her family as shown in Table 15-4.

TABLE 15-4   Nursing care plan for Margaret T and her family

Assessment	Nursing diagnosis	Plan/intervention	Evaluation
Physical	Lack of knowledge and financial resources related to following diabetic regimen	Identify knowledge of self-care regarding diabetes mellitus; encourage call to welfare for help with food stamps and medical supplies.	Client will verbalize principles of self-care and will secure funds for needed food and supplies.
Behavioral patterns	Ineffective family coping related to alcohol abuse	Implement plan of secondary intervention as discussed above.	Family members will avoid use of alcohol.
Social system	Potential ineffective family coping related to wife and child abuse	Implement plan of secondary intervention as discussed above.	Family members will avoid use of violence to express feelings.

SUMMARY

Caring for a dysfunctional family is a challenge for community health nurses. It requires nurses to confront their own feelings and thoughts regarding parenting, violence, frustration, and substance abuse. It also requires nurses to have patience, determination, and an ability to move at the family's pace. In addition, it requires nurses to seek help to resolve their feelings of frustration, hopelessness, and uselessness as these emotions arise during their relationships with these families. Nurses may find support through meetings with their peers or supervisors.

Community health nurses must act as advocates for all citizens by working with lay and professional groups in primary prevention programs to alleviate many of the problems that confront dysfunctional families. These include policy changes to decrease the incidence of violence within society. Nurses need to become involved in the promotion of these changes.

Community health nurses need to recognize that their care for these families will result in helping the families overcome their dysfunctional behaviors and ultimately will improve the level of wellness of the community at large by making it a safer place for all residents.

CHAPTER HIGHLIGHTS

- Dysfunctional families are those that experience severe levels of anxiety and often perceive a crisis as an overwhelming burden. Other characteristics include a tendency to encourage dependency and learned helplessness and to be suspicious of outsiders.
- Dysfunctional behaviors within a family include alcoholism, drug abuse, violence, hostility, overly rigid spiritual beliefs, and unrealistic expectations of other family members.
- The nurse must be aware of his or her own attitudes toward a dysfunctional family and not let these attitudes affect the care given.

- Enmeshment is a dysfunctional interaction pattern in which sharing among family members is extreme and individuality is viewed negatively.
- Disengagement is a pattern in which family interactions seem unresponsive and unconnected.
- Scapegoating occurs when one family member is blamed for the family's problems.
- Enabling is behavior by one family member that encourages another family member to act in a dysfunctional manner.
- Stressors that affect a family may be intrafamily, interfamily, and extrafamily stressors.
- In a dysfunctional family the flexible line of defense is not functioning effectively, which places constant pressure on the family's normal line of defense.
- The NANDA-approved nursing diagnosis that describes dysfunctional families is ineffective family coping.
- In formulating a care plan, the nurse should engage the family in care, capitalize on the strengths of the family system, empathize with the family's predicament, encourage realistic goal setting, allow all members to participate in discussions, and view all members as victims.
- The nurse uses primary, secondary, and tertiary prevention in implementing the plan of care.
- The nurse should become involved politically and socially to decrease the stressors that cause dysfunctional behaviors in families.

STUDY QUESTIONS

1. Describe three behaviors that may occur in dysfunctional families.
2. Discuss the influence of substance abuse in precipitating family violence.
3. Describe the role of the nurse in a suspected case of child abuse.
4. Using the nursing process, write a care plan for a family with a nursing diagnosis of ineffective coping related to family violence.

REFERENCES

Amundson, M. J. (1989). Family crisis care: A home-based intervention program for child abuse. *Issues in Mental Health Nursing, 10*, 285-296.

Anderson, L., and Thobaben, M. (1984). Clients in crisis: When should the nurse step in? *Journal of Gerontological Nursing, 10*(12), 6-10.

Bruss, C. (1988). Nursing diagnosis of hopelessness. *Journal of Psychosocial Nursing, 26*(3), 28-31.

Campbell, J. (1984). Abuse of female partners. In J. Campbell and J. Humphreys (Eds.), *Nursing care of victims of family violence* (pp. 74-118). Reston, VA: Reston.

Campbell, J. (1984). Nursing care of families using violence. In J. Campbell and J. Humphreys (Eds.), *Nursing care of victims of family violence* (pp. 216-245). Reston, VA: Reston.

Campbell, J. (1984). Theories of violence. In J. Campbell and J. Humphreys (Eds.), *Nursing care of victims of family violence* (pp. 13-52). Reston, VA: Reston.

Carpenito, L. (1989). *Nursing diagnosis—Application to clinical practice.* Philadelphia: Lippincott.

Carson, R., Butcher, J., and Coleman, J. (1988). *Abnormal psychology and modern life.* Boston: Scott, Foresman and Co.

Feigenbaum, J. (1986). Utilizing the nursing process with patients who abuse drugs and alcohol. In M. Mathewson (Ed.), *Pharmacotherapeutics: A nursing process approach* (pp. 119-136). Philadelphia: Davis.

Fleischman, M., Home, A., and Arthur, J. (1983). *Troubled families: A treatment approach.* Champaign, IL: Research Press Co.

Flynn, J. (1977). Recent findings related to wife abuse. *Social Casework, 58,* 13-21.

Foley, T., and Grimes, B. (1987). Nursing intervention in family abuse and violence. In G. Stuart and S. Sundeen (Eds.), *Principles and practices of psychiatric nursing* (pp. 925-970). St. Louis: Mosby.

Friedman, E. H. (1985). *Generation to generation.* New York: Guilford Press.

Fulmer, T., and Cahill, V. (1984). Assessing elder abuse:

A study. *Journal of Gerontological Nursing, 10*(12), 16-20.

Gelles, R., and Cornell, C. (1985). *Intimate violence in families*. Beverly Hills, CA: Sage.

Hallowitz, D. (1980). The problem-solving component in family therapy. In C. Munson (Ed.), *Social work with families: Theory and practice* (pp. 228-239). New York: The Free Press.

Hanson, J. (1984). The family. In C. Roy (Ed.), *Introduction to nursing: An adaptation model* (pp. 519-533). Englewood Cliffs, NJ: Prentice-Hall.

Humphreys, J., and Campbell, J. (1984). Introduction: Nursing and family violence. In J. Campbell and J. Humphreys (Eds.), *Nursing care of victims of family violence* (pp. 1-12). Reston, VA: Reston.

Hunka, C., O'Toole, A., and O'Toole, R. (1985). Self-help therapy in Parents Anonymous. *Journal of Psychosocial Nursing, 23*(7), 24-31.

Kelley, S. (1985). Interviewing the sexually abused child: Principles and techniques. *Journal of Emergency Nursing, 11,* 234-241.

Kneisl, C. and Petit, M. (1988). Applying the nursing process with families. In H. Wilson and C. Kneisl (Eds.), *Psychiatric nursing* (pp. 890-915). Menlo Park, CA: Addison-Wesley.

Leavitt, Maribelle. (1982). *Families at risk*. Boston: Little, Brown and Co.

Levinson, D. (1988). Family violence in cross-cultural perspective. In V. Van Hasselt et al. (Eds.), *Handbook of family violence* (pp. 435-456). New York, Plenum Press.

Limandri, B. (1987). The therapeutic relationship with abused women. *Journal of Psychosocial Nursing, 25*(2), 8-16.

McKinney, G. (1976). Adapting family therapy to multideficit families. In F. J. Turner (Ed.), *Differential diagnosis and therapy in social work* (pp. 109-118). New York: The Free Press.

Meister, S. (1984). Family well-being. In J. Campbell and J. Humphreys (Eds.), *Nursing care of victims of family violence* (pp. 53-73). Reston, VA: Reston.

Miller, J. (1983). Inspiring hope. In J. Miller (Ed.), *Coping with chronic illness: Overcoming powerlessness* (pp. 287-299). Philadelphia: Davis.

Millor, G. (1981). A theoretical framework for nursing research in child abuse and neglect. *Nursing Research, 30*(2), 78-83.

Munro, J. (1984). The nurse and the legal system: Dealing with abused children. In J. Campbell and J. Humphreys (Eds.), *Nursing care of victims of family violence* (pp. 384-402). Reston, VA: Reston.

Nelsen, J. (1983). *Family therapy—An integrative approach*. Englewood Cliffs, NJ: Prentice-Hall.

Neuman, B. (1983). Family intervention using the Betty Neuman health-care systems model. In I. Clements and F. Roberts (Eds.), *Family health: A theoretical approach to nursing care* (pp. 239-254). New York: Wiley.

Neuman, B. (1988, August 23). *The Neuman systems model workshop*. Paper presented at the Nursing Theory Congress, Toronto, Ontario.

Reed, K. (1982). The Neuman systems model: A basis for family psychosocial assessment and intervention. In B. Neuman (Ed.), *The Neuman systems model: application to nursing education and practice* (pp. 188-195). East Norwalk, CT: Appleton-Century-Crofts.

Rhodes, A. (1987). Identifying and reporting child abuse. *Maternal-Child Nursing Journal, 12*(6), 399.

Shealy, A. (1988). Family therapy. In C. K. Beck, R. P. Rawlins, and S. Williams (Eds.), *Mental health—psychiatric nursing* (2nd ed.) (pp. 543-575). St. Louis: Mosby.

Swift, C. (1986). Preventing family violence: Family-focused programs. In M. Lystad (Ed.), *Violence in the home: Interdisciplinary perspectives* (pp. 219-249). New York: Brunner/Mazel.

Tilden, V. (1989). Response of the health care delivery system to battered women. *Issues in Mental Health Nursing, 10,* 309-320.

Tripp-Reimer, T. and Lively, S. (1988). Cultural considerations in therapy. In C. Beck, R. Rawlins, and S. Williams (Eds.), *Mental health—psychiatric nursing* (2nd ed.). St. Louis: Mosby.

Weitzman, J. (1985). Engaging the severely dysfunctional family in treatment: Basic considerations. *Family Process, 24,* 473-485.

Wilson, H. & Kneisl, C. (1988). *Psychiatric Nursing*. Menlo Park, CA: Addison-Wesley.

Home Health Care

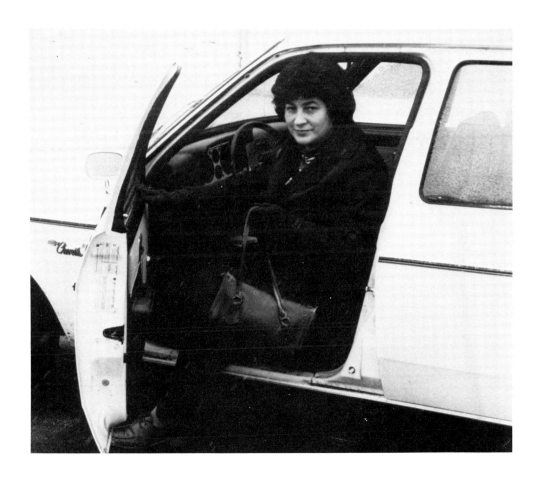

This unit focuses on the care of the client in the home. Demographical changes in client population, modern technology, and the increased cost of health care have altered the needs of the consumer and challenged the expertise and creativity of the nurse who plans and gives health care to the client in the home. This unit provides the student with a broad picture of contemporary home health care.

Chapter 16 describes what home care nursing is and identifies the professionals other than the nurse who practice in the home care setting. Various types of home care agencies and some sources of third-party payment are discussed.

Chapter 17 explains the role of the nurse as discharge planner and home care co-ordinator within the health care system.

Chapter 18 introduces the concept of modern technology and its use in the home. Selected therapies that nurses administer in the home, client eligibility for these services, and some of the legal issues involved are clarified.

Chapter 19 discusses the expanded role of the nurse in caring for the chronically ill client. Definitions of chronicity are presented, and the concept of trajectory as applied to chronic illness is explained. Several case studies are included.

Home Health Service Agencies

JOAN M. COOKFAIR

*Much that now strikes us as incomprehensible would be far less so
if we took a look at the racing rate of change that makes reality
seem, sometimes, like a kaleidoscope run wild.*

ALVIN TOFFLER

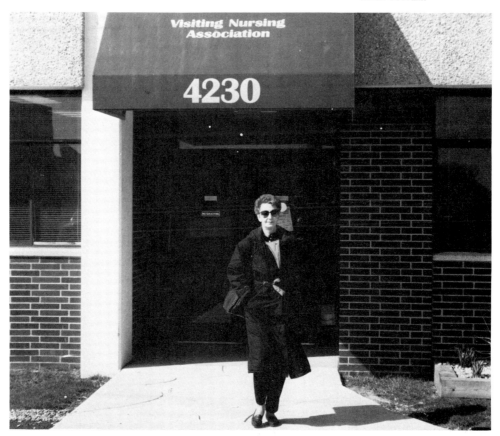

OBJECTIVES

At the conclusion of this chapter the student will be able to:
1. Define the key terms listed
2. Describe what home care is
3. Identify the various disciplines involved in home care
4. Describe various home care provider agencies
5. Discuss the financing of home care services
6. Discuss future trends in home health care
7. Identify the role of the nurse in home care

KEY TERMS

Home health agency   Palliative care
Home health aide   Proprietary agency
Home health care   Reimbursement
Hospice   Skilled nursing
Official agencies   Visiting Nurse Association

The National Association for Home Care (NAHC) defines home care as "services for recovering, disabled, or chronically ill persons; providing treatment and/or effective functioning in the home environment" (Moore, 1988, p. 225). The NAHC represents the National Association of Home Health Agencies, the National League for Nursing's Council of Home Health Agencies, and Community Nursing Services. These organizations were merged in 1982 to form the NAHC (Moore, 1988).

The demands of the 1990s for cost containment, an aging population, and altered family patterns are bringing about a change in health care delivery systems and the types of clients who need home care. The changing economy and the altered roles of women in contemporary society have reduced the number of individuals available to assume the role of primary support persons in the home (Moore, 1988).

Home care in the future will have to include a combination of services such as the following:

1. Assisting clients to recover from acute illness
2. Providing care during exacerbations of chronic illness
3. Developing plans to maintain persons in the home who need ongoing care and supervision
4. Assisting families in the care of terminally ill clients who need palliative care

CLIENTS WHO REQUIRE HOME CARE
Acutely Ill Clients

In 1983 the need for cost containment in the institutional setting led to the Medicare prospective payment system in the United States. This in turn has precipitated the discharge of clients from the hospital when the allotted payment for the particular altered health state runs out rather than after a long recuperative period. At times clients are sent home directly from an intensive care unit. The result has been to increase the number of acutely ill clients who require the services of skilled professionals and paraprofessionals in their homes.

Mentally Ill Clients

Hospitals are more inclined to discharge mentally ill clients into the community whenever possible because they cannot justify reimbursement for maintenance care in the institutional setting under the prospective payment system. These individuals may need daily supervision to ensure proper medication, and they often require various forms of assistance to survive in society.

Clients With Acquired Immunodeficiency Syndrome

Some geographical areas such as New York City have experienced an influx of patients with acquired immunodeficiency syndrome (AIDS) who require highly specialized kinds of intervention in the home setting. Elsie Griffith, Chief Executive Officer of the Visiting Nurse Service of New York stated in 1988, "The city had predicted that we would receive five new AIDS cases a week; in reality we received five a day" (Griffith, 1988, p. 272).

An Aging Client Population

Demographical trends indicate an increasing number of elderly persons in the general population. On the basis of the U.S. Bureau of the Census statistics predictions, by the year 2030, 20% of the total population in the United States will be 65 years of age or older. The consequent implications in terms of long-term care related to health problems of the aging are described in Chapter 12.

PROFESSIONALS INVOLVED IN PLANNING HOME CARE
Nurses

Historically nursing care has been the foundation of home care (see Chapter 1). The nurse traditionally has collaborated with a physician and a specific agency to coordinate client care, with focus on the family unit. Teaching health promotion and maintenance in the home has been an inherent part of providing direct care to a sick client. Although nursing care remains the hub of the wheel in home-based care, changing reimbursement systems, different client populations, and altered family patterns have necessitated a reassessment of nursing care plans and health care delivery.

Physicians

Many clients are referred to home health care providers by physicians. It is the responsibility of the physician who makes a referral to communicate necessary information to other members of the health care team. In the United States federal regulations require that a physician certify plans of care for clients in the home before the client is eligible for Medicare third-party payment. Some private insurance companies have similar criteria.

Physical Therapists

Most home care agencies use physical therapists to evaluate neuromuscular and functional ability. Physical therapists, who emphasize restorative therapy, frequently are involved in home care when clients have difficulty in ambulation or mobility (Stewart, 1979).

Social Workers

Social workers were among the first professionals to join nurses in home-based care. They help clients with social, intellectual, and emotional factors that affect their well-being

(Stewart, 1979), they assist clients to contact available community resources, and they provide advocacy in a variety of ways. Some social workers are specifically trained in counseling techniques and health-related problems.

Speech Pathologists

Speech pathologists focus on restorative therapy. They treat clients with communication and swallowing problems related to speech, language, and hearing.

Nutritionists

Nutritionists join the interdisciplinary team both through direct diet counseling to clients and through staff consultations. They frequently are asked to assist in team conferences to prescribe a therapeutic diet for individual clients. Much of the nutritionist's role in the home involves consultation with nurses and other care providers to assist them in giving nutritional guidance to clients (Stewart, 1979).

Occupational Therapists

Occupational therapists concentrate on the restoration of small motor coordination. They frequently are involved in enabling cllients who have lost the use of their hands or the ability to coordinate finer body movements to function at their highest level of ability.

Home Health Aides

Home health aide is a specific term, which is used by Medicare reimbursement funding programs in the United States, to designate a paraprofessional who assists in the home with a client's personal care. Home health aides also may perform some light housekeeping duties. Their services are provided to clients only as long as skilled nursing services are needed in the home, and for Medicare reimbursement they must be supervised by a registered nurse.

Miscellaneous Providers

Many agencies in the private sector employ paraprofessional aides to care for clients in the home. Some families employ personal caregivers on a private basis, and these aides become part of the family unit for which the nurse is caring.

In addition to these professionals, many volunteer agencies and services are available to assist clients in the home, such as Meals on Wheels, Friendly Visitors, and transportation services. Their accessibility depends on the local community's ability to provide them.

Vendors of durable medical equipment provide families with items that can withstand repeated usage, such as hospital beds, walking aids, ventilators, IV equipment, and wheelchairs. DME vendors work with the family and the home care nurse to determine the support necessary for the client who is being maintained in the home (Haddad, 1987).

An increasingly complex competitive interdisciplinary system requires flexibility and collaboration on the part of the nurse. The role of the nurse is to remain client-family centered as a plan of care is coordinated. At times it may be necessary for the nurse to function as family advocate when many disciplines are involved in client care.

TYPES OF AGENCIES THAT PROVIDE HOME CARE
Official Agencies

Official agencies are governmentally operated. In the United States federal agencies are under the control of the Department of Health and Human Services. Many official state agencies act only in a supervisory capacity and leave direct provision of care to local county and city governments. Most official local agencies, which are publicly funded, provide home care, well-child clinics, disease prevention programs, and health education.

In Canada, the Ministry of Health cooperates with provincial and local governments to implement official health programs.

Private Agencies

Visiting Nurse Association. From the early 1900s until the present the Visiting Nurse Association (VNA) had provided a broader spectrum of care. It originally was founded to give care and health education to the sick poor, establishing prenatal classes, providing health care to school children, and conducting school visits (Keating & Kelmann, 1988). VNAs were nonprofit voluntary health organizations financed by charitable contributions and fees for service. They focused primarily on indigent populations. Each VNA is autonomous, with its own board of directors and dependence on the visiting nurse as its main health provider. In the 1960s, in the United States, the advent of Medicare and Medicaid spawned a number of competing agencies that offered services to the public on a fee-for-service basis. Many of these became Medicare-certified and received third-party payment. In order to survive, some VNAs became Medicare-certified and combined services with other agencies. Some, like the Chicago VNA, have had to alter their programs dramatically (see box).

The problems of the VNA in Chicago represent the plight of not-for-profit agencies across the country. No longer able to cope with the increased needs of indigent clients, the need to compete for clients who can pay, and the need to maintain standards dictated by the federal government—which may or may not apply to individual situations—the VNAs must find new ways to survive or place the burden for care of the indigent on official agencies.

THE CHICAGO STORY

In May of 1986 the VNA in Chicago severly limited its free care visits (free care was provided to clients who had no reimbursement source). The VNA at that time provided 47% of the free care in the city of Chicago. The 1986 restriction completely reversed its philosophy and mission statement, which was "to provide professional and supportive health care to people of all ages and income levels" (p. 435).

The VNA, founded in 1889, had a long history of providing health and social services to residents of Chicago, particularly the indigent. A nonprofit voluntary agency, it focused on a family-centered approach, combining technical services with health promotion and prevention. Funding was provided by charitable organizations, endowments, and, since 1965, Medicare and Medicaid.

The first factor that influenced the VNA decision to limit free care visits was the cutback in social services at the federal, state, and local levels. The second factor was the necessity to compete with proprietary organizations who were providing care only to those who could pay. In fact, from 1982 to 1986, proprietary agencies transferred many clients to the VNA when the clients ran out of reimbursement sources. Hospitals referred medically indigent recipients to the VNA while referring private insurance and Medicare clients to proprietary home health agencies. Cutbacks in social services on federal, state, and local levels increased the need for home health services to the medically indigent. Unfortunately, they were not reimbursable and the Chicago VNA faced extinction.

From "The demise of free care: The Visiting Nurse Association of Chicago," 1988, by K. Kilbane and B. Blacksin, *Nursing Clinics of North America* 23, pp. 435-442. Copyright 1988.

Private agencies may be either nonprofit or profit making. Private, nonprofit agencies are tax exempt and organized to assist in the delivery of health services. If they are not Medicare-certified (as VNAs are), they may be funded by such charitable organizations as the United Way. Meals on Wheels and the American Cancer Society are examples of nonprofit agencies funded by charitable organizations.

Independent Proprietary Agencies

Private agencies, which operate for profit, are not tax exempt and may or may not be Medicare-certified. They generally are referred to as *proprietary* agencies. As the name implies, their goal is to make a profit. They may receive third-party payment or be paid directly by the client. Some sell equipment for special treatments whereas others coordinate their services with vendors of such equipment. They do not stress health promotion or prevention, and they do not provide care to those who cannot pay or otherwise reimburse them. Many services are delivered through paraprofessionals and technical staff members under the supervision of a registered nurse. Proprietary agencies frequently contract out the services of their nonprofessional staff members to VNAs, hospitals, and health departments.

Hospital-Based Agencies

Hospital-based home health agencies are controlled administratively by a hospital. Service, policies, and standards of care are determined by the institution (Stewart, 1979). The hospital itself may be proprietary, nonprofit, voluntary, or official. Many hospitals have developed home-based programs to direct follow-up care and control its implementation. Although the prospective payment system requires hospitals to discharge clients early, they still are morally responsible and legally liable for the client's recovery. It became necessary to develop a referral system that was efficient and responsive to patients' needs, and existing agencies were not always able to assist them. The problem is illustrated by the following examples:

Example 1. A patient made a rapid recovery from abdominal surgery and wished to be discharged on a Friday afternoon. Placement of a drain made dressing changes necessary over the weekend. A call to existing home health agencies resulted in a request for a written referral and notification that personnel were unavailable until the following Monday. The patient had to stay in the hospital 2 extra days. The hospital lost money, and the patient was unhappy.

Example 2. A patient who was dependent on a respirator was discharged to home care pending the availability of around-the-clock nursing care. A call to an agency resulted in the information that the few staff members who were able to function independently in the home with a patient with these needs were currently unavailable. The patient waited 2 weeks for discharge, and the hospital lost money. The hospital board believed it had a legal and moral obligation to delay discharge in the absence of a viable plan of care for the patient. At the same time the board had to find a way to remain fiscally sound.

As a consequence of these problems, it has become necessary for hospitals to devise plans that enable them to perform the following tasks:

1. Discharge patients within diagnosis-related group time limits
2. Facilitate care efficiently
3. Control the quality of care
4. Coordinate care
5. Develop an integrated program

Home care agencies based in the hospital have the advantage of providing good continuity of care between hospital and home through the hospital's discharge planner. Most are Medicare-certified.

Hospice Care

Hospice is a word that denotes a calm vision of death. It provides a time during which the dying spend their final days in the comfort of their home surrounded by friends and relatives (Paradis, 1985). A goal of most hospice programs is to keep the client in the home. A hospice program frequently operates in close association with a hospital that can provide the client with special treatment when needed through a hospice unit, which also may provide a family with respite services.

The hospice concept is fairly new in the United States, although it has been in existence in England since the 1800s and the idea spread to other countries in the United Kingdom. The goal of a hospice program is to keep the terminally ill client pain free and symptom free. The emphasis is on palliative rather than restorative care. Clients must be aware of their diagnosis and agree to the process.

FINANCING OF HOME HEALTH SERVICES

Historically home health care has been provided by socially conscious men and women with a sincere desire to help the sick poor. Early VNAs, for example, provided home care to those who requested it, charging fees on a sliding scale and receiving financial assistance from charitable organizations. When Medicare was enacted, the federal government included a provision that mandated medical supervision of Medicare recipients. The result was a subtle change in the nurse's role and the loss of much of nursing's autonomy. Care in the home also became medically oriented under the supervision of physicians.

Part of the nurse's role is to assist clients in locating funding sources. The client's ability to pay for services must be carefully assessed before services are provided. Clients must be fully informed as to the resources available to them and the costs they will have to assume personally. They can, if given adequate information, choose a plan of care appropriate to the services needed and to their ability to pay. The policies of Medicare, Medicaid, the Civilian Health and Medical Program of Uniformed Services (CHAMPUS), Veterans' Administration, and private insurance should be fully explored and explained.

Medicare

Medicare is a federally funded program that is available to most clients who are older than 65 years of age (Chapter 2). To receive Medicare benefits in the home a client must be considered "homebound." The law defines a homebound individual as one who cannot leave the home without assistance and for whom physical effort is taxing and difficult. A physician must certify the need for each service and recertify this need every 60 days. Criteria for reimbursement of home care services include the need for skilled personnel and for intermittent and medically necessary care. Primary skilled services are considered those provided by registered nurses, physical therapists, and speech therapists. If one of these services is provided in the home, so-called secondary services—provided by occupational therapists, social workers, home health aides, or nutritionists—may be reimbursed. Intermittent services required because of an exacerbation of a chronic illness may be covered, but long-term services to chronically ill clients are not reimbursable by Medicare.

Medicaid

Medicaid is a federally funded program that is available to clients with low incomes (see Chapter 2). It pays for skilled nursing services provided by a Medicaid-certified agency and ordered by a physician. Although physical therapy and speech therapy may be reimbursed, visits by social workers and occupational therapists are not; home health aide visits are limited. Coverage varies from state to state. Each state has a responsibility to match federal funds by 50%, but some provide more assistance than do others.

Private Insurance

Private insurance, whether purchased by individuals or provided by employers, generally covers home health care on a yearly deductible basis. Clarification with the client as to what home care services will be reimbursed should be included in the nurse's initial visit and plan of care for a client/family. For example, some plans underwrite home care services only if these services are in lieu of acute care hospitalization.

Benefits for Military Personnel

The Veterans' Administration covers home health services if the disability is related to service in the military or if the services are required after discharge from a veterans' hospital.

The Civilian Health and Medical Program of Uniformed Services (CHAMPUS) provides home health care for spouses and children of servicemen in the United States and during the period when they are stationed out of the country (Stanhope & Lancaster, 1988).

Nurses who coordinate and plan home care must be aware of the constraints placed on the client and the providers of care by the client's available resources. Teaching self-care when possible, referring to volunteer services, and eliciting help from family members when funding is limited can be helpful. Continued research (see box above) in alternative methods of payment for home care is needed.

LOGISTICAL ASPECTS OF HOME HEALTH CARE

The initiation of home health services generally begins with a referral from a physician, a hospital discharge planner, or a request from a client or family. A home health agency receives basic information, which will include, if the referral source is the physician or discharge planner, a diagnosis and a physician's specific order for service. A nurse is assigned to the case and contacts the client to arrange a home visit.

In contrast to hospital nursing, the home health nurse must consider factors other than the nursing care itself in the planning and providing of services. These factors include travel time, weather conditions, and personal safety, and the home health nurse may discover that the logistics of care delivery are more complex than the actual client care.

Geographical Considerations

The home health agency's service area is affected by physical geography, weather conditions, parking availability, traffic patterns, personal and property safety factors, and physical access to the client residence. Response time to initiate service, to deliver ongoing care, and to meet subacute home emergencies is not controlled entirely by staff availability. In addition to the logistics of time of day (or night) and day of the week, the community health nurse must consider other factors in organizing the day's schedule of client services. In urban areas community events such as a street fair, a 10-kilometer run, or other major sporting events usually are known in advance. However, unpredictable road closings, police activities, fire-fighting operations, protests and demonstrations, and traffic accidents can interrupt the best of plans for service delivery. The experienced community health nurse who works in an urban area stays tuned to traffic reports.

In some parts of the country the weather report becomes a paramount factor, for example, listening for flash flood warnings in the low desert of the Southwest, the snow conditions in Tahoe or Stowe, tornado watches in the Texas panhandle and the Midwest, and emergency plans for tropical storms in the Gulf states. Some home care companies are located in snowbelt areas, which requires staff members to have four-wheel drive vehicles and the ability to cross-country ski. Horseback riding skills may be needed in some remote rural areas; island areas off the coast require access to ferry or boat transport.

Safety Considerations

Assurance of personal and property safety requires additional preparation strategies. Many metropolitan-based providers use community aides to accompany staff members in high-crime areas during the daylight hours. Unarmed escort or guard services are employed for after-dark service visits. It is important that the community health nurse have practical "street smarts" and always comply with the employer's safety guidelines (see box below). Such guidelines have been standard in community health home care since the early 1960s. These precautions are based on the reality of conditions in many neighborhoods; for example, the presence of drug or gang-related activities cannot be ignored.

Text continued on p. 365.

SAFETY TIPS FOR HOME HEALTH NURSES

- Do not wear conspicuous jewelry or watches.
- Do not display wallet or purse.
- Carry only necessary identification and pocket cash.
- Secure personal belongings in the trunk of your car before leaving your residence for the day.
- Dress professionally in a manner appropriate to the work.
- Do not label boxes with the client's name, address, and contents (e.g., sterile syringes).
- If the parking area appears unsafe, drive to a convenience store or service station with a telephone and contact your supervisor.
- Maintain your automobile in good condition, and keep an active automobile club membership for emergency road service.

HOME HEALTH CARE AGENCY
HOME HEALTH CARE CLIENT NURSING ASSESSMENT

I. General information (please complete below)

_____ 1. Name of client

_____ 2. Address of client:

_____   city, state, zip code

_____ 3. Telephone number of client

_____ 4. Client clinical record number

_____ 5. Birthdate of client

_____ 6. Age of client

_____ 7. Sex of client

_____ 8. Date of client admission

_____ 9. Name of individual referring client to
                                            the home health care agency

_____ 10. Name of agency referring client to the
                                            home health care agency

_____ 11. Discharge date of client's most recent
                                            hospitalizations

_____ 12. Name of hospital from which client most
                                            recently discharged

_____ 13. Address of hospital from which client
_____   most recently discharged: city, state,
                                            zip code

_____ 14. Other

II. Social information (please complete below)

_____ 1. Name of client's informal caregiver

_____ 2. Address of client's informal caregiver:

_____   city, state, zip code

_____ 3. Telephone number of client's informal
Home   Work   caregiver

FIG. 16-1 Nursing assessment for client receiving home health care. *(Adapted from* Administrative policies and procedures for home health care *(pp. 71, 72, and 75) by J. Bulau, 1986, Rockville, MD: Aspen. Copyright 1986 by Aspen Publishers. Reprinted by permission.)*

_____ 4. Name of client's closest relative

_____ 5. Address of client's closest relative:

_____ 6. Telephone number of client's closest
Home   Work   relative
_____   city, state, zip code

_____ 7. Other

III. Medical information (please complete below)

_____ 1. Principal diagnosis of client

_____ 2. Secondary diagnosis(es) of client

_____ 3. Significant identified problem(s) of
_____   client

_____ 4. Significant current medical history of
_____   client

_____

_____ 5. Significant past medical history of client

_____

_____ 6. Name, dose, and administration times of
_____   medications client currently taking

_____

_____

_____ 7. Medication allergies of client

_____ 8. Food allergies of client

_____ 9. Other allergies of client

_____ 10. Name of client's attending physician

_____ 11. Address of client's attending physician:

_____   city, state, zip code
Home   Work

Continued.

FIG. 16-1, cont'd Nursing assessment for client receiving home health care.

_____ 12. Telephone number of client's attending
                                            physician

_____ a. Registered nurse   13. Type of home health care service re-
                                                    quired for client (please check [✔] one)
_____ b. Home health aide

_____ c. Other (please describe) _____

_____ a. Registered nurse   14. Frequency of home health care services
                                                    required for client (please fill in)
_____ b. Home health aide

_____ c. Other (please describe) _____

_____ Yes (please describe) _____ No   15. Equipment required for client (please
                                                    check [✔] one)
_____

_____ 16. Other

IV. Financial information (please complete below)

_____ a. Employment   1. Income source of applicant (Please check
                                         [✔] as indicated)
_____ b. Social Security

_____ c. Pension (please describe)   _____

_____ d. Other (please describe)   _____

_____ a. Employment   2. Amount of income source of applicant
                                         (please complete as indicated)
_____ b. Social Security

_____ c. Pension _____ d. Other _____

                                      3. Medical insurance information

Insurance coverage	Type of coverage	Name of policyholder	Group number	Contract number	Insurance verified		Comments
					Yes	No	
1. Medicare							
2. Medicaid							
3. Commercial insurance							
4. Worker's private							
5. Other							

FIG. 16-1, cont'd Nursing assessment for client receiving home health care.

_____   4. Name of individual responsible for client's bill

_____   5. Address of individual responsible for client's bill

_____

_____   6. Telephone number of individual responsible for client's bill

Work   Home

_____   7. Other

_____
Signature of client / responsible person   _____
                                                            Date of signature

V. Assessment of applicant for appropriate admission to home health care (please check [✓] one in each category)

Admission criteria	Admission criteria met		
	Yes	No	Comments
1. Applicant confined to applicant's place of residence: homebound.			
2. Applicant under care of a physician.			
3. Applicant needs part-time or intermittent skilled nursing services and at least one other therapeutic service, e.g., physical or occupational therapy.			
4. Reasonable expectation exists that the applicant's medical, nursing and social needs can be met adequately by the home health care agency in the applicant's place of residence.			
5. The home health care services are necessary and reasonable to the treatment of the applicant's illness or injury.			
6. Applicant is 16 years of age or older.			

_____ a. Yes   _____ b. No (Please explain)

_____

7. Applicant meets admission criteria and is appropriate for admission to the home health care agency (please check [✓] one)

_____

_____
Signature of home health care registered nurse
responsible for applicant assessment

_____
Date of signature

FIG. 16-1, cont'd   Nursing assessment for client receiving home health care.

HOME HEALTH CARE AGENCY
CLIENT EVALUATION OF HOME HEALTH CARE SERVICES

The Home Health Care Agency staff is dedicated to providing quality home health care for clients that is consistent with the Home Health Care Agency philosophy. As a recent client who has received our home health care services, you are being asked to complete this survey form. The information you give us on your completed survey form will be assessed to measure how well we have provided quality home health care services to you and ways in which we can improve the same service to you. Please promptly complete and return this form to the Administrator or Director of Nursing of Home Health Care.

Thank you for your assistance in our continuing effort to provide quality home health care services to you.

ITEM	IMPORTANCE OF EACH ITEM TO YOU				YOUR SATISFACTION WITH EACH ITEM				
	NOT IMPORTANT	IMPORTANT	VERY IMPORTANT	NOT APPLICABLE	NOT SATISFIED	SATISFIED	VERY SATISFIED	NOT APPLICABLE	
I. Referral to the home health care agency									
A. I was given a timely response from the home health care agency regarding my request for home health care services.									
B. I was given adequate information regarding the home health care agency policies and procedures.									
C. I was given adequate information regarding the home health care agency charges for services, including my eligibility for third party reimbursement.									
II. Admission to the home health care agency									
A. I was given adequate information about my rights and responsibilities for receiving home health care services.									
III. Home health care services									
A. I was treated with courtesy by all who provided home health care services to me.									
B. I was treated with respect by all who provided home health care services to me.									
C. I was given privacy by all who provided home health care services to me.									
D. I was given proper identification by name and title of everyone who provided home health care services to me.									
E. I was given a quality plan of home health care, that was developed with my participation, to meet my unique health care needs.									

F. I was given quality medical care.												
G. I was given quality skilled nursing care.												
H. I was given quality home health side care.												
I. I was given quality physical therapy care.												
J. I was given quality occupational therapy care.												
K. I was given quality social service care.												
L. I was given quality nutritional support.												
M. I was given quality laboratory services.												
N. I was given quality rehabilitation care.												
O. I was given quality mental health care.												
P. I was given prompt adequate responses to my needs, concerns and problems.												
Q. I was given adequate information about the home health care services I received.												
R. I was given adequate explanations about any questions and concerns I expressed to the home health care staff.												
S. I was given adequated information about my medical diagnosis, treatment, alternatives, risks and progress in terms and language I could understand.												
T. I was given adequate assistance in having my family participate in my care.												

Continued.

FIG. 16-2 Evaluation of home health care services provided by agency. *(From Administrative policies and procedures for home health care (pp. 16-18) by J. Bulau, 1986, Rockville, MD: Aspen. Copyright 1986 by Aspen Publishers. Reprinted by permission.)*

ITEM	IMPORTANCE OF EACH ITEM TO YOU				YOUR SATISFACTION WITH EACH ITEM			
	NOT IMPORTANT	IMPORTANT	VERY IMPORTANT	NOT APPLICABLE	NOT SATISFIED	SATISFIED	VERY SATISFIED	NOT APPLICABLE
IV. Discharge from the home health care agency								
A. I was given adequate assistance in developing discharge plans for my care and treatment in anticipation of my discharge from the home health care agency.								
B. I was given adequate information regarding the financial status of my home health care bill.								
C. My discharge from the home health care agency was efficient.								

V. Other

A. I would use the home health care services from the home health care agency in the future, if necessary. (Please check [✓] one below.)

    _____ 1. Yes.

    _____ 2. No. Please explain. _____

B. I would recommend the home health care agency to other individuals. (Please check [✓] one below.)

    _____ 1. Yes.

    _____ 2. No. Please explain. _____

VI. Comments (Please fill in the blanks.)

_____

_____

_____

VII. Optional information

A. Your name (please fill in blank) _____

B. Your address (please fill in blank) _____

C. Your sex (please check [✓] one) _____ Male _____ Female

D. Your age (please check [✓] one) _____ 17-35 _____ 36-50 _____ 50+

E. Length of time your received services from the home health care agency (please fill in the blank) _____

FIG. 16-2, cont'd Evaluation of home health care services provided by agency.

It is important to keep the risks in perspective without becoming an alarmist. The experienced community health nurse is alert and careful but does not report anecdotes to family or friends that may exaggerate their concerns for his or her safety. The presence of Neighborhood Watch and other community-sponsored safety awareness programs generally improves the safety and security of these neighborhoods.

The Nurse's Initial Visit

Most agencies use the nursing process as a framework for practice. On the first visit, the nurse collects necessary data, analyzes the data, and formulates a nursing diagnosis. The information collected must include the social, medical, and financial status of the client. (Fig. 16-1 provides a sample initial assessment tool). The nursing diagnosis must include the significant identified problems of the client *(Item III, 3)*, as well as an assessment of the necessity for services from other members of the health care team. In addition to facilitating the implementation of plan of care, the nurse has the responsibility of evaluating the care both as it is being given and at the time the client is being discharged (Fig. 16-2). If a home health aide is assigned, the nurse is responsible for supervising that person. If the client is receiving interdisciplinary services, the nurse may wish to schedule team meetings to coordinate the plan of care.

The nurse's role in the home should reflect the health provider's policy and mission statement, as well as the nurse's personal philosophy and theory base. It also should be consistent with the American Nurses' Association's standards of community health nursing practice.

FUTURE TRENDS IN HOME HEALTH CARE

Because of the success of DRGs in controlling costs in acute care settings, the Department of Health and Human Services (DHHS) wants to establish a prospective payment system for home health agencies. If it is implemented, the agencies will have to structure services to fit within guidelines to qualify for reimbursement. Nurses and other home care providers are seeing more acutely ill clients than ever before, and the rules that govern reimbursement of care are becoming more complex (Griffith, 1988). Increased medical control of nursing functions, brought about by criteria established for Medicare reimbursement, has mandated a collaborative relationship that must be factored into client care.

The number of home health care agencies has risen sharply since the passage of Public Law 89-97 (Medicare and Medicaid legislation; see Chapter 2), with proprietary agencies showing the greatest growth. There is a need for clarification of home care nursing practice both for the sake of the consumer and for the profession itself.

The needs of the frail elderly cannot be ignored. Advocacy for this target group must continue to be a nursing priority.

There remains the possibility that some form of national health insurance will become a reality in the near future in the United States. As more people become aware of the inequities in health care in this country, public pressure may grow to support legislation to provide health care for all (Williams & Williams, 1988).

Home health care nurses must develop the skills necessary to operate high-technology equipment in the home. At the same time they must not lose the holistic perspective that has long been uniquely theirs.

Although many uncertainties remain, it is clear that home health care providers will have to respond to the needs of the consumer. Agencies will have to be market-oriented, competitive, and business wise. The placement of health care managers within the agency framework who are nurses and who understand both client needs and marketing techniques may be the trend of the future (Williams & Williams, 1988).

SUMMARY

Home care provides services for clients in the home. It is rapidly becoming an interdisciplinary, interagency service that requires a collaborative, well-coordinated effort on the part of the health care team. Changes in the client population that requests and needs care have influenced health provider agencies. The constraints placed on health providers in terms of cost containment have ushered in a new era of fiscal responsibility. In planning care, the nurse must assess not only the client's needs but also the client's willingness and ability to pay. The nurse remains the "hub of the wheel" in home care. Assessing, diagnosing, planning, and implementing care, as well as evaluating the effects of the care, are all a part of the nurse's role.

CHAPTER HIGHLIGHTS

- Home care has been defined by NAHC as services for recovering, disabled, or chronically ill persons; it provides treatment and facilitates effective functioning in the home environment.
- Clients who require care in the home include those who are acutely ill, who are mentally ill, who have AIDS, who are elderly, and who are chronically ill.
- Professionals involved in providing home care include nurses, physicians, physical therapists, occupational therapists, social workers, speech pathologists, nutritionists, and home health aides.
- The nurse usually functions as the coordinator of the home care team.
- Agencies that provide home care services may be official (government operated) agencies, VNAs, independent proprietary agencies, and hospital-based agencies.
- In recent years proprietary agencies have proliferated and provided services to clients with the financial resources to pay. As a result voluntary agencies have faced financial difficulties as an increasing proportion of their clientele requires free services.
- Hospice care provides palliative care in the home to terminally ill clients.
- Home care may be financed through private insurance, Medicare, Medicaid, and the client's private payments. The nurse assesses the client's ability to pay for services and helps to locate additional sources of funding if necessary.
- It is possible that in the future, prospective payment systems will be established for home health services.

STUDY QUESTIONS

1. Describe the role of the community health nurse in the provision of health care.
2. Identify those disciplines that are considered skilled and primary by the federal government.
3. Describe four different sources of third-party reimbursement.
4. The following is the information received by one VNA 1 day before the hospital was to discharge a person who had had a cerebrovascular accident. On the basis of the assessment plan shown in Fig. 16-1, formulate a preliminary plan of care for your visit with the client the next day.

Name of client:	Mrs. R. Jones (lives alone)
Address:	27 Peach St.
Telephone:	832-6468
Clinical Record	
Birth date:	5/1/31
Referred by:	Dorothy Kline, discharge planner from St. Josephs Hospital
Nearest relative:	Janice Jones (daughter) who lives out of town; telephone: (123) 922-3800
Medical diagnosis:	Cerebrovascular accident with resulting hemiplegia
Medications:	Furosemide P.O., 40 mg Q.D., Nefedipine 10 mg, P.O., TID A.C. (Skidmore-Roth, 1990).
Physicians' order:	Skilled nursing care, home health aide, physiotherapy twice weekly, occupational therapy, nutritionist to see; monitor vital signs daily, supervise medications
Insurance coverage:	Medicare, Medicaid

REFERENCES

American Nurses' Association. (1974). *Standards for community health practice.* Kansas City, MO: Author.

Bulau, J. (1986). *Administrative policies and procedures for home health care.* Rockville, MD: Aspen.

Burwell, B. (1976, August 25). Shared obligations: Public policy influences on family care for the elderly. *Medicaid Program Evaluation Working Paper 2.1, 41*(166):35847. Washington, DC: Urban Institute Press.

Griffith, E. I. (1988). Home care in crisis: Turning it around. *Nursing Outlook, 36,* 272-274.

Haddad, A. (1987). *High-tech home care: A practical guide.* Rockville, MD: Aspen.

Home Health Services. (1982). *Commerce clearinghouse, Medicare and Medicaid Guide* (Paragraph 1401). Washington, DC: Department of Health and Human Services.

Keating, S. B., and Kelman, G. (1988). *Home health care nursing: Concepts and practice.* Philadelphia: Lippincott.

Kilbane, K., and Blacksin, B. (1988). The demise of free care: The Visiting Nurse Association of Chicago. *Nursing Clinics of North America, 23,* 435-442.

Moore, F. (1988). *Homemaker–home health aid to services: Script policies and practices.* Owings Mills, MD: National Health Publishing.

Paradis, L. (1985). *Hospice handbook: A guide for managers and planners.* Rockville, MD: Aspen.

Pasquale, D. K. A. (1987). A basis for prospective payment for home care. *Image: The Journal of Nursing Scholarship, 19,* 186-191.

Skidmore-Roth, L. (1990). *Mosby's nursing drug reference.* St. Louis: Mosby-Year Book, Inc.

Stanhope, M., and Lancaster, J. (1988). *Community health nursing: Process and practice for promoting health* (2nd ed.). St. Louis: Mosby.

Stewart, J. (1979). *Home health care.* St. Louis: Mosby.

Toffler A. (1970). *Future shock.* New York: Random House.

Williams, S., and Williams, J. (1988). *How to market home health services.* New York: Wiley.

Discharge Planning

PATRICIA A. O'HARE

Discharge planning aims to ensure continuity of care, helps sick and well persons and their families to find the best solutions to their health problems, at the right time, from the appropriate source, at the best price and on a continuous basis for the required period of time.

N.L.N., 1985, p. 9

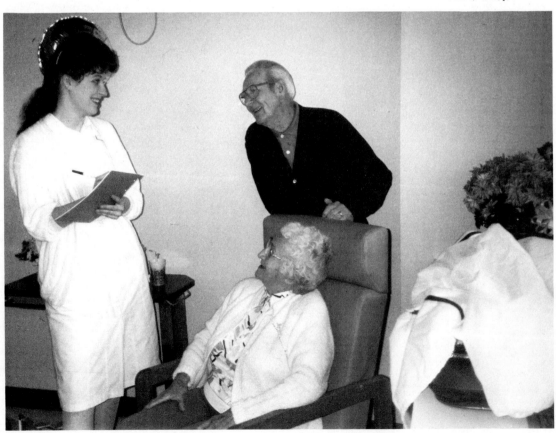

OBJECTIVES

At the conclusion of this chapter the student will be able to:
1. Define the key terms listed
2. Discuss the role of discharge planning in the overall delivery of health care today
3. Discuss the discharge planning process
4. Discuss the components for providing continuity of care
5. Analyze the nurse's role in discharge planning for continuity of care
6. Describe the role of the community health nurse as home care coordinator

KEY TERMS

Activities of daily living
Continuing care
Continuity of care
Continuum of care
Discharge planning

Instrumental activities of daily living
Levels of care
Referral
Uniform needs assessment instrument

Discharge planning for the provision of continuing care is one of the major elements in the overall delivery of health care today. It is the interorganizational link from the hospital to the community for continuity of care. Discharge planning needs to be carried out in all settings involved in the continuum of care, such as hospitals, home health agencies, nursing homes, physicians' offices, ambulatory care settings, health maintenance organizations (HMOs), and adult day-care centers.

HISTORICAL PERSPECTIVE

The concept of assessing needs and planning for ongoing care is not new. *Charities and the Commons,* a publication of Bellevue Hospital in New York City in 1906-1907 refers to "a nurse whose entire time and care is given to befriending those about to be discharged. She inquires into their circumstances, finds out whether they have home or friends to return to; if necessary, secures admission for them into some other curative or consolatory refuge."

Some referral systems for continuity of nursing care began as early as 1910 (Smith, 1962). One study (Carn & Mole, 1949), conducted by a joint committee of the National Organization for Public Health Nursing and the National League of Nursing Education, reported that 30 public health nursing agencies throughout the United States had liaison referral systems in conjunction with 43 hospitals. Another report (Smith, 1962) noted the increased interest in follow-up nursing services for patients after their discharge from the hospital in the period between 1946 and 1961. This study also identified the need for nursing involvement in discharge planning. Knowing which clients to assess for ongoing needs was considered the critical first step.

A follow-up publication, *Nursing Service Without Walls* (Wensley, 1963, p. 38), presented criteria that would be useful in alerting hospital staff members to client needs for referrals to community services. These criteria were as follows:

- The complexity of a procedure, such as administration of a medicine or a treatment, that requires professional assistance in the home

- An indication that a patient and/or family are unable to give care or do not understand directions for follow-up care
- Signs that the patient and/or family are unable to accept or are disturbed by some aspect of the condition or care.
- Evidence of need for reinforcement and clarification of instruction started in the hospital
- The expressed needs of patients for follow-up nursing service when professional personnel have corroborated the appropriateness of public health nursing to meet the needs
- Some aspect of the physical or social environment at home and outside the hospital that may interfere with a patient's satisfactory self-care, for instance, an elderly patient living alone or with an elderly spouse, or at a distance from the hospital that makes frequent trips to the clinic difficult

These criteria are as relevant today as they were in 1963. Indeed, the need always has existed for nurses to be involved in the planning for continuing care needs of clients. That need is even greater today, given the dynamics of the health care delivery system and societal and demographical changes. This chapter explores the concept of discharge planning, why it is important today, and the nurse's role in the process. Although discharge planning needs to be carried out in all settings, the examples in this chapter focus on the hospital because it is where the majority of nurses practice.

CURRENT PERSPECTIVES
Definitions of Discharge Planning

The American Nurses' Association (ANA) in 1975 stated that "Discharge planning is the part of the continuity of care process which is designed to prepare the patient or client for the next phase of care and to assist in making any necessary arrangements for that phase of care, whether it be self-care, care by family members, or care by an organized health care provider" (ANA, 1975, p. 3). The purpose of discharge planning is twofold: (1) continuity of care—coordinated delivery of services on a continuous bases as needed and (2) cost-effective care, that is, to move the person to the appropriate level of care as quickly as possible. Level of care is determined by client needs and may be designated as acute, subacute, skilled, intermediate, custodial/domiciliary, or chronic.

In 1985 the National League for Nursing (NLN) defined discharge planning as that "which aims to ensure continuity of care, helps sick and well persons and their families find the best solutions to their health problems, at the right time, from the appropriate source, at the best price, and on a continuous basis for the required period of time" (NLN, 1985, p. 9). Discharge planning is not an end point; it is a process, a linking mechanism that requires collaboration, communication, and coordination among the client and family and all other members of the health care team. By nature it is interdisciplinary because no one discipline can provide all services to the client.

Legislation Affecting Discharge Planning

The 1985 definition of discharge planning differs from the 1975 definition in that for the first time the economics of care are addressed. The "price" of care has become a major concern worldwide. In the United States the Social Security Act amendments of 1983 provided sweeping changes in the area of hospital reimbursement for Medicare patients. Public Law (P.L.) 98-21, Title VI, ushered in prospective payment for hospitals for services to Medicare patients on the basis of diagnosis-related groups (DRGs) (P.L. 98-21, 1983).

This legislation provided a major impetus for hospitals to review their admissions and to reduce the length of hospitalization, with major implications for the public at large and for health care delivery in general.

Recent Changes Affecting Health Care Delivery

The present importance of discharge planning in providing continuity of care is a result of the following changes in health care delivery:

1. The prospective payment system, with its 473 DRGs for Medicare reimbursement to hospitals resulted in a decrease in the average length of stay (ALOS). Because of early discharge, the client's follow-up needs are more complex.
2. Fiscal austerity in all sectors of the health care environment has resulted in decreased resources, not only in acute care but also in home care and long-term care.
3. Changing demographical patterns such as the "graying of America" have resulted in an expanding aging population, the fastest-growing segment of which is the group aged 85 years and older, an increase of 65% in the last decade (United States Department of Health and Human Services [USDHHS], 1987). Those older than 85 years often are frail and have chronic health problems that require ongoing care. Although persons aged 65 years and older represented only 12% of the United States' population in 1984, it is projected that this group will account for 31% of total personal health care expenditures (American Association of Retired Persons [AARP], 1988).

THE PROCESS OF DISCHARGE PLANNING

It is becoming increasingly important for nurses in all settings to be involved in planning for ongoing care. The hospital is part of the community, as are such settings as the home, the nursing home, and the adult day-care center. Regardless of where the nurse practices, it is necessary to view the client from a holistic perspective as a member of a family and of a community. Clients cannot be separated from their environments, and the nurse cannot be concerned with meeting only immediate needs. It is essential to know where the person came from, the place he or she is going to, who is available to help, what other responsibilities that care giver has, what resources are available in the community, what the eligibility requirements are for those services/resources, and how to gain access to them.

The discharge planning process for ensuring continuity of care parallels the nursing process. The components of the discharge planning process are as follows:

- Assessment of needs
- Analysis and diagnosis of needs
- A plan for how to meet those needs
- Implementation of the plan
- Evaluation of the outcome(s) of the plan

Assessment and Analysis

Assessment is the initial step. It involves data collection to identify and validate needs to diagnose current and continuing care need or needs. Assessment is an ongoing process with constant addition of new data and the change of plans as necessary. In addition, the impact of the illness or health problem on the client and family requires attention (Fig. 17-1).

Clients with high-risk factors such as living alone, being without insurance, being elderly (65 years or older), having specific diagnoses (e.g., cancer, stroke, confusion, and amputation, and having frequent hospital readmissions usually are screened in the hospital for continuing care needs. What may be overlooked, however, is the level of the client's functioning before hospitalization and the projected level of functioning as services are provided and care is received. Level of functioning needs to be defined to include not

GUIDELINES FOR HOSPITAL DISCHARGE PLANNING TO BE UTILIZED BY HOSPITAL NURSE

Section I: overview

Refer to basic information already on the admission fact sheet of the chart which includes: name, address, phone number, age, sex, marital status, occupation, place of employment, admitting diagnosis, insurance, and person to contact in emergency. The nurse would question whether this person would be available to help if assistance was needed after discharge. The nurse is trying to determine the patient's personal support system; that is, who the patient can and does depend on.

Section II: interaction/impact

Looking at the patient, family and diagnosis(es), consider the following:

What *concerns* does the patient and family have about the hospitalization, diagnosis or treatment?

Lifestyle—How do the diagnoses, treatments and their implications, if any, affect the patient and family lifestyle?

Will the condition interfere with the patient's present occupation or profession now or in the future? Is the situation short-term or long-term?

Assistance

Can the patient care for him/herself?
If the patient cannot care for self, who can assist him?
What other responsibilities does this person have?
Is professional assistance needed?
Is assistance needed continuously or periodically?
What about insurance coverage for financial considerations?

Section III: home needs

Consider the *home environment* in terms of space, stairs, location of toilet, etc.
Supplies or equipment need in the home:

What supplies will the patient be taking home from the hospital with him, e.g., irrigating equipment, dressings, walker, etc.?

What equipment will the family need to have in the home when the patient comes home, e.g., hospital bed, commode chair, wheelchair, etc.?

Referal for follow-up nursing in the home. Was the patient known to a Community Nursing/Home Health Agency before admission? Does the community health nurse know that the patient is in the hospital?

Is the form on the chart for referral to the Community Nursing/Home Health Agency?

Transfer or discharge to another facility

If the patient was in a nursing home before admission, is the nursing home holding the bed for him or must he reapply for admission?

If the patient is to be discharged to a nursing home or a community residential facility is the "Patient Transfer Form" on the chart? This form needs to be completed and sent with the patient to the facility.

Section IV: health teaching re: diagnoses and implications

Specific teaching as indicated looking at the physiological and psycholological changes in terms of resulting needs

Physical care required—mobility, continence, etc.

Dressings
Catheters
Special diets
Therapies—physical, occupational, speech

With the information elicited by means of these guidelines, the nurse has a data base for anticipating needs and planning with the patient/family/significant other and other diciplines for continuity of care during hospitalization and after discharge.

From "Factors affecting the hospital nurse in planning for patient discharge and continuity of care" by P.A. O'Hare, December 1975, Unpublished manuscript. Copyright 1975 by Patricia A. O'Hare. Reprinted by permission.

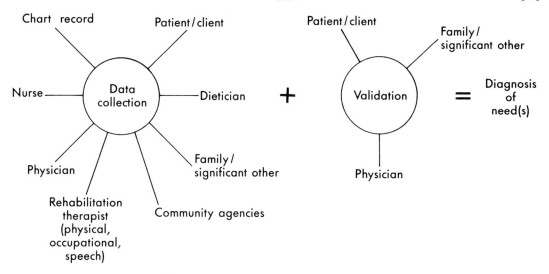

FIG. 17-1 Assessment process components.

only the activities of daily living (ADL), such as bathing, dressing, toileting, transfer, continence, and feeding) but also the instrumental ADL, which include shopping, light housekeeping, taking medications, handling finances, and using the telephone and transportation. The Manitoba Longitudinal Study on Aging (Shapiro, 1986) found that one of the best predictors of home care use, after age, is the client's level of difficulty in coping with instrumental ADL.

Assessment includes consideration as to whether the client is dealing with a short-term or a long-term illness and the possible changes in life-style or role that may occur as a result of the problem. Also assessed are specific home care needs in terms of both client and environment. The box on p. 372 provides a framework that is useful for all nurses in hospital discharge planning.

A nursing history obtained as part of the admission data base also is used. This nursing history provides the initial data for interacting with the client and family in planning care. This information and the current treatment needs of the client are shared by the nurse on the unit with the other members of the interdisciplinary team. This team can include the physician, social worker, discharge planner or continuing care coordinator, dietitian, rehabilitation therapists, and others. Sharing of this information might take place at weekly discharge planning rounds or patient care rounds. These rounds provide a mechanism for case finding and assessment for the discharge planner, with input from the staff nurse as an essential part of appropriate planning. The data are analyzed, diagnoses of current and continuing care needs are determined, and plans are made with the client, the family, and relevant health care providers to meet those needs.

Planning and Implementation: Teaching and Referral

Teaching and referral are part of the discharge plan. As noted in "Guidelines for Hospital Discharge Planning to be Utilized by Hospital Nurse," health teaching, or client and family teaching, is an integral part of discharge planning. In the current hospital environment of shortened lengths of stay, it is not possible, nor may it ever have been possible, for all teaching to be completed by the time of discharge from the acute care hospital. It is critical that all teaching be documented and recorded in terms of client/family ability to perform procedures, to state names and purposes of drugs, and so forth. It also is essential that plans be made for continued teaching in the community through referral to the community health nurse.

Referrals to home health agencies must include an account of teaching to date and those objectives still to be achieved. Whether the discharge planner or the staff nurse makes the referral to the home health agency, the staff nurse is responsible for documenting on the referral form the care provided to the client during hospitalization. This care includes the teaching content and an assessment of that teaching in terms of client/family learning and their ability to perform the care activities. For example, if a family has been taught decubitus care, the nurse would do the following:

- Describe the stage and condition of the decubitus ulcer
- Describe the ulcer care procedure
- State how many times, or even if, the family or caregiver has observed the procedure
- State how many times, or if, they have returned the demonstration
- State their understanding of what to do and why
- State their overall ability and willingness to do the procedure at home
- State the supplies or equipment needed in the home and whether they have been obtained or ordered

It is important that the community nurse receive this information so that continuing care can be maintained.

Evaluation

Although the discharge plan for the posthospitalization period can be evaluated by the discharge planner and can occur at a place other than the hospital unit, the discharge planning nurse needs to be informed of outcomes of referrals to home health agencies. This feedback from the nurse in the community includes the effect of teaching begun in the hospital, as well as the ability of the client or family, or both, to provide the care. It allows the unit nurse to integrate what has been learned from this client situation into future nursing interventions with other clients and families. Information from the agency can be communicated either in writing or through a follow-up telephone call, depending on the protocol established by the hospital and the agency.

COMPONENTS FOR PROVIDING CONTINUITY OF CARE

The major components for providing continuity of care are the care plan, education of the client and family, and the referral.

The Care Plan

The discharge plan should be identified specifically as part of the care plan. Not every client requires referral to another agency or facility, but every client should be assessed for continuing care needs. All nursing diagnoses require review from the perspective of ongoing needs. For example, if the nurse finds any unresolved nursing diagnoses at the time of discharge, it is critical to determine what that means in terms of continuing care needs and ongoing planning. A revision has been proposed of NANDA'S taxonomy of conditions that necessitate nursing care (Fitzpatrick, Kerr, Saba, Hoskins, Hurley, Mills, Rottcamp, Warren, & Capinito, 1989), which provides several possible examples. Under the category *Human Response Pattern: Moving* is the nursing diagnosis "physical mobility, impaired." If this alteration or impairment in physical mobility is an unresolved problem at the time of discharge, the nurse needs to incorporate this problem into the discharge plan. It may mean that a referral for physical therapy after hospitalization is indicated, or it may mean that equipment such as a wheelchair is needed, or both. Basically, all nursing diagnoses require review from the standpoint of possible implications for interventions for meeting continuing care needs.

Education of the Client and Family

Education involves the assessment of learning needs, readiness for learning, and level of understanding, as well as the use of principles of teaching and learning. It involves cognizance of the effects of stress on learning and the importance of repetition and return demonstration. It also involves assessment of continuing care needs and evaluation of client learning.

The Referral

Referrals are made as needed for home care or services such as those provided by a social worker, a dietitian, or rehabilitation therapists. Referrals need to be thought of as mechanisms for communication, coordination, and collaboration between and among care settings and disciplines.

REVIEW OF CRITICAL PROCESS INFORMATION

The information needed in carrying out the discharge planning process in any setting includes the following:

- Knowledge of the client's prior health status
- Current level of care needed
- Projected level of care needed
- Projected time frame for moving the client to the next level of care
- Therapy(ies) and teaching that should be accomplished before moving the client to the next level of care
- Ability and willingness of family or caregiver to provide care
- Financial resources of the client
- Available community resources and eligibility requirements

In all settings the client and family need to be involved in decision making regarding ongoing care. Yet the problem remains concerning the assurance of consistent assessment in all settings.

Uniform Needs Assessment Instrument

There is a need in health care today for an assessment tool or tools that can be used across care settings. The Omnibus Budget Reconciliation Act (OBRA) of 1986 attempts to address this identified need. OBRA '86 mandated that the Secretary of the Department of Health and Human Services develop a "uniform needs assessment instrument" that does the following (U.S. Congress, 1986):

(A) evaluates
  (i) the functional capacity of an individual
  (ii) the nursing and other care requirements of the individual to meet health care needs and to assist with functional incapacities, and
  (iii) the social and familial resources available to the individual to meet those requirements; and
(B) can be used by discharge planners, hospitals, nursing facilities, other health care providers, and fiscal intermediaries in evaluating an individual's need for posthospital extended care services, home health services, and long-term care services of a health related or supportive nature.

Case study A: a simple discharge plan*

Assessment and analysis

Mr. J is an 81-year-old man admitted to the hospital with a diagnosis of laryngeal cancer. He lives alone in a one-level house in a large senior citizens' housing complex in the suburbs of a metropolitan area. He has two adult children, a son and daughter, who live in the metropolitan area. A laryngectomy was performed 10 days previously, and Mr. J is medically ready for discharge. His son and daughter have visited fairly frequently during this hospitalization and have expressed to the primary nurse a willingness to assist their father with his posthospital care. Mr. J is a small, frail-looking man, but he is able to perform his ADL independently and has been in good health most of his life. He is hard of hearing, which he describes as "worse since this surgery." He does not use a hearing aid. He wears glasses for near vision activities. He has a postlaryngectomy stoma that requires care. Mr. J is able to clear his secretions but requires infrequent suctioning. His appetite is poor, but he is able to eat. He is unable to speak and communicates by writing. He shakes his head "no" vigorously when questioned about his son and daughter assisting him after he is discharged.

Planning and implementation

The primary nurse institutes the following activities:

1. Assesses Mr. J's feelings about his discharge and the need for follow-up care
2. Teaches Mr. J how to care for the stoma, self-suctioning, and skin care
   Teaches Mr. J about the role of adequate nutrition in the healing process. Explores with him how he will go grocery shopping and prepare meals at home. Talks with the dietitian about Mr. J's poor appetite. The dietitian discusses with Mr. J his food likes and dislikes and helps him plan his diet
3. Organizes a case conference with Mr. J, the social worker, and Mr. J's physician to discuss concerns about Mr. J's continuing care needs. Mr. J's son and daughter join the group later in the discussion. The primary nurse is especially concerned about Mr. J's safety in going home alone because of his inability to speak, his hearing deficit, and his inability to perform self-suctioning independently at this time. Mr. J agrees to go to his daughter's house immediately after discharge. He also agrees to allow her to assist with his care until he becomes more independent and is able to go to his own home. In addition, it is agreed that a hearing evaluation will be arranged
4. Begins to teach the daughter stoma care, skin care, and suctioning. The primary emphasis is on the suctioning
5. Discusses with the physician Mr. J's equipment needs, that is, suction machine, suction catheters, supplies for cleaning the stoma, and stoma covers
6. Arranges with the equipment company for delivery of the equipment and supplies to the daughter's home
7. Refers Mr. J to a certified home health agency for follow-up nursing services in the home and requests a visit on the day of hospital discharge to assess that needed equipment and supplies are in the home and that Mr. J and his daughter know how to operate the suction machine. In addition, the home health nurse/visiting nurse/community health nurse will evaluate Mr. J's and his daughter's ability to do the suctioning and will continue the teaching in the home

Evaluation and discussion

Mr. J's case is considered a simple discharge planning situation. However, the expectation is that the primary nurse would be supported by the hospital's continuing care clinician in carrying out this discharge planning process. The continuing care clinician in this situation assisted the primary nurse not only in counseling Mr. J but also including his son and daughter in the assessment and care planning. The continuing care clinician also was the catalyst for the organized care conference, at which time definitive, workable plans were made. It also was critical that the primary nurse make telephone contact with the nurse in the community, in addition to sending a written referral. It is expected that if care questions arise, the community nurse, who has the name and telephone number of the primary nurse in the hospital, will call for additional information and also provide feedback. This is the system that needs to be fostered so that continuing care is provided.

CASE STUDY

Case study B: a complex discharge plan
Assessment and analysis

Ms. M is a 38-year-old woman admitted to the hospital with a diagnosis of *Pneumocystis carinii* pneumonia (PCP). Human immunodeficiency virus (HIV) positivity had been diagnosed 2 months previously. Ms. M is divorced, works as a waitress, and has one child, a 20-year-old daughter who lives out of town. Her marriage ended 18 months previously. It was a difficult marriage that included violent sexual abuse. Ms. M is an intelligent, physically fit woman who lives alone in a city apartment, but has many friends for support. She was treated initially with sulfamethoxazole (Bactrim) intravenously, with poor response. Pentamidine, 180 mg per day, was then begun intravenously for 14 days, which Ms. M tolerated without difficulty. After 2 days on this regimen, the physician indicated that she was ready for discharge and was to continue the course of treatment at home. After the initial respiratory difficulty, Ms. M spent her days in the hospital in a darkened room, occasionally watching television. She refused to talk with a social worker or to have a psychiatric consultation. Ms. M was physically but not psychologically ready for discharge.

Planning and implementation

The primary nurse focused on providing support for Ms. M and making her aware of where she could obtain additional support when she was ready. The primary nurse also instituted the following actions:

1. Assessing Ms. M's response to the anticipated discharge and her willingness and ability to perform self-care regarding the medication schedule and needed monitoring
2. Teaching Ms. M about her disease process and about the medication, diet, the need to increase her fluid intake and initiating some limited discussion of sexual practices. Care of blood spills was discussed (use of Clorax and water at a 1:10 dilution) because Ms. M was to be discharged with peripheral intravenous access in place for administering the medication and also for performing finger sticks
3. Working with other members of the team such as the continuing care clinician, social worker, physician, and nurse from the infusion company to make arrangements for Ms. M to receive pentamidine intravenously at home
4. Discussing Ms. M's situation with the nurse from the home infusion company, who was to administer and monitor the medication after the client's discharge from the hospital

Evaluation and discussion

The continuing care clinician again was a resource and support person for the primary nurse during this care process. Feedback from the nurse employed by the home infusion company after Ms. M's hospitalization indicated that the client was responding positively to the medication and ongoing care. Although Ms. M at this time has not sought additional support from the AIDS support group, she is aware of its availability.

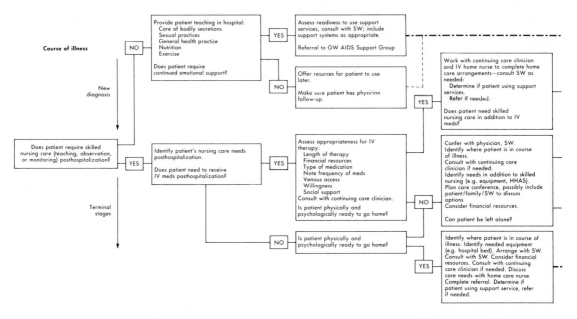

FIG. 17-2 Discharge planning decisions made by the primary nurse caring for a patient with AIDS. *(Copyright Irene Paige, R.N., M.S.N., Continuing Care Clinician. Reprinted by permission.)*

Progress is being made on this task. A draft entitled "Assessment of Needs for Continuing Care" was reviewed by a stratified sample of providers that included hospitals, nursing homes, home health agencies, and other organizations and individuals with expertise in needs assessment. The final meeting of the advisory panel on the development of the uniform needs assessment instrument was held in July 1989. The panel revised the draft instrument on the basis of a summary and analysis of comments from the stratified sample of providers and other experts in health care. The panel also developed recommendations regarding the use of the needs assessment instrument as follows (McBroom, 1989, p. 1, 3):

1. The primary purpose should be to determine a patient's need for continuing care and it is not intended to represent a comprehensive geriatric or functional assessment or a care plan.
2. Its was developed to evaluate needs for continuing care across various health care settings and is intended as a means of establishing consistency and communicating care needs in the post-acute care community.

When the form is fully developed, field tested, and implemented, the nurse in the acute care unit will be expected to contribute information and to assist in completing it even though the designated assessor may be the discharge planner. Therefore it is critical that the nurse be aware that such an instrument is being considered for future use.

DISCHARGE PLANNING ROLES
The Home Care Coordinator

A hospital may have a home care coordinator either from its own hospital-based home health agency or from a community-based home health agency. The primary role of the

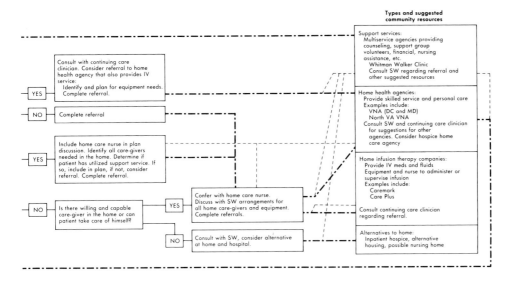

Types and suggested community resources

Support services:
Multiservice agencies providing counseling, support group volunteers, financial, nursing assistance, etc.
Whitman Walker Clinic
Consult SW regarding referral and other suggested resources

Home health agencies:
Provide skilled service and personal care
Examples include:
VNA (DC and MD)
North VA VNA
Consult SW and continuing care clinician for suggestions for other agencies. Consider hospice home care agency

Home infusion therapy companies:
Provide IV meds and fluids
Equipment and nurse to administer or supervise infusion
Examples include:
Caremark
Care Plus

Consult continuing care clinician regarding referral.

Alternatives to home:
Inpatient hospice, alternative housing, possible nursing home

YES — Consult with continuing care clinician. Consider referral to home health agency that also provides IV service:
Identify and plan for equipment needs. Complete referral.

NO — Complete referral

YES — Include home care nurse in plan discussion. Identify all care-givers needed in the home. Determine if patient has utilized support service. If so, include in plan, if not, consider referral. Complete referral.

NO — Is there willing and capable care-giver in the home or can patient take care of himself?

YES — Confer with home care nurse. Discuss with SW arrangements for all home care-givers and equipment. Complete referrals.

NO — Consult with SW, consider alternative at home and hospital.

home care coordinator is to facilitate coordination of home care referrals. Medicare will not reimburse home health agencies for discharge planning activities in the hospital. However, once the patient's physician has decided that home health services are required and the specific home health agency has been chosen, then reimbursable "coordination" includes the following postreferral activities by the home care coordinator (Lasater, 1983):

1. Explaining agency policies and procedures to the patient and family
2. Establishing a home care plan before discharge
3. Ensuring that the agency can meet the patient's needs

The home care coordinator attends hospital discharge planning meetings and suggests follow-up care services. In addition, the home care coordinator is a primary resource person in the education of physicians and hospital staff members as to what is involved in home care and the kinds of services that can be provided in the home setting. The home care coordinator's knowledge of the community and community resources is invaluable, especially when the diversity of backgrounds involved and the experience of the discharge planner are recognized.

The Discharge Planner and the Primary Nurse

The discharge planner may be a nurse, a social worker, or in some facilities even a clerical person. It is critical for the nurse to know the discharge planning process that is followed in the facility. OBRA '86 included a mandate to hospitals to provide the discharge planning process as a condition of participation for Medicare. Hospitals, however, may or may not have discharge planning programs in place to implement the process.

Each professional nurse has the responsibility for continuity of care planning as an integral part of professional nursing practice. The degree of nursing involvement depends on the structure in place in the facility inasmuch as a knowledge of the policies and procedures for discharge planning is required for continuity of care.

The hospital discharge planner may have one of many titles: discharge planner, continuing care coordinator, disposition coordinator, admission/discharge coordinator, RN discharge coordinator, coordinator of assessments, discharge coordinator, public health coordinator, community health nurse coordinator, or director of patient and family services. It also is possible that the designated person is responsible for both utilization review and discharge planning or quality assurance and discharge planning or utilization review, quality assurance, and discharge planning.

The role of the staff nurse may vary, depending on whether the continuing care needs of the patient and family are simple or complex. The simple discharge plan includes patient and family teaching and referral; the primary nurse can be expected to coordinate this discharge plan. Complex continuing care needs involve multiple disciplines and resources because of complex physical and perhaps financial and social problems. The staff nurse provides input and is involved in the planning but is not responsible for the coordination of the complex discharge plan. Two case studies are presented on pp. 376-377 to depict the role of the primary nurse in the discharge planning process. Fig. 17-2, shown on pp. 378-379, provides an additional example, one that shows the nurse using the decision-making process to care for a patient with acquired immunodeficiency syndrome (AIDS).

SUMMARY

The ideal qualifications for the person who plans the continuing care needs of patients include a background in physiology, psychology, pharmacology, medicine, and nursing, as well as an understanding of cultures and a broad perspective of the health care delivery system and reimbursement mechanisms in the United States today. The designated discharge planner may or may not possess this comprehensive knowledge base. Therefore all nurses should be prepared to function in this capacity, with a basic understanding of what continuity of care means and the role they must play in the process to meet the goals of effective continuity of care.

CHAPTER HIGHLIGHTS

- Discharge planning is the process of assessing needs and arranging or coordinating services for clients as they move through the health care system.
- Discharge planning should be carried out in all health care settings, including hospitals, home health agencies, nursing homes, physicians' offices, and ambulatory care centers.
- Criteria that indicate the need for further services include complexity of the procedures to be performed, inability of the client and/or caregiver to provide care, and environmental factors that interfere with a client's care.
- The implementation of the prospective payment system in 1983 led to a decreased ALOS in hospitals and an increased need for follow-up care.
- The discharge planning process begins with an assessment of the client's needs, including an assessment of the client's level of functioning before hospitalization.
- Health teaching, which is an integral component of discharge planning, should be documented in detail to ensure continuity after discharge.
- Referrals are mechanisms for communication, coordination, and collaboration between and among care settings and disciplines. The information communicated should include the client's prior health status, the level of care needed, therapies and teaching to be

accomplished, availability of care givers, financial resources, and available community resources.

- The uniform needs assessment instrument, currently in development, will allow for determination of a client's need for continuing care across various health care settings.
- Continuing care needs may be either simple or complex. A simple discharge plan can be coordinated by the primary nurse, whereas a complex plan involves health care providers from multiple disciplines.
- Each professional nurse is responsible for continuity of care planning as an integral part of professional nursing practice.

STUDY QUESTIONS

1. How has the implementation of DRGs and the prospective payment system influenced the role of the discharge planner?
2. What are the criteria that indicate a need for referral to community-based services?
3. List the information that should be included in a referral. Why is each piece of information important?
4. Differentiate between a simple and a complex discharge plan, and give an example of each.

REFERENCES

A field nurse for old Bellevue. (1906-07). *Charities and the Commons, 17,* 125.

American Association of Retired Persons. (1988). *A profile of older Americans.* Washington, DC: Author.

American Nurses' Association. (1975). *Statement on continuity of care and discharge planning programs in institutions and community agencies.* Kansas City, MO: Author.

Carn, I., & Mole, E. W. (1949). Continuity of nursing care: An analysis of referral systems with recommended practice. *American Journal of Nursing, 49,* 388-390.

Fitzpatrick, J., Kerr, M., Saba, V.K., Hoskins, L.M., Hurley, M.E., Mills, W.E., Rottcamp, B.E., Warren, J., & Capinito, L.J. (1989). Translating nursing diagnosis into ICD code. *American Journal of Nursing, 89,* 493-495.

Hartigan, E. G., and Brown, D. J. (Eds.). (1985). *Discharge planning for continuity of care.* New York: National League for Nursing.

Lasater, N. (1983). Nurse coordinator reimbursement. *Caring, 89,* 14-16.

McBroom, A. (1989). Advisory panel on uniform needs assessment instrument completes recommendations. *Access, 7*(3), 1, 3.

Public Law 98-21, Title VI. (1983). *Prospective payment for Medicare in-patient hospital services.* Washington, DC: U.S. Government Printing Office.

Shapiro, E. (1986). Patterns and predictors of home care use by the elderly when need is the sole basis for admission. *Home Health Care Services Quarterly, 7*(1): 29-44.

Smith, L.C. (1962). *Factors influencing continuity of nursing service.* New York: National League for Nursing.

Wensley, E. (1963). *Nursing service without walls.* New York: National League for Nursing, p. 38.

U.S. Congress. House. (1986, October 17). *Omnibus Budget Reconciliation Act: Report to Accompany H.R. 5300.* 99th Cong., sect. 9305.

U.S. Department of Health and Human Services. (1987). *Aging America: Trends and projections* (1987-1989 ed.). Washington, DC: U.S. Government Printing Office.

Home Health Care and Advanced Technology

MARY K. DETE

We are moving in the dual directions of high tech/high touch, matching each new technology with a compensatory human response.

JOHN NAISBITT

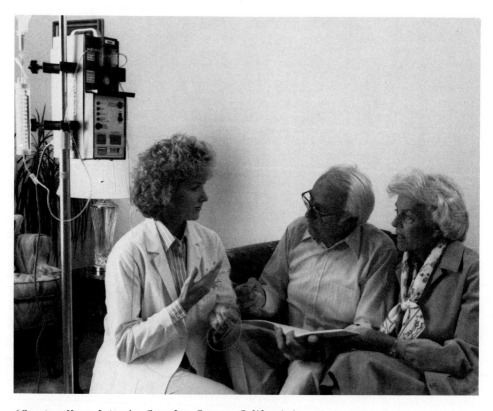

(Courtesy Home Intensive Care, Inc. Cypress, California.)

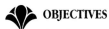 **OBJECTIVES**

At the conclusion of this chapter the student will be able to:

1. Define the key terms listed
2. Describe high-tech and high-touch home care, and discuss the relationship between them
3. Identify the role of the home care nurse in advanced technology home care
4. Identify the responsibilities of the infusion therapy company
5. Identify the various disciplines involved in advanced technology home care
6. Identify the key aspects of client and client family preadmission assessment
7. Identify key elements in client learning assessment
8. Describe the relationship of reimbursement to therapy selection
9. Describe the denial/appeal process
10. Discuss the importance of home care discharge planning
11. List the criteria for admission to a home phototherapy program

KEY TERMS

Admission criteria	High-tech care
Apnea monitoring	High-touch care
Client communication	Informed consent
Client eligibility	Infusion therapy
Clinical indicators	Noncompliance
Denial/appeals	Phototherapy
Discharge planning	Ventilator care

Each year technological advances in the home care setting make it possible for the acutely ill client who requires specialized services to be cared for at home. Virtually all community or home health care companies are prepared either directly or by arrangement with other companies to provide even the most complex of care when the clinical need arises and client and client family are in agreement. (Although the person assisting the client in providing care in the home is referred to here as a family member, the author recognizes that a family member may not always be available to assist the client. The care giver may instead be a friend, neighbor, or other individual.)

The community health nurse who chooses a role in home health care will have ever-increasing opportunities for skill development and clinical practice challenge. This chapter focuses on the role of the community health nurse in the delivery of "high-tech/high-touch" care to clients in their homes. Service models, team composition, team member roles and responsibilities, and service delivery systems are examined. Client and client family profiles for service eligibility are presented. Client teaching guidelines and identification of desired outcomes are highlighted. In addition, resources for further study and references to national standards are noted.

The phrase "high touch" entered the nursing lexicon in the late 1980s to denote those elements of care that are the results of therapeutic relationships among client, client family, and care team members. High touch is embodied in the display of empathy, warmth, sensitivity, and human understanding, and the community health nurse learns to recognize these attributes in his or her therapeutic use of self. Technical care without comfort is sterile both psychologically and medically.

The concepts of "high touch" and "high tech" are discussed separately only for purposes of discussion and education. Unless these elements of care are delivered as a unit, neither is complete. The nature of high technology brought with it client fears of isolation and dependence. High touch removes the barrier created by a mechanical device simply by its existence in the client and client family's lives. Through high touch the community health nurse assists the client in demystifying equipment and procedures. Humor, playfulness, and appropriate irreverence can dispel the intimidation experienced by the client and care partner when first confronted by the products of advanced technology.

SERVICES AND SERVICE MODELS

Advanced technology in the home care setting includes any of the following services: apnea monitoring, aerosolized antibiotic therapy, chemotherapy, enteral therapy, hydration therapy, hyperalimentation, investigational drug therapy, pain management through patient controlled analgesia (PCA), parenteral therapy, phototherapy, and ventilator therapy.

This service listing is certain to expand annually as medical advances occur. Each of these therapies or modalities is delivered to the client in the home through the combined efforts of several product teams. The total service package includes the physical product being administered, the equipment necessary for the therapy, the soft goods or disposable supplies, the clinical managers, and the hands-on care givers. These components can all be provided in one of the following ways: by one agency, several cooperating agencies, or one agency acting as a coordinator of services. The type of service that the community health nurse encounters is the result of a variety of factors: health care corporation designs, local community traditions, available companies, payer contract preferences, physician preferences, and company client admission capabilities.

TEAM MEMBERS AND ROLES

Central to every health care team are the client and an available care giver. Because of the needs of acute illness, they are joined by an attending physician and one or more consulting physicians such as an oncologist, a surgeon, an anesthesiologist, or an infectious disease specialist. The community health nurse, clinical pharmacist, medical social worker, nutritionist, laboratory technician, medical equipment specialist, enteral/parenteral supplier, and delivery personnel complete the team.

Community Health Nurse

The community health nurse who uses high-technology equipment in the home setting has developed proficiency in the care of a variety of parenteral therapy infusion devices, as well as in the use of pumps, monitors, and ventilators. This nurse specialist is cross-trained in community health, oncology care, adult and pediatric care, and enteral and parenteral therapy. The high-tech nurse is a client teacher par excellence as well as client advocate. Other high-priority skills include thoroughness in documentation and clarity in verbal communication to provide telephone support and to make service calls to the client and care giver at home. The community health nurse's basic background will be enhanced by ongoing education to continue to develop skills in client assessment, education, and outcome measurement. Courses that develop adult education (androgogical) skills are particularly valuable (see Chapter 5). In the home the nurse becomes a confidante, a guide, a role model, and a teacher. The nursing role is one of collaborator, not controller.

Client assessments are expressed in the language of nursing diagnosis, and the nurse is alert to risk factors and the client's perception of them.

The community health nurse on the high-tech team is one of the main coordinators of care planning and delivery. The nurse coordinates the service visits, arranges for emergency or unscheduled visits, maintains supply inventory checks, obtains laboratory specimens, verifies the transmission of laboratory results, and keeps the client and client family updated on any therapy changes. Flexibility and the ability to improvise are key skills for this nurse.

Primary Physician

The primary physician has the ultimate responsibility for selecting the most efficacious therapy and presenting it to the client and client family for their approval. The physician is aided in this selection by conferring with either the acute hospital high-tech team or the home care specialist group. The findings and recommendations of the pharmacist and nutritionist are balanced with the assessments of the clinical nurse specialist and/or the medical social worker. The ready availability of the physician and the clinical coordination by the community nurse professional are central to the smooth functioning of any high-technology team. It is of central importance that the client and/or care giver be involved at the very start of therapy plan development.

Pharmacist

The pharmacist, on the basis of the therapy selected, is actively involved in making recommendations for therapeutic doses and methods of administration adjustments. Prompt receipt of and response to laboratory reports enable the physician and pharmacist to prevent treatment delays. Successful clinical pharmacists are skilled in team communication. They continually plan ahead and are watchful for opportunities to provide the client with economical choices. The pharmacist is a key advisor in developing dose schedules that balance the client's need for therapeutic drug levels with the need for rest.

Medical Social Worker

The medical social worker on the high-tech team pays particular attention to the assessment of the client's understanding of the goals of the therapy and of the client and client care partner suitability and ability to participate in the care being planned. The therapy may represent a disruption in family roles, in wage earning, or in the family or household routine. The medical social worker and the community health nurse often experience role-blurring. Both need to be attentive to their respective contributions on the team and candid with one another in planning their respective ongoing responsibilities to each client. One of the keys to success in intrateam communication is the willingness of each member to be responsible for very specific aspects of the client care plan. The client and client care giver usually choose specific team members to become their spokespersons. These choices may be altered at any time, depending on which topic the client or care partner considers of most importance. This intrateam communication is discussed further in the case studies.

Nutritionist

The nutritionist can be an active team member who works directly with the client or care giver or can function as a consultant. Some clients require diet planning for oral nutrition while hyperalimentation is being tapered. Others may need specific nutritional counseling to develop a diet that promotes wound healing or weight gain or that complies with specific intake restrictions such as the amount of protein per day or the amount of sodium per meal. Each type of high-technology care has a corresponding nutritional component. The community health nurse also must be mindful of the nutritional needs of the patient care giver.

Home Health Aide

The high-technology team may include a home health aide who provides personal-care assistance to the client. The aide also might assist the client with ambulation, exercises, and a skin care program. At times the aide may provide much-needed respite time for the client care giver. As a nonlicensed person on the team, the aide may be viewed by the client as a less threatening and more accessible person. The aide can contribute helpful perspectives on the client's experience of the therapy and can respond to some specific fears and questions.

On-Call Support

The community health nurse and physician have the main responsibility for on-call support of the client and care partner receiving high-tech services. Several nurses probably share this responsibility for 24-hour, 7-day-a-week support. In one staffing model, one or two nurses receive all the client's telephone calls. If telephone guidance is insufficient to meet the client's after-hour needs, the triage nurse contacts a nurse who is prepared to make a home visit. In another staffing model the triage and home visit roles are performed by the same on-call nurse. In either model the triage nurse is skilled in the clinical and equipment management aspects of the care. When equipment malfunctions occur, the nurse is expected to function as a trouble-shooter, as well as to arrange for any replacements. Patients who are dependent on ventilators, for example, should have very specific back-up systems in place before home therapy begins.

After-hours calls can reveal a great deal about the strengths and weaknesses of the client and client family, including knowledge deficits, ineffective coping mechanisms, and physical/emotional exhaustion. Previously unexpressed anxieties and misconceptions, self-doubt, spiritual distress, or alterations in thought process can surface in these late hours. The on-call nurse requires a unique blend of technical knowledge, warmth, and perception. The "after hours" assessments and interventions must be communicated promptly to the day team. Their content must be attended to carefully and thoroughly. It is a common temptation to view a nighttime panic call from a family member as "just testing the system." In reality the situation may be more involved and sometimes is relieved by the nurse guiding the care partner in expressing the natural fears experienced by any person in this role. By encouraging the verbalization of these fears, the nurse can work with the individual to develop responses to reduce the fears or control their potential source.

PLANNING FOR THE USE OF ADVANCED TECHNOLOGY IN THE HOME

The following is a partial listing of points to be considered in planning for the use of advanced technology in the home:

A. Complete information regarding the proposed therapy

- Purpose, desired therapeutic effect
- Classification by drug category and route of administration when applicable
- Experimental status of therapy; availability of complete protocol; client's informed consent
- Precautions; safety considerations for client client family and staff
- Special handling instructions; method of disposal of used products

B. Review of community standards, the record of the provider agency, and members' staff experience with the therapy
C. Evaluation of risks, untoward outcomes
D. Client and family eligibility criteria
E. Client discharge criteria
F. Client and family education components
G. Procedure for administration of therapy
H. Staff education program
I. Identification of equipment and materials required and their source
J. Reimbursement plans available and reimbursement experiences of other companies and insurers
K. Timetable for program and development and its implementation
L. Method of monitoring and evaluating the program

Attention is paid to each component to develop and deliver a therapy that promotes a therapeutic regimen for the client, satisfies community standards review, keeps risk to a minimum, and reduces the possibility of error or untoward outcome.

Company Development Support Staff

High-tech programs are enhanced by the ongoing support of program development staff members. This staff might include a nurse, a pharmacist, and a physician who are responsible for the preparation of care policies and procedures and, when appropriate, continuing revision. In addition, staff members create educational materials for the client and the client care partner. They may develop documentation systems, clinical record forms, and quality assurance audit tools. They pay particular attention to results of outcome-oriented documentation systems. Whenever a new clinical therapy is proposed, the program development staff evaluates the therapy for its suitability for home administration.

The community health nurse on the program development staff is both a nursing and a client advocate. On behalf of the nursing staff this nurse reviews all proposed procedures that use advanced technology to ensure their adherence to the following criteria:

- Congruity with the Nurse Practice Act
- Consistence with Community Standards of Practice for home care nursing
- Safeguards required to protect the nurse's physical safety
- Type of learning experiences required to develop or adapt present clinical skills to the delivery of the needed technology
- Means to determine clinical competency of staff
- Method of selecting clinical staff for implementation of technology
- System of annual review of clinical competency of staff

The maintenance of high-quality program development is costly. Some home care agencies elect to purchase development assistance as needed from a consulting service. Program manuals also can be purchased and adapted to local community practices. Another resource option is to maintain an in-house staff. Some teaching institutions and large or highly specialized physician groups collaborate in program development activities with drug manufacturers or home care companies as part of their work in research.

Clinical Laboratory Services

The high-technology teams' choice of clinical laboratories affects the community health nurse in several ways. As a general rule, laboratories are first selected by physicians and payers. Ideally both select on the basis of reliability of the testing results and the competitiveness of the pricing. Some laboratories offer a specimen pick-up service, which saves the nurse transportation time and may offer increased safety and efficiency in specimen handling. The community health nurse receives from the laboratory directions regarding collection procedures, specimen labeling, and storage instructions. Knowledge of all appropriate infection control measures is essential. The community health nurse is responsible for follow-up to obtain the laboratory results and to verify that physician and pharmacist (if a pharmacist is providing therapy consultation) receive these results. The home care company may use trained clerks to assist in this communication and documentation activity—among the most time-consuming and vexing aspects of the care delivery process. Time spent initially to ensure that each person understands and accepts his or her respective responsibilities in this area saves hours of time later. It also greatly reduces the possibility of error or reporting delays. Certainly the client at home will not appreciate learning when the nurse arrives that therapy cannot be administered because of delayed communication of laboratory results, which then requires the client to wait an additional period for pharmacy delivery.

Service Area Logistics

Chapter 16 discusses the need for the home health nurse to consider geographical and safety factors in planning and making home visits. When a client is being considered for admission to a high-technology program, these factors require even closer consideration. Time-specific high-technology therapies take additional planning to allow for service response time, both to initiate and to continue therapy. An interesting aspect is the nurse's discovery that the logistics of care delivery are more complex than the client care itself. If the therapy has been initiated in the acute care hospital, dosage times may have been set in terms of the therapeutic requirements and the hospital staffing plans. Transition to the home, however, may require alterations in the scheduling the day of transfer to accommodate the multiple factors of client arrival, care partner availability, supply and equipment delivery, and of high-tech availability personnel. It is not uncommon for the community health nurse to discover that the client and care giver are too exhausted by the trip home and their individual anxieties to be receptive to any but the most minimal of teaching periods when they first arrive home. This may leave them more dependent on the community health nurse for the initial care. These factors also can alter the amount of staff support that will be necessary in the first 72 hours of home care.

Once treatment has begun, it is imperative that the high-technology team continue to be cognizant of the local factors that can exercise rigid physical control over their service delivery and response systems. Contingency plans must be developed before emergency situations occur. Client and care giver must be instructed in measures to protect client safety.

Assessment of Client Eligibility

Admission of clients to a high-technology home program requires careful client and care giver assessment, as well as a thorough exchange of information among the high-tech team members. Although each type of therapy has unique specific admission critiera, some criteria for client selection can be generalized. It is important to note that selection criteria are an integral and essential part of any quality assurance program for the high-technology provider. Selection criteria are intended to ensure appropriate selection of clients, to reduce risk, to identify payment sources, and to comply with accepted community standards of practice. The criteria merit respect and acceptance by all parties in the care planning and delivery systems.

The community health nurse is the primary client advocate in the eligibility review process and reviews the client assessment data to ensure their validity. Overstatements of client ability or desire for the home care setting can result in the client's premature hospital discharge.

If the client arrives home before the client and care partner are cleared for acceptance by the high-tech team, a "catch up" state will exist. The dangers of this state include the following:

- Delayed learning by the client and/or care giver
- Confusion about responsibilities
- Added expectations of the on-call staff
- Possible gaps in the product and/or equipment set-up times

Client and care giver communication. Client assessment is concerned with the communication abilities of both client and care giver. If team members are not fluent in the client's primary language, appropriate written instructions and translators should be available to promote adequate explanation of and education for the particular therapy and/or equipment.

Client communication also includes consideration of physical and cognitive abilities such as sight, hearing, speech, and learning. Significant speech, vision, or hearing deficits can preclude the client's eligibility for a particular therapy unless the care partner is able to compensate for the client's deficits.

The delivery of home care may depend on a network of care givers that uses the skills and availabilities of several care givers. A young child may be able to receive care through the collaboration of one or both parents, a grandparent or neighbor, and an older sibling. One key to success with multiple care givers is the use of written task schedules and assignments. A daily diary of tasks performed can be kept by all parties to ensure the completion of the necessary tasks. A calendar such as the one shown in Table 18-1 can be developed and kept in the home. The more specific the calendar, times, days, and person responsible, the more likely the tasks will be performed and recorded. A calendar can free the client and care giver of the anxiety of wondering who is doing or who did the particular task. The community health nurse keeps a copy of the calendar as part of the medical record for guidance in planning service visits and for noting unscheduled visits or services. This type of record keeping can be invaluable when untoward outcomes

TABLE 18-1   Calendar kept by care givers

Day	Task	Person responsible
Monday	Blood work	Community health nurse
	Dressing change	Sue
	Infusions: 8 AM and 2 PM	Mom
Tuesday	Dressing change	Sue
Wednesday	Dressing change	Sue
	Cannula change	Community health nurse
Thursday	Blood work	Community health nurse
	Infusions: 8 AM and 2 PM	Community health nurse

occur. The trail of who did what when is best "mapped out" daily. Any changes in task, timetable, or person must be noted. This record is also of great importance to the on-call nurse.

Telephone access. Telephone access is of great importance to the client and care giver. This is a vital link in summoning assistance, in calling for additional supplies, and in informing the high-technology team coordinator of client absences for medical appointments. Because the client may need to request emergency assistance at any time, the ability to deliver high-technology care in a home without telephone access is unlikely. A simple thing such as placing the telephone near the patient is easily overlooked, and the use of answering devices must be checked to ensure that the client can answer the telephone.

Client learning assessment and teaching. The client assessment includes an evaluation of the client's problem-solving skills and ability to anticipate or prevent problems. The client's level of anxiety, emotional involvement in his or her own care, self-confidence, and manner of expressing needs, fears, and frustrations are assessed. The community health nurse will find that to be an effective teacher, one first must be a good learner. The nurse will be attune to his or her own learning style and expectations of others. Thus the nurse's goal is to obtain the following information:

- Does the client learn best by reading or by hands-on practice with the equipment and products?
- Does the client want a large amount of theory?
- Does the client prefer written or verbal cues?
- Does the client want to make notes and checklists or rely only on printed materials?
- Does the client readily ask questions and seek information?
- Does the client make light of more complex or serious aspects of care?
- Does the client have previous experience with home care?
- Does the client expect to succeed in learning new tasks?
- Does the client have great doubts about own ability or that of any of team members?
- Does client express anger, hostility, or powerlessness?
- Does client appear passive or overly submissive?
- Does client make excessive or inappropriate demands of care giver, nurse, or other team member?
- Does client appear to play one member of the team against another?

The community health nurse who begins any client teaching session will be sorting out all of the aforementioned client information. The nurse learns to identify behaviors, to seek explanations of their cause, and to validate findings with the client, client family, or other team member. Whatever occurs that impedes the learning must be considered in an effort to reduce or remove these roadblocks. Often the nurse will be involved in a "what if" exercise:

"What if the nurse is delayed in traffic. . . ?" The client should know how to reach a family member or a neighbor or simply to turn off a pump or call the on-call nurse.

"What if supply delivery is incomplete. . . ?" If the supply inventory is performed daily and a backup of items is already known, then the client can turn to the backup supplier and remedy the situation.

"What if I'm not well enough to do my part. . . ?" The nurse anticipates this very real fear and has contingency plans: temporary coverage by the nurse, by a family member or primary care giver, or by the physician's office nurse during a regularly scheduled office visit.

"What if I develop an infection? Who will I call. . . ?"

Therapy administration route. Client selection involves careful attention to the therapy administration route. Consideration should be given to the client activity level and to the type and duration of therapy. Venous access devices can provide long-term service with minimum discomfort and controlled risk of infection when the protocols are followed. If peripheral therapy is desired, adequate venous access must be available. Venous peripheral sites are changed every 48 to 72 hours unless there is reason to permit a longer period. Peripheral venous access is the route of choice for short-term therapy via a heparin lock to allow for intermittent drug administration.

Most often parenteral therapy is initiated in the acute hospital setting. Once client tolerance to the drug and drug dosage is determined and a therapeutic effect is being obtained, discharge to the home can be planned. The client's response to therapy should demonstrate that a continued stable clinical status can be anticipated after the client is home. With the use of appropriate diagnostic monitoring, such as urinalysis, white blood cell counts, and peak and trough drug levels, the client's condition can be assessed and evaluated for home care. Before discharge the client on a parenteral medication regimen should receive that medication for a sufficient number of dosages to demonstrate a positive treatment response and a lack of uncontrollable adverse side effects. The client and client family are counting on a smooth course of care once implementation of the discharge plan begins.

Guidelines for determining a significant therapeutic response include but are not limited to the following conditions:

- Lack of fever for 24 to 48 hours
- Decreased sedimentation rate
- Decreased white blood cell count
- Decreased tissue inflammation if present at the start of therapy
- Medication blood levels within the normal therapeutic range before patient is discharged for home care

The high-technology home care team has the responsibility for communicating these factors to the inpatient care team well in advance of the discharge date determination. Plans for discharge from an acute hospital should begin on the day of admission to hospital.

For the client receiving hyperalimentation, either parenteral or enteral, glucose and insulin balance and documented lipid metabolism should be stable before the discharge is set in motion. Home monitoring methods must be chosen and established.

A number of clinical situations can develop after the client is at home that may call for the initiation of parenteral therapy in the home without a visit to the physician's office or outpatient clinic. Therapy can be ordered by the physician on the basis of the nurse's assessment or laboratory findings, or both. The following situations provide examples:

- Influenza accompanied by severe diarrhea may require hydration and electrolyte replacement.
- A child with cystic fibrosis who has a recurrent respiratory infection may require a course of antibiotic therapy and additional pulmonary care measures.
- A young adult with multiple sclerosis and a persistent urinary tract infection may require continuous bladder irrigations with antibiotic solutions.
- A person with acquired immune deficiency syndrome (AIDS) with recurrent pneumonia may require hydration, intravenous antibiotics, and aerosolized treatments.
- A terminally ill client may require hydration or pain control, or both.

These examples point out the variety of conditions and ages of clients. Many already will have had one or more courses of parenteral antibiotic therapy. The community health nurse researches the client's prior history and response to the previous therapies. For some clients therapy is delivered at school or at a work site, as well as at home.

Drug therapy restrictions. The majority of high-technology teams have specific limitations regarding which drugs can be initiated in the home setting. Certainly a client with a history of allergies to one or several antibiotics would not be a candidate for the initial dosage of an antibiotic to be administered in the home. For specific drugs the first dosage requires administration in a supervised setting such as the hospital outpatient clinic, emergency room, or physician's office. The box below lists the parenteral antibiotics that require first-dosage administration in a controlled setting for signs of an allergic reaction (type one antibiotics) and those that can be initiated in the home without prior administration in a controlled setting (type two antibiotics). In these cases the acceptable standard of community practice is for the community health nurse to remain in the home for at least 30 minutes after completing the infusion of medication, with an anaphylaxis kit at hand. Follow-up doses may be prescribed that continue for more than 2-hour periods.

In many cases of terminal illness, it would be inappropriate to transfer the client to the hospital to administer the first dose of parenteral morphine. Community health nurses who work in the specialty field of hospice or terminal care are trained specifically in the initiation of and ongoing use of morphine therapy. The boxes on p. 393-394 summarizes the elements of client selection, physician orders, community health nurse competency, and treatment protocol discussed in this chapter.

Medication and solution storage. Plans for storing medications and fluids that require

---

TYPE ONE AND TYPE TWO ANTIBIOTICS

Type one antibiotics (must be initiated in a supervised setting)

Amphotericin B
Ampicillin
Azlocillin
Bactrim
Carbenicillin
Cefamandole
Cefazolin
Cefonicid
Cefoperazone
Cefotan
Cefotaxime
Cefoxitin
Ceftazidime
Ceftizoxime
Ceftriaxone
Cefuroxime
Cephalothin
Cephapirin
Cephradine
Erythromycin
Imipen–cilastatin sodium (Primaxin)
Kanamycin
Methicillin
Metronidazole (Flagyl)

Mezlocillin
Monocid
Moxalactam
Nafcillin
Oxacillin
Penicillin G
Piperacillin
Sulfamethoxazole
Ticarcillin (Timentin)
Trimethoprim
Unasyn

Type two antibiotics (may be initiated in client's home)

Acyclovir
Amikacin
Aztreonam
Chloramphenicol
Clindamycin
Gentamicin
Netilmicin
Pentamidine (Pentam)
Streptomycin
Tobramycin
Vancomycin
Vibramycin

STANDARDIZED PROCEDURE FOR INTRAVENOUS AND CONTINUOUS SUBCUTANEOUS ADMINISTRATION OF OPIATES AND NARCAN

Policy

A. The following procedures are performed as part of the standardized procedure for intravenous and continuous subcutaneous administration of opiates and Narcan:
   1. Venipuncture for IV cannula insertion.
   2. IV infusion through cannula.
   3. Heparinization of IV cannula.
   4. Removal of IV cannula.
   5. IV infusion through Broviac/Hickman catheter.
   6. Heparinization of Broviac/Hickman catheter.
   7. Care and maintenance of subclavian catheter central venous line.
   8. Administration of IV medication through a Port-A-Cath Subcutaneous Injection Port.
   9. Administration of opiates via continuous IV drip.
   10. Administration of opiates via IV push.
   11. Administration of continuous subcutaneous opiates.
   12. Administration of intravenous Narcan.
   13. Administration of subcutaneous Narcan.

B. Administration of intravenous and continuous subcutaneous opiates shall be limited to morphine sulfate and Dilaudid.

C. Only registered nurses who have satisfactorily completed all educational and performance criteria listed in the IV manual and who have received written approval from the agency may perform this procedure.

D. Intravenous/continuous subcutaneous opiates and Narcan may be administered by certified registered nurses only under the following conditions:
   1. The patient shall meet the general criteria for admission to the agency.
   2. Patients will have a malignant condition with limited life expectancy.
   3. Under most circumstances other methods of pain control have proven ineffective.
   4a. Patient and family desires for resuscitation have been discussed with them and their resuscitation wishes are documented.
   4b. The physician confirms either "do not resuscitate" status (requiring documentation by RN on the treatment plan or on a supplemental MD order) or "resuscitate" status (not requiring supplemental MD order).
   5. IV or continuous subcutaneous opiate therapy shall be initiated when possible in the hospital setting and the patient should be on a controlled dosage for 24 hours prior to discharge, subject to the exceptions listed below:
      a. An agency-certified private duty RN is available in the home during administration of IV or continuous subcutaneous opiates for the first 24 hours *and*
      b. The patient has been managed previously with optimum doses of class II narcotics without evidence of adverse reaction.
   6. The patient must have a competent full-time primary caregiver or 24-hour/day agency-certified private duty RN in the home subject to exceptions listed below (the competency of the patient caregiver shall be determined by agency personnel):

Courtesy Hospital Home Health Care Agency of California.

Continued.

STANDARDIZED PROCEDURE FOR INTRAVENOUS AND CONTINUOUS SUBCUTANEOUS ADMINISTRATION OF OPIATES AND NARCAN—cont'd

   a. Agency staff have assessed patient and caregiver independence in procedure of IV/continuous subcutaneous administration of opiates and Narcan at home *and*
   b. This patient caregiver is present for a significant portion of every day *and*
   c. The patient's pain is controlled on a relatively stable opiate dose for 24-48 hours *and*
   d. The patient is not experiencing clinically significant adverse effects to the opiate.
      NOTE: Should the opiate require significant titrations at any time while on service, or should the patient's condition deteriorate, the agency reserves the right to again require the 24-hour presence in the home of a responsible caregiver.

 7a. The home care RN must make daily visits to assess ongoing patient status and patient caregiver compliance with instructions by agency personnel, unless there is a 24-hour/day certified private duty RN in the home, until the patient caregiver can perform independent return demonstrations of all necessary procedures.

 7b. Telephone contact by the RN must be made daily until the patient's desired level of analgesia is achieved, unless there is an agency-certified private duty RN in the patient's home 24 hours/day.

  8. Hospice and agency-certified private duty RNs may titrate IV and continuous subcutaneous opiates within a range prescribed by the patient's physician.

  9. Medical/surgical registered nurses must have specific MD orders each time intravenous or continuous subcutaneous opiates require adjustment.

 10. Narcan, and orders for Narcan administration, including dosage parameters per agency procedure, must be in the home prior to initiating IV/continuous subcutaneous opiates unless:
      a. An order not to resuscitate is obtained from the attending MD *and*
      b. An order not to give Narcan is obtained from the attending MD *and*
      c. The patient and family are in agreement with the above.

E. A physician must be notified under the following circumstances:
   1. If the patient's primary care giver is determined to be incapable of monitoring the safe administration of IV or continuous subcutaneous opiates.
   2. Pain control is not effective and a change in orders is required.
   3. When the patient or PCG [patient care giver] titrates pain medication upward beyond MD orders obtained by nurse.
   4. When an adverse reaction is suspected, i.e., *sudden, unexpected, acute, clinically significant changes* such as cyanosis, decreased respirations, changes in mental status, drop in blood pressure, cardiac irregularities.
   5a. When opiate toxicity is suspected, i.e., *sudden, unexpected, acute, clinically significant changes* such as coma, severe respiratory depression, skeletal muscle flaccidity, hypotension, bradycardia, convulsions (in infants and children), and cardiac arrest.
   5b. When Narcan is administered.

refrigeration or protection from light need to be developed before delivery can be made. Many medical supply or infusion therapy companies provide under-the-counter refrigerator units for drug and solution storage in the home.

   Drug therapy dosage schedules. The client and client family will be interviewed by the community health nurse to verbalize their preference regarding drug therapy time tables. Their need for rest, privacy, and handling of other responsibilities is to be considered before a drug therapy schedule is established.

A 6 AM to noon and 6 PM to midnight schedule usually is preferable to an 8 AM to 2 PM and 8 PM to 2 AM schedule, which would result in the client being awakened in the middle of the night for the 2 AM dose. Some drug regimens can combine nighttime dosages of an oral antibiotic and daytime infusion dosages. The community health nurse as the client advocate must remain sensitive to this area of client and care partner consideration.

Criteria exceptions

Exceptions request procedure. Many high-technology programs maintain an exceptions request procedure to review request for waiver of one or more admission criteria. This review process is intended to allow preapproved flexibility when it can be established that a substitute arrangement accomplishes the intent of the original criterion—for example, waiving the requirement that a community health nurse be present in the home for the first 24-hour period if the patient is receiving total parenteral nutrition (TPN) for the first time. This exception could be made if it can be verified, for example, that the client's sister and neighbor have had recent TPN administration experience as registered nurses at the local hospital and will be taking turns attending the client during the first 24-hour period at home. The intent of the admission standard is to respect the degree of risk to the client when TPN is initiated in the home. The unpredictable timing of an untoward reaction to the therapy supports the policy of requiring the presence of the experienced nurse for the first 24 hours.

Client with history of substance abuse. Eligibility criteria include assessment of any substance abuse in the client who is being considered for home parenteral therapy. Consider, for example, the client with a gunshot wound to the abdomen who has a documented history of parenteral drug abuse. The physician is considering client discharge to the home with a venous access device in place and a remaining 10- to 21-day course of intravenous antibiotic therapy.

A preadmission protocol would be developed for such a client as follows:

1. Physician or home care company is required to inform client of the following:
   - Any evidence of illicit use of the venous access device will be cause for immediate discharge from home care.
   - Any evidence of illicit use of prescribed or nonprescribed drugs will be cause for immediate discharge from home care.
   - Weekly supervised urine specimen collection will be required during the course of the therapy.
   - Client will sign a contract agreeing to these stipulations.

2. Home care team will receive copy of the signed client contract and will carry out its responsibilities for client assessment, specimen collection, and physician notification of any untoward findings.

Such a protocol is designed to protect the home infusion program and to promote client compliance with these safeguards. The intention of high-technology programs is not to tell clients how to live but to deliver a clear message concerning acceptable client behavior for admission to the home infusion program. As one physician expressed it, "The client is free to choose to honor the contract . . . or to break the contract and thereby choose not to receive the therapy."

Many community health nurses find it difficult to accept the right of clients with a history of substance abuse to home care under any circumstances. The nurse must realize that a client history of undesirable behavior should not be the basis for discrimination.

In the event that the client does not honor the contract, the nurse will document the facts and inform the physician and client of the client's discharge. If the physician requests that the nurse remove the client's venous access device, this is done only with the client's consent. If the client refuses, the nurse documents this refusal and informs the physician and infusion company.

Frequently the client with a history of substance abuse lives in a neighborhood of questionable safety. For some nurses, concern for their personal safety is the larger issue.

Payment for High-Technology Home Care

High-technology teams and the community health nurse are well versed in the limitations of insurance coverage and the client's potential financial liability for nonreimbursable care and services. The three main types of insurance that address the expense of high-technology care in the home are private insurance (includes employer-paid group health, client paid individual policy, preferred provider organizations, and health maintenance organizations), Medicare, and Medicaid (MediCal in California).

Each of these payment sources has its own eligibility criteria, payment authorization system, medical record review process, benefits exclusions, payment denial, and appeal mechanisms. The community health nurse needs to know how these apply to each client, in order to answer client questions and to be aware of the financial factors that can limit future technological applications for each client.

Private insurance policies rarely provide coverage for the administration of experimental drug therapy even when the drug manufacturer makes the drug available at no cost. If the dose or route of administration of the drug is deemed experimental, this may negate insurance reimbursement.

Medicare. Medicare provides the following types of coverage for high-technology home care:

- Approved total parenteral nutrition
- Drugs and solutions as part of an approved plan of treatment for an enrollee qualified to receive hospice benefits (only those drugs and solutions related to the terminal condition)
- Home care nursing services for approved physician-ordered enteral and parenteral therapies *excluding* the cost of drugs and most solutions and all biological agents
- Disposable supplies such as tubings used in these therapies

The Medicare Conditions of Participation require that the provider of intravenous medications must use only the services of registered nurses who meet specified requirements in terms of education, experience, and proficiency. These requirements are consistent with the standards of practice for general home care issued by the Intravenous Nursing Society (INS) and are similar to the Nurse Practice Act requirements of most states. Community health nurses can be confident that these minimum standards are not only high but will stand the test of time.

Acute care hospitals faced with reimbursement restrictions established by the diagnosis-related group payment formula occasionally elect to bear the expense of drug therapy in the home to enable earlier discharge of the client. This arrangement spares the Medicare beneficiary the cost of the drugs and solutions, and the Medicare home-care benefit covers the cost of the home therapy administration visits by community health nurses. The hospital then is saved the high cost of continuing acute care room and board.

TPN has been a Medicare-reimbursable service since the late 1970s. Medicare coverage requires that the beneficiary have a permanently inoperative or malfunctional internal body organ. The test of permanence will be met if at the initiation of treatment, the medical record indicates that the condition is not temporary; that is, the functional impairment will extend beyond 3 months. The test of permanence is also considered to be met if a terminally ill client's medical record indicates that the condition is neither temporary nor reversible on the basis of the facts of the particular case. Daily parenteral nutrition is considered reasonable and necessary for a client with a severe pathological condition of the alimentary tract that does not allow absorption of sufficient nutrients to maintain weight and strength commensurate with the client's general condition. These diagnoses may include short bowel syndrome, major bowel resection, mesenteric infarction, radiation enteritis, inflammatory bowel syndrome, intestinal obstruction, or motility disorders. These same tests are used by most private insurance plans to determine coverage for TPN and parental enteral nutrition (PEN).

Since its inception in 1965, Medicare has been modified by congressional action almost annually. The community health nurse should work actively for the continual monitoring and modification of the Medicare benefit package to ensure that it keeps pace with the technological developments of health care.

Medicaid. Medicaid covers only those medications on its approved drug list and only at its levels of payment rates. It also covers minimal quantities of supplies and only generic types of equipment. Home care companies are not required to accept Medicaid clients. Most high-technology agencies, however, do accept either all Medicaid referrals or a percentage based on a number that their operating margins will permit. Medicaid historically never pays true cost. The operating loss must be recouped from other payers or funding sources or absorbed by the agency.

Again, the community health nurse needs to be mindful of the client's reimbursement source so as to jeopardize neither the client's nor the provider's economic rights. Any client payment responsibility must be disclosed to the client before the initiation of the therapy.

Health maintenance organizations. Most high-technology therapies and equipment are fully reimbursed if the enrollee in the health maintenance organization (HMO) has the necessary medical condition and physician certification. The HMO enrollee enters a type of health care bartering system, exchanging increased levels of coverage and decreased out-of-pocket expenses for a reduction of choices in providers (physician, facilities, and pharmacies). The HMO enrollee usually is required to have at least one second opinion for surgeries and high-cost therapies. There may be waiting periods or required trial periods with alternative therapies before programs such as in-home TPN can be initiated.

Private insurance and managed care. Managed care in its ideal form is a system in which the payer has an identified service utilization unit that includes knowledgeable community health nurses who are responsible for identifying care operations and for performing prior authorizations for services to be performed by contracted health care companies. Managed care offers the community health nurse in home care another area of responsibility. This community health nurse will prepare reports for the managed care representatives and also may supply weekly or monthly summaries of client care status. These summaries may be both verbal and written and may include reports from the entire team. The high-technology team usually reviews the overall plan of treatment and these progress reports, whereas the community health nurse may be the person designated to track the prior authorizations received for the ongoing client care.

Legal Issues

National standards of practice for high-technology home care provide methods for reducing legal liabilities for companies, their personnel, and the client. Company policies and procedures are companion pieces that serve to ensure safe practice and to define the responsibilities of the high-technology team member, as well as those of the client and care partner.

Informed consent. The informed consent document and its presentation to the client for signature must not be completed in haste. The client must have the opportunity to ask questions and to receive answers to all of them. The client's rights and responsibilities should be presented at the time that informed consent is being obtained. A generic form is available for purchase from the National Association for Home Care.

The community health nurse usually is one of the first persons who earns the client's trust. In this relationship the nurse encourages the proper exploration of information regarding treatment ramifications and alternatives on behalf of the client. It must be stressed that no treatment can be initiated before the informed consent is signed. Frequently this requires advance planning to ensure that the care partner or significant other is present in the home for initial visit by the high-technology company's representative to the prospective client. It never is acceptable for the nurse to yield to the client's request that care be given inasmuch as "my daughter will sign the consent when she comes tomorrow."

Proper validation is required if the client's care decisions are under the control of a care partner who has received the client's durable power of attorney for health care. State laws concerning this practice vary.

"Do not resuscitate" orders. It is wise to determine the client's desires regarding resuscitation and/or intubation interventions. This issue requires skillful handling. Most high-technology team members profit from role-playing sessions to develop the necessary interpersonal skills for presenting this area to the client for decision making. It is much less alarming to discuss this with the client when a life-threatening situation is not imminent. Ideally, the client's physician would discuss this matter at the beginning of their relationship, not at a crisis point in the client's care. The signed physician's order regarding the resuscitation plan must be included in the client's medical record, and a copy should be readily available in the client's home.

Noncompliance. Client or care partner noncompliance must be addressed during the preadmission period. This is the time for the community health nurse or other team member to identify examples of noncompliance and their consequences. If noncompliance alters the therapeutic outcome or threatens any involved party's safety, the consequence usually is cessation of the therapy and discharge of the client from the home care service.

The community health nurse has a responsibility to investigate any episodes of noncompliance by the client and/or care partner to determine the risk established by the noncompliance. Examples of noncompliance include the following:

- Cancellation of needed laboratory work; refusal to permit specimen collection
- Refusal to safeguard supplies; unexplained shortages in sensitive areas of supply count (e.g., syringes and drugs)
- Refusal to perform dressing changes as taught and/or as frequently as taught
- Failure to report missed intravenous antibiotics (IVABX) doses by self or family member
- Failure to keep appointments with physician

Payer denials and client appeals. Third-party payer limits may present areas of legal liability and conflict. The client's right to be informed of any and all financial liabilities must be attended to before any financial liability occurs for the client. Most payers have a provision that allows them to deny reimbursement on the basis of medical reviews that determine whether rendered services are clinically appropriate. There usually is a process

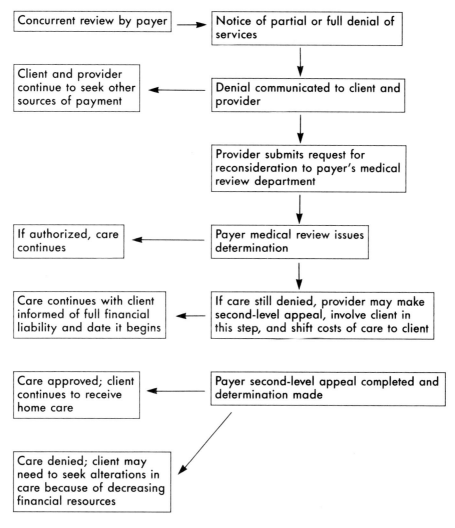

FIG. 18-1 Denials and appeals process.

to request a reconsideration if a denial is made (Fig. 18-1). The continuance of service during the appeal may place both client and company in a position of financial jeopardy. The client should be informed of the company's method of handling appeals and the policy regarding delivery of services while an appeal is under consideration. It is the unknown and the unclear that sets up grounds for legal action. Again, the high-technology team must plan ahead and inform the client in a timely manner at all times. This includes informing the client at the time of admission regarding the program's policy on appeals and denials.

The client can dispute either the high-technology company's plan and/or the medical plan for client discharge. The client's own avenue of appeal must be known by the client and duly carried out. This process could involve an internal committee review, for example, by the company's utilization review committee or by an independent party.

DIAGNOSES APPROPRIATE FOR HOME INFUSION THERAPY

Home antibiotic therapy

Abscess
AIDS-related opportunistic infections
Acute leukemia
Bacteremia
Bacterial endocarditis
Candidal endocarditis
Cellulitis
Chronic urinary tract infections
Cystic fibrosis
Fungal infections (local and systemic)
Otitis media
Osteomyelitis
Pelvic inflammatory disease
Peritonitis
Pneumonia
Prostatis
Pyelonephritis
Sepsis
Septic arthritis
Sinusitis
Wound infection

Home parenteral nutrition

AIDS-related enteropathy
Biliary atresia
Biliary cirrhosis
Bowel obstruction
Cancer:
    Abdomen
    Bladder
    Colon
    Liver
    Pancreas
    Stomach
Chronic renal failure
Colitis
Congenital bowel malfunction
Crohn's disease
Cystic fibrosis
Enterocutaneous fistula
Failure to thrive
Gastroenteritis
Hirschsprung's disease
Hyperemesis gravidarum
Inflammatory bowel disease
Intractable diarrhea
Ischemic bowel disease
Malnutrition
Motility disorders

Pancreatitis
Pseudoobstruction
Short bowel syndrome
Sprue

Home chemotherapy

Carcinoma:
    Breast, esophagus, lung, pancreas
    Gastrointestinal tract (colorectal, anal, gastric)
    Head, neck, lung, cervix
    Ovaries, testicles
    Germ cell neoplasms
Histoplasmosis
Leukemias
Lymphomas
Sarcomas
Small cell carcinoma of the lung
Squamous cell carcinoma of the lung, cervix, head,
    or neck

Home pain management

Chronic intractable pain caused by:
    Carcinomas and lymphomas (combined with
        chemotherapy)
    AIDS and related diagnoses
    End-stage cardiac disease and related angina

Home hydration therapy

Fluid and electrolyte imbalance caused by:
    Dehydration in terminal care
    Gastroenteritis
    Gastrointestinal dysfunction
    Hyperemesis
    Intractable diarrhea
    Short bowel syndrome

Intravenous drug therapy

AIDS-related opportunistic infections
Cardiac retention—end-stage renal disease
End-stage cardiac disease (dobutamine, furose-
    mide [Lasix])
High-risk pregnancy
Methcillin resistant staph aureous (MSRA)
Multiple sclerosis

Transfusion therapy

Anemia
Ante partum
Hemophilia
Leukemia

The national network of peer review organizations provides an independent mechanism to which a client can appeal for review of care or discharge actions.

Client discharge. The company and the community health nurse are cognizant of the client or care partner's inclination to view service discharge actions as "client abandonment." This interpretation is less apt to occur if the nurse has kept the client informed of the nature, frequency, and duration of the services to be provided. Adequate time must be given to the preparation of the client and care partner for client discharge.

It is advisable to put the discharge plan in writing. The plan must document ongoing arrangements for care, if needed, source of equipment, supplies, and physician responsible for medical care. The payer frequently requests a copy of this plan.

High Technology in Home Care

Infusion therapy

General indications. Home infusion therapy may be initiated for a wide variety of conditions, as shown in the box on p. 400. Types of infusion therapy include antibiotic therapy, TPN, chemotherapy, pain management, hydration therapy, transfusion therapy, and intravenous drug therapy. The indications for infusion therapy and client eligibility factors to consider were discussed earlier in this chapter.

Client education. The community health nurse, after determining the type of infusion therapy to be initiated, should assess the knowledge base of the client and client family concerning the procedure. The following elements must be clearly understood before the procedure can begin without 24-hour supervision by a registered nurse:

1. The preparation and administration of the IV medication or fluid
2. The care and storage of the equipment and medication
3. Maintenance of a clean environment in the area surrounding the client
4. Maintenance of a sterile environment while during the procedure around the administration site
5. Any complications that might develop during therapy

In addition, the community health nurse must stress the importance of contacting the 24-hour, on call IV nurse if a problem arises. The telephone number of the local hospital emergency room should also be given to the client and client family.

Apnea monitoring

General indications. This therapy is designed to monitor the client (usually an infant) in whom autonomic respiratory regularity is absent or delayed. Apneic episodes can trigger cardiac arrest or irreversible cardiac arrythmia, or both, which will result in cardiopulmonary arrest and death (see box on p. 402).

Client education. If the client is an infant or a toddler, the recipient of education is the parent or other family member such as a grandparent or baby sitter. The following elements must be addressed in the education program:

1. Care and use of the apnea monitor
2. Electrical safety; battery checks; equipment maintenance
3. Respiratory assessment; early detection of signs and symptoms of infection
4. Correct application of the monitor; use of event-recording devices
5. Demonstration of competency; independence in one- or two-person cardiopulmonary resuscitation (CPR)
6. Reports to physician, pediatrician, etc.
7. Travel precautions

CRITERIA FOR ADMISSION TO THE APNEA MONITORING PROGRAM

1. Patient resides in geographic area served by Hospital Home Health Care Agency of California and meets the general criteria for admission.
2. Apnea monitoring must be prescribed by the patient's physician.
3. Parents are able and willing to comply with monitoring program.
4. Parents must demonstrate independence in infant cardiopulmonary resuscitation (CPR).
5. Parents must have previous instruction in use and maintenance of monitoring device.
6. Parents must have a telephone in the home.

Courtesy Hospital Home Health Care Agency of California.

The community health nurse who serves clients who require apnea monitoring will receive education from the supplier of the apnea monitor. Each monitor has certain unique characteristics and comes with an instruction manual.

Because apneic episodes are potentially life threatening, the community health nurse will be sensitive to the emotional burden on the care giver, especially when this person is a parent or grandparent. In addition to providing opportunities to express fears, the nurse may suggest that the parent consider membership in a parent support group. This can provide additional education, emotional support, and even child care networking.

The nurse also helps the care partners find ways to balance their many responsibilities to family, to other children, to work, and to client care. Frequently the family needs permission not to do it all themselves. The nurse can help arrange for respite care.

One point must be stressed: all involved in the care must know exactly when the client is to be monitored. No one can be allowed to break the rules. For example, Grandma cannot remove the monitor just to take the child next door or to someone else's home if continuous monitoring is required.

Many infants will progress developmentally and thus outgrow their need for continuous monitoring. Generally there is need only for sleep-time monitoring by the age of 12 or 16 months.

Phototherapy

General indications. The infant who has neonatal jaundice may require phototherapy in the hospital, as well as for a brief period in the home. A reliable adult care giver must be present during the administration of the therapy in the home (see box on p. 403).

Client education. The community health nurse will be educating the client's (child) parents or other designated care giver. If the parents are absent during the day, the nurse will ensure that parents have an "authorization to trust" consent form on file at the nearest emergency room and at the attending physician's office, and a copy must be available to the home phototherapy staff.

The education of the client family addresses the set up of the equipment, the preparation of the infant, the application of protective eye coverings and removal of all clothing, including diaper, and the amount of time to be spent under the phototherapy lights.

A relatively new device, the Wallaby, is a fiber-optic device that eliminates the need for eye coverings and infant nudity. While wrapped in the Wallaby blanket, the infant can be held and/or fed. This device is an excellent example of the melding of high-tech and high-touch elements of care to achieve an effective therapeutic response.

CRITERIA FOR ADMISSION TO THE HOME PHOTOTHERAPY PROGRAM

1. The infant must meet the Hospital Home Health Care Agency of California's general criteria.
   a. Physician's order
   b. Source of payment
   c. Resides in geographic area served by the Agency
2. A reliable and compliant caregiver must be present in the home, providing constant supervision of the infant under phototherapy.
3. The infant must have undergone a standard clinical and laboratory evaluation to rule out pathologic jaundice and a diagnosis of physiologic jaundice must have been made by the physician.
4. The caregiver must be free of significant language barrier. For example, if not English speaking must have translator present during nursing visits.
5. The caregiver must have access to a telephone.
6. The infant must be full-term and appropriate for gestational age of 37 weeks or greater by obstetrical dating and a weight ranging between 4 and 10 pounds.
7. Five-minute Apgar score of 7 or greater.
8. The infant must have normal findings on physical examination.
9. The infant must be actively feeding.
10. The infant must have stooled and voided by 36 hours of age.
11. The infant must be greater than 48 hours of age, but less than 7 days of age at the initiation of phototherapy.
12. Serum bilirubin levels at the initiation of therapy must fall within the following levels:
    a. 10-15 mgm/100 ml at age 2 days
    b. 13-17 mgm/100 ml at age 3 days
    c. 14-18 mgm/100 ml at age 4 days
    d. 15-18 mgm/100 between the ages of 5 and 7 days

Courtesy Hospital Home Health Care Agency of California.

Ventilator therapy

General indications. The home care client may require ventilator-assisted care for any of the following conditions: lung failure, chronic dypsnea, respiratory arrest, fibrosis, complex pneumonia, emphysema, pulmonary edema of cardiac or noncardiac origin, chest wall defects, central degeneration, pulmonary parenchymal diseases, and spinal cord defects.

Clinical findings suggesting that a client is a candidate for home care management include the following:

- Ventilator settings are unchanged (or relatively unchanged during the previous week).
- Blood gas levels and acid-base studies show minimal fluctuations.
- Pulmonary function is unchanged; that is, client is able to maintain spontaneous ventilatory parameters.
- Infection is absent.
- Client's other conditions are stable.
- Client's functional abilities are not deteriorating.
- Client has demonstrated a balance in self-dependence and has a reliable care partner.

Client education. The community health nurse builds on the teaching plan begun in the hospital for the client and care partner (see box on p. 404).One key interface in

---

VENTILATOR HOME CARE TEACHING TOPICS

Goal of ventilator therapy
Disease process
Medications
Early detection of complications (infection, bronchospasm, excessive secretions)
Breathing control
Work simplification and energy conservation
Nutrition and hydration
Equipment maintenance
Suctioning, tracheostomy care
Support groups

---

the process is the final learner evaluation prepared by the hospital staff. Ideally, the community health nurse will make one or more hospital visits before discharge to meet the client and care partner(s); to become familiar with the specific elements of the client's care and specific equipment to be used in the home; and to validate the preparedness for the initiation of home care.

The client's psychological, emotional, social, and physical needs will continue to be intertwined at home, just as they were in the hospital. The client family will have related needs, as well as a life of their own. It is the community health nurse's task to keep the care plan evolving in a way that acknowledges and responds to all of these complex needs. Teaching plan goals include (1) prevention of potential infections caused by loss of normal airway clearance mechanisms and (2) client/care giver independence in tracheostomy care, ventilator checks, ventilator troubleshooting, suctioning manual resuscitation, and equipment cleaning.

APPLICATION OF THE NURSING PROCESS
Case Study Assessment

Vincent is a 45-year-old, married man with three children. Diagnoses are metastatic carcinoma of the right jaw, scalp, and lungs; and primary fibrosarcoma of the left thigh 2 years ago.

When the community health nurse received this profile, she was informed that Vincent was to leave the acute care hospital in 2 days with a Hickman catheter in place for future chemotherapy. His prognosis is listed as fair. Reimbursement is from employer-sponsored private insurance, which uses a case management firm to broker the health benefits.

The physical assessment indicates that the client has no fever. His heart rate is 80 beats per minute and blood pressure is 120/82 mm Hg; he has a regular respiration rate of 20 breaths per minute. Vincent is experiencing poor endurance; ambulation of about 30 feet leaves him weak and fatigued. His bowel movements are irregular, his appetite fair, and he describes his digestion as bothersome. He rates his generalized pain as a 6 on a scale of 1 to 10. Sleep is "so-so" in his words.

Nursing Diagnosis

On the basis of this assessment, the nurse formulated the following nursing diagnoses:

- Alteration in self-concept, powerlessness
- Alteration in family process
- Alteration in parenting

- Realization of future loss—grieving
- Spiritual distress
- Impaired social interaction
- Alteration in comfort—risk for acute and chronic pain
- Alteration in bowel elimination
- Potential for alteration in sexual function
- Risk for alteration in skin integrity
- Alteration in nutritional ability

Planning

The nurse who performed the initial visit develped the following care plan:

1. Nurse to assess all vital signs, to inspect Hickman site each visit, and to report significant abnormalities to the physician
2. Nurse to instruct/evaluate client and care partner in one or more of the following areas each visit until they can verbalize adequate knowledge:
   A. Hickman catheter care per agency protocol
   B. Medication regimen, including purpose, dose, and side effects
   C. Side effects of chemotherapy
   D. Self-management of pain control techniques
   E. Bowel regimen
   F. Daily food and fluid intake

Implementation

The nurse will develop a client and care giver teaching plan to cover these items and to measure their proficiency. The on-call system will be explained and demonstrated. The client can expect two or more visits the first week to focus on the teaching and to confirm the client's baseline data. The physical therapist will be asked to evaluate the client and to develop a simple home exercise program to promote energy conservation, to attempt endurance improvement, and to promote safety in ambulation and transfers.

The psychosocial, spiritual assessment may be initiated on the first client and client family contact. The plan of care to address their respective needs will evolve in the team planning conferences.

Mundane tasks such as supply and equipment deliveries and inventories need attention during the first visit. A support telephone call within 12 hours of the first home visit helps the client and care partner to settle in and to clarify their short-term expectations of the high-technology program.

Evaluation

At the end of the first month of home care, the client's condition appeared to have stabilized. The Hickman site was patent and free of infection. Vital signs were as follows: blood pressure, 120/80 mm Hg; pulse, 80 beats per minute; and respirations, 18 per minute and unlabored. The client had no fever, and the skin was intact. Vincent ambulated independently within his residence, and he needed standby assistance only on stairs and with car transfer. Pain was controlled by oral analgesics, was rated as 3 on a scale of 1 to 10. Vincent reported sleeping 5 to 6 hours without waking. Bowel evacuation is regular every other day, and he controls flatulence with slightly increased activity in the home. The client summed up his status in the following words: "I'm living on borrowed time and holding my own." Chemotherapy was to begin in 1 week if laboratory values were determined as being acceptable.

SUMMARY

The delivery of advanced technology care in the home relies on the skills and ingenuity of community health nurses. The nurse's ability to perform thorough client and care giver assessments and to provide effective client and care giver education are the keystones to the safe delivery of home infusion therapy, apnea monitoring, phototherapy, ventilator care, and other forms of advanced technology.

CHAPTER HIGHLIGHTS

- The integration of high touch in high-technology care is accomplished by the community health nurse who understands the inseparability of the two.
- The home can be the site of choice for ventilator care, apnea monitoring, phototherapy, and infusion care, including chemotherapy, enteral therapy, hyperalimentation, and patient-controlled analgesia.
- The components of high-technology care include the actual product being administered, the equipment, the supplies, and the care givers. All may be provided by a single agency or by several cooperating agencies or companies.
- Use of advanced technology in the home requires a multidisciplinary effort. The community health nurse plays a central role in the field of advanced technology care in the home. Other team members include the physician, pharmacist, medical social worker, nutritionist, and home health aide.
- In planning for high-tech home care, the community health nurse must balance a variety of factors such as geography, safety, client appropriateness, clinical variables, care partner education, and communication skills.
- Multiple funding sources are available for advanced-technology care in the home. The nurse should be familiar with any limitations in the client's insurance coverage and inform the client of his or her financial responsibilities before treatment is begun.
- Legal issues with which the community health nurse should be familiar include informed consent, "do not resuscitate" orders, client noncompliance, payer denials, client appeals, and client discharge.

STUDY QUESTIONS

1. List the members of the high-technology health care team, and describe their roles in providing client care.
2. Review the points to be considered in planning for the use of new technology in the home. How would these differ for (a) a 7-year-old with cystic fibrosis who lives with both parents and (b) an elderly client with pneumonia who lives alone and suffers from arthritis?
3. List and discuss the components of client and care partner communication that should be assessed in considering admission to a home care program.

REFERENCES

Ahman, E. (1986). *Home care for the high risk infant.* Rockville, MD: Aspen.

Aucamp, V. & Show, R. (1989). *Nursing care plans for adult home health clients.* East Norwalk, CT: Appleton & Lange.

Bernstein, L., Grieco, A., & Dete, M. (1987). *Primary care in the home.* Philadelphia: Lippincott.

Bullough, B. & Bullough, V. (1990). *Nursing in the community.* St. Louis: Mosby.

Carpenito, L. J. (1987). *Handbook of nursing diagnosis.* (2nd. ed.). Philadelphia: Lippincott.

Dete, M. (1987). Managed care—The executive nurse's view. *Home health management advisor,* 2(4), 5-8.

Gould, E. J., & Wargo, J. (1987). *Home health nursing care plans.* Rockville, MD: Aspen.

Intravenous Nurses Society. (1984). *Intravenous nursing standards of practice: General, home, and TPN* (Rev. ed.). Baltimore: Author.

Jackson, J. E. (1988). *Patient education in home care.* Rockville, MD: Aspen.

Johndrow, P. D. (1988, October). Making your patient and his family feel at home with T.P.N. *Nursing 88,* 65-69.

Johnson, D. L., Giovannoni, R.M., & Driscoll, S.A. (1986). *Ventilator-assisted patient care.* Rockville, MD: Aspen.

Kruzic, P., Grundfast, D., Stites, L., & John, E. (1987). *Home care I.V. therapy manual.* Rockville, MD: Aspen.

Meisenheimer, C. (1989). *Quality assurance for home health care.* Rockville, MD: Aspen.

Morris, A. P., Marshall III, J.W., & Muszynski Jr., I.L. (1989). Patient care decisions and employer liability. *Caring, 8* (9), 56-58.

Patient teaching care manual. (1985). Home I.V. therapy. Torrance, CA, Hospital Home Health Care Agency of California.

Randall D. A. (1989). Legal liability in the home care setting: New technology and new reality. *Journal of Home Health Care Practice, 1* (3), 27-36.

Ritter, M. (1989, Winter). Assisting staff nurses in patient teaching. *Ostomy/Wound Management, 25,* 25-29.

Strandell, (1988). *Client studies in home health care nursing,* Rockville, MD: Aspen.

Home Health Care and Chronic Illness

JOAN M. COOKFAIR

The solid meaning of life is always the same eternal thing—the marriage, namely of some unhabitual ideal, however special, with some fidelity, courage and endurance, with some man's or women's pains.

WILLIAM JAMES

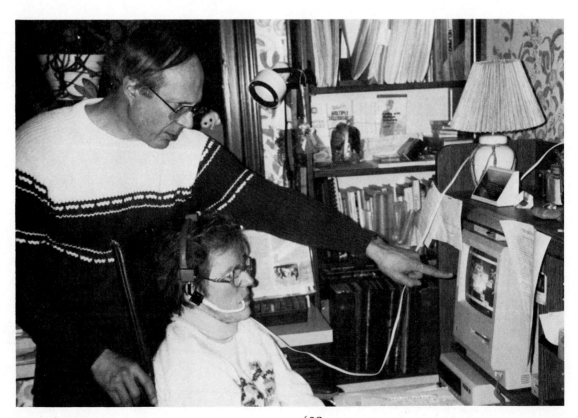

OBJECTIVES

At the conclusion of this chapter the student will be able to:
1. Define the key terms listed
2. Using Erikson's stages, discuss the effects of chronic illness on personality development
3. Identify selected chronic illnesses common to children and adults and discuss appropriate interventions
4. Discuss the use of the nursing process in the care of the chronically ill in the home
5. Identify some future trends in home care

KEY TERMS

Alzheimer's disease
Chronic illness
Chronicity
Cystic fibrosis

Hospice
Multiple sclerosis
Trajectory of chronic illness

The need to provide home care to chronically ill clients has become an increasingly major challenge to health professionals. The impact on families and communities faced with the necessity to provide services to this aggregate is profound. There are many reasons for the growing incidence of long-term illness, particularly in developed countries.

Because of improved technology and modern medical science, today many newborns at high risk survive, who a decade ago would have died. Chronic developmental disabilities related to prematurity, birth trauma, drug-addicted mothers, and other problems develop in some of these children.

Developments in the fields of bacteriology, pharmacology, and immunology have contributed to an increase in the life expectancy of many chronically ill children and adults. Successful public health programs worldwide have contributed to a decline in the mortality rate from infectious diseases in these populations.

Further, advanced technology and increased knowledge have resulted in increased longevity. Aging, however, frequently is accompanied by some type of chronic illness. Estimates by the U.S. Department of Commerce (1980) indicate that nearly half of all adults older than 65 years of age have some type of chronic illness.

DEFINITIONS OF CHRONICITY

The National Conference on Care of the Long-Term Patient reported the criterion for a condition to be designated chronic: hospitalization in excess of 30 days or the need for supervision or rehabilitation in excess of 3 months. (Roberts, 1954).

One author states that "the issue of chronicity is not the long-term nature of the disease and whether it is curable. Rather the concern is the unending, often uncontrollable, stress of illness and treatment—a stress worsened by uncertainty" (Bennett, 1988, p. 731).

Chronic illness can be defined in other ways: clinically, personally, and socially. The way in which a condition is defined influences the manner in which the family and the community respond to the individual with that condition.

Clinical definitions, which target the level of impairment or disability, are necessary for some types of financial assistance, such as workmen's compensation, disability insurance, and other medical insurances. For example, an employee who sustains a back injury on the job needs a confirmed medical diagnosis to be eligible for workmen's compensation or disability insurance.

Personal definitions by the individual affected have an impact on the person's response to an illness. This self-definition is influenced by several factors related to age, sex, and cultural and social expectations. The degree of visibility of the condition and the stigma attached, the nature of the onset (sudden or gradual), and the prognosis are factors that influence this type of definition (Dimond & Jones, 1983). For example, a young unmarried woman who requires a radical mastectomy may be more affected emotionally by it than would be an older woman who is past childbearing age and who has a secure relationship with her husband.

Social definitions, or the way a community and family respond to an ill individual, strongly influence the affected individual's response to a disability. For example, the client with acquired immunodeficiency syndrome (AIDS) may have difficulty in continuing employment because of the social stigma of this disease. By contrast, an employer may help the client with cancer continue to work if it seems desirable.

For purposes of this text chronicity is an ongoing process that requires intervention to maintain the highest level of wellness possible or to restore the highest level of functioning.

EFFECTS OF CHRONIC ILLNESS ON STAGES OF PERSONALITY DEVELOPMENT

Erik Erikson theorizes that each developmental stage is a building block to the next. Serious disruption at one stage averts normal progression and creates an alteration in the personality. An awareness of developmental stages can assist the home care nurse to plan appropriate interventions.

Trust versus mistrust. The first developmental stage occurs in infancy when the child learns to trust the environment or to be wary of it. If the environment is comfortable, mothering is adequate, and the infant's needs are reasonably met, a child tends to become a trusting person. On the other hand, the child whose environment is altered by constant discomfort and painful procedures may have difficulty establishing trusting relationships later in life.

Autonomy versus shame. The toddler stage produces a need for independence and exploration. The child who is unable to move because of congenital defects or whose physical development is delayed because of activity limitation cannot fully develop a sense of autonomy and may move toward shame and doubt.

Initiative versus guilt. Many children who are chronically ill during early childhood do not develop initiative because of minimal social interaction with peers. Reliance on parents as their chief companions allows few opportunities to make individual decisions; thus they become excessively dependent.

Industry versus inferiority. Middle childhood is a busy time for children. Most want to do everything, all the time, and run everywhere. Some chronically ill children are so frustrated by the curtailment of activities that they begin to feel inferior to their peers.

Identity versus diffusion. The adolescent with a negative self-image because of pain, disability, or chronic illness may have difficulty establishing a firm identity. Stigmatizing characteristics such as the loss of hair from chemotherapy can arouse feelings of self-doubt in an adolescent and thus damage self-esteem.

Intimacy versus isolation. The young adult who is beginning to move toward close relationships with significant others experiences serious developmental impairment by a sudden plunge into a life-threatening struggle, for example, with AIDS. Altered sexual patterns, the stigma attached to the disease, and its ultimate outcome may result in isolation and despair.

Generativity versus stagnation. This stage of life, characterized by productivity and responsibility, may be completely altered by the progressive disabling effects of a disease such as multiple sclerosis. "Multiple sclerosis is an inflammatory disease of the central nervous system that affects the myelin sheath of nerves. The disease is an exacerbating-remitting type, which manifests itself in progressive neurologic dysfunction. The average duration is 30 years" (Tabor's, 1989, p. 1157). Some affected persons may become completely self-absorbed and preoccupied with their illness.

Integrity versus despair. A person who is approaching retirement may look forward to a time of reflection and travel. If this stage is cut short by a severely crippling heart attack or terminal cancer, despair and depression can follow.

According to Erikson, even short-term disruptions can alter personality. Most certainly long-term chronic illness affects the ultimate development of an individual's cognitive and emotional skills.

CHRONIC ILLNESS ACROSS THE LIFE SPAN
Infancy and Childhood

Some common illnesses of childhood significantly shorten the life span of the child. Others greatly alter the quality of life. Congenital malformations such as meningocele, cleft palate, and Down's syndrome are apparent at birth and require immediate nursing intervention, both in the hospital and for follow-up home care. Illnesses caused by an inherited genetic trait such as Tay-Sachs disease, sickle cell anemia, muscular dystrophy, and cystic fibrosis are not apparent at birth but require nursing intervention as clinical symptoms develop. "Cystic fibrosis is a disease of the exocrine glands affecting primarily the pancreas and respiratory system. Prognosis is poor, but judicious use of antibiotics and modified life-style can prolong the life span of many patients" (Tabor's, 1989, p.447). In the case of Tay-Sachs disease, it is particularly important to initiate anticipatory grieving because the child will not live much beyond the age of 3 or 4 years and will become increasingly unresponsive to the family. Some illnesses such as AIDS, which are transmitted during pregnancy or shortly thereafter, may require in-depth nursing intervention in the home. Further information concerning these and other chronic diseases of childhood can be found in a medical, surgical, or pediatric text.

Older children who are chronically ill should be involved in the plan of care so that their cooperation can be ensured. The case study on p. 412 of a child with cystic fibrosis is an example of such client-centered care.

Young and Middle Adulthood

Some chronic illnesses in the adult years alter life goals and also may be life threatening. Because they occur at a time when most persons are beginning careers and starting families, they require special kinds of intervention.

CASE STUDY: CYSTIC FIBROSIS

Assessment and diagnosis

Tommey S is the only child of Howard and Darlene S, aged 28 and 27 years, respectively. Tommey is 7 years old and was diagnosed as having cystic fibrosis at the age of 6 months. A recent hospitalization for respiratory distress has prompted a home visit from a public health nurse. She finds Darlene and Tommey at home. The child seems well enough to return to school, according to his mother, but he insists that he isn't ready to return. During the initial assessment the nurse asks Tommey if he likes school. He replies that he doesn't like school because the other children make fun of his constant coughing. She asks if his appetite is good. He replies he could eat if he didn't have to take so many pills. When her son left the room to get a toy, the mother confided that Tommey was beginning to object to the daily pulmonary hygiene techniques although he liked doing his exercises when he wasn't too tired. She also said that Tommey did not like to leave her to go to school or for any other reason. The nursing diagnosis included Tommey's fear of school related to separation anxiety and fear of ridicule, potential for infection related to insufficient pulmonary hygiene, and alteration in nutrition related to prescribed chemotherapy.

Planning and implementation

Nursing goals were to encourage the mother to request a parent-teacher conference to explain Tommey's illness to the teacher. The nurse also suggested that Darlene ask the school nurse to meet with Tommey to let him know that help is available if he doesn't feel well while at school. The nurse also encouraged the parents to make necessary pulmonary hygiene a pleasant time for Tommey. A nutrition consultant was suggested to explore ways to cook for Tommey that would encourage him to eat.

The following actions were taken:

1. A parent/teacher conference was scheduled.
2. The school nurse met with Tommey to reassure him of her concern.
3. The parents were encouraged to allow Tommey to listen to tapes and watch videos while pulmonary hygiene was being performed.
4. Tommey's menu was reviewed. His mother was encouraged to give him small meals and nutritious snacks between meals. She also kept a food diary to ensure that Tommey was eating foods from all groups.

Evaluation

Expected outcomes of these interventions (actions taken) were that Tommey would begin to enjoy school, he would cooperate with the pulmonary hygiene regimen, and his nutrition would improve.

Illnesses such as brain or spinal trauma occur suddenly and without warning and may leave the individual in life-threatening circumstances, both physically and emotionally. Others, which begin insidiously, such as diabetes mellitus, rheumatoid arthritis, lupus erythematosus, and chronic fatigue syndrome, may be met with initial denial by the young adult, who has difficulty modifying behavior and adapting to the altered health state. At the onset of life-threatening illnesses such as leukemia, Hodgkin's disease, and AIDS, the client may react with total disbelief.

Assisting young and middle-aged adults to adapt to an altered health state may include family counseling as well as physical care. The following case study of an adult with multiple sclerosis provides an example.

CASE STUDY: MULTIPLE SCLEROSIS

In her midthirties Mrs. T was diagnosed as having multiple sclerosis. Weakness in her hands and intermittent visual problems were followed by weakness in her legs and difficulty in ambulation. Several years after the initial diagnosis Mrs. T found herself wheelchair bound, unable to continue in her teaching job, and dependent on her husband and two teen-aged daughters for physical care. The family seemed to be coping with Mrs. T's altered health state until the oldest daughter became ill with anorexia nervosa. There was some indication that the daughter's condition, in part, developed as a result of increased stress. As a developing adolescent it was difficult to deal with all of the aspects of her mother's illness. Mrs. T began to give lectures about multiple sclerosis, for which she was paid. This enabled her to hire a full-time aide to assist her in personal care. Eventually the daughter made a complete recovery.

Eighteen years after her diagnosis Mrs. T is wheelchair bound and has quadriplegia. She is troubled by constant leg cramps but, with the assistance of her aide, still lectures and maintains control of her life.

Mrs. T's positive motivation has assisted her in adapting to her altered life-style. Suggested nursing interventions include the following:

1. To monitor Mrs. T's skin in areas at greatest risk for extended pressure and breakdown
2. To monitor Mrs. T's extremities for contractures and fluid retention
3. To encourage continuing social outreach and interactions to maintain positive outlook

Positive outcomes would be that Mrs. T maintain skin integrity, that pain from contractures would be minimal, and that both Mrs. T and her family will maintain a functional coping pattern.

Older Adulthood

Chronic illness in an older adult may not only alter the life-style of the affected individual, but place stress on the health of the primary caretaker, who often is older. Their illness also may disrupt the family system. Osteoarthritis, cardiovascular disease, diabetes mellitus, and malignant neoplasms can cause increasing disability and can shorten the life span.

As longevity increases, Alzheimer's disease, a debilitating dementia of unknown etiology, is requiring increasing intervention in the home. Although death may not occur for many years, the disability is profound. Nursing intervention should be focused not only on the client but on the family, as shown in the case study on p. 414.

It is important that the nurse, in planning interventions for care, give attention to the care-giving environment to assessing the level of support within the family, to providing needed assistance, and to balancing that assistance with family involvement (Given, Collins & Collins, 1988).

CASE STUDY: ALZHEIMER'S DISEASE

Mrs. D. began having difficulty remembering things, missing time at work, and appearing in public in an untidy state at the age of 64 years. A widow who lived alone, she began calling her three adult children at odd hours of the day and night. Convinced that their mother was ill, the three (all daughters) insisted that she visit their family physician. After extensive testing they were told that their mother had Alzheimer's disease, that it was progressive, and that ultimately she would have to be institutionalized. Appalled, one unmarried daughter offered to move in with her mother and supervise her care.

Because Mrs. D.'s condition seemed to progress rapidly, the physician ordered a home visit by a public health nurse. When the nurse arrived, she found Mrs. D clean and well cared for, but the daughter complained of exhaustion and of getting very little help from her sisters. She also said she was afraid to go to work because her mother wandered away.

The nursing diagnosis was ineffective family coping related to care-giver fatigue. The actions taken were (1) to arrange for a family conference to assess family resources and (2) to place a full-time home health aide in the home so that the daughter could return to work. There would be an attempt to provide evening respite. When a family conference was held, it became apparent that the daughters living out of the home were not aware of the burden placed on their sister. They agreed to provide evening respite on alternate days and to assist with their mother's care. A full-time home health aide was placed in the home, and the daughter returned to work.

A positive outlook would be that despite the stress of their mother's illness, the family would remain intact and continue to cope in a functional way.

TRAJECTORY OF CHRONIC ILLNESS

In the planning of care for chronically ill clients in the home, thoughts of the final outcome cannot be ignored. The course of an illness can be viewed as possessing a trajectory or path of progression that is predictable. The perceptions of the nurse, the client, and the family may differ in terms of the ultimate outcome. The impact of the illness on the family may change over time. Chronically ill persons and their caretakers should be given as much information as possible about the progression and management of their disease. Trajectories show forward movement but at different rates of speed. Management or shaping of events may influence the course of the illness and its effect on a family in a positive way. Shaping may include management of the entire household and family. Nowhere is this more true than when the nurse is working with a terminally ill client. The trajectories of pain and the dying process can allow a thoughtful ordering of events and alter the course of the events in a positive way (Lubkin, 1986).

As a client progresses along a dying trajectory, it may be of value to recommend hospice care. The hospice concept is based on relief of pain, as well as the client and family's understanding that the ultimate outcome of the illness will be death. It emphasizes the quality of the dying person's life and the control of the symptoms of the disease. The following case study is an example of home hospice care.

Mr. H, a 64-year-old man with intractable pain as a result of advanced cancer of the prostate that has metastasized, was admitted to a hospice program. A hospice nurse visit was scheduled on a day when his wife and daughter were at home. Although Mr. H's chief complaint to the nurse was his excruciating pain, he also complained of anorexia and inability to get out of bed. He understands that he will not get well and emphasizes that he wishes to be free of pain. His wife and daughter (aged 59 and 23 years, respectively) both live with him and show obvious concern; Mr. H's wife denies that he will not get well. Both women work and believe that for financial reasons they cannot give up their positions. The nurse explains that Mr. H's eligibility for the hospice program depends on the availability of someone at home to assist with his care at all times. The daughter agrees to arrange her schedule so that she can be there when her mother is at work or, when both are at work, she will employ a personal care aide for her father. Table 19-1 provides a care plan for Mr. H and shows the nursing diagnoses that were formulated for him, along with the goal, intervention, and outcome for each.

TABLE 19-1   Care plan for Mr. H

Nursing diagnosis	Goal	Intervention	Outcome
1. Altered comfort, chronic pain	Mr. H will be free of pain.	Analgesics will be administered around the clock at the client's request.	Client was relatively pain free.
2. Altered nutrition	Mr. H will be able to ingest more each day.	Antinausea therapy in conjunction with small frequent meals will be offered.	Carl's caloric intake increased.
3. Impaired physical mobility	Mr. H will be able to transfer to a wheelchair and move around the house.	A wheelchair was provided to facilitate mobility.	Carl was able to sit in his room for short periods each day.
4. Self-care deficit (all areas)	Mr. H will receive assistance in self-care.	Personal care aide was provided.	Carl received assistance in self-care.
5. Anticipatory grieving	Family will communicate their concerns.	The family was referred for grief counseling.	Family received help in working through their acceptance of Carl's death.

Shortly before Mr. H's death he confided to the nurse that time had caught up with him and his life goals had not been met, but as a result of pain control he had been able to say good-by to friends and family. He felt that pain had made him a prisoner and that relief from it had made him a whole person again.

His death was quiet. His wife and daughter were there, as was the nurse. The nurse assisted Mrs. H in the arrangements for Mr. H's funeral and spent some time each day with the family as friends came to call.

Hospice bereavement follow-up spanned a year. Mrs. H met regularly with a support group to which she was referred, indicating that she did not want to be a burden to her daughter, but after 40 years of marriage she was incredibly lonely. The family was discharged 1 year after Mr. H's death.

In the case of dying children, parents must be informed concerning what to expect and what their role can be. Very young children fear separation from parents. The presence of a parent and, if possible, the holding by the parent of the child as death occurs can be of great comfort to the small child. Although school-aged children fear death in a personal way, a parent's presence can still be of consolation to them. Adolescents exhibit denial and anger; sometimes they become deeply depressed. Compassion and empathy are helpful, as is allowing the adolescent to ventilate his or her fears (Carroll, 1985).

The young adult who is dying tends to try to maintain some control over his or her life, which is more possible in the home than in the hospital environment. This is particularly true for the client who is dying of AIDS or cancer. Palliative and supportive home care and hospice programs offer invaluable resources and an alternative to hospitalization for those with AIDS and for their families. Other valuable services for these clients include Meals on Wheels, transportation to and from the hospital, counseling, and assistance from personal care aides (Bennett, 1988).

NURSING PROCESS

The use of the nursing process in the home allows the nurse to plan care that is appropriate, objective, and easily evaluated. Assessment is necessary to determine those factors that can be modified by an intervention and those that cannot. For example, it may not be possible to prevent a client's death or even prolong life, but it may be possible to enhance the quality of the client's remaining life by various interventions. (see case study on terminal carcinoma).

Assessment includes an objective and realistic analysis. All possible relevant data should be collected before any nursing diagnosis is attempted.

The nursing diagnosis should be client centered, and every effort should be made to include the client's and the family's participation in the plan of care.

Goals and outcomes, if they are to be effective, also must be client focused. Ongoing evaluation and assessment determine the most appropriate level of client and family participation.

CURRENT ISSUES IN HOME CARE OF THE CHRONICALLY ILL

There is an absence of financial assistance to the chronically ill in the United States. Medicare and Medicaid primarily finance short-term acute care, although some states provide additional assistance through their Medicaid program. Most insurance companies also are geared to assisting the acutely ill. Some provision is made for exacerbation of symptoms, but generally the cost for providing long-term assistance in the home is the family's responsibility. It takes very little time for a middle-class family to lose financial stability when challenged by the expenses that accompany long-term illness. Some insurance companies are beginning to sell policies to cover long-term care, as well as allowing terminally ill clients to cash in life insurance policies to help pay expenses.

In Canada the national government provides funds to the provinces to finance home care. The system has worked fairly well and is especially helpful in providing homemaker service benefits (Moore, 1988).

With the increase in the number of chronically ill persons in the home, a need exists to reassess the present system of federal assistance. A beneficent society is morally bound to respond to the needs of the chronically ill and the dying. Advances in medical science and technology have enabled the chronically ill to live longer and the population as a whole to reach a greater age. We must now be concerned with the quality of their lives.

FUTURE TRENDS

It is hoped that the person who is chronically ill views the illness as part of a life pattern rather than a foreign entity that has taken over his or her body. A nursing goal is for a client to achieve maximum satisfaction by living life to its fullest and functioning to the optimum at all stages.

Society must begin to view the chronically ill and disabled as participating members of the community. The extra care that may be required to permit a fuller participation would improve the quality of everyone's life and benefit the community as well as the individual. This is the hope of both professional health care providers and affected lay-persons for the future.

SUMMARY

The incidence and prevalence of chronic illness in the community are increasing. To plan effective care home care nurses must consider the effects of chronic illness on personality development and must be familiar with specific illnesses that occur in selected age-groups. The perception of a chronic illness as a family illness is important in that it enables the nurse to assist families to avoid secondary stress related to emotional dysfunctions and/ or care-giver fatigue. The future trend in home care of the chronically ill may include a concern for their quality of life as well as their quality of care.

CHAPTER HIGHLIGHTS

- Advances in health care are allowing people to live longer and to recover partially from acute diseases that once were fatal. As a result, chronic illness has become an increasing problem in society.
- A chronic illness is one that is permanent, leaves a residual disability, causes a nonreversible pathological condition, and requires long-term rehabilitation or supervision.
- Chronic illness may be viewed in terms of a clinical definition, a personal definition, or a social definition. The way in which the illness is defined influences the manner in which the individual, family, and community respond to the illness.
- The presence of a chronic illness may affect personality because it can prevent the individual from progressing normally through Erikson's stages of development.
- Chronic illness may occur in any age-group.
- In planning care for a chronically ill client, the nurse must consider the eventual outcome(s) of the client's disease.
- Hospice care allows the terminally ill client to remain at home; its emphasis is on palliative care.
- The nursing process may be used to plan care for the chronically ill client at home.

STUDY QUESTIONS

1. Define chronicity. Compare and contrast the definitions of chronic illnesses presented in this chapter.
2. Discuss the effect of chronic illness on the personality development of the young child.
3. Identify and plan care for a chronic illness common to (a) young children, (b) young adults, and (c) older adults.
4. Choose and discuss one issue in the health care of the chronically ill.

REFERENCES

Bennett, J. (1988). "Helping people with AIDS live well at home. *Nursing Clinics of North America, 23(4), 731.*

Carroll, D. (1985). *Living with dying: A loving guide for family and close friends,* New York: McGraw-Hill.

Dimond, M. & Jones, M. (1982). *Chronic illness across the life span.* East Norwalk, Appleton & Lange.

Erikson, E. (1963). *Childhood and society,* New York: Norton.

Given, W., Collins, C., & Given, B. (1988). Sources of stress among families caring for relatives with Alzheimer's disease. *Nursing Clinics of North America, 23,* 69-82.

Goode, W. (1960). A theory of role strain. *American Sociological Review, 25,* 483-496.

James, W. (1981). *The principles of psychology* (Vol. 1), Cambridge, MA: Harvard University Press.

Lubkin, I. (1986). *Chronic illness: Impact and interventions.* Boston: Jones & Bartlett.

Moch, S. (1989). Health within illness: Conceptual evolution and practice possibilities, *Advances in Nursing Science, 11,* 23-31.

Moore, F. (1988). *Homemaker–home health aide services: Policies and practices.* Owings Mills, MD: National Health Publishing.

Neuman, B.N. (1989). *The Neuman systems model: Application to nursing education and practice* (2nd ed.). East Norwalk, CT: Appleton & Lange.

Newman, M.H. (1984). Nursing diagnosis: Looking at the whole. *American Journal of Nursing, 84,* 1496-1499.

Pasquale, D. (1988). Characteristics of Medicare-eligible home care clients. *Public Health Nursing, 5(3),* 129-124.

Roberts, D. (1954). *The over-all picture of long-term illness.* Paper presented at a conference on problems of aging, School of Public Health, Harvard University, Cambridge, MA.

Ross, M. & Helmer, H. (1988). A comparative analysis of Neuman's model using individual and family as units of care. *Public Health Nursing, 5* (1), 30-36.

Stoff, J. & Pellegrino, C. (1988). *Chronic fatigue syndrome.* New York: Random House.

Tabor's Cyclopedic Medical Dictionary. (1989). L.T. Clayton (Ed), (16th ed.). Philadelphia, Texas: F.A. Davis Co.

U.S. Department of Commerce. (1980). *Statistical Abstract for the United States* (101st ed.), Series P-25, pp. 802, 888. Washington, DC: U.S. Government Printing Office.

Practice Roles and Settings

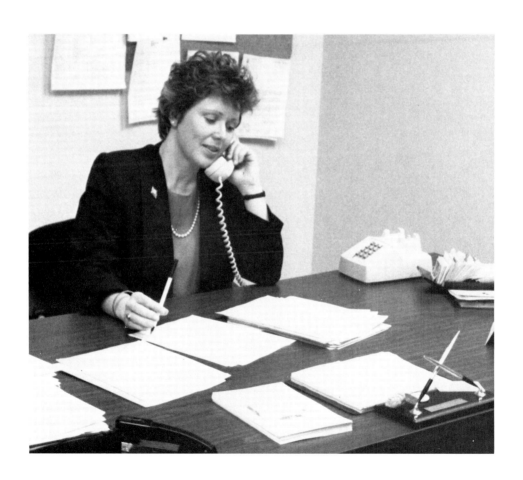

This unit describes the nurse's role in the workplace, high-risk aggregates within the practice setting, and the nurse's role in the prevention of communicable disease at primary, secondary, and tertiary levels. It also helps the student visualize and understand the expanded role of the nurse in the community.

Chapter 20 provides a discussion of the responsibility of the occupational nurse and identifies specific hazards in the workplace. The evolution of this particular specialty is traced historically and the importance of promoting a high level of wellness in the adult working population is emphasized.

Chapter 21 describes some of the aggregates at risk for increased illness in developed countries. The reader is introduced to the idea of the nurse as advocate. The following topics are discussed: factors that contribute to high infant mortality in some communities, conditions that predispose incarcerated persons to a low level of wellness, and events that lead to the phenomenon of a homeless population that is at high risk for illness. Suggestions are presented concerning what the nurse in the community can do to assist these groups as well as other high-risk aggregates.

Common communicable diseases are outlined in Chapter 22, in which agent, mode of transmission, incubation period, clinical symptoms, interventions, and methods of prevention are described. In addition, the complexities involved in dealing with clients with acquired immunodeficiency syndrome (AIDS) in the community are discussed in some detail. The concept of AIDS as a family disease is introduced.

Occupational Health Nursing

MARY K. SALAZAR, WILLIAM E. WILKINSON, and CHRISTINE L. RUBADUE

This act is passed to assure so far as possible every working man and woman in the nation safe and healthful working conditions and to preserve our human resources.

OCCUPATIONAL SAFETY AND HEALTH ADMINISTRATION (1970)

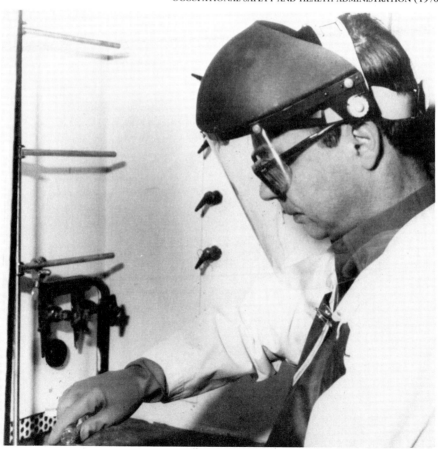

OBJECTIVES

At the conclusion of this chapter the student will be able to:
1. Define the key terms listed
2. List types of health and safety hazards that exist in the occupational setting
3. Relate the importance of considering the client's work environment in conducting a nursing assessment and in planning and implementing nursing interventions
4. Discuss some of the major governmental bodies that affect health and safety legislation
5. Outline the major occupational hazards to health care workers
6. Describe a conceptual model of occupational health nursing as a specialty area of community health nursing practice
7. Use the nursing process to apply occupational health concepts to the practice of nursing regardless of the practice setting

KEY TERMS

American Association of Occupational
  Health Nurses
Biological hazards
Chemical hazards
Educational resource centers
Ergonomics
Hazard
National Institute of Occupational Safety
  and Health
Occupational health
Occupational health history
Occupational health nursing

Occupational illness
Occupational injury
Occupational Safety and Health Act
Occupational Safety and Health
  Administration
Physical hazards
Psychological hazards
Risk
Teratogenic effects
Toxicology
Workmen's compensation

Occupational health nursing is an area of practice and research within the field of community health nursing. It has a specialized interest: the health care and safety of the adult working population. Working adults essentially are the backbone of the world's economy inasmuch as, through the organization and management of their labor, they produce and distribute virtually all goods and services. Indeed, the years spent working cover the major portion of most life spans. Occupational health nursing focuses on workers between the ages of 18 to 70 years, providing continuous and high-quality health care during what often is a 50-year period.

Knowledge, attitudes, and psychomotor skills related to occupational health have in many cases been neglected in nursing education. Yet inherent hazards to workers in the occupational setting can potentially affect the health of a large portion of our population. Clearly, it is essential that nurses who choose to work in the field of occupational health nursing be proficient and knowledgeable about this specialty area. Less clear, perhaps, is the importance of this knowledge to all nurses in related and diverse practice areas. To appreciate the potential effects of hazards in the occupational setting, consider that the majority of the adult population in North America is employed and that unemployed persons are likely to be living with someone who is a worker. Almost every job involves some degree of health hazard. Thus almost every client, whether in the work setting or not, is potentially affected by occupational injury or illness. Understanding the work environment is just as essential as understanding other environmental systems in which persons perform a nursing assessment or plan and implement intervention. Consequently, nurses must consider the various effects of occupational exposure (Salazar, 1987).

The purpose of this chapter is to introduce the reader to the field of occupational health nursing and to suggest some practical ways that this knowledge can be useful in nursing practice, regardless of the practice setting. In addition, some discussion about the special hazards that health care workers themselves face in their work setting is included in various sections, which can help the reader who is a health care provider better understand occupational health from a worker's perspective.

HISTORY

Interest in the health of workers first was noted in the early eighteenth century when an Italian professor of medicine, Bernardino Ramazzini, often considered the "father of occupational medicine," wrote his treatise *Diseases of Tradesmen* (1703). Despite Ramazzini's contribution and the ongoing efforts of many other health providers, much abuse and neglect continued to occur in the workplace. Injuries and illnesses associated with certain types of occupations were—and in many cases continue to be—considered "acceptable" risks, and neither the employee nor the employer may pay much attention when they occur. For example, it is well known and virtually accepted that coal miners eventually acquire "black lung" disease, that construction workers frequently are afflicted with chronic back pain, and that tree fellers may be killed by a falling tree.

A Century of Promoting Worker Health

Occupational health nurses (formerly called industrial nurses) have been a part of the industrial setting in both Europe and the United States for more than a century. During this period they have made many valuable contributions to the health of workers. Betty Moulder generally is recognized as the first occupational health nurse (OHN) in the United States. She was hired by a group of Pennsylvania coal-mining companies in 1888 to provide health care for the coal miners and their families. Ada Mayo Stewart, another important OHN from these early years, was hired by the president of the Vermont Marble Company who, unlike many of his collegues, had an interest in the health of his workers. Like Moulder, Stewart provided health services not only to the workers but also to their families. These early OHNs provided most of their services in the home setting.

The early twentieth century saw a broad expansion of occupational health services by nurses. As early as 1900 there are records of OHNs being employed in department stores and other retail operations on the West Coast. Of interest is the fact that in 1909 the Milwaukee Visiting Nurse Association "placed the first nurse in a local industrial plant for the purpose of demonstrating to the employer the economic value" of an OHN (Kowalke, 1930, p. 615). With the passage of workmen's compensation laws in 1911, occupational health nursing began to focus more on workers' injuries in the occupational health setting than on family health services in the home. A significant expansion of occupational health nursing services occurred during World War I. By 1918 there were 1213 OHNs, and by 1930 the Census of Population by Occupation reported that 3189 nurses were employed in industrial settings. Another huge expansion of OHNs occurred during World War II partly because of the industrial expansion that occurred during the war but also because of an ongoing expansion that resulted when the Social Security Act of 1935 granted federal funds for occupational health services at state levels. By 1943 it was estimated that 11,000 OHNs were working in industrial settings in the United States (Rogers, 1988).

As the number of occupational health nurses increased, interest in forming a national association developed among practicing industrial nurses, and in 1942 the American Association of Industrial Nurses (AAIN) was established. The purpose of the association was to improve occupational health nursing services and to offer opportunities for nurses interested in this area of practice. In 1977 the association changed its name to the American Association of Occupational Health Nurses (AAOHN).

Educational Resource Centers

After World War II there was a lull in interest in occupational health and safety, and the number of injuries in the occupational setting began to rise. Ultimately, this resulted in the passage of the Occupational Safety and Health Act in 1970, which, in turn, resulted in a resurgence of attention to health and safety problems that were occurring in the workplace. After the passage of this act, many businesses introduced occupational health programs for the first time and the role of the occupational health nurse began to expand. Because of the recognized need for more hightly trained and skilled occupational health professionals, the National Institute for Occupational Safety and Health (NIOSH) developed Educational Resource Centers (ERCs) in 1977. One purpose of these ERCs is to provide graduate-level education for the following professionals: occupational health physicians, occupational health nurses, safety managers, and industrial hygienists. There also is provision for continuing education, as well as for research in the field of occupational health. Currently, there are 14 ERCs in the continental United States, at least one in each federal service region. The University of Washingon in Seattle has an NIOSH-sponsored ERC, the Northwest Center of Occupational Safety and Health. It has graduate programs in occupational health nursing both at the master's and doctoral levels, an industrial hygiene program leading to a master's degree, and an occupational medicine program for practicing physicians. It also has an active continuing education program.

According to the most recent estimates available (1984) about 28,000 OHNs practice in the United States (Ossler, 1985). This number is increasing steadily as the demand for nurses with special knowledge and training in the field of occupational health continues to grow. Today employers are recognizing the importance of protecting the health and safety of their employees. Workers and employers now are asking occupational health care providers probing questions about exposure, safety, and health issues related to their work environment and about job-related health hazards to themselves and their families. The scope and range of services provided by the OHN today has greatly expanded since the early years.

Government Involvement

The Occupational Safety and Health Act (OSHAct) of 1970 was passed "to assure so far as possible every working man and woman in the nation safe and healthful working conditions and to preserve our human resources." The OSHAct created the Occupational Safety and Health Administration (OSHA) and established the National Institute of Occupational Safety and Health.

OSHA, which is part of the Department of Labor, encourages employers and employees to reduce hazards and to improve safety and health programs in the workplace by educating workers and by promulgating and enforcing standards and regulations (McCunney, 1988, p. 47):

> It [OSHA] accomplishes its mission by setting health and safety standards, enforcing these standards by the use of intermittent worksite inspections, and assisting employers in solving various worksite problems by offering consultation through state OSHA agencies. Through the on-site consultation program, hazardous conditions can be corrected without OSHA's relying on its enforcement powers.

The National Institute of Occupational Safety and Health (NIOSH) was established as a branch of the United States Public Health Service's Centers for Disease Control (USPHS/ CDC) within the Department of Health and Human Services (DHHS). NIOSH has greatly expanded epidemiological and laboratory research into the causes of occupational disease and injuries and the methods of preventing them. The "major responsibilities of NIOSH include investigating the incidence of workplace illness and accidents and determining the present or potential hazard of a substance, practice, or condition" (U.S. Government Printing Office, 1977 p. 1) NIOSH publishes many reports and materials detailing occupational hazards and ways of preventing or controlling them.

Workmen's compensation laws are a series of state and federal laws established to shift some of the costs of occupational injuries and illnesses from the worker to the employer. These laws generally require employers or their insurance companies to reimburse a portion of injured workers' lost wages and all their medical rehabilitation expenses. Workmen's compensation laws include both federal and state statutes, in which generally state statutes establish the extent of employer liability, that is, the amount of money payable to a worker for lost wages as a result of occupational injury and/or disease and the circumstances under which the employer is responsible for the medical care (Brown, 1981; Wilkinson & Wilkinson, 1982).

One of the most recent standards passed by OSHA is called, The Hazard Communicating Standard. This is sometimes referred to as The Worker's Right to Know Act. This standard requires all manufacturers and distributors of hazardous chemicals to provide material safety data sheets (MSDSs) that identify the potential effects of the chemicals with which their employees work. It also requires that all employees who handle or are in contact with hazardous chemicals be properly trained and that employers keep a file for each employee that identifies the chemicals to which they are exposed and the dose of their exposure (McCunney, 1988, p.25).

> In addition, under the 1986 amendments reauthorizing the "Superfund" Act (SARA amendments), MSDSs or a list of the chemicals for which the company has MSDSs must be supplied to local emergency planning committees, state emergency planning committees, fire departments, and state emergency response commissions. In addition, inventories on hazardous chemicals must be submitted to these state and local agencies. Any citizen who requests that information from the state or local authorities is entitled to receive it with certain trade secret exceptions.

Other Mandates

The federal Coal and Mine Safety Act of 1969 was passed to establish coal mine health standards, to provide benefit payments to coal miners disabled by black lung disease, and to initiate research. This legislation was initiated by the death of 78 miners in a coal mine explosion in Farmington, West Virginia, in 1968. In 1976 the Toxic Substances Control Act (TOSCA) was established to regulate commerce and to protect human health and the environment. This Act, legislated in an attempt to control some of the chemical hazards in industry, requires testing and restricts the use of certain chemical substances.

WORK-RELATED INJURIES AND ILLNESS

Statistics

It has been estimated that as many as 20 million injuries and 390,000 new work-related illnesses occur each year (Levy & Wegman, 1988). However, according to the most recent data available from the Bureau of Labor Statistics (U.S. Department of Labor, 1988), the total number of reported cases of injury and illnesses in 1987 was slightly more than 5,600,000. (This figure was obtained from the private sector, which represents approximately 75% of the total working population. Assuming that injuries and illnesses in the public sector are reported at a similar rate, the total number would still be considerably lower than the estimated figure.) In 1987 work-related injuries were reported at the rate of 8 per 100 full-time workers, which represents a slight increase from the previous year. Nearly half these injuries involved lost workdays (U.S. Department of Labor, 1988). In the same year 190,000 new cases of occupational illnesses were reported, 70% of which were related to repeated trauma (e.g., noise-induced hearing loss and carpal tunnel syndrome) or to skin diseases.

Another frequently cited estimate first noted by the President's Report on Occupational Safety and Health in 1972, is that approximately 100,000 deaths occur annually as a result of cancer, lung conditions, or other diseases that may be a result of long-term work exposure. This figure may, in fact, be underestimated. Nevertheless, only 3400 work-related fatalities were recorded in 1987, according to the Bureau of Labor Statistics (U.S. Department of Labor, 1988).

On the basis of such discrepancies as these, it is easy to see how the current statistical information may be inadequate. The reason for this is twofold: First, many occupational health problems do not come to the attention of the health care provider or employer and therefore are not included in the record keeping of occupational injuries and illnesses. Second, many occupational health problems that come to the attention of the health care provider or employer are not recognized as work-related. Despite difficulties in determining the precise frequency of their occurrence, it is clear from either report or estimated information that occupationally related injuries and illnesses may pose a serious threat to the population.

Definitions

The terms *occupational injury* and *occupational illness* require definition. Occupational injury is an injury that results from an acute episode and usually is easily identifiable in terms of its cause and effects. It includes such incidents as cuts, fractures, and sprains that result from an accident in the work environment. Injuries constitute approximately 95% of all compensable accidents in the workplace. Occupational illness, on the other hand, often is difficult to diagnose because it tends to be subtle and frequently manifests as a long-term condition indistinguishable from chronic conditions of a nonoccupational origin. Occupational illnesses include abnormal conditions or disorders that are caused by exposures to environmental factors associated with employment. These illnesses can result from inhalation, absorption, ingestion, or direct contact.

Manifestations

Occupational illnesses are revealed in a variety of ways. By far the greatest number of reported occupational illnesses occur as skin disease. It is estimated that skin diseases constitute 35% to 50% of all job-related illnesses in this country (Storrs, 1988). Several contributing factors are responsible. For one, the skin is exposed directly to the occupational environment and therefore is susceptible to a number of dermatological injuries. For another, like injuries, the presence of skin disease is more readily apparent than are many other occupationally related illnesses. Usually the symptoms can be easily related to the actual exposure. In many cases the skin problem is a result of an immediate adverse reaction to brief exposure to a toxic agent (CDC, 1986).

The results of many long-term exposures to chemical or biological substances at the work site frequently are less clear. For example, exposures to occupational hazards may have any of the following adverse effects:

1. Reproductive and teratological effects, including sterility (both men and women), spontaneous abortion, and birth defects
2. Cancers, including respiratory and skin cancer and leukemia
3. Cardiovascular disease, including coronary heart disease

Impact

The effect of occupational injury or illness on the employee, the employee's family, the employer, and on society may vary but, in general, is significant. The employee and the employee's family may suffer both tangible and intangible consequences of work site incidences. The injury or illness may disrupt family life and in some instances may be responsible for the breakup of families. The loss of earnings plus expenses for care related to the incident can cause problems far beyond those noted at work. Stress may be a direct or an indirect result of the multiple problems associated with the actual injury or illness, including the loss of wages and concern about future employment. Stress is likely to be especially profound if the employee is the sole wage earner. Another important consideration to both employee and family is the pain and suffering that may accompany the injury or illness.

The employer may experience a loss of productivity, a turnover in staff, high absenteeism, and possibly a lowered employee morale level as a result of workplace incidents. Society pays for the extra costs involved in workmen's compensation and other employer losses by paying higher prices for goods and services. Also, society loses revenue from taxes that are not being paid by an unemployed person, as well as the loss of that employee's contribution to society.

MAINTENANCE OF HEALTH IN THE WORKPLACE
Effects of Environment

To determine the relationship of work to health it is important to understand the type and nature of hazards in the work environment. Approximately one fourth to one third of the working individual's day is spent at the workplace. Adults in this country are likely to spend 40 years or longer in their work environment, which affects their health and their attitudes about health during a large portion of their lives.

The health of the worker in the workplace is the central theme of occupational health care. Measuring and evaluating occupational exposures must be considered in terms of their effects on workers. Among the greatest challenges to occupational health professionals is the continual delineation and identification of occupational health risks as new technological advances and new work hazards emerge. The identification of risk factors involves constant surveillance and monitoring of the work environment.

Attitudes Toward Health

The work environment is profoundly affected by attitudes about occupational health. To create successful occupational health programs both employer and employee must be actively interested and involved in health, safety, and education. Employers, specifically those at the highest levels of management, must be interested in a healthy and safe work environment; they must communicate that health is a high priority; and they must enforce policies regarding employee health at lower levels of management. Enforcement can include mandatory participation in health and safety activities, with evaluation of participation to be included in performance appraisals. Employees must want to stay healthy and must take an active role in maintaining a healthy work environment. They also must feel that management is concerned and supportive of their efforts to maintain an optimum level of health.

Health and safety professionals in the occupational setting are an essential part of any good occupational health program. These individuals must be committed to working with the various members of the health team, with the management, and with the employees to maintain a healthy work force. A key feature of occupational injury and illness is that in many cases it is *preventable.* Implementing engineering controls, providing safer materials, identifying health hazards, and educating the work force inevitably will lead to a healthier and safer environment. The occupational health professional must be constantly aware of the hazards that may jeopardize the well-being of the worker.

MAJOR CATEGORIES OF HAZARDS IN THE WORKPLACE

A tremendous array of occupations is represented by the more than 120 million people working in the United States, and American workers are exposed to a variety of potential health hazards in the course of their workday. The injuries and illnesses that result from work-site exposure can cause pain and hardship for these employees. Most hazards that occur in the occupational setting can be classified as physical, ergonomic, chemical, biological, or psychological.

Physical

The majority of reported occupational injuries are a result of physical hazards that result in injuries with a wide range of causes and effects. Physical factors that contribute to the occurrence of injury include the structure of the work space, the equipment used, the temperature in the work environment, the presence of radiation, the lighting, and noise levels. The most commonly reported injuries include strains and sprains, lacerations, contusions, scratches, and abrasions. By far the most commonly reported type of injury that occurs in work settings is musculosketetal, particularly back injury. More than 1 million workers suffer back injuries each year, and back injuries account for one of every five reported workplace injuries (U.S. Department of Labor, 1987).

The physical factors of noise and radiation have received much attention in the last 10 years. Both these factors are more insidious in nature than many other physical factors, and the health effects that result from prolonged exposure can be devastating. In recent years there has been an increasing number of legal claims as a result of hearing loss. (This increase may be due more to the recognition of hearing loss as an acceptable, reportable, and compensable injury than to an increased number of these injuries.) Noise-induced hearing loss is incurable and irreversible. The most common cause of occupational hearing loss is unprotected exposure to loud noise over an extended period of time. In view of the disabling effects of occupational hearing loss, the importance of prevention cannot be overemphasized.

As with noise, injury because of radiation most frequently is a result of unprotected exposure over an extended period of time. Some radiation generates unstable, highly reactive ions as the energy from this radiation moves through living tissue. This is called *ionizing* radiation. The most serious damage from ionizing radiation occurs within the nuclei of living cells where chemical changes to deoxyribonucleic acid (DNA)—the heredity unit of the cell—may occur. Low doses of radiation over prolonged periods can lead to cancers, tumors, fetal birth defects, and mutations in offspring (Holum, 1978). Recently there has been concern about the ionizing radiation emitted from video display terminals (VDTs). Reports indicate an increase in incidences of spontaneous abortions among VDT users. Follow-up investigations of these reports, however, have failed to confirm an association (National Academy of Sciences, 1983). Many studies on VDTs currently are in progress. In addition to the effects of exposure to ionizing radiation, there is concern about muscle strain and ocular effects associated with it. It is estimated that more than 1 million persons are exposed occupationally to ionizing radiation each year (Office of Technology Assessment, 1985). Because industrial use of ionizing radiation is expanding, more workers are likely to be exposed to its harmful effects.

The biological effects of nonionizing radiation are different from those of ionizing radiation. Nonionizing radiation includes ultraviolet, infrared, and laser radiation, as well as microwave radiation. Exposure to ultraviolet, infrared, and laser radiation may cause burns, and ultraviolet radiation is regarded as a cause of skin cancer. The primary effect of exposure to microwave radiation is tissue heating. Studies that have examined the mutagenic effects of exposure to microwaves are inconsistent and conflicting (Saunders, Darby, & Kowalczuk, 1983). However, testicular degeneration in men has been associated with microwave dosages capable of causing tissue heating (Council on Scientific Affairs, 1984; Lebovitz & Johnson, 1983; Saunders & Kowalczuk, 1981). Investigative research on the effects on female reproductive organs have not provided clear evidence of pathological damage or reproductive failure. There continues to be disagreement among investigators about both thermal and nonthermal effects of nonionizing radiation; therefore additional studies are necessary to establish safe exposure levels.

Ergonomic

Many injuries that occur in the work setting are the result of the poor use of the principles of ergonomics. The word *ergonomics* is derived from the Greek words, *ergo*, which means work, and *nomos,* which means law. Occupational ergonomics is a discipline that attempts to establish the best fit between the human and the imposed job conditions in order to maximize the health and well-being, as well as the productivity, of the worker. The guiding principle of ergonomics is to adapt the work site to the worker rather than the worker to the work site. Inadequate attention to ergonomics can result in stress to two major body systems, the musculoskeletal and the peripheral nervous systems. The most common musculoskeletal complaint that results from an inadequate "fit" between the human and the work environment is muscle strain and fatigue, frequent results of static muscle work. Cumulative trauma disorders frequently affect the peripheral nervous systems, for example, carpal tunnel syndrome, radial nerve entrapment, and digital neuritis. These conditions are associated with tasks that require repetitive motions. Primary risk factors for these disorders are the frequency with which the tasks are performed and the force and posture required when performing the tasks (Fig. 20-1) (Frederick, 1984).

Chemical

More than 60,000 chemicals were commonly used in industry in the 80s (Omenn, 1986), and it is estimated that 1000 new synthetic chemicals are introduced each year. An

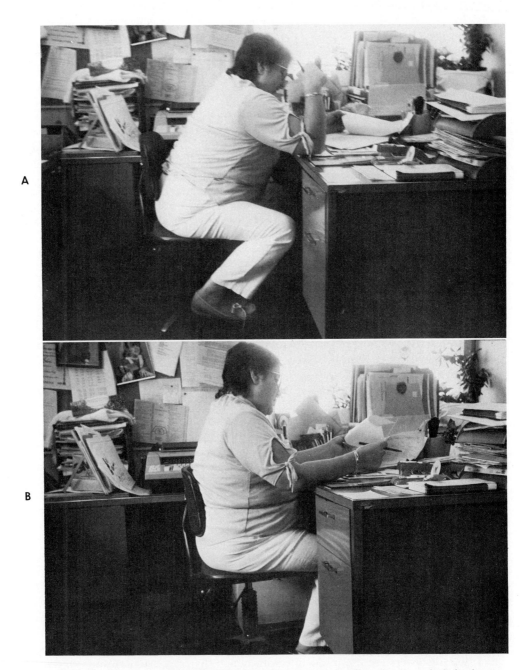

FIG. 20-1 The fit between the worker and the environment can affect the musculoskeletal system. **A,** Example of poor body alignment; **B,** Example of good body alignment.

TABLE 20-1 Some diseases caused by exposure to chemicals

Chemical	Occupation	Disease
Gasoline	Filling station attendant	Chemical pneumonitis
	Motor transport worker	Pulmonary edema
	Refinery worker	
Coal tar derivatives	Dry cleaners	Leukoplenia
	Refinery workers	Leukemia
	Varnish makers	
	Stainers	
	Painters	
Asbestos	Textile makers	Mesothelioma
	Auto brake repairers	Asbestosis
	Construction workers	
	Insulation workers	
Chromium/chromates	Copper etchers	Lung cancer
	Electroplaters	Squamous cell cancer
	Photoengravers	
	Stainless steel workers	
Ethylene oxide	Detergent makers	Dermatitis
	Grain elevator workers	Pulmonary edema
	Hospital workers (CS)	
Vinyl chloride	Resin makers	Raynaud's disease
	Rubber makers	Hepatic damage
	Organic chemical synthesizers	Angiosarcoma
Trichloroethylene	Dry cleaners	CNS depression
	Perfume makers	Peripheral neuropathy
	Textile cleaners	Liver tumors
	Printers	
Carbon disulfide	Degreasers	Behavioral disorders
	Electroplaters	Polyneuritis
	Painters	Atherosclerosis
	Rayon makers	Heart disease
	Wax processors	

Data from *Occupational diseases: A guide to their recognition* by USPHS/CDC, NIOSH, DHEW, 1977.

increasing concern for workers who are exposed to chemicals was reflected in the surgeon general's report (U.S. Department of Health, Education, and Welfare, 1979).

Chemicals in the workplace exist in the form of gases, dusts, mists, vapors, and solvents. Effects from chemicals range from acute (such as chemical burns) to chronic (such as silicosis). In addition to carcinogenic effects, teratogenic effects, which cause incomplete or improper fetal development, have been attributed to chemical exposure in the workplace. Samples of some common chemical exposures and related diseases are listed in Table 20-1.

The three primary routes of exposure to chemical agents are through inhalation, ingestion, and skin absorption. Inhalation is the major route of entry for gases, vapors, mists, and airborne particulate matter. One disease caused by inhalation of a chemical is mesothelioma, a lung cancer that results from exposure to asbestos. Ingestion is a less common route of exposure. It can, however, occur; a chemical on the hands, such as lead, may be ingested when an employee eats or smokes. Skin absorption most frequently occurs through epidermal cells or through hair follicles and sebaceous glands; a number of factors affect percutaneous absorption of chemicals, including the condition of the skin and the nature of the chemical. The effects from skin absorption may be local or systemic. An example of a local effect is an eczema like syndrome that results from exposure to nickel. Liver disease is a potential systemic effect of skin absorption of polychlorinated biphenyls (PCBs).

Toxicology is the science that studies the harmful biological effects of chemicals. Currently very few of the 60,000 chemicals being used have been scrutinized by scientists. What scientists have discovered over recent years, however, is that most chemicals, even the most innocuous, when taken into the body in sufficient amounts, can lead to undesirable health effects. Conversely, even the most harmful substance, when taken in a sufficiently minute amount, will be harmless. In other words, the harmfulness or safety of a chemical compound is related to the amount of that compound that is present in the body. Toxicologists attempt to determine the amount of a chemical to which one can be exposed without suffering any harmful effects (Loomis, 1978). It also must be noted, however, that even low levels of exposure to a chemical over extended periods of time can result in serious health effects.

There is great concern in the occupational health community about the lack of specific knowledge about so many chemicals. Although it is known that many chemicals are harmful to humans, the link between exposure and occurrence of disease is ambiguous. One reason is that the disease process often is slow and insidious. Another reason is that many of the diseases that are related to chemicals have multifactorial causes. The identification of a single exposure or cause is next to impossible. The problems associated with occupational diseases are discussed in further detail in a later section.

Biological

Biological hazards result from infection-producing organisms that are found in the workplace. Examples of biological agents are bacteria, viruses, molds, fungi, and parasites. Biological hazards vary, depending on the work site. Agricultural workers, for example, sometimes are exposed to fungi-contaminated grain dust, which may cause a respiratory disorder known as farmer's lung (Richard & Spradley, 1985); cotton mill workers are susceptible to a fungus disease, coccidioidomycosis; animal trappers may be exposed to rabies, a virus; and the bacterium that causes salmonellosis can infect food processing workers (Levy & Wegman, 1988).

It is well documented that health care workers are especially vulnerable to infectious disease (Clever & Omenn, 1988; Levy & Wegman, 1988; Omenn and Morris, 1984; Wilkinson, 1987). Hospital employees are exposed to staphylococcal and streptococcal infections, hepatitis, tuberculosis, viral infections, and many other infectious diseases. Of recent concern are health care workers' exposure to the human immunodeficiency virus (HIV) that causes acquired immunodeficiency syndrome (AIDS), cytomegalovirus, herpes virus, and scabies (Omenn & Morris, 1984). Physicians, nurses, dentists, and laboratory workers are at particularly high risk for viral hepatitis, type B, which probably is the most common and most fatal work-related infectious disease in the United States. It is spread primarily through contact with blood products, often as a result of an accidental puncture with a contaminated needle or other medical instruments. Like hepatitis B, the main source of the HIV virus, for which there is no vaccine, is blood or blood products. Fortunately, an excellent vaccine for the hepatitis B virus is available and should be administered to health care workers who come into contact with blood or blood products. To maximize protection from these and other infectious diseases, the Centers for Disease Control (CDC) developed recommendations for universal precautions among hospital employees (CDC, 1987). Universal precautions include any precaution a health care worker would take when caring for a patient, such as the use of gloves in handling blood or body fluids and adequate hand washing after patient contact. The difference between universal precautions and the routine precautions nurses take in the course of their work when a known communicable disease is present is that universal precautions are used with all patients regardless of known pathogens, inasmuch as the presence of infectious disease is not always apparent (CDC, 1988). In 1989 OSHA drafted a proposed standard to regulate worker exposure to blood-borne pathogens and to require, among other things, that universal precautions be implemented in health care settings.

Health care workers represent a substantial portion of the American work force. There has been a particularly rapid growth of these workers in both hospitals and community settings in the last two decades. The Bureau of Labor Statistics (1981) projected a growth from 4.6 million health care workers in 1970 to 11 million in 1990. In the last 10 years much has been written about the many hazards to which workers are exposed. Thus increasing attention has been given to their health and safety. Guidelines for safe work practices have been established by the American Hospital Association (AHA), by the National Institute for Occupational Safety and Health (NIOSH), and now by OSHA. There is a continuing need for more research in this area, however, so that compliance with recommendations can be assessed and even more definitive guidelines can be established.

Psychological

Psychological injuries and illnesses are the most difficult to identify because they are the least tangible. They include stress and fatigue, muscular tension, apathy, and depression. Psychological conditions result from the worker's response to the work environment. Work that depends on meeting deadlines or that conflicts with one's personal values can cause a great deal of stress. Loneliness and boredom have been associated with monotonous tasks. Work sites that have some type of monitoring system frequently create paranoid reactions; some environments cause feelings of alienation, social isolation, and lack of privacy (Slutzker, 1985). Other conditions that may result in psychological hazards are shift work, high workload, an unstable work environment (as may be present with corporate takeovers), job rotation, and poor leadership. The emotional energy required in caring for ill people and in meeting the emotional needs of patients and families poses an additional occupational hazard for members of the nursing profession.

Frequently, manifestations of stress are not recognized as being related to the individual's occupation. Family disharmony or marital problems can be a result of poor working conditions. Low self-esteem because of feelings of inadequacy related to the job may lead to self-destructive behaviors such as substance abuse or overeating. Subtle destructive changes in attitudes and behavior that diminish the general quality of life may be an indirect although powerful consequence of an unsatisfactory work environment.

Clearly, occupational stress is a diffuse and complex phenomenon. It often is difficult if not impossible to identify and quantify exposure to stress. It is known, however, that in addition to the psychological conditions already identified, physical conditions often result from excessive stress. These include coronary disease, hypertension, ulcers, and a variety of nervous conditions. Furthermore, many existing conditions, such as diabetes mellitus and arthritis, may be aggravated by stress. Frequently studies approach stress from the worker's perspective, and they may suggest that the attitudes and behaviors of the worker must change to decrease stress. A shift of emphasis from the worker to the workplace conditions may, in fact, be more beneficial to the mental health of the employees. Research to identify workplace stressors is an important step toward designing modifications of the workplace so that these stressors can be reduced or eliminated.

• • •

Each of these hazards in the work environment can result in a variety of injuries or illnesses. Frequently an overlap exists among the five identified categories; for example, many physical injuries may be by-products of psychological problems in the workplace. As mentioned in an earlier section, the most commonly reported and recorded health events in the occupational health setting are related to injury. Insidious occupational illnesses generally represent 5% or less of workmen's compensation claims received by the Department of Labor and Industries. Obviously injuries, which account for the other 95%, usually result from an acute episode and are easily identifiable, whereas illnesses often are the result of chronic exposures and the manifestations are more subtle.

As of 1989 there were nearly 7 million health care workers in this country. Despite the fact that their main mission is to care for others, it is clear from existing evidence that they frequently are at risk for a variety of injuries and illnesses as a result of their work-site exposure. The box on the opposite page provides an overview of some of the occupational health hazards to which hospital employees are exposed.

ROLES AND FUNCTIONS OF THE OCCUPATIONAL HEALTH NURSE

Occupational health nursing is the application of nursing principles to help workers achieve and maintain the highest level of wellness throughout their lives. This specialized practice area is devoted to promoting health in the workplace by preventing employee injury and illness. The emphasis of occupational health is wellness, life-style change, and risk reduction whereas the practice of occupational health nursing involves primary, secondary, and tertiary prevention.

Although the primary focus of occupational health nursing is the worker, the target population also includes the family of the worker, which in many situations also is affected by workplace hazards of the employee. For example, persons who work with lead may bring lead dust home on their clothes, thus exposing their families to this heavy metal toxin, which could result in the illness of family members as a result of lead poisoning. The consequent effects of this work-related exposure to the family are not likely to be recorded as work-related.

The occupational health nurse has a body of knowledge different from that of other nursing specialists. Special skills required by the OHN include training in safety hazards, disaster planning, familiarity with safety equipment, and accurate and up-to-date knowledge of current legal standards and laws that affect the working population. The OHN has specialized knowledge in the areas of toxicology, epidemiology, and the environmental sciences.

Occupational health nursing has several other unique features. The OHN often works in isolation from other registered nurses and frequently from other health care personnel. In addition, the OHN frequently is the only health care provider in an organization. Many OHNs create their own jobs and job descriptions. Although they perform according to some set of predetermined guidelines established by the profession itself and by the management of the company, the OHN determines the priorities appropriate to the situation, establishes goals and objectives, and determines the appropriate course of action.

OCCUPATIONAL HEALTH HAZARDS TO HOSPITAL EMPLOYEES

Physical

Physical hazards have a wide range of causes and effects. Statistics indicate that this category poses the greatest threat to hospital employees, with the most common injuries as follows:

- Puncture wounds from needles and sharps
- Burns and scalds
- Abrasions, lacerations, and contusions
- Hearing loss from overexposure to noise
- Possible genetic damage from exposure to radiation

Ergonomic

An inadequate "fit" between the individual and the work environment is creating an increasing number of hazards for hospital employees. The most common injury in this category is sprain and strain, particularly to the back.

Chemical

The potential for exposure to chemical hazards exists in many parts of the hospital. Chemicals themselves are present in a variety of forms and can manifest toxicity in a number of ways. Among the most common chemicals in the hospital setting are ethylene oxide, anesthetic gases, mercury, and various drugs, detergents, and disinfectants. The most common effect of chemical exposure is a dermatological reaction. Other potential effects are chromosomal aberration, miscarriages, sterility, and cancer.

Biological

Biological hazards are the most obvious and, therefore, the most studied class of hazards to hospital personnel. Among the most common biological hazards are the following:

- Respiratory viral infections
- Streptococcal, staphylococcal, and enteric infections
- Childhood infections such as rubella, varicella, or mumps
- Hepatitis B or AIDS (rare) via needlestick
- Cytomegalovirus (CMV)
- Tuberculosis

Psychological

Although stress sometimes is less tangible than other hazards, it is a very real and important factor in the consideration of work-related health problems among hospital employees. The impact of stress can be manifested in a number of ways.

Physiological manifestations
- Headaches
- Fatigue, muscular tension
- Ulcers
- Coronary heart disease

Psychological manifestations
- Apathy
- Depression
- Inability to concentrate
- Suicide

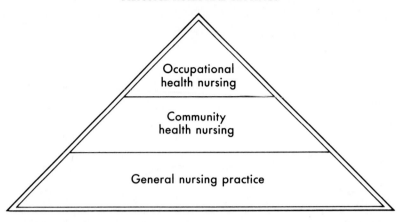

FIG. 20-2 Relationship among general nursing practice, community health nursing, and occupational health nursing.

In contrast to many other nursing specialties, the focus of occupational health nursing frequently is primary prevention, although secondary and tertiary prevention also may constitute part of the OHN's practice.

A strong relationship between community and occupational health has always existed. Fig. 20-2 illustrates how occupational health nursing fits within general nursing practice and community health nursing. Although the OHN's "community" is primarily the workers, she or he also influences the health of the family and the extended community. The OHN serves as a consultant to community health agencies, and some health departments have OHNs on their staff. Ensuring the health of the community frequently requires collaboration among many members of the health community.

Wilkinson (1990) has developed a conceptual model of occupational health nursing called the Wilkinson windmill model, which uses a windmill (Fig. 20-3) to describe how occupational health nursing is implemented in the occupational setting. The model has five main components. The core of this windmill is composed of the workers in the organization; the hub represents the OHN; the four blades represent the work environment, the management group in the organization, the other members of the health team, and the occupational health programs. These blades are propelled by the external "winds of influence," which have an impact on the workings of the organization. The winds of influence include social values, laws and regulations, political influences, health care trends, and economic influences. The base of the windmill consists of bricks, which represent the knowledge, the special qualities and skills, and the professional preparation of the OHN.

The roles and functions of the OHN include the duties described in the following section.

Primary care provider. The OHN is a primary care provider for occupational illnesses that are evaluated by means of nursing assessments and diagnoses. This role includes health screening and early detection of disease. The OHN may provide emergency services, preplacement and routine physical examinations, return-to-work assessments, and medical monitoring. Such monitoring includes audiometric testing, vision testing, pulmonary function testing, and any other testing appropriate to specific workplace conditions.

Counselor. The OHN counsels distressed employees and assists in personal and emotional problems. The OHN may be required to provide mental health and crises intervention for employees.

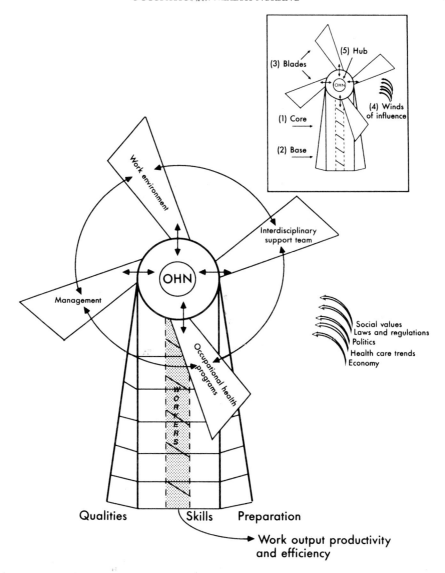

FIG. 20-3 The Wilkinson windmill model of occupational health nursing. *(From* A conceptual model of occupational health nursing *by W.E. Wilkinson, 1990,* AAOHN Journal, 38 *(2), p. 71. Copyright William E. Wilkinson. Reprinted by permission.)*

Advocate/liaison. The OHN frequently is a middleman between the employer and management. She or he brings worker problems to the attention of management and works with management to bring about solutions. Although the OHN is hired by management and works for management, her or his primary responsibility is to the employee. The professional objectives of the OHN may be different from those of management.

Manager/administrator. The OHN designs and implements a nursing service within the company that will ensure quality service to the employees. This requires skills in decision making, problem solving, and independent nursing judgment and communication. The OHN often participates in periodic interdisciplinary meetings to coordinate program activities and promote communication. The OHN determines the priorities appropriate to the situation, establishes his or her own goals and objectives, and determines the appropriate course of action.

Teacher/educator. The OHN teaches employees about good health and safety and motivates individuals to improve their health and safety practices. She or he educates the community and the workers about occupational health and safety issues.

Assessor/monitor. The OHN assesses and monitors workers who are exposed to potentially harmful substances or procedures, assesses and monitors the workplace for potential health or safety problems, and develops strategies to minimize the risk to the workers.

Professional member of the health team. The health team in the occupational setting includes the safety manager, the industrial hygienist, and the physician. The OHN collaborates with these members of the health team in exploring ways to promote environmental surveillance, to problem solve, and to advise management about the health and safety needs of the employees.

Researcher. The OHN systematically and continuously collects data concerning the health status of the worker and the real or potential health hazards in the work environment.

• • •

The OHN may function in all or only some of the capacities summarized here. The actual job description of any OHN varies, depending on the particular work site. In most smaller industries the OHN may be the only health professional at the site. Further, the composition of the health team depends on the individual company's perceived and actual need for occupational health services. Because OHNs are "revenue saving" and not "revenue producing," they frequently are required to "prove" their cost effectiveness to convince management that their services are beneficial to the company.

The Occupational Health History

It is not unusual for clients' symptoms to be related to workplace exposures. Each health history therefore should have an occupational health component. The goal of the U.S. Department of health and Human Services (1989) is that by the year 2000 at least 75 percent of primary health providers should routinely elicit occupational health exposures as part of the patient's health history. The occupational health history is an excellent means of obtaining information about the possible relationship of an individual's health to workplace conditions. Through the occupational health history the health care professional may be able to identify actual or potential hazards in the work setting and to counsel the patient regarding measures that can be taken to minimize any health risk.

In evaluating a health problem, the health care provider always should consider the symptoms in the context of the client's work (Ginetti & Greig, 1981). Included in the occupational health history is, at the least, information about each of the following items:

- Description of all jobs held
- Known work exposures and protection from them
- Nonwork environmental exposures
- Presence of symptoms and relation to work
- Patterns of symptoms or illnesses among other workers

The occupational health history can be used at four levels. The *basic* level identifies the employee's current occupation and the possible health implications, for example,

Date:_____

Interviewer:_____

EMPLOYEE HEALTH HISTORY

Name:_____ Sex: M ☐ F ☐

Address:_____

Phone: (Home)_____ (Work)_____

SS Number:_____ Occupation:_____

Marital status: S ☐ M ☐ D ☐ W ☐ Date of birth:_____ Race:_____

Allergies: Y ☐ N ☐ If yes, describe:_____

Physician's name:_____

      Address:_____

Date of last physical exam:_____

In case of emergency, please contact:_____

      Address:_____ Phone:_____

MEDICAL HISTORY

A. Hospitalizations (date, surgeries, illnesses, accidents, etc.):_____

_____

B. Past illnesses:_____

C. Current state of health:_____

D. Current medications: (Name and dose if known)_____

_____

FAMILY HISTORY

Describe any hereditary illnesses among parents or siblings_____

_____

_____

Continued.

FIG. 20-4 Employee health history form.

HEALTH HABITS (do you use the following?)

A. Tobacco? Y ☐ N ☐ Type_____ Amount_____

B. Alcohol? Y ☐ N ☐ Type_____ Amt/day_____

C. Caffeine? Y ☐ N ☐ Type_____ Amt/day_____

D. Sleep pattern_____ Amt/24 hours_____

OCCUPATIONAL HISTORY

Job title:_____ _____

Description of duties:_____

Date of hire:_____ How long in current position?_____

A. Do you feel that there any health risks or hazards associated with your job?   Y ☐ N ☐

If yes, please describe (Include symptoms):_____

B. Do you wear protective equipment on the job? Y ☐ N ☐. If yes, please indicate which of

the following: ☐ Gloves ☐ Coveralls/apron ☐ Safety glasses ☐ Mask ☐Respirator

☐ Hearing protection   ☐ Other _____

C. In the past, have you ever experienced an illness or an injury which you think may have

related to your job? Y ☐ N ☐. If yes, explain below._____

_____

ENVIRONMENTAL HISTORY

A. Have you ever been required to change your residence because
of health problems? Y ☐ N ☐.

B. Do you have a hobby or craft that may expose you to chemicals, metals or other substances?

Y ☐ N ☐. Describe:_____
C. Do you live near any type of industrial plant? Y ☐ N ☐
D. Does your spouse or any other member of your household have contact with dusts or
chemicals at work or during leisure activities? Y ☐ N ☐
E. Do you use pesticides around your home or garden? Y ☐ N ☐
F. Are there any other work, recreational, or domestic exposures that you feel are potentially
hazardous? Y ☐ N ☐ If yes, please describe._____

_____

FIG. 20-4, cont'd Employee health history form.

Date: _____

Interviewer: _____

ACUTE EPISODE FORM

Name: _____ Sex: M ☐ F ☐

Address: _____

Phone: (Home) _____ (Work) _____

Social Security Number: _____ Department: _____

Reason for visit (Include complete description of symptoms): _____

_____

Date of onset of symptoms: _____

Have these symptoms occurred in the past? Y ☐ N ☐ If yes, describe circumstances: _____

_____

How long have you worked in your current position? _____

Do you feel that your job duties contributed to your symptoms? Y ☐ N ☐

If yes, describe: _____

If you use any protective equipment, does it fit and work properly? Y ☐ N ☐

If no, explain: _____

Are there any other employees in your department experiencing similar symptoms? Y ☐ N ☐

If yes, please describe as completely as possible: _____

_____

Have there been any changes in your work environment in the last year? Yes ☐ No ☐

If yes, please explain when the changes occurred and what they were: _____

_____

Does your condition change when you are away from the work site? Y ☐ N ☐ How? _____

_____

Any other comments? _____

FIG. 20-5 Acute episode form.

how a diagnosis of laryngitis may affect a teacher's return to work. At the *diagnostic* level there is an investigation of the possible link between the patient's job and a current illness. For example, an occupational health nurse might question if a warehouse worker's back pain is caused by lifting heavy items at the work site. At the level of *screening* a client regularly is evaluated for the occurrence of symptoms related to known workplace exposures; for example, employees exposed to a high noise level will be given a regular hearing test. Finally, on the *comprehensive* level occupational health history is used for the investigation of complex medical problems. Researchers might explore the possible relationship between the work environment and a patient's diagnosis of bladder cancer (Occupational and Environmental Health Committee, 1983).

It is not unusual for the occupational health history to be entirely omitted from a health history. Yet few clinicians would omit information about the patient's family history. Because the client may spend one third of a lifetime in the job setting, the health implications of occupational exposures cannot be overlooked. The relationship between many chronic conditions and exposures at the workplace is becoming increasingly apparent, but all too often this connection is missed by the health professional. Although physical findings and laboratory tests may raise suspicions that a condition is occupationally related, it is the occupational health history that ultimately will prove the work relatedness of a medical problem. Fig. 20-4 provides an example of a form that can be used to obtain an employee's health history, and Fig. 20-5 shows an acute episode form for use when a single incident occurs at the work site. The following case studies show how an occupational health history can furnish a health care provider with invaluable information.

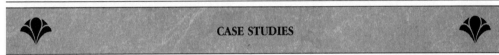

CASE STUDIES

Case 1

A 28-year-old male assembly line worker in a plywood manufacturing plant complained that his eyes constantly burned and that it hurt him to breathe. An investigation into the possible cause revealed that he was exposed to toluene diisocyanate, which was present in the glues used in manufacturing plywood. He had not been wearing a respirator regularly.

Case 2

A 53-year-old printer and lithographer reported to his health care provider that he had multiple episodes of falls and trauma in the previous several weeks. An investigation revealed that he also suffered from memory loss and episodes of syncope. Upon investigation it was discovered that this client's symptoms were caused by chronic exposure to organic tin, resulting in irreversible damage to his central nervous system.

Case 3

A 34-year-old male bridge worker complained of generalized weakness, abdominal cramps and diarrhea, and a recent 20-pound weight loss. A further examination revealed the presence of neuromuscular, central nervous system, and renal symptoms. Just before a scheduled exploratory laparotomy, an astute nurse questioned the patient about his job. Upon discovering that he had been in the process of removing paint from a large city bridge, the nurse decided to obtain a blood lead level. Results showed that the client was suffering from lead poisoning, and when he was removed from the source of exposure, the symptoms disappeared.

Occupational Disease: Difficulties in Determination

Traditionally, occupational health programs have emphasized the prevention of injury, with little or no concern about the prevention of occupational disease. As was pointed out in the section on the occupational health history, it is vitally important that clinicians be attuned to the possible relationships between workplace exposures and the occurrence of disease. Four primary reasons are responsible for this missed relationship:

1. The lag time between exposure to an agent and the onset of symptoms
2. The multifactorial origin of many diseases
3. The additive effect of some workplace conditions in conjunction with other exposures or life-style behaviors
4. Difficulty in evaluating the contributing role of the workplace

In addition, problems often are inherent in the reporting systems. Frequently employers, health care providers, or even the employees themselves fail to recognize the occupational relationship of a disease. Many primary care physicians have inadequate training in occupational medicine. Further, an effort to restrict the cost of workmen's compensation may lead to a failure to connect a disease with conditions in the workplace. It has been estimated that the true incidence of occupational illnesses may be 10 to 50 times greater than reported (Mathias, 1985).

Although more and more data are being accumulated that demonstrate the relationship between occupational exposures and human diseases, studies still are sparse and inconclusive. An important defense against the occurrence of occupational illness is continued epidemiological research that explores the relationship of illnesses to exposures and conditions in the work environment. On the basis of resultant findings, work sites can be altered to decrease the risks to the employee. In addition, health care professionals need to be taught to recognize occupational disease. Again, the occupational health history is an invaluable tool that allows primary care providers to make the connection between the disease process and the client's occupational exposures.

The Nursing Process in the Occupational Setting

The occupational community, in contrast to many other communities of interest to the health professional, consists of an essentially well population. The primary objective of occupational health nursing is to maintain and enhance the health of the workers and to prevent injury and illness that could occur as a result of occupational exposures. The community health nursing process described in Chapter 3 provides an excellent framework for accomplishing this objective. The case study on pp. 444-445 illustrates how this nursing process might be used in the occupational setting.

Occupational Safety and Health Programs

Phenomenal growth has occurred in occupational health and safety programs in the last two decades, partly as a result of a national movement toward primary and secondary prevention. This trend is reflected by the publication of the surgeon general's report, *Healthy People,* in 1979, followed by *Promoting Health/Preventing Disease: Objectives for the Nation* (U.S. Department of Health and Human Services) published in 1980. In addition, the passage of the Occupational Safety and Health Act in 1970 focused attention on the need to improve the health and safety of the working population in this country.

Because of the great variation of work sites and the diversity of jobs, the potential hazards and the type of programs also are considerably varied. Safety and health programs in the occupational setting can be broadly divided into two categories: those that focus

CASE STUDY

Earl is the chief occupational health nurse for a busy telephone company. It is a typical Friday morning in the health unit. Earl is reviewing the health unit logs for the past month. These logs summarize all employee visits to the health unit, including the reason for the visit and the action taken. A certain pattern over this last month captures Earl's attention. He notices that eight employees from the North office have visited the health unit complaining of a headache during this period, some of them visiting the unit twice. Earl checks the previous month's log and notes that there were five similar visits during that month. A further check reveals that during the two previous months, there were no visits. Earl decides that a thorough investigation of the situation is warranted. He calls the administrator of the North office to tell him that he will visit that building early this afternoon.

Assessment

For the assessment phase of the community health nursing process, Earl will perform the following actions:

1. Review the charts of the employees who visited the health unit with the complaint of a headache to determine the exact job responsibilities of the employee and to obtain a more detailed description of the visit
2. Interview the administrator of the North office to determine if there have been any changes in office equipment, procedures, or other during the last 2 months
3. Walk around the work environment to identify any potential risk factors
4. Interview a sampling of the employees with headache to determine if the symptoms persist
5. Interivew employees who work in the same environment who did not visit the health unit to determine if any of them had similar symptoms
6. Confer with the industrial hygienist, occupational physician, and safety manager to determine if they have any information to contribute to Earl's assessment

Through this assessment the following facts were revealed. In addition to the headache, several of the employees complained of blurred vision. This office building, which is only 6 months old, has no windows that open and it faces the afternoon sun. A check with the building engineer indicates that no ventilation problems have been identified. The entire office was equipped with new video display terminals (VDTs) a little more than 2 months ago. The employees who visited the health unit continue to have the headaches and occasional blurred vision, but they have managed to keep them at a tolerable level through the use of over-the-counter analgesics such as acetaminophen or aspirin. It was discovered that several employees with similar symptoms had not reported them to the health unit. In all cases the headaches are less pronounced or disappear altogether on the weekends. All affected employees are regular VDT users and work on the west side of the building near the windows. The employees generally agreed that their work is fast paced and relatively demanding.

Nursing diagnosis

The community health nurse considers the following three components: the health problem, the population characteristics, and the environmental characteristics. In this case the health problem is the regular occurrence of headache and blurred vision during the working week. The population consists of adult persons who are otherwise healthy and who spend more than half their workday using VDTs. The environment in which the health problem occurs is on the west side of the North office, near a bank of windows that cannot be opened. In addition, it was determined that although this area has sufficient lighting for general work, glares on the VDT screen and otherwise inadequate lighting make close work and the reading of the screen difficult. In view of these findings, Earl makes the following diagnosis: risk of decreased quality of work life, decreased productivity, and lowered employee morale among VDT operators in the North office of the Ring-a-Ding Telephone Company related to the regular use of VDT equipment, inadequate

CASE STUDY—cont'd

lighting and screen glare, and a fast-paced work environment, as demonstrated by the regular occurrence of headaches and blurred vision. Earl considers that the symptoms may be related to the physical environment or to stress that results from the demands of this job.

Planning and implementation

Earl's primary goal for this population is to decrease the occurrence of headache and blurred vision through the alteration of the environment. He discusses his findings and his diagnosis with the administrator in the North office and the safety engineer, and together they plan appropriate strategies to address the identified problems. As a result of this meeting, the following changes were implemented:

1. Antiglare screens were purchased for all VDT operators.
2. The lighting system was assessed and revised so that close work and screen reading could be accomplished without eye strain.

3. All VDT operators were encouraged to break up their work day so that they never spent more than 1 hour at the screen during a single sitting.
4. Shades were placed on the windows to prevent direct sunlight from entering the west section of the building.
5. A stress management class was developed and offered to all employees in this office. The adminstrator, recognizing the significance of the problem, has agreed to allow employees to participate in the class during work hours.

Evaluation

Earl will carefully monitor this population to determine if there is a decrease of symptoms as a result of the changes that were made. He will not rely on health unit visits. He will make periodic visits to the North office so that he can interview the employees, particularly those who work on the west side of the building. He will ask the administrator to inform him if he becomes aware of any other complaints.

on occupational safety and health issues and those that focus on health promotion outside the workplace. The first group of programs include those on safety education, health surveillance such as hearing-conservation training in handling materials, and communication concerning hazards. They include, of course, treatment of occupational injuries and illnesses. Programs that are not occupationally related may or may not be a part of a company's total health program. In addition to treatment of injuries or illnesses unrelated to the work site, programs can include a variety of health promotion activities such as hypertension screening and follow-up, cancer screening and education, cholesterol screening, smoking cessation, automobile safety, and substance abuse programs. The purpose of any safety and health program is to provide a safe and healthy work environment and to promote the personal health behaviors of employees to maintain a healthy and productive work force.

Occupational health programs generally include preventive health care as well as health maintenance. The basic objectives of an occupational health and safety program can be described as follows: (1) to identify health hazards in the work environment and to eliminate or control them, (2) to provide curative care and rehabilitation for people who have been injured or who become ill from work-connected causes, (3) to provide services that ensure maximum compatibility between the worker's capabilities and limitations and the physical, mental, and emotional demands of the job, and (4) to promote and protect workers' health (Brown, 1981).

Health and safety programs at the work site can make a significant contribution to the health of the adult population of this country. In addition to the direct health effects, these programs often result in increased job performance and job satisfaction of workers. Studies have indicated that well-planned health and safety programs increase productivity and decrease absenteeism and turnover among employees. Ongoing research in this area will assist occupational health providers in developing effective and efficient programs that will provide the maximum benefit to the working population.

SUMMARY

Occupational health nursing comprises (or should comprise) at least a small part and sometimes a large part of every nurse's practice. Although the OHN requires special training in environmental health principles, toxicology, epidemiology, and industrial hygiene, each nurse should be alert to and aware of possible occupationally related health and safety problems of his or her clients. Occupational health is the responsibility of every health professional, and general training in occupational health nursing should be included within the community health nursing curriculum of all baccalaureate and graduate nursing programs.

CHAPTER HIGHLIGHTS

- OHNs have worked in industrial settings in the United States and Europe for more than 100 years and have made many valuable contributions to the health of workers.
- Educational resource centers, of which there are 14 in the continental United States, provide education and research in the field of occupational health nursing.
- The actual number of illnesses and injuries with occupational causes is difficult to estimate because many do not come to the attention of occupational health professionals or are not recognized as work related.
- An occupational injury is an injury that results from an acute episode and is usually easily identifiable in cause and effect.
- An occupational illness is an abnormal condition or disorder caused by exposure to environmental factors associated with employment.
- In many cases occupational injury and illness are preventable.
- Governmental involvement in improving safety in the workplace includes the passage of the Occupational Safety and Health Act and the establishment of the Occupational Safety and Health Administration and the National Institute of Occupational Safety and Health.
- Most hazards that occur in the workplace may be classified as physical, ergonomic, chemical, biological, or psychological.
- Health care workers, who represent a large portion of the work force, are particularly vulnerable to occupational illness as a result of exposure to infectious diseases.
- The OHN, whose focus tends to be on primary prevention, frequently is the only health professional in the work setting.
- The roles and functions of the occupational health nurse include primary care provider, counselor, advocate/liaison, manager/administrator, teacher/educator, assessor/monitor, professional member of the health team, and researcher.
- All health care providers should include an occupational health component as part of a general health history by obtaining information such as the following: a description of all jobs held, known work exposures and protection from them, environmental

exposures unrelated to the workplace, the presence of symptoms and their relation to work, and patterns of symptoms or illnesses among other workers.

- Occupational illnesses often are difficult to diagnose because the cause and effect may not be closely related.
- As a result of a national movement toward primary and secondary prevention, the number of occupational health and safety programs has grown dramatically.
- Occupational health and safety programs can contribute greatly to the general health of the adult population, as well as increase job satisfaction and productivity.

STUDY QUESTIONS

1. What is the relationship between an individual's work and health? How do employers' and employees' attitudes toward health affect the work environment?
2. Discuss the impact of the Occupational Safety and Health Act on safety in the workplace.
3. List the five major categories of occupational hazards. For each, name one example of a hazard and the type of worker likely to be affected by it.
4. Using the Wilkinson windmill model, describe how occupational health nursing is implemented in the work setting.
5. What information should be obtained as part of an occupational health history? Why is this information important?

REFERENCES

American Medical Association. (1972). *Scope, objectives, and functions of occupational health programs.* Chicago: Author.

Brown, M. L. (1981). *Occupational health nursing.* New York: Springer.

Centers for Disease Control. (1986). Leading work-related diseases and injuries. *Morbidity and Mortality Weekly Report, 35*(35), 561-563.

Centers for Disease Control. (1987). Human immunodeficiency virus infection in the United States: A review of current knowledge. *Morbidity and Mortality Weekly Report, 36*(49) 1-48.

Centers for Disease Control. (1988). Update: Universal precautions for prevention of transmission of human immunodeficiency virus, hepatitis B virus, and other bloodborne pathogens in health-care settings. *Morbidity and Mortality Weekly Report, 37*(24), 377-391.

Clever, L. H., & Omenn, G. S. (1988). Hazards for health care workers. *Annual Review of Public Health, 9,* 273-303.

Council on Scientific Affairs. (1984). Effects of physical forces on the reproductive cycle. *Journal of the American Medical Association, 251,* 247-250.

Frederick, L. (1984). An introduction to the principles of occupational ergonomics. *Occupational Health Nursing, 32*(12), 643-645.

Ginnetti, J., & Greig, A. E. (1981). The occupational health history. *Nurse Practitioner, 6* (5), 12-13.

Holum, J. R. (1978). *Fundamentals of general, organic, and biologic chemistry.* New York: Wiley.

Kowalke, E. (1930). Industrial nursing service provided by public health nursing association. *The Public Health Nurse, 22,* 615-617.

Lebovitz, R. M., & Johnson, L. (1983). Testicular function of rats following exposure to microwave radiation. *Bioelectromagnetics, 4,* 107-114.

Levy, B. S., & Wegman, D. H. (1988). *Occupational health: Recognizing and preventing work-related disease.* Boston: Little, Brown & Co.

Loomis, T. A. (1978). *Essentials of toxicology.* Philadelphia: Lea & Febiger.

Mathias, C. G. (1985). The cost of occupational skin disease [Editorial]. *Archives of Dermatology, 121,* 332-334.

McCunney, R. J. (1988). *Handbook of occupational medicine.* Boston: Little, Brown & Co.

National Academy of Sciences. (1983). *Video displays: Work and vision.* Washington, DC: National Academy Press.

Occupational and Environmental Health Committee. (1983). Taking the occupational history. *Annals of Internal Medicine, 99,* 641-651.

Office of Technology Assessment. (1985). *Reproductive health hazards in the workplace,* Washington, DC: Author.

Omenn, G. S. (1986). A framework for risk assessment for environmental chemicals. *Washington Public Health, 6* (Summer), 2-6.

Omenn, G. S., & Morris, S. L. (1984). Occupational hazards to health care workers: Report of a conference. *American Journal of Industrial Medicine, 6,* 129-137.

Ossler, C. (1985). *Distributive nursing practice in occupational health and safety. Distributive nursing practice: a systems approach to community health.* (2nd ed.). J. Hall and B. Weaver (Eds.), Philadelphia: J.B. Lippincott.

Rogers, B. (1988). Perspective in occupational health nursing. *AAOHN Journal, 36*(4), 151-155.

Spradley, B. W. (1985). Health of the working population. In *Community health nursing: concepts and practice* (2nd ed.). Boston: Little, Brown & Co.

Salazar, M. K. (1987). Occupational health nursing as a component of baccalaureate nursing education. *Nursing Education, 26,* 255-257.

Saunders, R. D., Darby, S. C., & Kowalczuk, C. I. (1983). Dominant lethal studies in male mice after exposure to 2.45 GHz microwave radiation. *Mutation Research, 117,* 345-356.

Saunders, R. D., & Kowalczuk, C. I. (1981). Effects of 2.45 GHz microwave radiation and heat on mouse spermatogenic epithelium. *International Journal of Radiation Biology. 40,* 623-632.

Slutzker, P. C. (1985). Ergonomics in microelectronic office technology. *Occupational Health Nursing, 33,* 610-614.

Storrs, F. J. (1988). Demographics of occupational skin disease. From *Recent developments in occupational medicine.* Course presented at Northwest Center for Occupational Health and Safety, University of Washington, Seattle.

Travers, P. H. (1987). *A comprehensive guide for establishing an occupational health service.* Atlanta: American Association of Occupational Health Nurses.

U.S. Bureau of Labor Statistics. (1981). The national industry-occupation matrix: 1970, 1978, and projected 1990 (Bulletin 2086, No. 2, pp. 490-494) Washington, DC: U.S. Government Printing Office.

U.S. Department of Health and Human Services.

(1989). *Promoting Health/Preventing Disease: year 2000 objectives for the nation* (draft for public review and comments). Public Health Service, Washington, DC.

U.S. Department of Health, Education and Welfare. (1973). *The industrial environment—Its evaluation and control.* Washington, DC: U.S. Government Printing Office.

U.S. Department of Health, Education and Welfare. (1978). *The new nurse in industry.* Washington, DC: U.S. Government Printing Office.

U.S. Department of Labor. (1987). Back injuries—Nation's number one workplace safety problem. (Fact Sheet No. OSHA 87-09.) Washington, DC: U.S. Government Printing Office.

U.S. Department of Labor. (1988). *BLS reports on survey of occupational injuries and illnesses in 1987* (USDL No. 88-562). Washington, DC: Bureau of Labor Statistics.

U.S. Government Printing Office. (1977). *An act Public Law 91-596.* 91st Congress, S. 2193, Dec. 29, 1970.

U.S. Public Health Service. (1980). Promoting health/ preventing disease: Objectives for the nation (GPO 017-001-00435-9). Washington, DC: U.S. Government Printing Office.

U.S. Public Health Service. (1983). *Health U.S. and preventive profile.* Hyatsville, Md: U.S. Department of Health and Human Services.

U.S. Department of Health, Education and Welfare. (1979). *Healthy people: The surgeon general's report on health promotion and disease prevention.* Washington, DC: DHEW: Publication No. 19-55071, Washington DC.

Wilkinson, W. E. (1987). Occupational injury at a midwestern health science center and teaching hospital. *AAOHN Journal. 35*(8), 367-376.

Wilkinson, W. E. (1990). A conceptual model of occupational health nursing. *AAOHN Journal, 38*(2), 71-75.

Wilkinson, W. E., & Wilkinson, C. S. (1982). Workers' compensation and the occupational health nurse. *Occupational Health Nursing, 30,* 22-24.

High-Risk Aggregates in the Community

JOAN M. COOKFAIR

Identifying aggregates within the population which are at high risk to illness, disability and premature death, and directing resources toward them is one of the most effective approaches for accomplishing the role of Public Health Nursing.

AMERICAN PUBLIC HEALTH ASSOCIATION

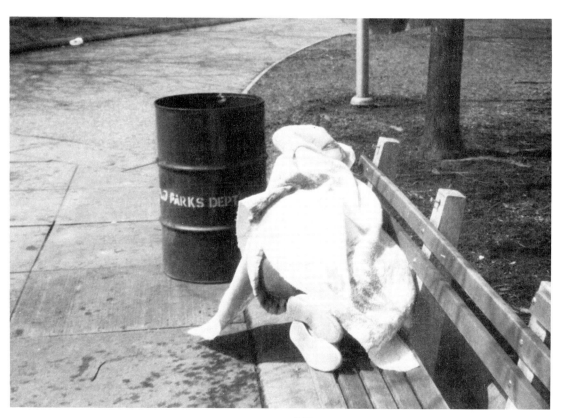

OBJECTIVES

At the conclusion of this chapter the student will be able to:
1. Define the key terms listed
2. Describe epidemiological methods to identify high-risk aggregates in the general population
3. Identify common characteristics or factors that place infants younger than 1 year of age at risk for death and disability
4. Identify common characteristics or factors that place incarcerated persons at risk for death and disability
5. Identify common characteristics or factors that place the homeless at risk for death and disability
6. Use the nursing process to plan care for high-risk aggregates in the community

KEY TERMS

Aggregate
Correctional institution
Deinstitutionalization
High-risk aggregate

Homeless Person's Survival Act
Homeless population
Infant mortality

Epidemiological surveys of large population groups frequently reveal common characteristics or factors in some members of those populations that place them at high risk for death, disease, and disability. Many studies of large population groups, for example, have identified a relationship between maternal cigarette smoking and low infant birth weight. Low birth weight increases the risk for infant mortality and disability. Therefore the infants of mothers who smoke may be considered an aggregate at risk for death and disability, with maternal smoking revealed as the common factor. An aggregate is a collection of individuals who share some similar characteristics.

A high-risk aggregate is a collection of individuals who share similar characteristics or who experience common factors that place them at risk for death and disability. This chapter describes some aggregates in the community that are at high risk for disability and disease.

INFANTS AT RISK

As discussed in Chapter 3, recording vital statistics in one selected community and converting them to relative numbers revealed a high infant mortality rate—20 per 1000—in that community. When this rate was compared with that of a neighboring community—7 per 1000— it was apparent that infants under 1 year in the first community were at higher risk for mortality than those in the second community. An in-depth assessment revealed some common characteristics and factors in the community with the high infant mortality rate that were not shared with the neighboring area in which the infant mortality was lower. One factor was the age of the mothers. There was a higher incidence of pregnancy among teen-agers in the community in which infants were at risk than in the compared area. Consequently, low birth weight, which is associated with pregnancy in teen-agers, may be one factor that places infants at higher risk of mortality and morbidity.

CASE STUDY

A nurse who worked in a special school for pregnant adolescents assessed their unique health problems in the following manner.

Assessment and diagnosis

To determine their students' specific needs and knowledge deficits the nurse met with each student as she entered the school and asked questions about her past and present health history and her source of prenatal care. If the student was not receiving prenatal care, she was referred to a provider. Students were made aware that the school nurse would be available for counseling while they were at the school and that a public health nurse would visit them after the baby's birth. The initial physical examination included determination of blood pressure and weight and a urinalysis.

The nursing diagnosis for the students included potential for high-risk pregnancy related to young age (teen-ager) and lack of prenatal care.

Planning and intervention

The goals of the program were to maintain the student's health during pregnancy and to en-

sure their delivery of healthy babies with normal birth weights.

In an effort to do as much preventive counseling and intervention as possible students were encouraged to weigh in frequently so that the nurse could talk with them. Also visual aids with important information about nutrition, infant development, exercise, and pregnancy were placed on bulletin boards in strategic locations throughout the building.

A nurse's group was formed for group counseling sessions. Some of the topics covered were physical and psychological changes of pregnancy, labor, delivery, and birth control. Much time was spent on nutrition.

Evaluation

Students who completed this program showed a lower incidence of low birth weight babies (5 pounds 8 ounces or less) than did population groups with similar demographical statistics served by the city health department's maternity clinics (Higgs & Gustafson, 1985, pp. 130, 131).

A second group, premature infants, is at high risk for infection because of immature immunological defenses. These infants also may have weak sucking and swallowing reflexes and may require gavage. Because the parents cannot hold or feed the baby, the bonding process may be delayed. An immature respiratory system can lead to respiratory distress, anoxia, and even death. Cerebral ischemia or other trauma can result in permanent neurological impairment. Careful monitoring and adequate postnatal care can make a positive difference.

Another risk factor that places children of teen-aged parents at high risk for death and disability stems from the fact that although the parents are physically mature, emotionally they are adolescents working through their own developmental needs. Unless they receive highly supportive family or social services, parenting may be a tremendous stressor for them, which places their children at high risk for abuse, untended physical problems, or abandonment.

Other factors identified in the community with high infant mortality were unemployment, lack of accessibility to prenatal and postnatal care, substandard housing, high incidence of drug abuse in the neighborhood, and a predominant Hispanic population that spoke and read English poorly.

Investigators were unable to identify one single factor that caused the high infant mortality rate in the community. Rather they hypothesized that multiple causes led to the phenomenon. A web of events that placed infants born in this community at risk is shown in Fig. 21-1.

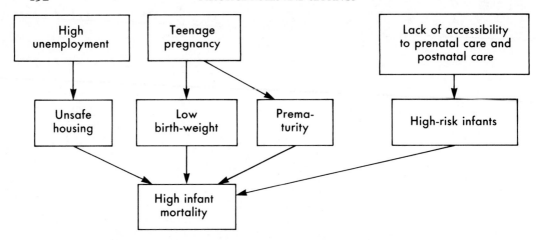

FIG. 21-1 Multiple factors leading to high infant mortality. (From Community as client: Application of nursing process. (p.41) *by E. Anderson, and J. McFarlane, 1988, Philadelphia: Lippincott. Copyright 1988 by the J.B. Lippincott Company. Modified by permission.*)

How the factors interacted was difficult to assess, but the elimination of any one of them should reduce the risk to infants younger than 1 year of age in the community. A nursing diagnosis of potential for injury to infants under 1 year related to multiple risk factors was made. The plan was to decrease the risk factors related to increased infant mortality at primary, secondary, and tertiary levels.

Primary prevention consisted of the following actions:

1. Submit the results of the assessment to local, state, and federal agencies with requests for grant funding to the area for job training, education, and medical care.
2. Meet with local community leaders to plan educational programs related to contraception and prenatal care.

Secondary prevention consisted of the following actions:

1. Educate pregnant teen-agers about proper nutrition and prenatal care to prevent prematurity and/or low birth weight.
2. Visit high-risk infants in the home to monitor progress and educate parents in parenting skills (i.e., anticipatory guidance).

Tertiary prevention consisted of the following actions:

1. Become an advocate for well-baby and sick-child clinics in the neighborhood.
2. Visit failure-to-thrive infants in the home to assess the cause and to implement appropriate interventions.
3. Visit infants in the home, if child abuse is suspected, to assess the situation and to implement intervention if appropriate.
4. Assess the infant's home environment, and plan appropriate interventions if the environment is unsafe.

Evaluation was effected in terms of the success of any of the interventions, that is, evidence of decrease in the infant mortality rate over time. Interventions would be altered and changed, depending on the success or failure of any of the factors.

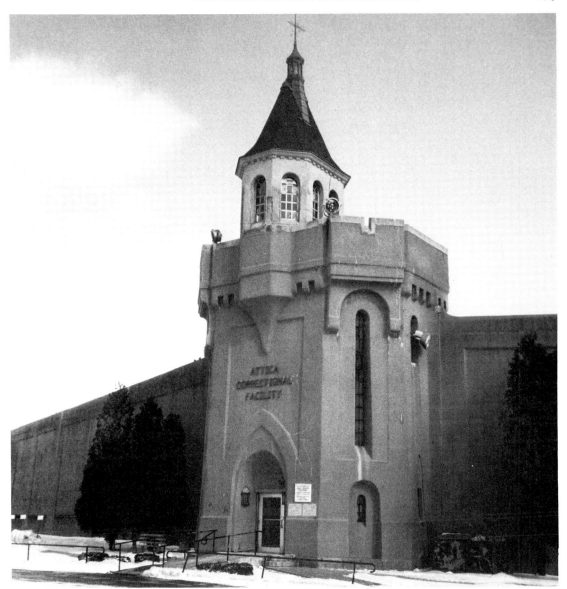

FIG. 21-2 Attica State Prison, Attica, NY.

THE PRISON POPULATION

National crime surveys show that a high percentage of prisoners are young, black, and unmarried and frequently have histories of dysfunctional family life and long-term unemployment.

In 1986 there were more than 400,000 male prisoners in state and federal prisons in the United States, which represents 200 per 100,000 population (0.2%) in the general male population of this country. Of the more than 420,000 (total number of prisoners in custody) at that time, only 20,000 (or 0.4%) were women. Statistics also showed a

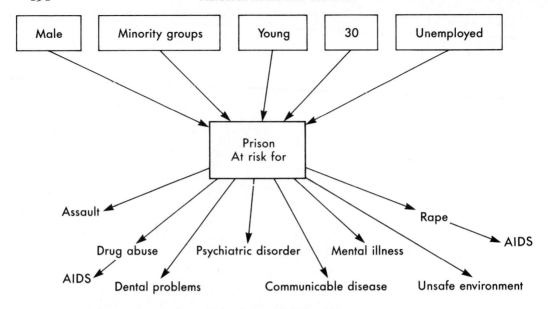

FIG. 21-3 Characteristics common to a majority of the prison population.

sharp increase in the number of incarcerated persons since 1980 (more than 200,000) (Sourcebook of Criminal Justice, 1988).

A study in New York State (Northrop & Kelly, 1987) described the prison population in that state as being at higher risk than the general population for drug abuse, assault, psychiatric disorders, seizures, asthma, venereal disease, tuberculosis, dental problems, and hypertension. Common factors or characteristics shared by the prisoners were that most were men (91%), young (75%) and members of minority groups (57% black and 24% Hispanic). Fig. 21-2 depicts the results of that study.

Maintaining a safe environment for the total prison population is part of the prison nurse's job. All correctional institutions are subject to the same sets of standards that apply to other public institutions. However, periodic lack of funding by federal, state, and county legislatures makes enforcement difficult. Requests for funding sometimes receive a low priority because of a lack of advocacy for the type of client housed in correctional institutions. The need for maximum security in some correctional facilities makes them so expensive to maintain that the provision of modern improvements becomes financially prohibitive.

Sexual assaults occur with alarming regularity. The same altered coping mechanisms that resulted in the prisoners' conviction for rapes, robberies, and other offenses can lead to acts of aggression and subjugation toward members of their own sex when other outlets are cut off (McCuen, 1973). It is believed that these assaults are not a result of sexual frustration but instead are manifestations of the anger and frustration that caused these offenses against society in the first place.

Nursing diagnoses appropriate to this group include the following: (1) self-esteem: chronic low, related to incarceration; (2) injury: potential for, related to unsafe environment; (3) violence, potential for, related to altered coping; and (4) potential for altered health state related to altered life-style).

Nursing goals for this population are to decrease the risk factors at primary, secondary, and tertiary levels.

NURSING PRACTICE IN CORRECTIONAL FACILITIES: STANDARDS OF CARE

Standard I. Organization of nursing services

Nursing services provided in correctional settings will be planned, organized, and administered by a professional registered nurse who has education and experience commensurate with responsibilities.

Standard II. Data collection

The nurse in the correctional setting accurately collects data pertinent to the health of the inmate in an organized and systematic manner.

Standard III. Diagnosis

The nurse in the correctional setting uses nursing diagnoses to express conclusions supported by health assessment data.

Standard IV. Planning

The nurse in the correctional setting develops a nursing plan with specific goals and interventions delineating nursing actions that contribute to the health and well-being of the inmate.

Standard V. Intervention

The nurse in the correctional setting intervenes as guided by the nursing care plan to implement nursing actions that promote, maintain, or restore health; prevent illness; and effect rehabilitation.

Standard V-A. Intervention: health education

The nurse in the correctional setting promotes individual and group well-being through health education activities, including health counseling, health teaching, and formal programs in health education.

Standard V-B. Intervention: suicide prevention

The nurse in the correctional setting uses current mental health concepts in the assessment of suicide risk and in the planning and coordination of interventions that prevent suicidal behavior in the correctional setting.

Standard V-C. Intervention: communicable disease control

The nurse in the correctional setting uses current principles of community health nursing to promote a healthful environment and reduce the incidence of communicable diseases within the correctional setting.

Standard V-D. Intervention: alcohol and drug rehabilitation

The nurse in the correctional setting participates with other members of the health care team in the treatment of inmates who have substance abuse problems.

Standard V-E. Intervention: somatic therapy

Administration of medications within the correctional setting shall be under the supervision of a registered nurse. The nurse shall supervise the adminstration of medications in accordance with state regulations and national standards for the practice of nursing and pharmacy.

Standard V-F. Intervention: psychosocial counseling

The nurse in the correctional setting uses clinical skills to provide inmates with crisis intervention and episodic and ongoing psychosocial counseling.

Standard V-G. Intervention: emergency care

The nurse in the correctional setting initiates emergency care as needed according to community standards of care.

Standard V-H. Intervention: environmental health

The nurse in the correctional setting regularly monitors the environment for conditions that would have a negative impact on health and safety within the facility and reports significant findings to the institution's management.

From Northrop, K. and Kelly M. (1989). Modified from *Standards of nursing practice in correctional facilities* by the American Nurses' Association, p. 255.

Continued.

NURSING PRACTICE IN CORRECTIONAL FACILITIES: STANDARDS OF CARE—cont'd

Standard VI. Evaluation

The nurse in the correctional setting periodically evaluates outcome of nursing actions and revises as necessary plan of care, data base, and nursing interventions.

Standard VII. Collaboration

The nurse in the correctional setting collaborates with other health care providers and colleagues in the facility in assessing, planning, implementing, evaluating, and coordinating health care services consistent with the needs of the institution's population.

Standard VIII. Continuing education

The nurse in the correctional setting shall increase knowledge and skills in nursing practice through participation in continuing education and professional development activities that include an understanding of the uniqueness of the correctional setting.

Standard IX. Professional conduct

The nurse working in the correctional setting must maintain a professional identity and consistently promote health and be an advocate in health promotion.

Standard X. Ethics

The nurse in the correctional setting shall use the code for nurses as established by the American Nurses' Association as a basis for practice.

Prevention

Primary. Each newly incarcerated person will receive an initial health assessment. This assessment shall include examination for possible sexually transmitted disease, drug use, tuberculosis, hypertension, dental problems, breathing disorders, other communicable disease, and mental disorders. The assessment and its findings shall result in a written plan and order to correct health deficits. No person will be admitted who is unconscious.

Secondary. Each correctional institution shall make available a range of health services beyond those that can be provided on an ambulatory basis. This shall include levels of care inside and outside the institution. Prison infirmaries shall meet the same requirements as university and college infirmaries.

Tertiary. Health services shall be provided in every correctional institution. Toothaches and functional impairment of broken and missing teeth shall be corrected with the consent of the inmate. Counseling and mental health services will be available.

Nurses who work in correctional facilities are advised by the American Nurses' Association to follow the standards of nursing practice in correctional facilities (see box on p. 455-456). Careful evaluation on the basis of accurate record keeping and constant monitoring of nursing outcomes provides data to reevaluate nursing interventions.

Evaluation

Evaluation will be based on accurate record keeping and constant monitoring of nursing outcomes. A decrease in the number of health problems reported and treated will be considered a positive outcome.

Society historically has endorsed a punitive attitude toward those who are incarcerated. Attempting to raise the level of wellness of the prisoners within the facility may be viewed as coddling by those outside the helping professions. In addition, prisoners, who are frequently disenfranchised when they enter the system, may become manipulative and feign illness to gain special privileges or a break from routine. Nurses who try to maintain the standards of nursing practice in this setting face a challenging and complex task as they attempt to cooperate with other professionals in the facility to work within the system.

THE HOMELESS POPULATION

The homeless are defined generally as any person whose primary nighttime residence is a public or private shelter, an emergency lodging, a park, a car, or an abandoned building. The homeless suffer from a lack of food, clothing, medical services, and social support.

Articles that romanticize the plight of "bag ladies," "street people," and "grate gentlemen" have tended to overlook the reality of their illnesses and lack of coping ability. A comparison of two principal groups in Philadelphia, the chronically ill and the episodic homeless, described the typical chronically homeless person as white, older than 40 years of age, whose diagnosis was schizophrenia, substance abuse, and other health problems (Arce A., Tadlock, M., Vergare, M.J., & Shapiro, S.,1983). A 1982 field study in New York City (Baxter and Hopper) assessed mental disability and service needs among the homeless on New York City streets. Results suggested as many as half suffer from serious psychiatric disorders. At the same time, however, these reports pointed out the necessity to account for the confounding effects of physical illness before a homeless person is diagnosed as being mentally ill.

Without safe refuge, the homeless are vulnerable to criminal acts such as robbery, assault, and rape. Persons whose faculties are impaired by alcohol abuse and mental illness are particularly susceptible to injury. Their recovery may be hampered by inadequate wound care, poor nutrition, and exposure.

Assessment

Demographical characteristics. It is difficult to estimate the actual number of homeless persons in the United States. Government estimates range from 250,000 to 1 million. Between 1970 and 1980 there was a shift from a homeless population composed largely of alcohol abusers to one with a significant number of persons who once had been diagnosed as mentally ill, disabled individuals, families with young children, and elderly persons.

One investigation (Leaf and Cohen, 1982) detailed the demographical and diagnostic changes in the population of New York City during this same decade (1970-1980). The researchers found significant changes in age and racial composition. Although abusers of alcohol and other substances still accounted for a large portion of the homeless population,

TABLE 21-1 Homelessness in major cities of the United States		
City	Estimated no. of homeless persons	Shelter beds available
Burlington, Vermont	75-120	60
Boston, Massachussets	5000-8000	1,400
Cincinnati, Ohio	1600	800
Dallas, Texas	14,000	1,000
Los Angeles, California	33,000-50,000	3,640
Miami, Florida	9000	350
New York City	60,000-80,000	22,000
Portland, Oregon	7000	2,000
St. Louis, Missouri	10,000-15,000	428
Tucson, Arizona	2000-3000	165

From U.S. Conference of Mayors. (1986). *Responding to homelessness in America's cities: A 13 city survey:* Washington, DC.

the group in 1980 was younger and had a relatively higher percentage of black and Hispanic persons.

As shown in Table 21-1, a study initiated by a 1986 conference of mayors in the United States reported the number of homeless persons in various areas of the country and the lack of facilities available to help them. Data compiled by this group also indicated the following pattern in the homeless category: 51% black, 33.3% white, 14.8% Hispanic, and some native Americans and Asian Americans (First & Arewa, 1988).

Common health problems. The incidence of episodic illness and chronic health problems is high among the homeless (Table 21-2). Physical problems that are chronic and are related to the homeless state include disorders of the lower leg and the feet, which occur to a disproportionate degree compared with cohorts in the general population because homeless persons sometimes have no place to lie down at night. Thus edema and loss of venous valve competence often result (Lamb 1984). Infestation occurs because of shared clothing and lack of sanitary living conditions. According to recent studies, the homeless also are at high risk for tuberculosis; once it has developed, recovery is slow because this population generally is of noncompliance with follow-up care.

Causes. The causes of homelessness include a critical lack of affordable housing, economic factors (including persisting high levels of unemployment), insufficient care for the mentally ill, and federal cutbacks of aid to the poor (Fig. 21-4) (National Coalition for the Homeless, 1988).

In the 1960s, in response to less than satisfactory conditions in mental institutions, a policy of releasing mental patients to halfway houses was begun. Although well intended, the policy, termed deinstitutionalization, resulted in the release of some individuals to the streets. Poor discharge planning and inadequate alternatives are blamed for the phenomenon of the mentally ill homeless. The concept of deinstitutionalization may have failed because halfway houses and planned supervised group homes were not established.

The budget cuts of the Reagan administration reduced aid to the poor from $32 billion to $7.6 billion. Demolition of public housing to make way for urban renewal drastically reduced the availability of housing for many low income persons. High unemployment and falling wages caused an increase in the number of poor Americans. Although the shift from an industrialized society to a service economy has created many new jobs, most of these pay very low wages.

Once a family that is on the edge of poverty loses its home because of a family crisis or the loss of job, finding a new job, registering for school, and applying for public assistance are almost impossible. The cycle of homelessness begins. Merely the deposit to rent an apartment becomes unattainable. Benefits to elderly and disabled persons were cut severely during the 1980s. For example, in 1985 some 491,300 persons with disabilities were dropped from the roles. Lengthy legal procedures reversed the process, but by that time many elderly and disabled persons already had become homeless. Since 1981 funding for Aid to Dependent Children and the food stamp program have been drastically reduced.

The Homeless Person's Survival Act. In October 1986 Congress passed the Homeless Person's Survival Act. It included the following provisions:

- Homeless persons living in shelters are now eligible for food stamps. In addition, food stamps may be used by homeless people to buy prepared meals served by nonprofit agencies.
- Federal agencies may not bar any person without a fixed address from receiving benefits from Supplemental Social Security Income, Medicaid, Aid to Dependent Children, or the Veterans Administration.

TABLE 21-2 Presenting medical diagnoses in 434 homeless patients seen in a free clinic in New York City

Diagnosis		No.
Acute or chronic alcoholism		160
Drug use, intravenous or subcutaneous		102
Trauma		80
Assault	32	
Accidental	38	
Burns	10	
Respiratory infection		76
Active pulmonary tuberculosis		54
Leg ulcer, cellulitis		41
Acute gastrointestinal disease		22
Seizure disorder		16
Jaundice or acites		15
Venereal disease		7
Gonorrhea	5	
Primary syphilis	2	
Osteomyelitis		2

From *Providing services for the homeless: The New York City program* (p. 82) by A. Leaf and M. Cohen, 1982, City of New York Human Resources Administration, December 1982.

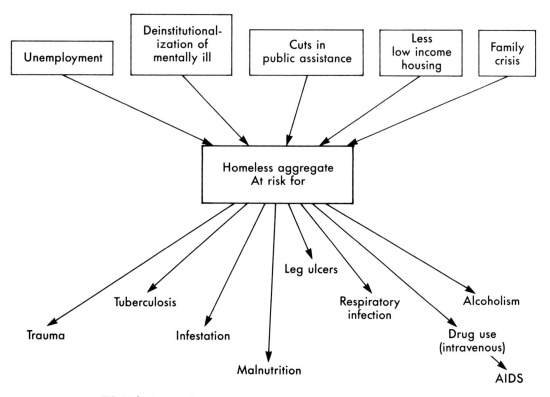

FIG. 21-4 Factors that contribute to homelessness and resulting risk factors.

- Homeless persons are specifically included in the Job Training Partnership Act.

Proposed solutions. The National Coalition for the Homeless is a privately funded group first organized in 1979; it has offices in New York City, Albany, New York, and Washington D.C. The goal of a paid staff of 30 persons and scores of volunteers is to ease the plight of the homeless by serving as their advocate and providing services to them. The organization has proposed the following solutions to the problems of this population (1988):

- Ensure that all persons have a base minimum of emergency shelter.
- Provide effective outreach so that homeless persons receive the federal benefits to which they are entitled.
- Provide special emergency assistance to homeless families, including shelters for families with infants.
- Prevent unnecessary evictions from subsidized and private housing.
- Preserve low-rent housing such as single-room-occupancy hotels.
- Modify Aid to Dependent Children eligibility requirements to discourage maintenance of extended-family living arrangements.
- Increase the number of federally subsidized housing units.
- Require local governments that receive federal funds to make vacant, tax-foreclosed buildings available to house the homeless.
- Develop community-based permanent residences for mentally ill homeless persons.

Nursing Diagnosis

Nursing diagnoses for the homeless include the following:
- Potential for injury related to unsafe environment
- Altered nutrition, less than body requirements
- Potential for infection related to shared clothing and lack of sanitation
- Altered peripheral perfusion related to lack of sleeping space
- Self-care deficit; bathing hygiene
- Powerlessness related to homelessness
- Ineffective coping related to substance abuse
- Ineffective coping related to mental state
- Ineffective family coping, compromised

Planning

Planning interventions to decrease homelessness requires the elimination of some of the harmful characteristics that increase the risk of disability and disease.

Implementation

Nursing outreach to the homeless is most likely to occur in the public shelters that provide medical assistance (Fig. 21-5) or in hospital emergency rooms where the homeless go for care.

Intervention: Prevention

Primary. Primary prevention of homelessness includes supporting legislation that helps the poor, needy families, and persons with mental illness. Writing or calling politicians may help to lower the incidence of homelessness.

Secondary. Secondary prevention measures include screening in shelters and emergency rooms for tuberculosis, infection, malnutrition, leg ulcers, trauma, and drug abuse and providing care as appropriate.

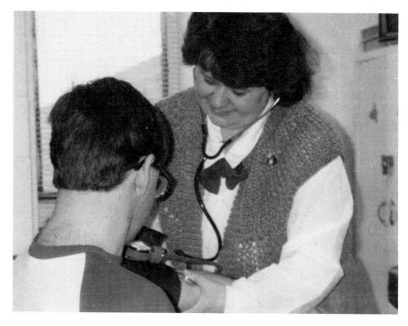

FIG. 21-5 A community health nurse performs a health assessment for a homeless client.

Tertiary. Tertiary prevention focuses on the facilitation of care for alterations in health states of the homeless. It includes counseling of families, as well as single persons, concerning the help that is available to them.

Evaluation

Crisis visits to emergency rooms would decrease, and studies would show that the health of the homeless was improving if these nursing interventions were effective.

SUMMARY

Epidemiological surveys and research studies can identify aggregates in populations that are at high risk for death and disability. A knowledge of the common characteristics and factors of these groups can assist the community health nurse to plan for their care. Specific interventions can be planned to raise the level of wellness in targeted populations at primary, secondary, and tertiary levels. Infants at high risk, prisoners, and the homeless are some high-risk aggregates. Abused children, battered women, and disabled and elderly persons are also at high risk and may require priority intervention and care. Raising the level of wellness of population aggregates in a community also can raise the level of health of the community in which these groups live.

 CHAPTER HIGHLIGHTS

- A high-risk aggregate is a group of individuals who share similar characteristics or experience common factors that place them at risk for disease, disability, or death.
- Aggregates at risk include low birth weight infants, prisoners, the homeless, the mentally ill, and persons with AIDS and their families.
- Health problems prevalent in the homeless population include lower leg disorders and tuberculosis.

- At one time the homeless population consisted primarily of single men who abused alcohol. Today this population includes families with children, the mentally ill, the elderly, and the disabled.
- Deinstitutionalization is the process of releasing mentally ill patients from psychiatric institutions to halfway houses or group homes. In many cases, however, discharge planning is inadequate and follow-up facilities are not available, resulting in increased homelessness.
- Community health nurses who work with high-risk aggregates use primary, secondary, and tertiary prevention strategies to promote optimum health and to minimize disease, disability, and death.

STUDY QUESTIONS

1. Define high-risk aggregate.
2. Describe the multiple causes that place infants younger than 1 year of age at high risk for death and disability.
3. Describe the nurse's role in the prison as outlined by the American Nurse's Association standards of nursing practice.
4. Describe the acute and chronic illnesses for which the homeless are at risk.

REFERENCES

American Public Health Association. (1976). *Standards for health services in correctional institutions.* Washington, DC: Author.

American Public Health Association. (1981). *The definition and role of public health nursing in the delivery of health care: A statement of the public nursing section.* Washington, DC: Author.

Anderson, E., & McFarlane, J. (1988). *Community as Client: Application of nursing process.* Philadelphia: Lippincott.

Anderson, L. & Thobaben, M. (1984) Clients in crisis: When should the nurse step in? *Journal of Gerontological Nursing, 10*(12), 6-10.

Arce, A., Tadlock M., Vergare M. J., & Shapiro, S. (1983). A psychiatric profile of street people admitted to an emergency shelter. *Hospital and Community Psychiatry, 34,* 812-217.

Baxter, E. & Hopper, K. (1981). *Private lives/public spaces: Homeless adults on the streets of New York City.* New York: Community Service Society.

Bruss, C. (1988). Nursing diagnosis of hopelessness. *Journal of Psychosocial Nursing, 6*(3), 28-31.

First, R. & Arewa, B. (1988). *Homelessness: Understanding the dimensions of the problem for minorities.* National Association of Social Workers, Inc. *33,* pp. 120-124.

Goldman H. H., Gattozzi, A., & Taube, A. (1981). Defining and counting the chronically mentally ill. Hospital and *Community Psychiatry, 32*(1), 17-27.

Hallowitz, D. (1980). The problem-solving component in family therapy. In C. Munson (Ed.), *Social work with families: Theory and practice* (pp. 228-239). New York: The Free Press.

Hartman, C. (1987). *The housing part of the homeless problem.* Boston: The Boston Foundation.

Higgs, Z., & Gustafson, D. (1985). *Community as client: Assessment and diagnosis:* Philadelphia: Davis.

Lamb, R. (1984). *The homeless mentally ill: A task force report of the American Psychiatric Association.* Washington, DC: American Psychiatric Association.

Leaf, A., & Cohen, M. (1982, December). *Providing services for the homeless: The New York City program.* City of New York Human Resources Administration, p. 82.

McCuen, G. (1973). *America's Prisons,* Mississippi. San Diego: Greenhaven Press.

National Coalition for the Homeless. (1988). New York: Author (105 East 22 St., New York, NY 10010).

Northrop, C. & Kelly, M. (1987). *Legal issues in nursing.* St. Louis: Mosby.

Sourcebook of Criminal Justice. (1988). (Bureau of Justice Statistics). T. Flanagan & K. Jamieson (Eds.). Washington, DC, copyright by Hindelang Criminal Justice Bureau.

U.S. Conference of Mayors. (1986). *Responding to homelessness in America's cities.* Washington, DC.

U.S. Department of Justice, Bureau of Justice Statistics. (1988). In Whaley, L. F., & Wong, D. L. (1987). *Nursing care of infants and children* (3rd ed.). St. Louis: Mosby.

Communicable Diseases

ROBERT J. PERELLI and JOAN M. COOKFAIR

The body's immune system can be thought of as flexible lines of resistance that help a person to defend against a stressor.

BETTY NEUMANN

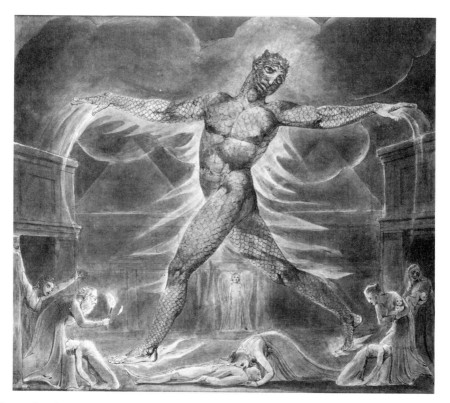

Pestilence: Death of the firstborn. *(Illustration to the Bible. William Blake, English, 1757-1827. Pen and watercolor on paper, ca. 1805, Height, 12 inches; Width, 13½ inches. Gift by subscription. Courtesy Museum of Fine Arts, Boston.)*

OBJECTIVES

At the conclusion of this chapter the student will be able to:

1. Define the key terms listed
2. Describe the concept of relevant immunity in individuals and populations
3. Discuss the impact of altered immunity on the incidence and prevalence of disease
4. Use selected epidemiological models in planning interventions against communicable disease
5. Describe some of the methods used to facilitate the surveillance of communicable disease in populations and groups
6. Identify and describe selected communicable diseases
7. Discuss some of the complex issues surrounding the nursing care of the client with acquired immunodeficiency syndrome (AIDS)

KEY TERMS

Acquired immunodeficiency syndrome
Active immunization
Artificial immunity
Chain of transmission
Direct transmission
Immunity
Immunization
Incubation period

Indirect transmission
Natural immunity
Opportunistic infection
Passive immunity
Period of communicability
Plague
Surveillance
Universal precautions

Immunity, or resistance to a particular disease or infection, can vary in an individual or in a population on a day-to-day basis, particularly in terms of resistance, or lack of resistance, to communicable diseases.

Two types of immunity are active and passive. Active immunity to a specific disease or infection can be heightened by the natural acquisition of antibodies as a result of a specific infection or by the acquisition of antibodies through immunization by injection with weakened or killed toxins. Passive immunity can be acquired naturally, passed from the mother to the fetus in utero. It also may be acquired by the injection of gamma globulin or antibodies to a specific disease. Passive immunity generally is not permanent (see Glossary).

An individual with active or passive immunity thus may respond adequately to prevent illness (clinical symptoms) if immunity is strong when an infection invades the body.

Immunity, however, is relative, and protection that had been adequate can be overcome by the excessive strength of an infectious agent. It can also be diminished by (1) some forms of immunosuppressive chemotherapy, (2) infection that has weakened cellular immunity, or (3) the aging process. The client's inherent belief system, values, and culture can affect his or her level of immunity. For example, the Amish, who do not believe in artificial immunization, recently experienced an outbreak of polio in Pennsylvania. Areas closeby where children (and sometimes adults) had been immunized against the disease were not affected.

Immunity can be diminished in an individual by exposure to extreme heat or cold or a prolonged disease state. Excessive stress, whether psychological, biological, or physical, can reduce an individual's immunity (Benensen, 1981). The stressors may be internal or external.

A population's resistance to disease is affected by the level of immunity of the majority of the population, the environment in which the population lives, and, in some measure, the socioeconomic level. It also can be affected by accessibility to health services. For example, teams of health professionals have vaccinated a sufficient number of people against smallpox (variola) so that since 1977 *no* cases have been reported anywhere in the world. Thus the disease has ceased to exist in human reservoirs, and in 1980 the World Health Organization declared global immunity to smallpox (Benensen, 1981). This is not to say that everyone in the world has been vaccinated against smallpox; in fact, immunization is not recommended anymore. At this time, one reported case of smallpox anywhere in the world probably would result in massive immunizations on a global scale.

APPLICATION OF BETTY NEUMAN'S SYSTEMS MODEL TO THE CONCEPT OF IMMUNITY

Betty Neuman's client systems model can be used to visualize the dynamics of relative immunity. (See Chapter 3 for an explanation of this model and its application to the level of wellness in a community.) As shown in Chapter 3, *the flexible lines of defense* are represented by the outer broken lines of the model. They form the outer boundary of the external influence on an individual or population group. According to Neuman, each line of defense contains similar elements related to five variables—physiological, psychological, developmental, sociocultural, and spiritual. Ideally the flexible lines of defense protect the client from stressor invasions. They are relative and can vary in individuals and populations depending on factors previously mentioned. Climate, developmental stage, socioeconomic group, culture, exposure to infection, accessibility to health care, level of air pollution, and effective public health services are some of the variables.

The normal line of defense is depicted by the solid larger circle in the model. It represents the individual's or the population's usual wellness state. If a stressor breaks through the normal state, lines of resistance are activated. The normal line of defense is influenced by coping patterns, life-style factors, developmental and spiritual influences, and culture. The normal line of defense, or usual wellness state, can remain the same, become reduced, or expand after treatment of a stressor reaction (Neuman, 1989).

The lines of resistance, shown by the inner broken concentric circles around the basic structure, are constantly changing. They represent known and unknown factors internal to the individual or group that become activated upon the invasion of a stressor. An example of an individual's line of resistance is the body's mobilization of white blood cells or immune system mechanisms upon the invasion of a biological stressor. In a community, on the other hand, local, state, and federal agencies would mobilize to combat a biological stressor that threatened to turn into an epidemic.

The basic structure, represented by the small inner circle, consists of survival factors common to the individual or population that preserve the basic integrity of the system, for example, innate genetic factors, strengths and weaknesses of system parts, and basic energy resources. Stressors that penetrate this inner circle can cause severe illness or death both in an individual and in the community.

EPIDEMIOLOGICAL TRIAD

The epidemiological triad (see Chapter 7) identifies the three components (agent, host, and environment) that are necessary for a communicable disease to spread. Identification

---

WATER-RELATED DISEASE OUTBREAK, 1985

An outbreak of typhoid fever *(Salmonella typhi)* occurred after cross-contamination between parallel sewer lines during maintenance procedures in 1985. All cases were associated with the drinking of chlorinated but unfiltered water. This outbreak of water-borne typhoid fever was the first to be reported in the United States or its territories since 1974.

From "Water-related disease outbreaks" by the Centers for Disease Control, June 1988, *MMWR. Morbidity and Mortality Weekly Report, 37,* 55-2, p. 16

---

and modification of any one of these can, theoretically, alter the incidence and prevalence of infectious disease.

The *agent* is most often viral, bacterial, fungal, or protozoal. Knowledge of the causative agent can help the nurse predict its method of transmission. For example, varicella (chickenpox) is caused by a virus that is transmitted by droplet infection or by direct contact with the drainage from the lesions it causes. Although the mortality rate is low, the disease is highly communicable. To prevent its spread individuals with chickenpox are advised to limit contact with others and to stay at home until all drainage from lesions has stopped.

The *host,* or person who may be infected by the agent, may or may not be vulnerable to it. As previously discussed, several factors may influence the host's level of immunity. In addition, some agents are more virulent in specific groups under specific conditions. For example, the effects of pertussis (whooping cough) are much more serious in children younger than 2 years of age than in older children. The susceptibility of the host decreases with age. Active artifical immunization is therefore seldom recommended for children older than 6 years.

The *environment* is another factor that can affect the incidence and prevalence of communicable disease. Before the advent of water purification, *Salmonella,* the bacteria responsible for a number of gastrointestinal diseases, including typhoid fever *(S. typhi),* was responsible for many deaths. The bacillus is excreted in the feces of infected persons and is spread by contaminated food and water (particularly shellfish). Even before the identification of the causative agent, epidemics were stopped in England by the discovery of the mode of transmission and subsequent water purification campaign (see Chapter 1). The disease still surfaces today in areas where water becomes contaminated (see box above). Modification of any component of the agent/host/environmental traid can eliminate or stop the spread of an infectious disease.

Mode of Transmission

The manner of transfer of an agent to a host sometimes is called the mode of transmission. *Direct transmission* occurs from human being to human being or from animal to animal by direct contact through some portal of entry. For example, tuberculosis, which is caused by a bacillus, is spread by droplet infection from the lungs through the upper respiratory tract. An infected person can pass it by such activities as sneezing, coughing, or even laughing. Gonorrhea, also caused by a bacteria, is spread through contaminated body fluid, most often through the reproductive tract. Systemic mycosis can be transmitted by clothing or bedding that is contaminated by fungus spores (Harrison, 1975).

Indirect transmission of disease occurs in the following ways (Benenson, 1981):

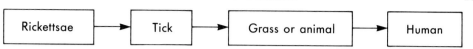

FIG. 22-1 Chain of transmission of Rocky Mountain spotted fever.

1. Vehicle borne, for example, *Salmonella* transmitted by contaminated food or water
2. Vector borne, for example, plague, which is transmitted by fleas
3. Airborne, for example, Legionnaires' disease, which is transmitted through contaminated air

Chain of Transmission

Some diseases have so complicated a mode of transmission that they are said to have a chain of transmission (Fig. 22-1). Rocky Mountain spotted fever is a febrile disease with a rash that resembles rubeola (measles). The causative agent is a minute bacterial organism called *Rickettsia,* which grows in the cells of ticks that then harbor the infection throughout their lifetime and become carriers. Ticks adhere to grass and small animals as well as to human beings, who contract Rocky Mountain spotted fever by the transfer of the *Rickettsia* organism through the bite of an infected tick. Interrupting the chain of transmission at any point can stop the spread of disease. Spraying infected grassy areas, wearing protective clothing in areas where ticks may be found, and daily inspection of house pets are all measures that can interrupt the chain of transmission.

Obviously this concept is similar to the agent/host/environment model depicted by the epidemiological triad whereby getting rid of the agent can stop the disease process, altering the environment can stop the disease process, and altering the susceptibility of the host can stop the incidence of disease.

SURVEILLANCE

Surveillance, or monitoring, of the incidence and prevalence of communicable diseases through accurate record keeping and data collection can alert health professionals to the possibility of dangerous outbreaks of disease in populations. For example, the results of ongoing surveillance of the incidence of plague in the United States showed the possible development of a serious epidemic of plague on a Navaho Indian reservation. In 1955 only two cases of plague were reported in the United States. Until seven cases of plague occurred on the Navaho reservation in 1965, cases continued to occur at the rate of 1 to 2 per year. Then an insidious increase began in the United States, with a peak of 40 cases in 1983 and 31 cases in 1984. A disproportionate number of cases occurred among the Navaho.

Of the 299 cases of plague reported from 1956 to 1987, 74 occurred on the Navaho reservation, which seemed to be the center of distribution (Table 22-1). The Navaho reservation encompasses a 26,000-square-mile area in northwestern New Mexico, northeastern Arizona, and southern Utah. The white and Hispanic persons who were infected were all from southwestern states that border the Navaho reservation. Of the 299 who were infected, 53 died; 20 of these victims were younger than 9 years old. It seems likely that plague, which is transmitted by infected fleas on rodents to human beings, is more likely to occur among persons who live in rural and semirural areas of the Southwest than in other parts of the country.

Historically plague has been prevalent in crowded and unsanitary conditions where rats transport infected fleas. In the case of the outbreak in the Southwest, researchers have

TABLE 22-1   Distribution of 299 human plague cases, by racial/ethnic group, United States, 1956-1987

Racial/ethnic group	No. cases	No. fatal cases
Caucasian	146	27
Caucasian-Hispanic	50	10
American Indian		
Navajo	74	14
Pueblo	12	1
Hopi	1	0
Mescalero Apache	2	0
Warm Springs	1	0
Southern Ute	1	0
Other*	2	1
TOTAL	299	53

From Centers for Disease Control: "Plague in American Indians 1956-1987" by the Centers for Disease Control, July 1988, *MMWR. Morbidity and Mortality Weekly Report, 37*, 55-3, p. 14.
*Other = 1 Japanese, died; 1 Iranian, survived.

found that a plague-susceptible rodent, the rock squirrel, probably is responsible. These squirrels live close to human activity, and the fleas they carry transport the disease effectively. Prairie dogs also are susceptible to infected fleas and are part of the chain of transmission that transports the fleas to human beings. The antelope ground squirrel can be a source of infection as well.

To stop the spread of the disease, insecticides and rodenticides have been used to kill vectors and carriers. Educational programs have been attempted by tribal community health workers and the federal government with some degree of success. The vastness of the area made the plague difficult to control, but by 1985 only 11 cases were reported. The threat of the spread of this very serious disease and the possibility of an epidemic pose a danger to the country and actually to the entire continent. Ongoing surveillance and monitoring continue (CDC, July 1988).

Prompt reporting to local health authorities of all communicable diseases in populations assists in ongoing monitoring and surveillance. Each health jurisdiction declares a list of reportable diseases (Benensen, 1983). After the information is given to local health authorities, the information is passed on to the district, state, or provincial level. Appropriate information is routed to national information centers. The collecting agency in the United States is the Centers for Disease Control; in Canada it is the Laboratory Center for Disease Control. National agencies report to the World Health Organization the incidence of diseases for which there may be global concerns (Benensen, 1983).

PREVENTION

Illness caused by a specific infective agent or its toxic products is said to be communicable. Community health nurses need a firm knowledge of the agent, the mode of transmission, the incubation period (the time from exposure to the agent until symptoms appear), and the period of communicability (the time when the disease can be spread). They also need to know the clinical symptoms and the appropriate nursing interventions to prevent disease and to plan secondary and tertiary care. Many common communicable diseases are listed in Table 22-2.

TABLE 22-2	Common communicable diseases						
Disease	Agent	Mode of transmission	Incubation period	Period of communicability	Clinical symptoms	Nursing intervention	Prevention
Diphtheria	Bacteria	Direct contact or articles soiled from lesions	2-5 days	2-4 wk	Lesions of tonsils, pharynx, and nose; serious in infants. High mortality rate in children under 2 yr	Symptomatic; possible tracheostomy care; monitor carefully	Immunization
Fifth disease (erythema infectiosum)	Unknown	Unknown	5-10 days	Unknown	Mild fever, erythema over face, generalized maculopapular rash	Acetaminophen for fever, fluids; treatment of symptoms	None
Mumps	Viral	Droplet infection	18 days	48 hours before swelling occurs	Mild fever, swelling of one or more salivary glands	Acetaminophen for fever, soft foods, liquids; limited activity, isolation	Immunization
Poliomyelitis	Viral	Direct contact (fecal/oral)	3-35 days	36 hours before symptoms, 72 hours after	Fever, headache, stiffness of neck, paralysis of muscles of neck and swallowing. Sometimes minor, sometimes fatal; may cause paralysis	Treat symptoms as they occur; appropriate isolation techniques	Immunization
Rubella	Viral	Droplet infection; crosses placental barrier	16-18 days	1 wk before and 4 days after onset of rash. Infants who have congenital rubella shed the virus for months after birth	Low-grade fever, headache, coryza, conjunctivitis, macular rash in some cases. Teratogenic effects in congenital rubella to the fetus in utero	Limited activity, acetaminophen for fever; fluids. Keep away from pregnant women	Immunization; immunoglobulin (Ig) serum to pregnant women exposed to rubella

Continued.

470 PRACTICE ROLES AND SETTINGS

TABLE 22-2 Common communicable diseases—cont'd

Disease	Agent	Mode of transmission	Incubation period	Period of communicability	Clinical symptoms	Nursing intervention	Prevention
Rubeola (red measles)	Viral	Droplet infection	8-13 days	Just before symptoms appear and about 4 days after the rash is gone	High fever, hacking cough, conjunctivitis, irregular red lesions (Koplik's spots) with blue-white centers in mucous membranes of mouth, red maculopapular rash, generalized malaise	Limited activity, acetaminophen for fever, cough syrup if needed. Protect eyes from light; soft diet, push fluids. Monitor carefully; isolation	Immunization
Scabies	Mite	Skin to skin, undergarments, soiled bed clothes	2-6 wk	Until treated	Tiny linear patches on skin that itch	Kwell	None
Scarlet fever	Streptococci	Direct or indirect	1-3 days	10-21 days	Fever, skin rash, strawberry tongue	Acetaminophen for fever, rest, antibiotics, soft foods, fluids	Limit spread
Shigellosis	Bacillus	Fecal, oral transmission; contaminated food	1-3 days	During acute infection and some time after	Severe diarrhea; often afebrile	Nonirritating diet, Kaopectate, etc.	Avoid contaminated water/food
Streptococcal sore throat	Streptococci	Direct or indirect through objects or hands	1-3 days	10-21 days	Fever, sore throat, cervical lymph nodes	Acetaminophen for fever, pain; fluids, limited activity, antibiotics	None

						Symptomatic	Immunization
Tetanus	Bacillus	Spores in soil, street dust, lacerations and burns	4-21 days	None	Painful muscular contractions of neck and trunk muscles; may be fatal		
Tinea capitis (ringworm)	Fungus	Direct or indirect contact	10-14 days	As long as lesions are present	Scaly patches and papules that spread; may itch, may cause baldness	Lindane (Kwell); advise to wash all contaminated clothing	None
Varicella (chickenpox)	Viral	Droplet infection	2-3 wk	1-2 days before rash, 6 days after appearance of vesicles	Slight fever, vesicular skin eruption	Acetaminophen for fever, limited activity, soft foods, fluids, baking soda baths	None
Venereal							
Chlamydial	Trachoma	Sexually transmitted	Unknown	Unknown	Urethritis, pelvic inflammatory disease	Medications as ordered, comfort measures	None
Gonorrhea	Gonococcus	Sexually transmitted	2-7 days	Until treated	Purulent discharge, pain	Antibodies	Education
Herpes	Viral	Intimate contact	2-12 days	When lesions are weeping	Painful, weepy vesicles in infected area	Burrow's soaks; keep dry and clean	Education
Syphilis	*Treponema pallidum*	Sexually transmitted	3 wk	Unless treated 2-4 yr	Primary lesion, rash, systemic effect	Antibodies	Education

Primary Prevention

Preventing the occurrence of a disease through active immunization is a method of primary prevention. The American Academy of Pediatrics has recommended a schedule of immunizations for infants and children (see Chapter 9).

Measles, mumps, and rubella may be combined into one injection, which usually is given at 15 months. Tetanus/diptheria is a combined immunization administered to children older than 6 years of age. A combined injection of diptheria/pertussis/tetanus is given to those younger than 6 years.

Immunizations that contain attenuated toxins should not be administered to pregnant women or to individuals in an altered immune state or given after recent injections of immunoglobulin serum. They should be postponed during an acute febrile illness, particularly in children, and screening for hyperactivity or allergy is recommended. A careful history should be taken before the adminstration of immunizations; for example, children with a history of seizures should not receive pertussis vaccine. Clients must be reassured, however, that the benefits far outweigh the risks to those for whom an immunization is not contraindicated.

Secondary Prevention

Preventing the manifestation of clinical symptoms by screening for the presence of an agent may enable the nurse to plan interventions before a client becomes ill.

Frequency of tuberculin testing depends on the client's risk of exposure and on the prevalence of tuberculosis in a population group. The tine test, or purified protein derivative (PPD), should not be given at the same time as the measles, mumps, rubella vaccine. It is not an immunization but rather a screening test to determine the presence of tuberculosis antibodies. If it is administered at the same time as an immunization against another disease, the result may be a false positive reaction to the test because of the body's immune response to a vaccine.

Tertiary Prevention

The prevention of disability after clinical symptoms have manifested can be accomplished by appropriate nursing intervention. A gonorrheal infection can cause pelvic inflammatory disease in a woman, which can lead to sterility. Appropriate adminstration of antibiotics to stop the spread of the infection can prevent the occurrence of both events.

COMMON COMMUNICABLE DISEASES
Hepatitis

Viral hepatitis is a serious communicable disease. Although the several viruses that cause this infectious disease have somewhat different characteristics, the result is a similar type of illness.

Viral hepatitis A is spread by the fecal-oral route. The incubation period is 15 to 50 days, and the period of greatest communicability is toward the end of the incubation period and during the first few days before the onset of jaundice. Symptoms include fever, malaise, anorexia, nausea, and abdominal discomfort. Jaundice usually is present at some stage. The disease can be mild to severe, but mortality is rare. Rest, multivitamins, and small appetizing meals are appropriate interventions. Good hand-washing technqiues, separate dishes or careful sterilization of utensils, and general enteric precautions are advised during the first stages of the disease. If water purification is impaired, the disease can be spread through the system via the fecal route.

Temporary heightened immunity can be given to individuals exposed to hepatitis A by the adminstration of immune globulin, 0.02 ml/kg of body weight. The best primary prevention is good sanitation and hygienic practices to reduce fecal contamination of food and water.

Viral hepatitis B is transmitted through body fluids and blood products. The incubation period is 45 to 160 days. The period of communicability remains throughout the course of the disease, and a chronic carrier state may develop. Symptoms include anorexia, abdominal discomfort, nausea, vomiting, and sometimes a rash. In some cases jaundice occurs. Nursing care includes rest, multivitamins, and small appetizing meals. Blood and body fluid precautions are essential to prevent transmission. Active artificial immunization is available by means of hepatitis B vaccine (Heptavax-B), which should be given to those at high risk for contracting the disease.

Viral hepatitis that is caused by unidentified agents is similar to hepatitis B in type and treatment. Some protection is provided by the hepatits B immunization.

Tuberculosis

Tuberculosis is caused by a bacillus. Most often it is transmitted by droplet infection and, without treatment, is communicable throughout the course of the disease. The agent is transmitted from host to host through infected sputum. The time period from infection to clinical symptoms is about 4 to 6 weeks. Fatigue, fever, and weight loss occur early. Cough, chest pain, hemoptysis, and hoarseness appear late in the disease.

Nursing intervention includes supervision to encourage compliance with the therapeutic regimen for persons being treated at home. Specific drug therapy may control infectiousness very rapidly; compliance can result in bacteria-free sputum within a few weeks. Infected persons must be taught to cover the mouth and nose with tissue when they cough, sneeze, or laugh. Proper disposal of the tissue also is important. Clients whose sputum is free of bacteria, who are not coughing, and who are medically compliant need not be isolated. Good hand-washing technique and housekeeping practices are adequate precautions in the home.

Prevention can be accomplished by investigation of contacts and routine tuberculin testing of large segments of the population. Positive tuberculin tests of contacts who show positive reactions but who have no clinical disease can be converted by chemotherapy in most cases.

Older persons who have been infected early in life but are symptom free should be made aware that a relapse is possible if an altered health state occurs and immunity is depressed.

Elimination of tuberculosis among dairy cattle and pasteurization of milk are other public health measures. Bovine tuberculosis, although rare, still can be a problem in underdeveloped countries where the bacillus can be spread through unpasteurized milk.

Tuberculosis is apt to be more of a problem in crowded, unsanitary living conditions than in well-ventilated, hygienically sound surroundings.

Lyme Disease

Lyme disease, first recognized in eastern Connecticut, is caused by a spirochete that is transmitted by an infected tick. The symptoms are fatigue, chills, and fever, plus a distinctive skin lesion referred to as erythema chronicum migrans (ECM). Arthritic symptoms follow in some cases. Symptoms can last as long as 2 years, with periods of remission.

Nursing intervention includes careful assessment of the client's objective and subjective history to facilitate proper medical diagnosis. A care plan should include a recomendation of limited activity and supervision of the medical regimen, such as the administration of salicylates, steroids, and antibiotics.

TABLE 22-3 Number of cases of AIDS reported to the World Health Organization, June 1988

Continent	No. of countries reporting one or more cases	No. of cases
Africa	43	11,530
The Americas	40	71,343
Asia	21	254
Europe	28	12,414
Oceania	4	892
TOTAL	136	96,433

From *Bulletin* (Vol. 23, 10) (p. 10) by the Pan American Health Organization, 1989, Washington, DC: Author. Copyright 1989 by the Pan American Health Organization. Reprinted by permission.

The prevalence of Lyme disease seems to be regional. Persons in areas where it is prevalent should be advised to wear protective clothing in tick-infested areas and to examine exposed skin for tick bites and unusual lesions (Pickering & Dupont, 1986).

Acquired Immunodeficiency Syndrome

Incidence and prevalence. In 1981, an outbreak of *Pneumocystis carinii* pneumonia occurred in San Francisco. All the affected individuals were young men with a history of homosexual activity and all died. At this time, the disease that we now know as acquired immunodeficiency syndrome (AIDS) has developed into a global pandemic. Although more knowledge about the disease now exists, it remains difficult to prevent and impossible to cure, and it always is fatal. Statistics show an increasing number of cases, which has led to worldwide concern. By June 1988, 96,433 cases of AIDS had been reported to the World Health Organization. Table 22-3 lists the number of cases per continent as of June 1988.

Recently a new statistic was reported from Rumania. Because of antiquated medical procedures performed on newborns and the use of outmoded medical supplies, of a total of 2084 children in Bucharest, Rumania, more than 700 have shown a positive reaction to human immunodeficiency virus. These children were born healthy; they did not contract the disease in utero. They were given contaminated blood and, as an economy measure, were immunized with reused needles. Rumanian officials have banned the practice of giving transfusions to healthy newborns and reusing needles. They also have begun to screen blood products. All the children infected in this new epidemic will die, victims of a health care delivery system that failed them. (Salholz, Waldrop, & Marshall, 1990).

As of December 1989, 117,781 cases of AIDS had been reported in the United States (Table 22-4). Homosexual and bisexual men remain at highest risk, with intravenous drug abusers second. Blood transfusion recipients and heterosexual persons also are at risk, as are children of parents with AIDS.

In Canada, as of June 1988, 2003 cases had been reported. The Laboratory Center for Disease Control in Canada has established a monitoring system for reporting what appears to be an emerging Canadian epidemic.

History of the AIDS epidemic. The first reported cases of AIDS in the United States were among young homosexual men. Soon cases of AIDS were reported in other populations, such as intravenous drug abusers and those with hemophilia who had received

TABLE 22-4 Reported cases of acquired immunodeficiency disease in the United States as of December 1989

	No.
Cummulative reported	117,781
Adult	115,786
Children under 13	1,995
Racial/ethnic	
White	66,881
Black	32,348
Hispanic	18,284
Asian	725
Indian	157
Unknown	285
Deaths (as of December 1989)	70,313
Adults	69,233
Children	1,080
Age-groups (yrs)	
Under 5	1,643
5-12	352
13-19	491
20-24	5,090
25-29	18,966
30-34	38,871
35-37	35,463
40-44	15
45-49	8,991
50-54	5,162
55-59	3,318
60-64	1,786
65 and older	1,718

From Centers for Disease Control. (1989). *Monthly surveillance report,* Atlanta, GA. Obtained verbally.

blood transfusions or blood products. Some individuals in the new population group shared none of the characteristics of the high-risk homosexual group. It seemed increasingly possible that the disease was infective in origin (DiVita, Hellman, & Rosenberg, 1988).

In 1983 researchers at the Pasteur Institute in Paris reported a retrovirus called *HIV* as the causative agent of the disease (Lewis, 1988). It became clear after the virus was identified that it was new to Western populations. At the same time it became apparent that AIDS was spreading throughout Central Africa in epidemic proportions (Fig. 22-2). Researchers found that it was a relatively new phenomenon in Africa as well. Further studies have suggested that the virus was not present in human beings until perhaps 50 to 100 years ago. In the case of the United States and Canada, current evidence suggests the absence of the virus until approximately 10 to 15 years ago (DeVita, Hellman, & Rosenberg, 1988). Wherever it came from, whatever the source, HIV is the established agent of AIDS and at this time, continues to be virulent and fatal once acquired.

Mode of transmission. HIV is transmitted directly through body fluids. Almost all cases in the United States have been contracted through four portals of entry: (1) sexual

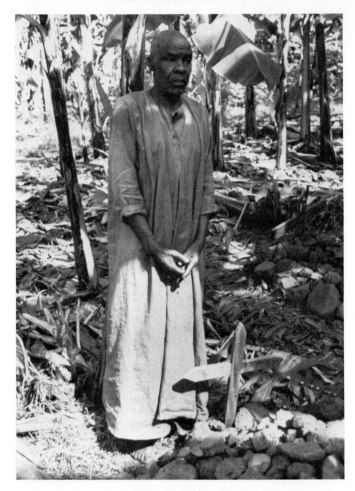

FIG. 22-2 AIDS has developed into a global pandemic. In an African village a grieving father prays by the graves of his seven children and grandchildren, all victims of AIDS. *(Photograph by E. Hooper.)*

contact, (2) intravenous drug administration with contaminated needles, (3) transfusion of blood or blood products, (4) passage of the virus from infected mothers to their newborns (Witt & Pharm, 1986).

Given the knowledge concerning the mode of transmission, it follows that the general population should be educated as to what constitutes high-risk sexual behavior. All blood products should be screened for HIV-positive antibodies. Women with HIV positivity should be warned that infection can be passed through the placenta during pregnancy and thus may cause HIV-positive reactions in their newborns. Users of intravenous drugs should be made aware that the infection can be passed through contaminated needles.

Nurses and other health professionals are at risk for occupationally acquired HIV infection as a result of needle-stick injuries and blood spills, as shown in the following examples:

Example 1: Seroconversion in a nursing student after a needle stick. A nursing student pricked the fleshy part of her index finger with a needle used to draw blood from a patient. There was no apparent injection of blood. A month later she showed HIV seronegativity, but within 4 months her test indicated seropositivity. Her husband's was seronegative. No other risk factors were involved. (DeVita, Hellman, & Rosenberg, 1988).

Example 2: Seroconversion in nurse after an incident involving skin-to-blood contact. During a resuscitation attempt a nurse applied direct pressure with her index finger for 20 minutes to an arterial line insert. She was not wearing gloves. At postmortem examination the patient was found to have AIDS. The nurse showed seroconversion 8 months later, but in the interim fever, malaise, lymphadenopathy, and a weight loss of 14 pounds occurred. There were no other risk factors (DeVita, Hellman, & Rosenberg, 1988).

Because of these and other isolated case studies the Centers for Disease Control recommended that health care workers follow universal precautions with all clients (see box on p. 478).

Incubation period. Knowledge of the incubation period of AIDS is essential to an understanding of the disease. A number of studies have shown varying results. For example, a cohort of 6700 homosexual and bisexual men has been followed up since 1983. Blood samples collected from the men as early as 1978 have been analyzed for HIV antibodies. After 88 months of verified sero positively, AIDS had developed in 36% of the group, and more than 40% had other signs and symptoms of HIV infection. Only 20% remained symptom free. On the basis of this study and others a mean estimated incubation period of 8 years is believed to be conservative; 10 years probably is closer (Benett & Searl, 1989). This prolonged incubation period, during which a symptom-free person is carrying and transmitting the disease, may be part of the reason why the disease is spreading so quickly.

Period of communicability. An ability to predict the period of communicability is necessary to forecast the possible future incidence and prevalence of the disease.

AIDS may be transmitted any time from the movement of seroconversion until the death of the infected person. Epidemiological studies have shown that increased number of sexual partners and receptive anal intercourse or other practices associated with rectal trauma increase the risk of the transfer of the virus.

Pathology. HIV is a retrovirus; that is, it is able to invade the nucleus of a receptive cell and remain there for the life of a cell. The receptive cell for the HIV virus, the T-lymphocyte helper cell, normally coordinates the body's immune response. HIV copies itself into the genetic material of the helper cell and eventually kills it. How this happens is not as yet clear. A person with a normal immune system has a balance of helper T cells (triggered into action by an invading stressor) and suppressor T cells (which turn off the immune response when it is no longer needed). In the person with AIDS the death of the helper T cells has occurred, but a full complement of suppressor T cells exists. Severe immunocompromise is present, and the person is susceptible to opportunistic infections and unusual malignancies (Lewis, 1988).

The early stages. The early stages of AIDS begin with one or more episodes of acute infection, before which and between which the person seems fairly well. At this time an antiviral drug, zidovudine (previously called azidothymidine [AZT]) is found to be useful. The FDA approved this drug for use in 1987. It can be prescribed for oral use on an outpatient basis. Clients must be monitored carefully because of the side effects. The most critical is that bone marrow suppression can cause severe anemia. Other side effects include nausea and vomiting, headaches and myalgia. Studies have shown that persons on a maintenance regimen of zidovudine remain well longer than those who are not (DeVita, Hellman, & Rosenberg, 1988). Clients whose T4 lymphocyte count is low can

UNIVERSAL BLOOD AND BODY FLUID PRECAUTIONS

Because medical history and examination cannot reliably identify all clients infected with HIV or other bloodborne pathogens, blood and body-fluid precautions should be used consistently for *all* clients. This approach, previously recommended by CDC, referred to as *universal blood and body-fluid precautions* or *universal precautions,* should be used in the care of *all* clients, especially including those in emergency-care settings in which the risk of blood exposure is increased and the client's infection status usually is unknown.

1. All health care workers should routinely use appropriate barrier precautions to prevent skin and mucous-membrane exposure when contact with blood or other body fluids of any client is anticipated. Gloves should be worn for touching blood and body fluid, mucous membranes, or non-intact skin of all clients; for handling items or surfaces soiled with blood or body fluids; and for performing venipuncture and other vascular access procedures. Gloves should be changed after contact with each client. To prevent exposure of mucous membranes of the mouth, nose, and eyes, masks and protective eye wear or face shields should be worn during procedures that are likely to generate droplets of blood or other body fluids. Gowns or aprons should be worn during procedures that are likely to generate splashes of blood or other body fluids.

2. Hands and other skin surfaces should be washed immediately and thoroughly if contaminated with blood or other body fluids. Hands should be washed immediately after gloves are removed.

3. All health care workers should take precautions to prevent injuries caused by needles, scalpels, and other sharp instruments or devices during procedures; when cleaning used instruments; during disposal of used needles; and when handling sharp instruments after procedures. To prevent needle-stick injuries, needles should not be recapped, purposely bent, or broken by hand, removed from disposable syringes, or otherwise manipulated by hand. After they are used, disposable syringes and needles, scalpel blades, and other sharp items should be placed in puncture-resistant containers for disposal; the puncture-resistant containers should be located as close as practical to the use area. Large-bore reusable needles should be placed in a puncture-resistant container for transport to the reprocessing area.

4. Although saliva has not been implicated in HIV transmission, to minimize the need for emergency mouth-to-mouth resuscitation bags, or other ventilation devices should be available for use in areas where the need for resuscitation is likely.

5. Health care workers who have exudative lesions or weeping dermatitis should refrain from all direct patient care and from handling equipment for patient care until the condition resolves.

6. Pregnant health care workers are not known to be at greater risk for contracting HIV infection than are health care workers who are not pregnant; however, if HIV infection develops during pregnancy, the infant is at risk of infection as a result of perinatal transmission. Because of this risk, pregnant health care workers should be especially familiar with and should strictly adhere to precautions to minimize the risk of HIV transmission.

Implementation of universal blood and body-fluid precautions for *all* clients eliminates the need for use of the isolation category of "blood and body fluid precautions" previously recommended by the CDC for clients known or suspected to be infected with bloodborne pathogens. Isolation precautions (e.g., for enteric and upper respiratory infections) should be used as necessary if associated conditions, such as infectious diarrhea or tuberculosis, are diagnosed or suspected.

These precautions should be used (1) in emergency departments and outpatient settings, including both physicians' and dentists' offices; (2) during cardiac catheterization and angiographic procedures, (3) during a vaginal or cesarean delivery or other invasive obstetrical procedure in which bleeding may occur, and (4) during the manipulation, cutting, or removal of any oral or perioral tissues, including tooth structure, in which bleeding occurs or the potential for bleeding exists. The universal blood and body-fluid precautions listed here should be the minimum precautions for *all* invasive procedures.

Modified from "Recommendations for prevention of HIV transmission in health-care settings" by the Centers for Disease Control, 1987, *MMWR. Morbidity and Mortality Weekly Report, 36*(Suppl. 2S [35-185]).

be helped by the administration of aerolized pentamidine to prevent *Pneumocytis carinii.* This drug also can be given on an outpatient basis and has few side effects.

Diagnosis. The Centers for Disease Control has established the following criteria for a diagnosis of AIDS:

1. The individual must have at least one of the following indicator diseases: *Pneumocystis carinii*, cytomegalovirus, Kaposi's sarcoma, multifocal leukoencephalopathy, or other evidence of opportunistic infection.

2. There must be laboratory evidence of HIV. A test called the *enzyme-linked immunosorbent assay* (ELISA) clearly identifies the antibody if it is present in the blood. The virus also may be isolated by the culturing of cellular or body fluid samples. In most persons infected with the virus, specific antibodies develop within a few weeks or months and persist throughout the disease. The ELISA test, however, is not always conclusive. The Western blot, or immunoblot, is another test that can detect the presence of individual HIV antibodies (DeVita, Hellman, & Rosenberg, 1988).

3. There must be an absence of other causes of immunodeficiency, such as long-term systemic corticosteroid therapy, Hodgkin's disease, multiple myeloma, immunosuppressive, or cytotoxic therapy, or congenital immunodeficiency syndrome.

Common infections. As immunocompromise increases over time, opportunistic infections, which are normally resisted by the helper T cells, occur.

Pneumocystis carinii pneumonia (PCP) is caused by a protozoan agent that infects the lungs, resulting in severe inflammation and illness. Persons with this infection have fever and dyspnea. The drug of choice is trimethoprim-sulfamethoxazole, which usually is administered intravenously.

Lymphomas related to AIDS occur in the central nervous system and in the bone marrow. Small malignant tumors, which can become large, develop in the lymphatic system, causing occlusion of vessels, pain, and discomfort. They also develop in the bone marrow. There is no standard treatment regimen, and the mortality rate is very high.

Cytomegalovirus, which is caused by a viral agent, can result in blindness from a retinal infection.

Herpes simplex is caused by a viral agent. Extremely painful lesions may break out in the mouth or in the genital or anal area.

Candidiasis is caused by a yeast organism that may be a normal flora in human beings. This condition is sometimes called thrush and results in lesions of the gastrointestinal tract, especially the mouth and esophagus. Treatment with nystatin often is effective.

Kaposi's sarcoma is a diffuse malignancy that results in multiple small tumors of the wall of the blood vessels throughout the body. The tumors may block lymphatic drainage and cause edema of the extremities or face.

● ● ●

Because of the stigma attached to a diagnosis of AIDS, the client's confidentiality must be respected. On the other hand, potential contacts should be informed, as must insurance companies that provide medical benefits and disability. Advocacy by a nurse can be helpful to the client at this stage of the disease.

Nutritional needs in AIDS. The ability to withstand infection is decreased by deficiencies in protein and calories. A high-protein, high-calorie diet with vitamin supplements, particularly vitamins A and E, may assist the client in fighting off opportunistic infections and in preventing tissue depletion as the disease progresses.

Children with AIDS. Most of the children who are infected with HIV have acquired it transplacentally or perineally from their mothers. In a few cases the virus has been transmitted through blood transfusions, intravenous drug abuse, and sexual abuse (DeVita, Hellman, & Rosenberg, 1988). It is estimated that by 1991 more than 10,000 children in the United States will be infected with the HIV virus (Lewis, 1988).

It is difficult to establish the antibody status of an infant born to a mother with HIV seropositivity, because the infant may carry passive antibodies in the serum for approximately 15 months. Those who are infected, however, have a 50% risk of progression to AIDS during a 2- to 3-year period, and symptoms are apt to develop at about 4 months. Neurological complications are more common in children than in adults.

Children with AIDS frequently are very ill. Planning home care for them is difficult because one or possibly both of their parents may be ill. In addition, the social stigma attached to the disease may extend to them. It may be necessary to arrange foster care for them, and families that find it difficult to give these children the kind of care they need may require nursing help and support.

Children, like adults, require supportive therapy. Guidelines for therapy include the following:

1. Boys with potential HIV seropositivity should not be circumcised.
2. These children should be isolated from children who have infectious diseases.
3. Infants who have HIV seropositivity should not be given live vaccines because of the danger of depressed immunity.
4. Children may be given low-maintenance doses of trimethoprim-sulfamethoxazole as prophylaxis for *Pneumocystis carnii* pneumonia.
5. Monthly intravenous injections of gamma globulin may be given to bolster the children's compromised immune system.

The family with AIDS. A family member's positive test reaction to HIV creates the kind of emotional crisis that can cause family dysfunction. The nurse who sees developing signs of dysfunctional behavior that is preventing the family from dealing with the crisis may be able to communicate those insights therapeutically and thus help family members avoid that dysfunctional behavior. The family of a client with AIDS must be viewed as a family with AIDS, even though other members of the family may not have HIV.

Family patterns become an important part of the therapeutic process. Therefore the goal is to look beyond the presenting problem and see issues in terms of the total family adaptation. This may include not only the nuclear family but the extended family as well. It also may include significant others, particularly those with whom the client has had intimate relationships.

John's story. In the case of a family with a homosexual son, the more the son's sexual preference is perceived as a stigma, the more difficult it may be to help the family to reconcile relationships.

At the age of 28 years, John was admitted to the hospital emergency room with a fever of 103°F, a pulse of 120 per minute, and a respiration rate of 44 per minute. His diagnosis was *Pneumocystis carinii* pneumonia and AIDS. His parents sat in a corner of the room huddled together, not speaking to their son or to each other. Until that day they had not known that John was ill or homosexual. They did not seem to be reacting appropriately; rather they were not outwardly reacting at all. They appeared to be in shock. Within 6 hours their son was breathing only with the help of a respirator. In 2 days he was dead. During that time, nurses noted the parents coming closer to their son and encouraged them to do so. At the end they held his hand and cried together. Reconciliation was painful but urgent and was assisted by nursing intervention.

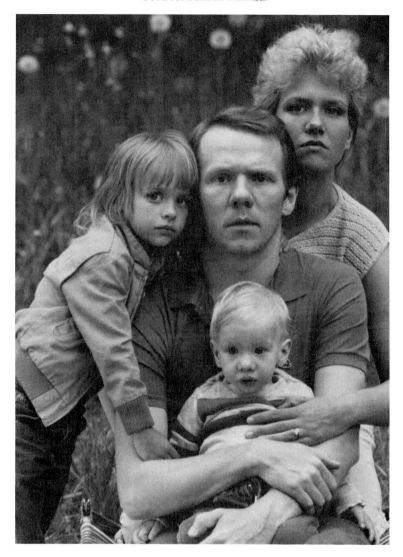

FIG. 22-3 The Burk family. *(Photograph by Lynn Johnson. Used by permission of Black Star.)*

The Burk family. One of the saddest stories about families with AIDS is that of the Burk family. Fig. 22-3 shows the family in 1985. The father, Patrick, had hemophilia and had contracted HIV from a transfusion. Before he was aware that he was infected, he had transmitted the virus to his wife, Lauren, who was pregnant with their second child. Patrick and Dwight, the son in utero at the time, have since died. The daughter, Nicole, was uninfected. Lauren's fate is unknown.

Michelle's story. Michelle, a 25-year-old woman, showed a positive HIV test reaction. Swollen lymph nodes developed in her neck, she lost 14 pounds, and she had persistent diarrhea. A blood analysis showed an unusually low number of helper T lymphocytes. Her physician suggested that she might be in the stage of infection called *AIDS-related complex (ARC).*

Michelle was experiencing a great deal of stress and was having an increasingly difficult time in handling her anxiety. She felt depressed because she thought that most, if not all, of the plans for the future (such as marriage and having a family) had been dashed by the onset of her disease. She was in a relationship with a young man whom she wanted to marry but was afraid to disclose her HIV status for fear he would abandon her. Michelle talked to her family of origin very infrequently; she was afraid to tell them about her illness because she thought they would disown her or, at best, treat her like a leper by keeping her nieces and nephews away from her.

Michelle believed that she must keep her condition a secret from everyone because she had heard that some persons with AIDS experienced discrimination by employers, landlords, and insurance companies, as well as physicians and dentists who refused to treat those with AIDS.

To make a bad situation worse, because of the lack of energy—concomitant of this disease—Michelle did not think that she would be able to hold her job much longer. If she continued working, her health would most likely deteriorate, but if she quit working, she would have no means of support. Although persons with a diagnosis of fully developed AIDS can apply for disability benefits, Michelle's physician maintained that her case had not yet reached that point.

Although Michelle had been away from her family of origin for 8 years, she realized that the only place where she might receive some of the support that she was going to need was from her family. Michelle's parents were divorced and both had remarried, but she felt that her mother might provide her with sufficient support to keep the stress of the disease at a manageable level.

Helping someone like Michelle disclose this disease status to family members and to those who may be infected by the virus can increase the quality and length of the person's life if the result is the receipt of financial and emotional support. Disclosure also can help someone like Michelle's boyfriend receive early counseling and treatment, if that is necessary.

SUMMARY

An understanding of the concept of immunity can assist the nurse in planning interventions at primary, secondary, and tertiary levels. The use of Betty Neuman's systems model can provide the nurse with a visualization of the various factors that influence an individual's or a population's relevant immunity. Some epidemiological concepts—for example, the epidemiological triad, the mode of transition, and the chain of transmission—can be helpful in understanding the way infections are spread. This understanding can enable the nurse to plan and implement programs of prevention. Surveillance of communicable diseases by the World Health Organization, the Centers for Disease Control, and the Laboratory Center for Disease Control provides a constant update on the incidence and prevalence of disease locally and worldwide. Community health nurses need a firm knowledge of the agent that causes a disease, the method of transmission to the host, the incubation period, and the period of communicability of specific diseases in order to plan health programs for populations to prevent the spread of infection where these diseases exist.

CHAPTER HIGHLIGHTS

- Immunity can be active or passive; it may be acquired naturally or artificially. The level of immunity in an individual or a population can vary, particularly with respect to communicable diseases.

- Betty Neuman's client systems model can be used to illustrate the concept of relative immunity.

- The epidemiological triad identifies the three factors necessary (host, agent, and environment) for the spread of communicable diseases. Modifying any or all of these factors can influence the spread of disease.

- Primary prevention of communicable diseases consists of immunizations whenever possible. Artificial active immunization given orally or by injection is available for many diseases, including poliomyelitis, measles, mumps, rubella, diphtheria, pertussis, and tetanus.

- Screening for communicable diseases allows the nurse to practice secondary prevention by planning interventions before a client exhibits symptoms of a disease.

- Tertiary prevention is used to limit disability after an individual has symptoms of a disease.

- Communicable diseases commonly encountered by the community health nurse include hepatitis, tuberculosis, Lyme disease, varicella (chickenpox), scarlet fever, and AIDS.

- Although the HIV first was prevalent only in young homosexual men, the virus has spread to the general population. Other groups at risk for AIDS are intravenous drug abusers and persons with hemophilia.

- AIDS is spread through direct contact of body fluids, which can occur by means of sexual activity, intravenous administration of drugs with contaminated needles, transfusions of contaminated blood or blood products, or transfer from mothers to infants in utero through the placenta or through breast-feeding.

- Because of compromised immunity, the patient with AIDS is susceptible to many infections that normally would be resisted by the body's immune system.

- There is no cure for AIDS, and the disease is always fatal.

- When a family member shows a positive test reaction for HIV, the family often is thrown into a crisis and must be treated as a unit.

STUDY QUESTIONS

1. Describe three factors that will alter the immunity of a population.
2. Discuss the difference between active and passive immunity.
3. With the use of Betty Neuman's systems model, appropriately place the three factors mentioned in question No. 1 in terms of the flexible lines of defense and the lines of resistance.
4. Plan interventions at primary, secondary, and tertiary levels to decrease the incidence and prevalence of plague among the Navaho Indians.
5. Write the nursing goals and expected outcomes for an ambulatory client with AIDS who is receiving long-term health care and who currently has a medical diagnosis of *Pneumocystis carinii* pneumonia. List the nursing diagnoses.

REFERENCES

American Academy of Pediatrics (1988). *Report of the Committee on Infectious Diseases* (21st ed.). Elk Grove Village, IL: Author.

Aronson, (1978). *Communicable disease nursing* [Nursing Outline Series]. Garden City, N.Y.: Medical Examination Publishing Co.

Benenson, (1981). *Control of communicable diseases in man* (13th ed.). Washington, DC: American Public Health Association.

Bennett, C. & Searl, S. (1982). *Communicable disease handbook*. New York: Wiley.

Braunwald E., Thorn, G., Adams, R., Isselbacker, K., & Petersdorf R. (Eds.). (1987). *Harrison's principles of internal medicine,* (11th ed.). New York: Mc-Graw-Hill. Isselbacker, Petersdorf (Eds.). (1987).

Pan American Health Association Bulletin. (1989). Vol. 23, ISSN 0085-4636, (10-13), Washington, DC: Author.

Campbell, J. M. (1987). *Medical evaluations of HIV infection.* Bay Area Physicians for Human Rights.

Centers for Disease Control (1982, November 5). Universal precautions for health care workers *MMWR. Morbidity and Mortality Weekly Report, 31* (43) 577-579.

Centers for Disease Control (1988, June). Water-related disease outbreaks, *MMWR. Morbidity and Mortality Weekly Report, 37* (55)

Centers for Disease Control (1988, July). Plague in American Indians, *MMWR. Morbidity and Mortality Weekly Report, 1956-1987, 37, (55)*

DeVita, V., Hellman, S. & Rosenberg, S. (1988). *AIDS: Etiology, diagnosis, treatment and prevention* (2nd ed.). Philadelphia: Lippincott.

Edison, T. (1988). *The AIDS caregiver's handbook.* New York: St. Martin's Press.

Hanson, J. (1984). The family. In C. Roy (Ed.), *Introduction to Nursing: An adaptation model* East Norwalk, CT: Appleton & Lange.

Leavitt, M. (1982). *Families at risk.* Boston: Little, Brown & Co.

Lewis, A. (1988). *Nursing care of the patient with AIDS/ARC* Rockville, MD: Aspen.

Neuman, B. (1989). *Application to nursing education and practice, The Neuman systems model:* (2nd ed.) East Norwalk, CT: Appleton & Lange.

Pickering, L. & Dupont, H. (1986). *Infectious diseases of children and adults.* Reading, MA: Addison-Wesley.

Salholz, E., Waldrop, T. & Marshell, R. (1990, February 19). Watching the babies die. *Newsweek,* p. 63.

Witt, M., & Pharm D. (1986). *AIDS and patient management: Legal, ethical and social issues.* Owings Mills, MD: Rynd Communications.

Developmentally Disabled Persons in the Community

THERESE M. MUDD and JOAN M. COOKFAIR

Monday's child is fair of face,
Tuesday's child is full of grace,
Wednesday's child is full of woe,
Thursday's child has far to go. . . .

UNKNOWN

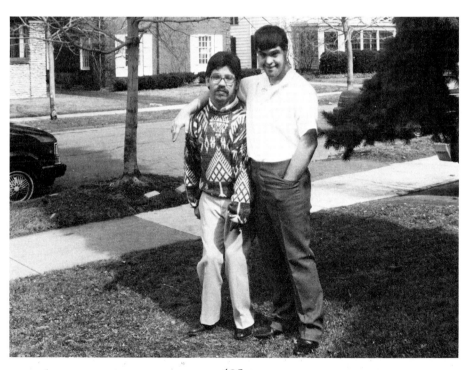

OBJECTIVES

At the conclusion of this chapter the student will be able to:
1. Define the key terms listed
2. Discuss the reasons developmentally disabled individuals are becoming more visible in the community
3. Describe the community health nurse's role in the care of the developmentally disabled
4. Identify selected developmental disabilities
5. Describe attitudinal changes in society that affect the health care of the developmentally disabled
6. Discuss developmental disabilities from a life-span perspective
7. Use the nursing process to address the needs of a disabled married couple
8. Discuss selected legal and ethical issues that apply to those with learning disabilities
9. Describe alternatives to institutional care

KEY TERMS

Autism
Blindness
Cerebral palsy
Deinstitutionalization
Developmental disability
Developmental model
Down's syndrome
Hearing loss
Intermediate care facility

Individuation
L'Arche community
Learning disability
Least restrictive environment
Mental retardation
Normalization
Public Law 94-142
Self-actualization

Over the years society has drastically altered its views toward the developmentally disabled. During ancient times and the Middle Ages deviation from the norm placed an individual at risk for early death, or confinement in prison, or both.

The first serious study of the mentally impaired was conducted by a French physician, Jean Stard, during his work with the "wild boy of Aveyron." His work and that of his protégé, Edward Sequin, during the early nineteenth century led to the beginnings of educational programs for individuals with mental impairments (Matson & Marchetti, 1988).

By the midnineteenth century residential schools and institutions for mentally handicapped children were established in North America. Primarily educational, their objective was to teach these youngsters life skills and to return them to their families. These initial attempts soon were thwarted by the difficulty of mainstreaming them back into society. An attitude evolved of protecting the mentally handicapped from society, and the schools became more custodial (Matson & Marchetti, 1988). By the midtwentieth century another attitude developed—that of protecting society from the mentally handicapped—and physicians often recommended "putting a disabled child away" so that the rest of the family could have a normal life and society did not have to see the "abnormal" child.

For many years it was believed that developmentally disabled, and in particular mentally retarded, persons were best cared for in an institutional setting. However, groups such as the National Association for Retarded Citizens, formed in 1950, and social reform efforts championed by President John F. Kennedy in the early 1960s began a change toward acceptance of these people into the community. Isolated pockets of enlightened individuals established special schools for the mentally impaired, but the trend toward institutionalization continued until the early 1970s, when Willowbrook, the world's largest institution for the retarded, located on Staten Island in New York City, was exposed by a few courageous staff members and some parents. The media showed shocking conditions that dehumanized the residents (Neier, 1980). The New York Civil Liberties Union brought suit against the institution on behalf of the residents. Other states began to investigate their own institutions and a new question was asked: Why the institution at all, why not the community? A movement called *deinstitutionalization,* which had a profound effect on societal attitudes, began. People began to have to deal with the reality of the disabled population. A developmentally disabled person, like any individual, may live in a number of different settings, hopefully in his or her own family home during childhood. Some disabled children may have been cared for in a family situation, with a personal care provider who acted as a foster parent and tended to their needs. Litigation addressing the rights of retarded citizens, and federal legislation created a special language that

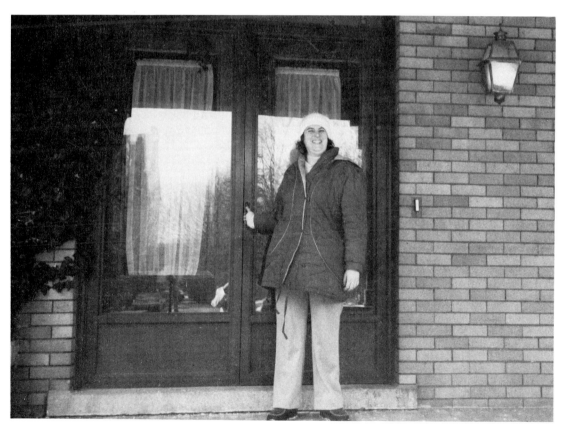

FIG. 23-1 Some mentally retarded adults are able to live in group homes in the community.

reflected a new way of viewing disability, for example, such terms as *normalization, developmental model, individuation,* and *self-actualization.* Normalization stresses the principle that disabled persons should live as normally as possible, and the developmental model reflects the capability of each individual to grow and develop. Individuation focuses on the uniqueness of each person and deemphasises the practice of labeling and categorizing individuals. Self-actualization maintains the right of each person to become all that he or she can be, regardless of any handicapping condition (Matson & Marchetti, 1988).

Some disabled adults live in community residences—home-like accommodations run by either a state or a private agency—that may house from 6 to 24 children and/or adults of both sexes (Webb, 1986). Others live in intermediate-care facilities (ICFs), which are about the same size as community residences, but that have the advantage of more complete medical services, usually provided by staff nurses, with additional personnel employed to cope with difficult behavior. This type of facility too may be run by a state or a private agency. Along the continuum from institutional to independent living, the disabled adult may live in supportive or supervised apartments (Fig. 23-1). In any of these cases the availability of community nursing services helps to facilitate life in the least restrictive environment.

Deinstitutionalization has not been accomplished without problems. Occasionally some individuals fail to adjust to community living simply because their new environment is not structured to meet their needs. Life outside an institution also can be restrictive if the clients do not have proper support services to help them.

ROLE OF THE COMMUNITY HEALTH NURSE

Community health nurses, who traditionally focus on providing health care to persons in their homes and other community settings, are highly involved with developmentally disabled clients. Nursing activities include educating other health providers, coordinating services, implementing prevention at primary, secondary, and tertiary levels, and consumer advocacy. Nurses serve on advisory boards and planning committees, calling attention to inadequate and unjust treatment. They help make the human service systems more aware of and responsive to the needs of this special population (Rubin, 1989).

The nurse's role in the community may begin with a posthospitalization home visit to an infant who is handicapped or at high risk. Focusing on the child while emphasizing his or her personality and not the disability can be helpful in assisting the parent to accept the child. The simple act of calling the child by his or her name instead of emphasizing technical terms can make a positive difference. The nurse will be better able to empathize with parents if there is an awareness that parents may react with anger, disbelief, and sadness as they mourn the child who might have been and begin to adjust to a new reality. Maximizing early intervention initiatives and infant stimulation can assist with the child's development.

As the child matures, the community health nurse remains a central figure, participating in health care in ambulatory care settings such as community health centers, hospital outpatient programs, local health departments, traveling health teams, native American reservations, and remote mountain villages. Some community health nurses establish individual private practices and work in cooperation with physicians, therapists, and other professionals as part of a network of community care. School health services make use of community health services; because children with special health problems are included under the Education for all handicapped children act (Public Law [P.L.] 94-

142), which states that all handicapped children have available to them a free public education which emphasizes special education and related services designed to meet their unique needs, to assure that the rights of handicapped children and their parents or guardians are protected, to assist states and localities to provide for the education of all handicapped children, and to assess and assure the effectiveness of efforts to educate handicapped children (United States Statutes at Large, 1975). With increasing frequency nurses in the schools are performing complex procedures and providing care to children with severe mental and physical disabilities.

Community health nurses must provide care for disabled employees, as well as serving in an advocacy role for them. Home health care and coordination of respite and other family support services also are facets of the nurse's role. In addition, nurses assume a primary role in the supervision of personnel employed in community settings such as group homes, family care, and residential communities in which developmentally disabled persons live. Increasingly, community health nurses are involved in health care, coordination of services, and advocacy for the developmentally disabled in the community.

DEFINITIONS OF DEVELOPMENTAL DISABILITY

A developmental disability is defined in P.L. 94-103 as a disability that has the following characteristics (United States Statutes at Large, 1975, p.497):

A1. is attributable to mental retardation, cerebral palsy, epilepsy, or autism.

  2. is attributable to any other condition of a person found to be closely related to mental retardation because such a condition results in similar impairment of general intellectual functioning or adaptive behavior similar to that of mentally retarded persons or requires treatment and services similar to those required for such persons; or

  3. is attributable to dyslexia resulting from a disability described in Numbers **1** or **2.**

B.   originates before such person is age 18;

C.   has continued or can be expected to continue indefinitely;

D.   constitutes a substantial handicap to such person's ability to function in society.

Further, the functional aspects of disability have been defined through federal law in the Amendments to the Rehabilitation, Comprehensive Services and Developmental Disabilities Act (P.L. 98-527) as a severe, chronic disability that has the following characteristics:

1. It is attributable to a mental or physical impairment or to a combination of mental and physical impairments.

2. It manifests before the person attains the age of 22 years.

3. It is likely to continue indefinitely.

4. It results in substantial functional limitations in three or more of the following areas of major life activity: self-care, receptive and expressive language, learning, mobility, self-direction, capacity for independent living, and economic self-sufficiency.

5. It reflects the person's need for a combination and sequence of special interdisciplinary or generic care, treatment, or other services that are of extended or lifelong duration and that require individual planning and coordination.

SELECTED DEVELOPMENTAL DISABILITIES
Cerebral Palsy

Cerebral palsy is a broad term used in reference to disorders of movement that result from damage to the brain. It manifests in severe or mild problems with muscle coordi-

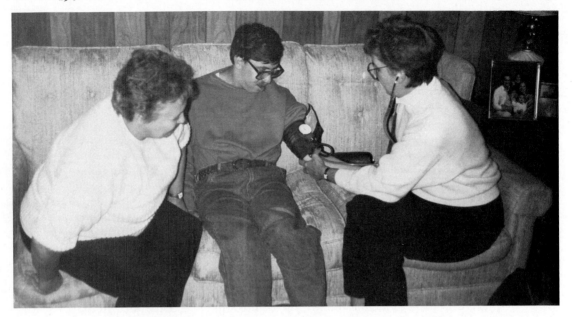

FIG. 23-2 The community health nurse uses a health assessment as an opportunity to teach a developmentally disabled young man and his mother.

nation. The severity of involvement relates to the location of the cerebral lesion and its extent (Gabel & Erikson, 1980). Although neonatal jaundice, birth trauma, and neonatal asphyxia play important roles in the etiology of cerebral palsy, in many cases the reason for the disorder is never known.

The incidence of cerebral palsy is believed to be approximately 1.5 to 2 per 1000 live births, (Pueschel, Bernier, & Weidenman, 1988). Generally it is not diagnosed until an infant attempts controlled movement and abnormal patterns are noted (usually at 12 to 18 months of age).

Nurses frequently become involved in assisting clients and primary caretakers as families attempt to accommodate the needs of persons with cerebral palsy in the home and at school. During home visits, either during or after illness, the nurse can take the opportunity to provide health care teaching to the family (Fig. 23-2).

There is no cure for cerebral palsy. Some individuals with this condition have a strong drive to achieve despite intense disability. They may or may not have below average intelligence (Gabel & Erikson, 1980).

Two common classifications of cerebral palsy are spastic and choreoathetoid. The former is manifested by increased muscle tone. The limbs may be drawn into abnormal positions by overactive muscles pulling against weak ones. The latter term is used when the individual has difficulty controlling body movements (Pueschel, et al., 1988).

A third, less common, type is ataxic cerebral palsy, which can occur by itself or can accompany other forms. It is characterized by weakness, lack of coordination, and difficulty with rapid or fine movement.

P.L. 94-103 recognizes cerebral palsy as a lifelong disability. Among the characteristics defined in P.L. 98-527 are severe chronic disability, which may continue indefinitely and result in functional limitations in three or more of the following areas (United States Statutes at Large, 1984, p. 2664):

1. Self-care
2. Receptive and expressive language usage
3. Learning
4. Mobility
5. Self-direction
6. Capacity for independent living
7. Economic self-sufficiency

Secondary effects stem primarily from difficulty in communication and lack of mobility, for example, problems with nutrition and elimination. Socialization problems almost always occur when communication is impaired. As profoundly affected persons age, parents may no longer be able to physically care for them, and placement becomes a problem. Thus lifelong nursing services and advocacy for this population may be required.

Down's Syndrome

Down's syndrome, first described by John L. H. Down in 1866, is a disorder that occurs as a result of an extra chromosome in cells of the affected person so that each cell contains 47 rather than 46 chromosomes. The incidence of Down's syndrome increases in children born to mothers older than 40 years of age. About 4% of the cases occur as a result of the translocation of chromosomes. This type usually is hereditary (Whaley & Wong, 1987).

Down syndrome is evident at birth. The back of the head often is flattened, skin folds at the inner corners of the eyes may be present, and there may be excess skin at the back of the neck. Muscle strength and tone are diminished. One third of the children have congenital heart disease and do not live to middle adulthood. Some, however, live well into their 50s and 60s. They generally are severely to moderately retarded although some achieve low average intelligence (Pueschel et al., 1988).

Assistance with feeding may be necessary because the large protruding tongue interferes with feeding, as does the tendency to be mouth breathers. Early stimulation programs enhance cognitive and physical development. Parents may be given a detailed outline that helps the child to develop his or her potential. Care of the skin is important because children with Down syndrome have soft pliable skin that is prone to infection (Whaley & Wong, 1987). Avoidance and/or early treatment of upper respiratory infection should be stressed.

From the beginning nursing intervention should focus on the family of the child and not the child in isolation. Emphasizing to the parents that they need respite and time for each other, as well as focusing on the child and not the disability, may better enable the parents to accept the child and diminish stress in the family.

When the child starts school, he or she should be placed in the least restrictive environment, as defined by P.L. 94-142 (United States at Large, 1975, p. 497). Some adolescents with this disability are emotionally labile. They can be very happy or very sad in a matter of minutes. They also can, at times, perseverate and be difficult to move on from a depressed or euphoric state. Teaching parents to implement a structured behavioral modification program is helpful to the child and to the family.

The adolescent and young adult with Down syndrome needs assistance to learn appropriate social behavior and, hopefully, to find work in a sheltered workshop. Because these persons sometimes live until 50 or 60 years of age, they may outlive their parents. Thus planned placement in a group home can ensure satisfactory adjustment.

This lifelong disorder is categorized as a disability in P.L. 94-103 (mental retardation) and as a severe chronic disability in P.L. 98-527. Given careful guidance and health care, some persons with Down syndrome become well-adjusted contributors to family life and to society.

Mental Retardation

"Mental retardation refers to significantly subaverage intellectual functioning existing concurrently with deficits in adaptive behavior and manifested during the developmental period" (Grossman, 1973, p. 11). Subaverage intellectual functioning presupposes an intelligence quotient (IQ) score of less than 68 or 70 on a standard intelligence list. Adaptive behavior refers to the skills needed for personal independence and social responsibility. The developmental period is defined as the time between birth and 22 years of age (Pueschel, et al., 1988).

Factors that cause mental retardation may occur in the prenatal, perinatal, and postnatal periods. These include chromosomal defects, genetic factors, congenital infections, drugs, and radiation. Many causes of mental retardation are unknown.

Categories vary from mild to profound. Some mildly retarded persons are indistinguishable from the average population and are able to function in school and employment with a minimum of assistance. Moderately retarded persons (IQ, 35 to 40) can learn the basic skills necessary for the activities of daily living and usually are employed, after schooling, in sheltered workshops or other supervised settings. Those who are severely mentally retarded (IQ, 20 to 25) may have motor and speech problems. They may be able to work in supervised workshops but require lifelong supervision. Profound mental retardation results in very low functioning. In addition, there may be motor impairments, speech and hearing loss, and severe health problems. Adults may require an institutional setting when parents can no longer help them.

Mental retardation is a lifelong condition that is recognized by law as a developmental disability. Parents need counseling concerning realistic expectations for the young child. Ideally, structured, well-supervised programs in workshops and social settings will be available during the adolescent and young adult years. Later, placement in the least restrictive environment for the aging mentally retarded population often becomes the responsibility of the community health nurse. To facilitate a satisfactory adjustment, it is important to assist families with such placement before the death or disability of parents.

Autism

Autism is a rare developmental disability that affects 4 to 5 of every 10,000 children. It manifests in the child's problems with receptive and expressive language. Children with autism have difficulty in establishing interpersonal relationships. The condition usually becomes evident by 30 months of age, although a trained observer may diagnose it earlier. There is no known cause for autism. The criteria for diagnosis are as follows (Pueschel et al., 1988):

1. The condition appears before 30 months of age.
2. The child is unresponsive to others, avoids eye contact, resists cuddling or physical contact, and may show inappropriate affective behavior.
3. Language development is severely impaired.

Language development is slow and painfully difficult. Organizing visual or auditory communication into anything meaningful seems to be difficult for the autistic individual. The stress in coping with what appears to be a completely disorganized existence manifests in ritualistic behavior and a need for structure in a nonthreatening, quiet environment. Outbursts and self-stimulation are common. This is believed to be a result of profound stress and frustration at not being able to make sense of the surrounding world. The ritualistic behavior can become a problem with nutrition inasmuch as affected individuals insist on eating only one kind of food in a repetitive way.

Autism, which is much more common in boys than in girls, may or may not be accompanied by retardation. There are no physical handicaps connected with autism, and a normal life span can be predicted.

Autism is one of the most difficult disabilities with which parents and teachers must cope. Only about one sixth of the children diagnosed with autism make a reasonable social adjustment. Most are severely handicapped throughout life. Respite for parents is difficult because taking autistic individuals anywhere can result in an emotional outburst because of their need for sameness. Often respite is arranged in the home rather than taking the child to another place. It is not uncommon for the parent of autistic children to experience stress that results in health problems and marital difficulties. Twenty-four-hour care of individuals with this disability is physically and emotionally draining. In addition, financial problems can occur in localities in which public services are unavailable.

As the autistic child approaches adolescence, nurses and other health professionals can help parents gain access to services to assist in the child's socialization. Advocacy in the community to gain acceptance and understanding of autistic behavior can be helpful. Education of parents, teachers, and significant others includes instructions to speak slowly in short sentences and to use concrete terms. Other valuable strategies are using repetition and structure in learning environments, promoting better communication by facing the individual, and gently taking the individual's hand. These techniques help others to cope and thus make the autistic person's life somewhat easier. Behavior modification techniques, patience, quiet, and structure are helpful, whereas authoritarian behavior, physical punishment, and denial of privileges may have disastrous results.

This lifelong disorder qualifies as a developmental disability. If placement in a group home is necessary as the parents age, great care is required in the transition from family care because autistic persons have a tenuous hold on reality and a tendency to withdraw into themselves.

Learning Disabilities

In 1981 the National Joint Committee on Learning Disabilities defined learning disabilities as "a generic term that refers to a heterogeneous group of disorders manifested in the acquisition and use of listening, speaking, reading, writing, reasoning or mathematical abilities. These disorders are intrinsic to the individual and presumed to be due to central nervous system dysfunction" (Selekman, Goldenthal, & Clark, 1988, p. 2). The definition differentiates learning disabilities from mental retardation, sensory deprivation, emotional disturbances, motor deficits, and environmental deficits. Learning disabilities frequently are classified as attention-deficit disorders.

The Association for Children and Adults with Learning Disabilities states that 20% of school-age children are learning disabled. Of these, 66% to 83% are boys.

There are many causes of learning disabilities, and research is ongoing. Lead poisoning, effects of cerebral insult, anoxia, and sequelae from meningitis are some possible causes. Early diagnosis is important because some behavioral problems may already be in place by the time the child is of school age.

Community health nurses in well-child clinics should refer a child for psychological testing if a parent complains of a toddler's hyperactivity, poor coordination, and lack of comprehension of simple requests. School nurses should refer for testing children who, according to their teachers, are performing below ability, are inattentive in class, or are constantly active and lack concentration. These children may speak well but with little comprehension of their own words. There may be difficulty in the ability to use and process information; there may be altered visual perception resulting in dyslexia, or a disturbance in the ability to read. There may be auditory perceptual problems, resulting in difficulty in listening and following directions, as well as in reading emotions into a speaker's tone of voice. There may be disorders of tactile perception that result in difficulty in perceiving body language and in performing psychomotor activity.

Early diagnosis can enable the nurse to assist parents and teachers to communicate effectively and to help the child to learn. Home visits may prevent family dysfunction as parents alter expectations and substitute realistic goal performance.

Multisensory teaching methods, visual cues, auditory prompts, memorization through repetitive writing, and rewriting to teach spelling can assist the learning process. Constant feedback to prevent misconceptions and to facilitate the intake of accurate information will decrease the child's stress level and thus result in fewer mistakes.

A learning disability is lifelong and affects the individual across the life span. Adolescents have difficulty with social skills and success in school. Earning a living wage is sometimes difficult because of communication problems and psychomotor deficits. Marriage and family raising can be frustrating for the same reasons.

Persons with learning disabilities usually have normal intelligence and with proper guidance and support may be able to compensate and overcome the problems caused by their disability. Educational services available to them through P.L. 94-142 can be invaluable. Local rehabilitative and vocational services can assist them to become independent and to accomplish life goals. As with other disabilities the nurse should perceive the family of a child with a learning disability as a learning-disabled family, guiding members in helpful methods to use with the child and alleviating stress caused by problems associated with the disability.

Sensory Disorders

Early detection of visual or hearing disorders is of primary importance in helping a child to avoid developmental delay in cognition. Blind children cannot learn from modeling or imitation. If blind from birth, they also will have difficulty in understanding spatial relationships. Nurses making home visits or performing physical examinations in well-baby clinics should be alert for ceaselessly roving eye movements (which may denote blindness). The so-called setting sun sign also is ominous; that is, only the upper part of the iris appears above the lower lid when the eye is at rest. The child should be referred for further testing. If the cornea of one eye is larger than the other, glaucoma may be present, and early treatment might prevent blindness. A milky film or clouding suggests cataracts, which are correctable. Nurses in the schools can detect near-sightedness or far-sightedness (acuity) by means of a Snellen chart that is age appropriate (see Chapter 10). Amblyopia, or lazy eye, should be detected early in well-child clinics and day-care settings to prevent loss of vision. Loss of vision sometimes can be prevented by early diagnosis and treatment, and promoting optimal vision can prevent developmental delay (Haynes, 1980). In cases of blindness the nurse can assist parents and teachers to substitute alternative methods for visual stimulation to facilitate learning.

Hearing loss can be detected in newborns if it is severe or profound. A newborn will become startled or open its eyes at a sudden new sound. A high risk for deafness or hearing loss should be considered if one or more of the following factors is present: (1) family history of hearing loss, (2) hyperbilirubinemia, (3) congenital rubella syndrome, (4) defects of the ears, nose, or throat, and (5) birth weight of 1500 gm or less (Haynes, 1980).

Nurses in well-child clinics and schools should refer for audiometric testing those children who exhibit difficulty in understanding speech or who have delayed speech patterns or behavior problems. They also may have problems with social interaction, and parents may complain of the children's inattentiveness and difficulty in following directions. If hearing loss is detected early, developmental delay and behavioral problems may be avoided. Early detection, prevention of hearing loss, and counseling of family and significant others are important to the satisfactory adjustment of these children. Approximately 1 in every 1000 children has some degree of hearing loss.

HISTORICAL BACKGROUND

Many legal definitions of the rights of handicapped individuals center around the concept of the "least restrictive environment." To determine the least restrictive environment it is necessary to consider how the person functions at home in daily living and in educational and vocational settings, as well as factors such as the person's sexual development, leisure activities, self-image, and any special needs that should be accommodated as much as possible within the normal environment.

A primary objective of the federal government for the rehabilitation of the developmentally disabled is the provision of alternatives that allow the person to achieve maximum independence and full and equal opportunities to live in the least restrictive environment. In 1971 the federal government amended the Social Security Act, with Title XIX establishing Medicaid payment to fund the intermediate-care facility. Such a facility allows developmentally disabled individuals with medical problems to live in the community but also to obtain the treatment needed for their physical needs. It provides care beyond room and board but less extensive care than a skilled nursing facility; 50% to 78% of the cost for such care is federally reimbursed if the facility is approved and its primary purpose is to provide health and rehabilitative services.

The 1971 regulations require the least restrictive alternative for a client in a facility that is rehabilitative rather than custodial. Normalization is a goal, and care is to be delivered on the basis of a developmental rather than a medical model. The developmental model (Center on Human Policy, Syracuse, 1981) stipulates that retardation is not a disease and that development is a lifetime priority that is superseded only by medical needs. Independence is fostered through programs more compatible with a home or school environment than that of a hospital. P.L. 94-142 helped parents of severely disabled children to keep them at home and to provide a life that was, to the greatest extent possible, normal. It stipulated that all handicapped children should have an individualized education plan and that the parent be a part of the committee responsible for the plan, along with the school nurse, the psychologist, and the child's teacher.

DEVELOPMENTAL DISABILITIES THROUGHOUT THE LIFE SPAN
Infants and Children

The individual with a developmental disability does indeed have "far to go." There has been a tendency to think only of the *child* who is "special" when developmental disabilities are discussed. This focus is, of course, important, particularly in terms of the nurse's role in the nursery for newborns and in visits to the home for in-depth assessments of infants at high risk. However, the family must be addressed as a unit. Family support services can begin with the diagnosis or discovery process, in which the specific nature of the child's disability is determined.

The birth of a disabled child is a major crisis that may affect family stability. Counseling is needed to assist families to understand the nature and implications of the disability.

Families can be helped to provide effective care for these children, and to integrate them into the family and community. Maintaining a disabled child in his or her natural home until maturity is the least costly and the most normal system of care.

Diagnosis and evaluation of a child's handicapping condition, information about services, out-of-home placement considerations, training to deal with a child's needs, and strategies to cope with general family strains suggest the scope of the problem and the needs of the family.

Early childhood (birth to 5 years) frequently is the time of the developmentally disabled child's greatest cognitive development. Infant stimulation programs and mobility training can take best advantage of this time period. Speech therapy, occupational therapy, and preschool education sometimes enable disabled children to attend regular classes by the time they enter grade school. Certainly it will assist them to make the most of their potential.

During later childhood (ages 6 to 12 years) the school is the primary agency helping the child. At this time the school nurse can provide liaison between the child, the parent, the teacher, and the administration.

Adolescence and Young Adulthood

Adolescence is a time that requires attention to appropriate social behavior and information regarding body changes and sexuality. Just as in general education, the handicapped individual needs an individualized plan so that sex education will be adapted to meet unique needs.

The young adult (18 to 21 years) must begin a transition into adulthood. This includes graduation from school, movement into a more independent setting such as an apartment or a group home, and even an intimate relationship and marriage. An understanding, when appropriate, of sexual activity, hygiene, and pleasure, as well as family planning and contraception, is necessary. Disabled persons sometimes are treated as asexual beings, which of course is an error. They should be advised not only about their sexuality but also about appropriate behavior as they mature.

Sexual activity may include dating and courtship and, for some, marriage and family planning. For persons with mild handicaps the process of meeting and mating and marrying may be no different than it is for able-bodied people. One important difference, however, should be noted. Handicapped teenagers and young adults are subject to the same cultural influences as are the rest of society. They expect to fall in love with beautiful girls or handsome men, not handicapped adults. Some achieve this dream. Others settle for something less ideal, perhaps someone who is similarly handicapped. Sometimes the mildly handicapped, rehabilitative, self-supporting person can make his or her way and find a suitable mate. Those with more severe disabilities face other difficulties. Parents frequently object to any kind of a mature relationship, and matters of independence can influence this issue. In the case of the mentally retarded the ability to undertake a marriage contract may be a factor.

A relationship between two individuals may not necessarily lead to marriage but can lead to pleasure, mutual growth, and long-term stability and mutual satisfaction. On the other hand, marriage can be highly satisfying for severely handicapped persons who are unable to participate in human endeavors such as work, which provide meaning to the lives of those who are able-bodied. In marriage they may find a meaning and purpose far beyond that which marriage holds for the average person. It is possible for two disabled persons to form a stronger, more binding union than usually is seen.

Some objections to marriage between handicapped individuals have to do with questions of support. Most handicapped persons who cannot support themselves are entitled to public assistance, whether married or not. Thus physical disability is not an insurmountable deterrent. Raising children is another issue that must be given careful thought, and individual decisions must be made on the basis of good advice.

Handicapped people are sexual beings, and parents, professionals, and the public should be helped to accept that fact. Community health nurses are in a position to facilitate understanding by communicating facts and to provide counseling in the area of sexuality in an empathic and fair manner to all concerned.

The Older Adult

Life between 55 and 75 years of age presents physiological and psychological changes that result in decreased functional abilities, increased physical frailty, and concomitant family stress. The age and needs of care givers become a problem in this period of development, if not sooner. After caring for the disabled person for most of his or her

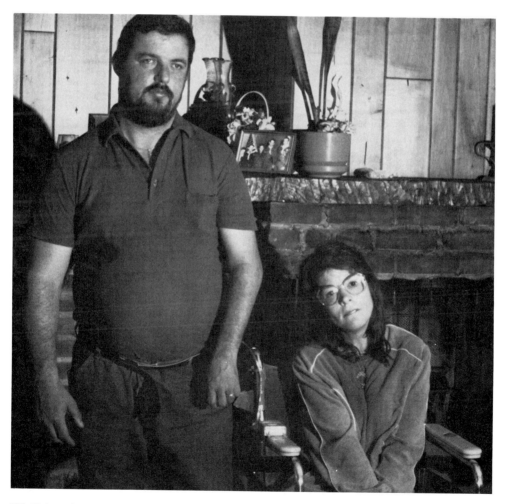

FIG. 23-3 A developmentally disabled couple lives independently in their own home and makes a contribution to the community.

life, parents, as they age, no longer are able to provide this care. Community nurses must be aware of the special needs and resources available to the developmentally disabled older person. The death of a parent may be a life-threatening loss to a disabled person who has been dependent on that parent for care. Sometimes disabled members are kept from the activities of the mourning family in a mistaken effort to shield them; however, they must be allowed to grieve. Careful and appropriate explanations as to the reason for the death, the plans being made for their care, and empathic understanding can be crucial to the handicapped person's survival at this time.

The Dying Handicapped Person

An appropriate death—one that occurs in comfort, without pain, and with loved ones around—is the right of a handicapped person as it is for those who are not handicapped. Hospice care, the choice to die at home, and the consideration of needs and wants can be facilitated by a community health nurse who recognizes this right.

Anticipatory and realistic planning for the handicapped person across the life span can make a significant difference in life adjustment. Particularly important is the education of family and clergy members concerning the need to prepare for the loss of significant others and even, perhaps, for the need for planning the handicapped person's own death.

Application of the Nursing Process

Although most developmentally disabled individuals are not ill, the community health nurse can use the nursing process to promote health and to assist clients in attaining a better quality of life than they might be able to by themselves. The following case study illustrates the use of the nursing process to assist a developmentally disabled couple that is living independently in the community (Fig. 23-3).

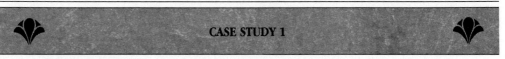

CASE STUDY 1

Assessment

Amy, 27 years of age, is severely handicapped with cerebral palsy. She has never been able to walk or talk. She converses by means of sounds uttered through clenched teeth. She spells many of her messages, but occasionally people can guess words to her satisfaction. She has always shown normal or above-normal intelligence in action even though school records show her as virtually untestable because of physical impairment. She lived at home with her family, which included younger brothers and sisters, and her life was filled with normal activity. She attended special schools in the area, was a Girl Scout, and attended sports events in which her brothers and sisters participated.

Her menstrual periods began when she was 14 years old. She is totally dependent on care givers for personal hygiene. She was given appropriate sexual information as she matured. She knew in advance of the onset of menses and understood her sexual development. She appreciated her own physical development, her breasts, her pubic hair, and her period.

At an early age she took great interest in boys. She fantasized love affairs and flirted whenever the opportunity occurred. In this area of development she was normal. She attended camps for the handicapped and would come home in love with various counselors each year, a typical teen-age reaction.

Bob is 35 years old and mildly retarded. He was raised at home and attended parochial

CASE STUDY 1—Cont'd

school until he switched to a trade school in the area. At the age of 21 years he entered a sheltered workshop. Although Bob has cerebral palsy that affects his entire left side, he is very strong. When he was 27 years old, he was hired by the county to do maintenance work. He was dependable and followed instructions well. Eventually he was given permanent civil service status.

All through his young adulthood Bob had girl friends. At one time he and a girl were found enjoying intimacy in the furnace room of his sheltered workshop. The matter was handled as if it were aberrant behavior, but Bob's feelings and the young lady's were normal. Their opportunity to express those feelings were much more limited than that of the average young couple. At another time Bob purchased a diamond ring because he wanted to become engaged to a girl he was seeing. His family insisted he break the engagement.

Until he was 33 years old, Bob lived at home, where he was sheltered by his family and treated as if he were a child. The family basically ignored his social development. Ultimately he chose to rent an apartment, a move in which his family assisted him. Although Bob considered cooking and cleaning odious tasks that his mother performed, he assumed these responsibilities to normalize his social life.

When Amy was 21 years old, she joined a young adult recreation group sponsored by the local cerebral palsy association, where she met Bob. The club gave adult handicapped individuals an opportunity to socialize. A few of the members paired off in couples, and Amy and Bob were one of the couples. Bob was able to lift Amy, handle her wheelchair, generally make her comfortable, and understand her. Soon, with the help of friends and family, Amy moved in with Bob.

Amy and Bob lived together for over a year, with the help of home care aides, and then they were married. The marriage was strongly opposed by Bob's parents, but less so by Amy's. Amy insisted on a tubal ligation before marriage because she did not feel she could raise a child independently. Although intimacy is a personal matter, the two have shared their success in enjoying a complete sex life by adaptive positions, understanding, and love. Originally Bob had had hygiene problems regarding matters of simple cleanliness, which his family had not been able to communicate to him. When Amy objected, he learned the proper procedures.

The marriage affected Amy's Social Security and Medicaid status, cutting off financial support and medical coverage. Bob's medical coverage, however, includes Amy's normal medical needs. Currently, they are attempting to obtain a new electric wheelchair for Amy because her present one is worn out and insurance coverage is uncertain.

The couple have made a down payment on a house, which has been adapted for Amy's wheelchair. Their siblings help them with the normal repair and upkeep of the house. An aide, whom they pay from their income, comes in once a week to clean the house and attend to Amy's needs.

Amy is employed at the local sheltered workshop operated by the United Cerebral Palsy Associations, where she uses a word processor with adaptive equipment. Bob's civil service job seems secure. However, life is not easy for the couple. Amy's parents think that Bob is inclined to drink more than he should. They worry about Amy's well-being. Bob's parents remain concerned that they do not handle money responsibly. In spite of this criticism, the union appears stable. Bob and Amy have achieved as much accord as people without handicapping conditions. They have received the respect and friendship of their neighbors and the admiration of all who watch their day-to-day normal activity. They can be seen on Saturdays shopping for food or running domestic errands.

Continued.

CASE STUDY 1—Cont'd

Nursing diagnosis

Nursing diagnoses appropriate for this couple include the following:
1. Altered family coping related to physical and mental disability
2. Impaired physical mobility related to developmental disability
3. Impaired social interaction related to physical disability
4. Income deficit related to decreased earning power

Planning and implementation

Nursing goals include the following actions:
1. To provide counseling for Bob and Amy concerning Bob's tendency to drink too much; to give Bob information about moderating and controlling this behavior and the reasons it would be a good idea to do so; and to counsel Amy in assisting Bob to deal with stress in some other way.
2. To assist Amy, perhaps through a local independent living center or some other source, to obtain an electric wheelchair and to investigate the possibility of funding from local government sources.
3. To advocate social programs for the couple and to assist in contacting supportive family members for transportation to social events and family gatherings.
4. To advise the couple on supplemental services available to them, for example, Supplemental Social Security or other government funding, home health aids, and other home care services.

Evaluation (outcomes)

The nurse will continue to visit the couple at regular intervals to monitor their emotional and physical well-being. In addition, the nurse will maintain weekly telephone contact with the couple and/or supportive family members.

The community health nurse's role in assisting young adults like Amy and Bob to live independently and as normally as possible can be crucial to their well-being.

LEGAL AND ETHICAL ISSUES
Right to Life

Perhaps the most important ethical issue in terms of the developmentally disabled individual is a very basic right to life. Humane treatment of such persons is becoming a reality in developed countries, but what of the child in utero? Defects such as Down's syndrome can be detected by amniocentesis during the second trimester of pregnancy (Haynes, 1980); parents can legally elect to terminate a pregnancy at this time. The ethical dilemma centers around the rights of the unborn child.

Right to Education

The right of handicapped children to an education through the age of 21 years is mandated by law in the United States and Canada. Assisting parents and teachers to choose the least restrictive environment appropriate for the child is an important part of the nurse's role in working with a family or in contributing a judgment to a committee for the handicapped in local school systems (Public Law 98-527).

Education in the least restrictive environment has not always been accessible to a physically handicapped child, and some parents, who are paying for public education, have seen their children assigned to home instruction. School nurses are in a position to enlighten other parents and teachers concerning the need to provide the best environment for the child.

A new dilemma, which requires careful thought, is finding the best environment for the child with acquired immunodeficiency syndrome (AIDS). At present, children with AIDS sometimes are denied access to schools because of objections by other parents. In some instances even siblings of children with AIDS are unwanted. Community health nurses who work in areas where AIDS is prevalent can help by educating parents and teachers concerning the method of transmission of the disease.

Right to Work

When a developmentally disabled person becomes 21 years old, the educational system no longer provides services. At this time the school or community nurse can inform the parents and the young adult of available options, for example, independent employment, sheltered employment, day treatment, day training, or day-care. There have been incidents of handicapped persons being forced to work in an institution or in a family without reimbursement and in a way that is damaging to their self-esteem. Thus it is important that nurses who help developmentally disabled individuals through the transition from school to work force inform them of the choices available to them.

Right to Sexual Expression

Handicapped persons have the same needs for sexual expression that other persons have, but sexuality in this group often is overlooked, and the result is that disabled persons tend to be treated as if they were asexual (without sexual needs). Generally, handicapping conditions that affect sexual expression can be divided into two categories, physical and mental (Nigro, 1973). In some cases sexual functioning is impaired by a condition such as a spinal cord injury. In other cases, for example cerebral palsy, it is believed that affected individuals generally are capable of completing the sex act.

Mentally retarded persons may have difficulty in understanding what is socially acceptable and appropriate behavior. Nurses can provide information (1) to parents concerning a disabled child's normal sexual desires and (2) to the disabled individual concerning sexual activity and preference, contraception, family planning, sexual hygiene, and pleasure. The nurse also can function as a buffer between the disabled individual and the community, educating the general population on the propriety of sexual identity and activity for the disabled individual.

"Sexuality encompasses not only actual intercourse but also love given and received in many ways" (Thompson, 1986, p. 135). Handicapped adults may need to learn alternate ways to express love. Some will never marry. Those who can may find that having children would be inadvisable. As with the general population sexual decisions are based on a number of factors, including matters of personal preference. Handicapped teenagers should be given the same knowledge and value base as their peers. They should have the opportunity to make decisions for themselves. The elements of responsibility for one's actions are a factor with the disabled individual, but not more so than with the general population.

Incest, homosexuality, and rape, as well as premarital intercourse, appropriate and inappropriate touching, AIDS, and personal hygiene are all subjects nurses in community settings should address when they work with the handicapped.

Right to Marry and Bear Children

A handicapped couple should have the right to marry and bear children within the limits of their capabilities. Some states in the United States have laws that limit the right to marry for those who have mental deficits. Some families oppose such unions. Guidance information and advocacy once again can be a part of the community health nurse's role.

Right to Leisure and Retirement

Concurrent with the increase in life expectancy for the population as a whole is an increase in the life expectancy of the developmentally disabled. Access to services that maintain their quality of life as they age can be facilitated by the community health nurse.

Right to an Appropriate Death

Anticipatory planning for a comfortable and pain-free death with family close by should be an option for handicapped people.

Rights Concerning Child Abuse

Child abuse is more frequent in families that experience high stress. Home visits by a community health nurse can identify children at risk and perhaps prevent neglect or trauma by aggressive intervention. Developmentally disabled children frequently cause a family stress the family cannot cope with. Family counseling, respite, and assistance with care are appropriate measures. In extreme cases a judgment of alternate placement may be required. Nurses can watch for signs of ambivalence toward the child's needs, depression, overwhelming and incapacitating anxiety, and excessive guilt on the part of the parent as warning signs for the need for intervention (Haynes, 1980). Obvious signs such as bruises, recurrent infection, altered nutrition, and lack of cleanliness are signs of the need for immediate intervention.

Rights Concerning Behavior Modification and Psychotropic Drugs

Matters regarding drugs used to control behavior always have had ethical implications, but they also have legal implications. Such drugs should not be used for the convenience of the caretaker and require documentation of therapeutic effects. Efforts to decrease the drug dosage to the minimum amount to maintain behavioral control must be shown by the caretaker.

Another issue that surrounds medication is that of informed consent. The client must participate in planning to the best of his or her ability. An adult client is considered competent until declared incompetent by the court. Competency is a very personal issue. Persons with disabilities function at differing levels for different activities. If medication is one of the issues about which the client is able to make a judgment, then he or she should participate in the planned usage or stoppage of medication.

One of the most important functions of the nurse who works in an intermediate-care facility or a community residence is the training of nonmedical personnel in the administration of medications. The nurse must certify that nonmedical personnel are competent and able to administer drugs. Conscience and discretion in this matter are of primary importance to the welfare of the client. Supervision and teaching families proper administration of drugs in the home also are part of the nurse's role.

Seizure medications are not in question ethically because individuals who have convulsive disorders as a part of their disability need them to stay well. It is crucial to the handicapped person's well-being that the primary caretaker have an understanding of proper dosages, the importance of regularity of administration, and side effects. If self-medication is chosen, then the nurse's responsibility is to teach handicapped persons at their level of understanding how to take their medications.

Psychostimulant drugs such as methylphenidate (Ritalin) and dextroamphetamine (Dexedrine) need careful monitoring. Studies have shown that these drugs sometimes increase a hyperactive child's ability to concentrate. Side effects include nervousness, nausea, dizziness, headache, talkativeness, moodiness, palpitations, and a possible slowing of the child's growth rate. School nurses in particular should closely observe a child who is taking psychostimulants to be able to make a judgment about the effectiveness of the medication and possible untoward effects. Family counseling, an appropriate classroom setting, and a quiet and consistent environment are all helpful to a child receiving drug therapy or to one who is not (Pueschel, Bernier, & Weidenman 1988).

Antipsychotic medications are used to control an aggressive behavior in children and adults. Chlorpromazine (Thorazine), thioridazine (Mellaril), thiothixene (Navane), haloperidol (Haldol), and benztropine mesylate (Cogentin) are commonly used. Side effects include lethargy, tardive dyskinesia, minor liver problems, and rapid heartbeat (Pueschel, et al., 1988). Administration of these drugs sometimes is questioned as a method of behavior control. They should not replace family counseling, appropriate placement, and individual psychiatric counseling. The same holds true for antidepressant medications such as amitriptyline (Elavil) and imipramine (Tofranil), which may cause dry mouth, nausea, and heartburn.

Nurses who supervise the administration of psychotropic drugs in the home, the institution, or the community are responsible for monitoring correct administration of the drugs and possible side effects. There also is a moral obligation to assess whether the drug is being administered in the interest of the handicapped person or simply for the convenience of the caretaker.

Right to Choose

Disabled individuals have the same right as others to fail or succeed; to suffer or experience joy; to curse or bless; and even to despair. To protect the disabled from these experiences is to deny them life. All persons have the right to honesty as a base on which to make decisions, including those who are disabled. Only they know what is possible for them. Others can assist by recognizing and motivating them to use their potential. Attentive nurses who are attuned to listening can facilitate and assist the disabled to become fully self-actualized.

The Right to Reach Full Potential

"Handicaps are made, not born" (Buscaglia, 1975). The attitude of society at large has far more impact on the disabled person's life than the disability itself. The manner in which persons with disabilities are treated has far more impact on their self-image, hence their ability, than any other force, including the disability itself. Society sets the limits, not the disability. According to Marc Gold, "mental retardation is most meaningfully conceptualized as a sociological phenomenon, existing within society, which can only be observed through limited performance of some of the individuals in society (1980, p. 6). Gold's alternative definition is a gentler, more optimistic characterization of the problem. Gold continues thus (p. 2):

> The mentally retarded person is characterized by the level of power needed in the training process required for them to learn, and not by the limitation of what they can learn. A retarded person's level of functioning is determined by the availability of training technology and the amount of resources society is willing to allocate and not by significant limitations in biological potential.

Gold developed a training system that provides a method of organizing training programs for special populations of workers that include strategies to enhance the abilities of severely disabled persons. The system is based on the premise that persons labeled "handicapped" respond best to a learning situation based on respect of their human worth and capabilities. They have the breadth and depth of capabilities to demonstrate competence, given training appropriate to their needs: "A lack of training in any particular situation should first be interpreted as an inappropriate or insufficient use of teaching strategy, rather than an inability on the part of the learner" (p. 5). Labeling is both unfair and unproductive.

These strategies are based on the following premises: (1) retardation does not affect every area of existence. There are many ways in which retarded persons function exactly as others in their age-group. (2) Many things can be learned if the educator adapts techniques rather than assumes that the student lacks ability. Persons who are retarded can learn to do a great deal if someone will take the time to teach them.

Learning is a lifelong phenomenon for the retarded as it is for others. No behavior defines potential. What can be learned depends on how it is taught. All persons can adapt their behaviors and, when motivated, do so. Training is much more useful than testing and does not lay failure on the client.

Learner and trainer find they must adapt to each other not only in terms of the learning process but also in terms of their human relationship. Quite simply, the relationship between a learner labeled handicapped and a trainer should be the same as any sound relationship between two persons working together toward learning a common task. "A basis of respect and recognition allows each person the freedom to be himself or herself, adapting only for the sake of the relationship or the common goal" (Gold, 1980, p. 4).

The Right to be Part of a Community of Love and Concern

In 1964 Jean Vanier, the son of the Governor General of Canada, founded the first L'Arche community in France. This movement (L'Arche Philosophy, 1987) was followed in the United States with similar communities. Vanier teaches that mutual relationships are the heart of human existence. His homes are based on an attitude of interdependence and mutual value.

The difference between these communities and ordinary community residences is a philosophy of giftedness. Vanier firmly believed that the men with whom he created a family had much to offer his community. The spirit of giftedness prevails in L'Arche communities today. Thus the administrator, the breadwinner, and the therapist all participate in a community in which their gifts of administration, therapy, and nursing are celebrated with the gifts of love and honesty and simple service that the retarded individuals offer the same community. So it is in an environment of human value that the residents of L'Arche mature.

Vanier's homes are more than residences. They are communities in which people with mental handicaps share life with those who might be thought of as helpers but who see the total situation in a context of mutuality. Life at L'Arche offers a sense of belonging.

For Vanier the weakest member of the community is the most important. The weakest member is the gift through whom all the others learn their own identity and their own weakness. The L'Arche experience indicates that growth in authentic human relationships is the most important value of any work with people with handicapping conditions.

The Right to Normalization

Wolf Wolfensberger is responsible for a concept known as *normalization.* Much of the responsibility for being "different" is placed not on the individual but on the society that has labeled that person "different."

Wolfensberger's concept of normalization in the vocabulary of the serving professions has a very special connotation. It stresses the imperative of making available to people with disabilities normal patterns of everyday life. Disabled persons should have the same options and opportunities that are the rights of everyone else, with support to enable them to take advantage of the options.

SUMMARY

The role of the nurse with the developmentally disabled in the community is rich and varied. It demands all the talents and skills of the profession.

Definitions of disabilities are changing from day to day. Means of caring for the disabled individual are in flux as they change from the days of Willowbrook and are being affected by the passage of federal laws. Community nursing has been greatly affected, especially by the advantages of interdisciplinary (team) treatment of disabled people.

Deinstitutionalization, normalization, the least restrictive environment, and refinements in definitions of disabilities all affect nursing procedures.

Federal regulations are being updated to protect the disabled, and the nursing community must keep abreast of them to adequately maintain residences and day-care facilities and to satisfy funding sources.

The traditional functions of prevention, early identification, education, and family counseling on health matters are properly in the domain of the nurse in the community.

Sexual needs of disabled persons in the form of education, intervention, family planning, and referral to genetic counseling and advocacy are relevant issues.

Criteria for adequate nursing procedures have been developed and are meant to be followed and refined.

The growth of a body of skills and a philosophy that affirms each human being's giftedness by defining the contributions that disabled persons can make to society will enable the nurse to assist the developmentally disabled population.

CHAPTER HIGHLIGHTS

- A shift in societal attitudes over the past two decades has led to an increased number of developmentally disabled persons in the community. Federal legislation has mandated such objectives as normalization, individuation, and placement in the least restrictive environment.
- Community health nurses are involved in the education of health providers, coordination of services, and prevention at primary, secondary, and tertiary levels, as well as active advocacy with this population.
- Developmental disabilities are defined by P.L. 94-103 as a disability that has the following characteristics:

  1. It is attributable to mental retardation, cerebral palsy, epilepsy, neurological impairment, or autism.
  2. It results in impairment of adaptive behavior and requires treatment similar to that of a retarded person.

3. It originates before the individual reaches 18 years of age.
4. It is expected to continue indefinitely.
5. It constitutes a substantial handicap that affects the individual's performance in society.

- Deinstitutionalization, or the placement of disabled persons in their own homes with support services, family care, group homes and community residences, is the result of heightened public awareness as to the inhumane treatment of the developmentally disabled in such institutions as Willowbrook on Staten Island.
- The developmental model of meeting the needs of the developmentally disabled takes into account the evolving needs of this population across the life span.
- P.L. 94-142 stipulates that all handicapped children should have an individualized education plan and that the parent should be a part of the committee responsible for the plan, along with the school nurse, the psychologist, and the child's teacher.
- Legal and ethical issues still surround the care and treatment of the developmentally disabled. Some of them are the right to life, the right to an education in the least restrictive environment, the right to work, the right to sexual expression, the right to marry and bear children, the right to leisure and retirement, freedom from abuse, ethical use of psychotropic drugs for behavior modification, and the right to an appropriate death.

STUDY QUESTIONS

1. What are the effects on community health nursing practice of the definitions of developmental disabilities in P.L. 94-103 and P.L. 98-527?
2. Choose two of the developmental disabilities discussed in this chapter. For each, how can the community health nurse assist a client to promote optimum health and to live as independently as possible?
3. What are some of the advantages and disadvantages of deinstitutionalization?
4. What are some of the needs of developmentally disabled young adults? How can the community health nurse assist the client in meeting these needs?

REFERENCES

ARC Newsletter reprint, (1972.) *Our children's voice, 24,* June 2. New York State association for Retarded Children.

Buscaglia, L. (1975). *The disabled and their parents: A counseling challenge.* Thorofare, NJ: Slack.

Byers, D. M. (1987). *Opening doors.* Ministry with persons with disabilities, Washington, DC: Center for Human Policy, Division of Special Education and Rehabilitation. (1981). Title XIX and Deinstitutionalization: Syracuse University. National Catholic Office for Persons with Disabilities.

Curry J. B., & Peppe, K. K. (Eds.). (1978). *Mental retardation: Nursing approaches to care.* St. Louis: Mosby.

Englehardt, K. F. (1978). Principles of normalization. In J. B. Curry & K. K. Peppe (Eds.), *Mental retardation: Nursing approaches to care* (pp. 33-41). St. Louis: Mosby.

Gabel, S., & Erikson, M. (1980). *Child development and developmental disabilities.* Boston: Little, Brown & Co.

Gold, M. W. (1980). *Try another way training manual.* Champaign, IL: Research Press.

Grossman, H. J. (Ed.). (1973). *Manual on terminology and classification in mental retardation* [Special Publication No. 2]. Washington, DC: American Association on Mental Deficiency.

Haynes, U. (1980). *A developmental approach to case finding among infants and children.* Rockville, MD: U.S. Dept. of Health, Education, and Welfare, pp. 34-35.

Human warehouse. (1972, February 14). *Time,* pp. 68-69.

Matson, J., & Marchetti, A. (1988). *Developmental disabilities: A life-span perspective.* Philadelphia: Grune & Stratton.

Neier, (1980, July 19). Willowbrook—Back to Bedlam. *Nation,* pp. 80-82.

New York State Commission on Quality of Care for the Mentally Disabled. (1982). *Your child's right to a free appropriate education.*

Nigro, J. (1973, November). Sexuality in the handicapped. *Speech Institute of Rehabilitation Medicine.*

Pattulo, A. W. (1978). Developing sexuality among people who are retarded. In J. B. Curry & K. K. Peppe (Eds.). *Mental retardation: Nursing approaches to care* (pp. 204-223). St. Louis: Mosby.

Pueschel, S., Bernier, J., & Weidenman, L. (1988). *The special child.* Baltimore: Brooks.

Rubin, L., & Crocker, A. (1989). *Developmental disabilities: Delivery of medical care for infants and Children.* Philadelphia: Lea & Febiger.

Scheenberger, R. C. (1976). *Deinstitutionalization and institutional reform.* Springfield, IL: Charles C. Thomas.

Selekman, J., Goldenthal, P., & Clark, K. (1988). The learning disabled child. *Holistic Nurse Practitioner, Feb. 2, pp. 1-10.*

Shaw, H. (1986). *Pathways to the future: Critical steps for 1986.* Family support services: Expanding alternatives for familes. Albany, NY: New York State Office of Mental Retardation and Developmental Disabilities.

Stanhope, M., & Lancaster, J. (1988). *Community health nursing: Process and practice for promoting health* (2nd. ed.) St. Louis: Mosby.

Summarah, A. (1987). L'Arche Philosophy and Ideology, *Mental Retardation, 24* (3), Summary.

Thompson, C. (1986). *Raising a handicapped child.* New York: Morrow.

United States Statutes at Large. (1975). *89,* p. 497, 775.

United States Statutes at Large. (1984). *98,* p. 2664.

Vessy, J. (1988). Care of hospitalized child with a cognitive developmental delay. *Holistic Nurse Practitioner,* Feb. 2, pp. 48-54.

Webb, A. (1986). *Strengthening the continuum 1887-1990,* Albany, NY: New York State Office of Mental Retardation and Developmental Disabilities.

Whaley, L. F., & Wong, D. L. (1987). *Nursing care of infants and children, (3rd ed.).* St. Louis: Mosby.

Wolfensberger, U. (1972). *The principle of normalization in human services.* Toronto: National Institute on Mental Retardation.

Issues and Concerns in Community Health Nursing

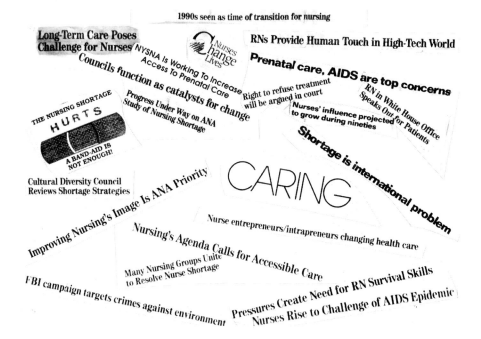

As nurses enter the 1990's they face uncertainties and challenges that are unique in the experience of humankind. Promoting and maintaining the health of clients now encompasses the total community. In addition, and expanded knowledge base requires the nurse to possess a degree of sophistication unheard of a generation ago.

Chapter 24 discusses the importance of good nutrition and its effect on the health of the individual across the life span. It also discusses methods of altering nutrition to the highest possible level of wellness in an individual already experiencing an altered health state.

Concern about the immediate environment surrounding a patient began with Florence Nightingale. This concern has expanded to include the total environment affecting the client and the client family. Chapter 25 outlines some of the problems associated with today's environment and describes actions the nurse can take to make the environment healthier. It also predicts some environmental hazards the nurse may encounter in the future.

The problem of substance abuse is addressed in Chapter 26. The tragedy and the challenge of addiction and dysfunction accompanying drug dependency is described. The nurse of the future may have to deal with drug abuse in epidemic proportions.

Advanced technology, and accelerating change have created legal and ethical issues not even imaginable a generation ago. Chapter 27 outlines some of those issues and makes suggestions about client advocacy, problem solving, and patient concerns. It is emphasized that many judgements are made in a gray area where there are no clear rights or wrongs and many decisions are made in the hope that they are the correct ones with no real certainty that this is so.

Finally, Chapter 28 describes professional issues confronting the community health nurse. The need for nurses to be aware of health policy issues of the present and future, to develop a theory base for community health practice, and to be accountable, are described.

The future of community health nursing is vague and uncertain. To be prepared for it, the nurse of the 90's would be well advised to begin with a strong theoretical base, and to develop a firm understanding of the technology necessary for practice. The nurse must be prepared to act as a client advocate and must be aware that the community health nurse has to function and practice in the total community.

Nutrition in the Community

EDWARD H. WEISS

Our daily diets can bring a substantial measure of better health to all Americans.

C. EVERETT KOOP, Surgeon General of the Public Health Services

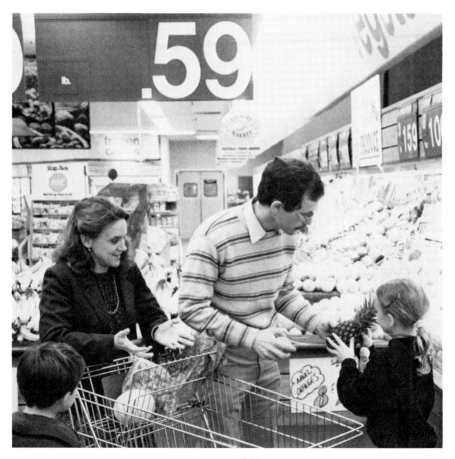

OBJECTIVES

At the conclusion of this chapter the student will be able to:
1. Discuss the health implications of the dietary guidelines for the general public and for specific at-risk groups
2. Outline nutritional concerns, assessment criteria, and recommendations within the stages of life (pregnancy, infancy, adulthood, aging)
3. Describe the development, format, and impact of a nutrition education program for an elderly audience
4. Identify, on the basis of the chapter's contents, the nutritional concerns and educational needs of an elderly person with non-insulin-dependent diabetes mellitus

KEY TERMS

Alcohol	Dietitian
Anthropometric measures	Fluoride
Body mass index	Iron
Breast-feeding	Nutrition
Calcium	Nutritional assessment
Calorie	Obesity
Cholesterol	Saturated fats
Complex carbohydrates	Sodium
Diet	

Good nutrition is not an end in itself but is one of many factors that have an impact on health. Research has shown that diet can play an important role in the prevention of chronic disease. Poor diet has been identified as a risk factor for coronary heart disease, some cancers, high blood pressure, stroke, dental disease, osteoporosis, diabetes mellitus, and obesity (*Surgeon General's Report*, 1988). Nutrition *alone* cannot be expected to alter the course of most diseases or to prevent them, but an individual's nutritional status can play a significant role in the treatment and prevention of some diseases.

WHAT IS A HEALTHY DIET?

In the United States diseases of dietary excess have replaced the problem of nutritional deficiencies (e.g., rickets, pellagra, and goiter). This change is largely a result of an improved variety of available foods and the fortification of foods with critical vitamins and minerals. The important relationship between nutrition and disease is demonstrated by the development of numerous dietary guidelines that offer recommendations on how adults should eat. The community health nurse should recognize the similarities among recommendations made by a number of diverse organizations, including the American Heart Association, the American Cancer Society, the American Diabetes Association, and Canada's Food Guide; Handbook (Table 24-1).

The similarity among dietary recommendations intended to reduce the risk of cancer,

TABLE 24-1   Comparison of surgeon general's diet recommendations (1988) with other dietary guidelines

Issues	USDA/USDHHS (1985)	Areas of agreement			
		American Heart Association (1988)	American Cancer Society (1984)	American Diabetes Association (1987)	Canada's food guide (1982)
1. Reduction of fat/cholesterol	X	X	X	X	X
2. Energy/weight control	X	X	X	X	X
3. Complex carbohydrates and fiber	X	X	X	X	
4. Sodium	X	X	X	X	X
5. Alcohol	X	X	X	X	X
6. Fluoride					
7. Limiting sugars	X			X	X
8. Increased calcium	X	X			X
9. Iron	X	X			X

USDA/USDHHS, U.S. Department of Agriculture/U.S. Department of Health and Human Services. (1988).

X, Identifies agreement with surgeon general's report on nutrition and health.

diabetes, and heart disease means that community education efforts to improve dietary behavior can be based on a common message. There are, however, limitations to these guidelines. All of these recommendations focus on the "typical" adult diet and its effect on the chronic diseases that are the leading cause of death in America. This diet is characterized by dietary excess, *not* hunger. Therefore these guidelines do not directly address the concerns of persons who do not have to an adequate diet.

An in-depth review of research supporting dietary guidelines for the public has resulted in the publication of the *Surgeon General's Report on Nutrition and Health* (1988). This report provides the community health nurse with a basis for answering the question, "What is a healthy diet?" The report offers a consensus on dietary recommendations that can guide community nutrition education efforts for adults. Individual differences in age, sex, income, ethnic background, health, and behavior must be considered in the use of these recommendations to guide individual behavior. Each of the nine recommendations in the surgeon general's report are discussed here.

DIETARY RECOMMENDATIONS FOR MOST PERSONS
Recommendation 1: Fats and Cholesterol

Reduce consumption of fat (especially saturated fat) and cholesterol. Choose foods relatively low in these substances, such as vegetables, fruits, whole grain foods, fish, poultry, lean meats, and low-fat dairy products. Use food preparation methods that add little or no fat (*Surgeon General*, 1988).

The reduction of dietary fat is recommended because of its importance as a risk factor for chronic diseases such as diabetes, cancer, and heart disease. Fat is a concentrated source of calories, and excess calories from fatty foods are linked to obesity and related health problems (e.g., hypertension and hyperlipidemia). In addition, reduced fat intake, along with increased activity levels, aids in weight management for non-insulin-dependent

---

HOW TO AVOID TOO MUCH FAT, SATURATED FAT, AND CHOLESTEROL

- Choose lean meat, fish, poultry, and dry beans and peas as protein sources
- Use skim or low-fat milk and milk products
- Moderate your use of egg yolks and organ meats
- Limit your intake of fats and oils, especially those high in saturated fat, such as butter, cream, lard, heavily hydrogenated fats (some margarines), shortenings, and foods containing palm and coconut oils
- Trim fat off meats
- Broil, bake, or boil rather than fry
- Moderate your use of foods that contain fat, such as breaded and deep-fried foods
- Read labels carefully to determine both amount and type of fat present in foods

USDA/USDHHS, 1985, p. 16.

---

diabetes mellitus (NIDDM). Both the American Heart Association and the American Diabetes Association recommend that total fat intake be less than 30% of all calories, that saturated fat be limited to 10% of total calories, and that dietary cholesterol should not exceed 300 mg/day. These recommendations are in direct contrast to the current American diet, which contains approximately 37% fat calories. Reduction of obesity, serum cholesterol, and blood pressure lowers the risk for cardiovascular disease and supports the management of diabetes mellitus.

How to reduce dietary fat. The box above lists some suggestions for reducing dietary fat. Dependence on "fast foods," which are typically high in fat and calories, can increase dietary fat. Saturated fats (solid fats) should be replaced with polyunsaturated fats (vegetable oils). Total fat intake can be measured by the use of computer nutrient analysis, food frequency records, or diabetic exchange lists (American Diabetes Association and American Diabetic Association, 1977).

Dietary concerns for special groups. A screening test for total serum cholesterol levels will identify individuals at risk. Persons with blood cholesterol levels of 200 mg/dl (6.0 mmol/L) (American Heart Association, 1988) or less should be asked to follow guidelines and have their cholesterol checked every 5 years. Persons with levels between 200 and 240 mg/dl are at moderate risk and should have a second cholesterol check to ensure an accurate measurement of this highly variable test. The treatment of choice for those at moderate risk includes (1) reaching and maintaining ideal body weight and (2) reducing dietary fat to 30% and decreasing saturated fat intake. The reduction of other risk factors, also is suggested (i.e., smoking, diabetes, hypertension, and obesity). More detailed testing and treatment methods are required for persons whose levels are above 240 mg/d[l] (7.2 mmol/L) (Hoeg, 1987).

Some clients can benefit from even greater reductions in dietary lipids. The American Diabetes Association (1987) recommends that persons with elevated cholesterol levels, especially elevated low-density lipoprotein (LDL), could benefit from a stricter fat-modified diet. Such restrictions require detailed instructions and the aid of a registered dietitian.

There are important differences in the feeding recommendation for infants and children (American Academy of Pediatrics, 1986). Because of the high rate of growth and development in this age-group, dietary fat should *not* be restricted during the first year of life. A moderate restriction in saturated fat and cholesterol is acceptable (30% to 40%

of calories) after 1 year of age. Children's diets should avoid extremes, offer variety, maintain ideal body weight, and support adequate growth and development.

Recommendation 2: Energy and Weight Control

Achieve and maintain a desirable body weight. To do so, choose a dietary pattern in which energy (caloric) intake is consistent with energy expenditure. To reduce energy intake, limit consumption of foods relatively high in calories, fats, and sugars, and minimize alcohol consumption. Increase energy expenditure through regular and sustained physical activity (*Surgeon General*, 1988).

A significant problem with this recommendation is the difficulty of identifying a person's "desirable weight." A number of methods have been used. Most involve measurements of height and weight in relation to life expectancy and health risks within a specific population. All methods are subject to limitations (as screening tools) in their ability to detect obesity (sensitivity) and to identify nonobesity (specificity). The National Institutes of Health (NIH) (1985) recommends that health professionals use one of the two following criteria to define obesity in adults: (1) desirable body weight for that person's height and weight on the basis of the 1959 or 1983 Metropolitan Life Insurance Company tables and (2) the body mass index (BMI).

The BMI is a useful expression of a person's weight-height relationship. It can be conveniently calculated by means of metric system measurements. A person's body weight (in kilograms) is divided by the square of the person's height (in meters), according to the following formula:

$$BMI = \frac{\text{Body weight in kg}}{(\text{height in m}^2)}$$

In clinical settings, the NIH consensus panel on obesity (1985) recommended that the BMI be used because it is simple and highly correlated with other estimates of percentage of body fat. The index tends to minimize errors across different heights and the redistribution of fat with aging. It also allows for comparisons among populations.

The nomogram shown in Fig. 24-1 provides a convenient means for calculating an individual's BMI. First locate the person's height in the left-hand column. Next, find the point at which the person's weight is shown in the column on the right. Then, using a straight edge, draw a line connecting the two points. The BMI then can be read directly at the point at which the line crosses the middle column. Thus, for example, using the nomograph to determine the BMI of a 5 foot 1 inch (i.e., 61 inches or 155 cm) woman, weighing 106 pounds (i.e., 48 Kg), a line drawn from the 155-cm point on the left column to the 48 Kg point on the right column would cross the center column at a point indicating a BMI of about 22 (a "desirable" BMI for a woman). The *Surgeon General's Report* (1988) defines "overweight" as a BMI over the 85th percentile and "severely overweight" as a BMI that exceeds the 95th percentile.

If height-weight tables are used, the nurse should recognize that the 1983 Metropolitan height and weight tables (versus the 1959 tables) offer slightly less conservative weight goals (see Chapter 11). Persons who weigh 20% more than their desirable weight should be advised to lose weight.

Obesity, or excess body fat, is recognized as a major health risk for coronary heart disease, stroke, high blood pressure, diabetes mellitus, gallbladder disease, and some cancers, as well as other types of illness. Reduction of total body fat to achieve desirable weight typically improves serum cholesterol levels and can help lower high blood pressure. A majority of persons with noninsulin–dependent diabetes mellitus (NIDDM) are 20% or more overweight and exhibit a relative insulin deficiency as a result of insulin resistance. The achievement of ideal body weight (IBW) typically controls plasma glucose toward normal levels and has been identified as the "most important treatment for those persons not requiring insulin" (ADA & ADA, 1977).

How to achieve and maintain desirable weight. Weight loss is the result of consuming fewer calories than needed. It requires the selection of lower-calorie foods and an increase in physical activity. The goal of any weight reduction program should be a slow and steady reduction in the percentage of body fat. Diets that result in rapid weight loss (greater than 2 pounds per week) cause undesirable loss of protein and water weight, not fat (Yang & VanItallie, 1976). Characteristics of a safe weight reduction program are as follows:

1. Supplies fewer calories than needed, resulting in a 1 to 2 pound loss per week
2. Offers a variety of foods (i.e., breads and cereals, milk products, protein sources, vegetables, and fruits)
3. Allows for recording and retraining eating behaviors
4. Is simple and easy to follow
5. Increases regular physical activity in step-wise increments according to ability

Dietary concerns for special groups. The prevalence of obese children in the United States is a major community health concern (Gortmaker, Dietz, Sobol, & Wehaler, 1987). It is a major concern because childhood obesity tends to become a lifelong problem. With childhood weight reduction programs, special efforts should be made to prevent severe calorie restrictions, which can arrest healthy development. Emphasis should be placed on increasing energy needs through regular physical activity (American Academy of Pediatrics, 1985).

Persons with diabetes mellitus who are asked to exercise should be reminded that activity can affect blood glucose levels. Persons who take sulfonylureas may be at risk for hypoglycemia, and those with insulin-dependent diabetes mellitus (IDDIU) usually must reduce their dosage. As adolescents with IDDM mature, they must be careful to reduce energy intake (and insulin dose) to reflect their changing needs, or they are at risk for obesity.

Recommendation 3: Complex Carbohydrates and Fiber

Increase consumption of whole grain foods and cereal products, vegetables (including dried beans and peas), and fruits (*Surgeon General*, 1988).

Dietary fiber is the undigestable material in plant foods and characteristically offers a rich source of vitamins and minerals; it also is low in fat and calories. There are many types of fiber, each with a unique chemical structure and different physiological properties.

Many health benefits have been suggested from increasing the variety and amount of fibers in the diet. High-fiber, low-fat diets have been linked with lower risks of diverticulosis, constipation, obesity, and some cancers. Intake of water-soluble fibers found in some fruits, oat bran, and legumes (beans and peas) has been correlated with reductions in blood glucose and lipids levels. Until more is known about the specific effects of fiber compounds, the best advice is to increase fiber by including a variety of plant foods in the diet (Connor, 1990).

How to increase fiber in the diet. The typical American diet is low in fiber and complex carbohydrates and is high in simple sugars. Increasing the amount of whole grain foods, legumes (beans, peas, lentils), nuts, fruits, and vegetables in the diet will supply a variety of fiber, plus many essential vitamins and minerals. Fiber-rich foods offer many more nutrients than are gained when processed bran is used to increase dietary fiber. Increased consumption of complex carbohydrates to 50% to 55% of the total day's intake is a common dietary recommendation (American Diabetes Association, 1987, and AHA, 1988). This increase is accomplished by emphasizing plant foods such as vegetables, fruits, and grains. Except for persons with diabetes, most dietary recommendations do not specify the exact amount of fiber required in the diet.

Some basic concepts need to be understood before clients attempt to increase the amount of fiber in their diets. The amount of fiber varies among individual foods and how much those foods are processed. For example, a fresh apple is a significant source of fiber, but apple juice is not. Whole grain wheat or oat cereals contain more fiber than products made from highly processed white flour. Detailed listings of high-fiber foods are available through many computerized diet analysis software, diabetes exchange lists, diabetic teaching nurses, or a registered dietitian.

Clients should be cautioned that the amount of fiber in the diet should be increased gradually to minimize potential side effects such as abdominal cramping and flatulence. An adequate intake of fluids also is needed; otherwise constipation problems can occur.

Dietary concerns for special groups. The American Diabetes Association (ADA) suggests that persons gradually increase fiber intake, with the general goal of doubling their consumption of fiber. The Association suggests that an intake of up to 40 g/day of fiber appears to be beneficial, with a maximim intake of 50 g/day. These levels contrast with the typical intake in the United States of 19 g/day and 13 g/day for adult men and women, respectively (ADA, 1987). Persons with diabetes should be cautioned that hypoglycemia may result when insulin dosages are not reduced after dramatic increase in fiber intake (ADA, 1987).

Recommendation 4: Sodium

Reduce intake of sodium by choosing foods relatively low in sodium and limiting the amount of salt added in food preparation and at the table (*Surgeon General*, 1988).

A majority of dietary guidelines suggest limiting sodium by moderating the intake of high-sodium foods and reducing the amount of salt added during cooking or at the table. Because of the association of salt-cured, smoked, and sodium nitrate–cured foods with some cancers (e.g., of the esophagus and stomach), moderation in the consumption of these products has been recommended (American Cancer Society, 1984; National Research Council, 1989).

Although sodium is an essential nutrient, Americans typically consume many times the levels of sodium considered to be safe and adequate by the National Research Council (1.1 to 3.3). Because of its major extracellular action, which can result in fluid retention, sodium intake is a risk factor for hypertension. At greatest risk are persons with a family history of hypertension.

The National Research Council suggests that the total daily intake of sodium be limited to 2.4 g. This is equivalent to 6 g sodium chloride (6 g equals about 12 average-size paper clips). Further restriction may be recommended for persons with hypertension (American Heart Assocation [AHA], 1988), although not all individuals with hypertension respond to sodium restriction. A trial diet currently is the only method of identifying who will benefit significantly.

How to reduce sodium intake. Approximately one third of dietary sodium is found naturally in food, one third is added during processing, and the remaining third is added during preparation or at the table. Two thirds of this intake can be reduced by limiting

---

HOW TO AVOID TOO MUCH SODIUM

- Learn to enjoy the flavors of unsalted foods
- Cook without salt or with only small amounts of added salt
- Try flavoring foods with herbs, spices, and lemon juice
- Add little or no salt to food at the table
- Limit your intake of salty foods such as potato chips, pretzels, salted nuts and popcorn, condiments (soy sauce, steak sauce, garlic salt), pickled foods, cured meats, some cheeses, and some canned vegetables and soups
- Read food labels carefully to determine the amount of sodium
- Use lower-sodium products, when available, to replace those you use that have higher sodium content

USDA/USDHHS, 1985.

---

sodium-rich processed foods and replacing salt with other spices or flavorings during home preparation (see box). Food labels offer an easy way to identify high-sodium foods. Sodium can be found in diet beverages (saccharin sodium), canned foods, gravies, condiments, frozen prepared meals, sandwich meats, and snacks.

Recommendation 5: Alcohol

> To reduce the risk for chronic disease, take alcohol only in moderation (no more than two drinks a day), if at all. Avoid drinking any alcohol before or while driving, operating machinery, taking medications, or engaging in any other activity requiring judgment. Avoid drinking alcohol while pregnant (*Surgeon General*, 1988).

No dietary guidelines actually recommend the consumption of alcohol, although several suggest that moderate consumption is acceptable. Moderate consumption has been defined as one or two drinks per day in the Dietary Guidelines for Americans (1980).

The problems associated with excess consumption of alcohol are well documented. These include liver disease, cancer, birth defects, accidents, antisocial behavior, suicides, homocides, and malnutrition. Alcohol contributes calories but provides few nutrients. Excess calories from alcohol can contribute to obesity while replacing other foods and can result in vitamin and mineral deficiencies.

Moderate consumption of alcohol has been linked to reduced risk of coronary heart disease by means of the elevation of high-density lipoproteins. However, no direct proof that alcohol will reduce vascular disease has yet been demonstrated (AHA, 1988). Therefore alcohol consumption has *not* been suggested as a method of disease prevention.

Recommendations for special groups. Women who are pregnant and those who are trying to conceive should avoid drinking alcohol (*Surgeon General*, 1988). Irreversible damage to the fetus (fetal alcohol syndrome) is reported to occur with as few as two drinks a day. The damage can occur during the first weeks of development, before the mother knows she is pregnant. Excessive consumption has been shown to cause physical and mental retardation, brain damage, and physical deformities in the newborn.

Persons with diabetes who choose to drink need to observe the same precautions (moderate consumption) with alcohol use as does the general public (American Diabetes. Association [ADA, 1987]), plus additional recommendations to control hypoglycemia, hyperlipidemia, and obesity. They should understand that alcohol will decrease blood glucose, decrease glycogen release, and reduce gluconeogenesis. Therefore alcoholic beverages must be consumed with food or after a meal.

Recommendation 6: Fluoride

> Community water systems should contain optimal levels for prevention of tooth decay. If such water is not available, use other appropriate sources of fluoride (*Surgeon General*, 1988).

A fluoride concentration of approximately one part per million has been shown to reduce the prevalence of dental cavities by more than 50% (*Surgeon General*, 1988). Fluoride incorporated into the tooth structure during development helps protect against the erosion of tooth enamel as a result of bacteria-produced acid.

An association between osteoporosis and fluoride intake has been reported, but the effect of fluoride in the prevention and/or treatment of osteoporosis has not yet been established conclusively (National Research Council, 1989).

Not all public drinking water contains the recommended amount of fluoride. The public health nurse can play an important role in educating the public about the benefits of fluoridation. Community leaders cannot act without broad support by a well-informed public. If community water supplies are inadequate, children should obtain a physician-prescribed supplemental source that meets their need. Breast-fed infants may be at risk, regardless of public water levels, because the fluoride content of human milk is quite low. Breast-fed infants often receive supplements of 0.25 mg fluoride/day after 2 weeks of age (Alpers, Clouse, & Stenson, 1983). Excessive fluoride intake should be avoided because of the risk of discoloring and mottling of permanent teeth even though this effect is only cosmetic (Alpers et al; 1983).

Recommendation 7: Sugars

> Those who are particularly vulnerable to dental caries (cavities), especially children, should limit their consumption and frequency of use of foods high in sugars (*Surgeon General*, 1988).

The association between sugar intake and dental disease is well recognized. Recommendations are to limit the amount and the use frequency of high-sugar foods (see box). Currently in the United States approximately 30% to 50% of carbohydrates consumed are simple sugars (AHA, 1988). High-sugar foods provide calories without needed nutrients, and this increase in total energy is linked to the risk of obesity and dental caries. The combination of acid-forming bacteria (*streptococcus mutans*) on tooth surfaces and sugary foods can result in loss of tooth surface enamel and eventually the tooth itself. Table sugar (sucrose) poses a unique risk because bacteria are able to convert sucrose into plaque, the sticky film that allows the organisms to adhere to the tooth enamel.

HOW TO AVOID TOO MUCH SUGAR

- Use less of all sugars and foods containing large amounts of sugars, including white sugar, brown sugar, raw sugar, honey, and syrups. Examples include soft drinks, candies, cakes, and cookies.
- Remember, how often you eat sugar and sugar-containing foods is as important to the health of your teeth as how much sugar you eat. It will help to avoid eating sweets between meals.
- Read food labels for clues on sugar content. If the name sugar, sucrose, glucose, maltose, dextrose, lactose, fructose, or syrups appears first, then there is a large amount of sugar.
- Select fresh fruits or fruits processed without syrup or with light, rather than heavy syrup.

USDA/USDHHS, 1985.

Dietary concerns for special groups. Persons with diabetes are counseled that *modest* amounts of simple sugars may be acceptable for most, but this is contingent on maintaining metabolic control and body weight (ADA, 1987). Diet counseling is required to match the unique needs of each person with his or her meal patterns, activity level, health status, and life-style.

Recommendation 8: Calcium

Adolescent girls and adult women should increase consumption of foods high in calcium, including low-fat dairy products (*Surgeon General*, 1988).

Although the direct relationship between dietary calcium and the development of osteoporosis remains questionable, the National Research Council (1989) suggests that higher intakes (1200 mg/day) through the age of 24 years will promote the development of a greater bone mass, reducing the impact of losses associated with aging.

How to increase calcium intake. The diet of a person who eats a variety of foods contains many sources of calcium, such as in dairy foods, green leafy vegetables, legumes, whole grains, canned fish, and eggs. Many low-fat dairy products that do not dramatically increase calories are rich sources of calcium. In addition to food sources, many antacid tablets contribute to the total intake of calcium. The consumption of calcium supplements above the recommended daily allowance (RDA) is not advocated inasmuch as high calcium supplement intakes can increase the risk for constipation and inhibit absorption of iron, zinc, and other needed minerals (National Research Council, 1989).

Dietary concerns for special groups. Calcium intakes of 1200 mg/day are recommended for pregnant and lactating women (NCR, 1989). Persons at greatest risk for bone loss are women who work in sedentary jobs and do not exercise.

Recommendation 9: Iron

Children, adolescents, and women of childbearing age should be sure to consume foods that are good sources of iron, such as lean red meats, fish, certain beans, and iron-enriched cereals and whole grain products. This issue is of special concern for low-income families (*Surgeon General*, 1988).

The typical diet in the United States is one of excess rather than deficiency. The intake of the essential mineral iron is an important exception. In the first health and nutrition survey (U.S. Public Health Services, 1974), iron was found to be the most common below-standard nutrient consumed by children (ages 1 to 5 years), adolescents (12 to 17 years), and women (18 to 44 years). In addition, low income was identified as a risk factor for low iron intake.

The second nationwide food consumption survey findings also identified low income as a concern (USDA, 1987). Average daily intakes of iron by women of low income (19 to 50 years) were only 57% of the RDA. Low iron is responsible for the most common type of anemia (microcytic anemia). Reduced iron status also is associated with depressed immune function, fatigue, and impaired wound healing (Hallberg, 1982).

How to select iron-rich food sources. To obtain and absorb needed levels requires planning. Iron-rich foods commonly consumed include liver, beans, beef, pork, poultry, lentils, soy beans, dried peaches, prune juice, raisins, spinach, asparagus, green peas, turnip greens, and enriched cereals.

Dietary concerns for special groups. Persons at greatest risk for iron overload include adult men and postmenopausal women. The body has an extremely limited ability to get rid of excess iron, and high iron levels are known to be toxic. For this reason, iron supplements are *not* recommended for these two groups.

Vegetarians who refrain from consuming meat, poultry, and fish will not obtain one of the most easily absorbed forms of iron, which is found in meat (heme iron). Careful selection of plant foods rich in iron and vitamin C will provide for the needs of this group.

Rapid growth during the first year of life places infants at risk for iron deficiency. It is estimated that full-term infants are born with sufficient iron stores for approximately 6 months. Iron-enriched cereals (plus other foods) supply needed iron after the infant reaches 6 months of age (Alpers, Clouse, & Stenson, 1983).

Iron needs increase dramatically during pregnancy. Absorption rates also increase with need; however, most diets typically cannot meet these increased needs. Oral supplements commonly are given to pregnant women (Alpers, Clouse, & Stenson, 1983).

NUTRITIONAL NEEDS THROUGH THE LIFE SPAN
Pregnancy

The increased nutritional needs during pregnancy result from fetal growth and the requirements of supportive maternal tissues. Nutritional needs reflect the rate of growth during various stages of pregnancy. Only a minimal increase in energy is needed during the first trimester. The higher rate of growth during the second and third trimesters is supported by a 15% increase in calories. The typical Western diet can adequately supply most nutrient needs during pregnancy, for example, the increased need for protein (30%). Women whose caloric intake is insufficient may be at risk because protein will be used to supply needed energy, which reduces the amount of protein available for the growth of fetal and maternal tissues.

Weight gain and energy needs. A 15% increase in basal energy requirements (approximately 300 calories) is needed during the second and third trimesters of pregnancy. This increase reflects the changes in growth rate and the metabolic demands of pregnancy. Both excessive and inadequate weight gains during pregnancy are associated with risks to the mother and fetus. Total weight gain for adult mothers normally is between 2 to 4 pounds for the first trimester, with an average increase of approximately 1 pound per week during the remaining pregnancy. If the mother is neither underweight nor overweight, a recommended gain of 25 to 30 pounds is common (Aflin-Slater, Aftergood, & Ashley, 1986). The pattern of weight gain appears to be of more importance than the exact amount. A typical pattern results in a slight increase during the first trimester, the most rapid growth during the second, and a slower but steady increase during the last trimester.

The selection of an adequate diet is made difficult because the nutrient needs rise at a much greater rate then energy needs. Thus it may be difficult to acquire the additionally needed nutrients without caloric overconsumption. Clients should be counseled to select nutrient-dense foods rather than simply to increase their normal intake. Most increased nutrient needs can be supplied within the average diet, with the possible exception of a few key ones. The review of a patient's dietary history should focus on those nutrients at risk; including iron, folic acid, and calcium.

Iron. The increased requirement for iron reflects the 20% to 30% growth in the maternal blood supply. Iron is required in the formation of the fetal red blood cells, iron stores, and muscles (Alpers, Clouse, & Stenson, 1983). As with most nutrients, absorption rates for iron will increase with need. Iron poses a unique risk because the typical Western diet, even a carefully planned one, will not supply the recommended levels during pregnancy. Women with initially low levels are at added risk. Low-iron status can result from poor intake or absorption, a recent pregnancy, a history of heavy menstrual flow, or another type of blood loss. The National Research Council (1989) found that the typical American diet cannot supply the increased requirements for iron and suggests the use of an iron supplement (30 to 60 mg) during pregnancy, and for 2 to 3 months afterward.

Supplements are of value only if they are taken. Problems with noncompliance can arise because of gastrointestinal side effects. These side effects and suggestions for preventing them should be discussed in advanced with clients. Commonly reported problems associated with iron supplements include heartburn, nausea, diarrhea, and constipation. Taking the iron supplement after a meal may help prevent these problems. The increased intake of fiber-rich foods is an effective method for reducing constipation. Clients should be made aware that antacids commonly used to treat heartburn can reduce stomach acidity and hinder the absorption of iron.

Folic acid.   The increased need for folic acid (over 100% increase) reflects its use in growth (DNA synthesis) and in the formation of red blood cells. Megaloblastic anemia resulting from severe folic acid deficiency is uncommon in the United States; however, depleted folic acid stores have been found in 25% to 30% of groups sampled (Alpers, Clouse, & Stenson, 1983; Butterworth & Tamura, 1989). There is no consensus on the recommendation of folic acid supplements during pregnancy. Modest amounts of folic acid (0.5 to 1.0 mg/day) appear to provide a "safety factor" for persons with potentially low levels while offering almost no risk (Alpers, Clouse, & Stenson, 1983).

Folic acid is easily available in foods such as green leafy vegetables, broccoli, and peanuts. Therefore most mothers can meet their increased needs if cautioned about overcooking foods, because folic acid can be easily destroyed during cooking or canning.

Calcium.   Formation of the fetal skeleton and tissues requires approximately 30 g of calcium. Although fetal bones do not begin to calcify early in the pregnancy, maternal calcium supplies should be supported by an intake of 1200 mg throughout pregnancy and lactation (National Research Council, 1989). Many women may not be able to consume significant amounts of milk or milk products because of an inability to digest lactose (milk sugar).

This lactose intolerance results in gastrointestinal distress, diarrhea, and flatulence. Low-lactose milk products are available, for example, cultured yogurt, hard cheeses (e.g., cheddar, swiss, and blue), buttermilk, and fresh milk. Lactaid, an enzyme product which can be added to fresh milk, is available from most pharmacies and "digests" the milk sugar. An increased consumption of whole milk and cheese may add unneeded fat calories, a potential problem for obese women. Low-fat milk, however, offers an important source of calcium without the extra calories.

Early prenatal care should include screening for nutritional risks. This includes a review of problems associated with past pregnancies (e.g., pregnancy-induced hypertension [PIH], low-birth-weight infant, and anemia), the client's current weight and weight history, and a brief dietary history that focuses on foods supplying key nutrients, alcohol use, and prescribed or over-the-counter medications. Table 24-2 offers an overview of nutritional risks and the screening methods used to assess them.

Maternal prepregnancy weight and weight gain during pregnancy have been shown to identify women at risk. The incidence of low birth weight (LBW) infants has been associated with both low prepregnancy weight and low maternal weight gain. Very young mothers pose a special concern for LBW infants because of the combined demands of adolescent growth and fetal development (*Surgeon General*, 1988).

Prepregnancy obesity and excessive weight gain have been linked with pregnancy-induced hypertension, gestational diabetes, and increased surgical risk. The risk factors

TABLE 24-2 Screening for nutritional risks during pregnancy	
Nutritional risk	**Screening method**
1. Prepregnancy underweight/overweight status (<85% or >120% IBW)	Weight for height tables
2. Inadequate (<2 lb/mo second and third trimester) or excessive (>2 lb/wk) rate of weight gain	Plot and compare weight gain to recommendations
3. Anemia	Hemoglobin/hematocrit below standard
4. History of gestational diabetes	Tests for ketones, glucose urea, protein urea
5. Multiple pregnancies within previous 2 yr	Client history
6. Prior oral contraceptive use	Client history
7. Poor diet resulting from extreme nutrient intake (high/low), excessive alcohol use, or lactose intolerance	Client history, food frequency, questionnaire
8. Strict vegetarian (potential deficiency for B_{12}, riboflavin)	History

Data from Alpers, et al., 1983; Little Brown & Co., 1984.
IBW, Ideal body weight.

associated with obesity are reduced if total weight gain is limited to no more than 24 pounds (*Surgeon General*, 1988). Women who are overweight before pregnancy should be cautioned against attempting to lose weight during pregnancy. Severe restriction of calories during pregnancy will reduce protein absorption and utilization. Reducing total intake increases the risk of not obtaining needed nutrients; severe caloric and carbohydrate restriction can result in ketosis. In addition, maternal ketonemia (resulting from starvation or diabetes) is a significant risk to fetal development.

The federal government has recognized the implications of improved nutrition during fetal development and its impact on maternal child health. This need has resulted in the creation of the Special Supplemental Food Program for Women, Infants, and Children (WIC). Studies (Edozien, Switzer, & Bryan, 1976) indicate that before participation in the WIC program, dietary intakes of "at risk" pregnant women were below the RDA for energy, calcium, iron, vitamin A, thiamin, riboflavin, and niacin.

Infancy and Toddler Period

The nutritional needs of infants are based on the developmental level of their gastrointestinal and neuromuscular systems, their high growth rates, limited reserves, and immature kidneys. The infant's high growth rate and metabolism relative to its limited nutritional reserves offers little room for error. The typical healthy infant will double in weight between birth and 4 months and will increase in length by 50% during the first year. This means that the comparison of individual growth rates with standardized charts can offer a sensitive screening tool to identify infants with potential nutritional problems.

An infant's diet can be divided into three distinct stages: nursing, transitional, and modified adult (American Academy of Pediatrics [AAP, 1985]). Fig. 24-1 describes these stages in the infant's diet over time. Both the high nutrient needs relative to body weight and the immature digestive and excretory systems place demands on the adequacy and digestibility of infant foods. These foods need to reflect the nutrient needs and the developmental level of the infant. Therefore, as infants and children develop, their diets must change.

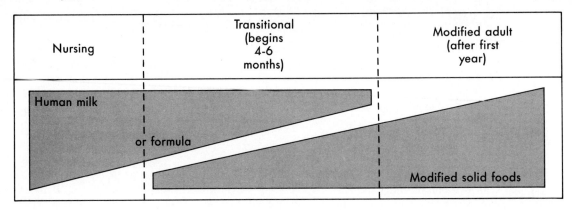

FIG. 24-1 Stages in infant diets.

Nursing. During the first 4 to 6 months of life, human milk or formula supplies all the nutrients the infant requires. The infant's ability to feed is limited to sucking and swallowing liquids because of the newborn's undeveloped neuromuscular system, which is incapable of chewing or swallowing solid foods. During the early months of life the child is unable to perform the complex tongue movements required to eat solid foods. Before 4 months of age the child's immature kidneys are less able to concentrate solutes; thus they are unable to handle an increased load of greater amounts of dietary protein or electrolytes (Alpers, Clouse, & Stenson, 1983).

Breast-feeding. The promotion of breast-feeding as the preferred method of infant feeding is widely supported (American Dietetic Association, 1987). This is reflected in the increase in breast-feeding from a low of 25% in 1971 to 60% in 1984 (American Dietetic Association, 1987). Successful breast-feeding requires a mother to obtain support and instruction both before and after the birth of her child. Most mothers have selected a method of infant feeding before the third trimester (Sarett, Bain, & O'Leary, 1983). Therefore the critical time for nursing intervention in the decision to breast-feed typically occurs before birth. The box summarizes the advantages and disadvantages of breast-feeding.

The community health nurse should recognize that although breast-feeding is a growing trend, many women lack the knowledge and support that are critical for success. Although it is a natural process, successful breast-feeding demands the mother's understanding of infant nutritional needs, feeding techniques, common problems, and their solutions. WIC, which advocates breast-feeding, can serve as an important resource for teaching materials on infant feeding (breast or bottle) and the introduction of solid foods. At no time should a mother feel she has failed if she cannot, or chooses not to, breast-feed her child. Contraindications for breast-feeding include (1) transfer of medications taken by the mother, (2) genetic inborn errors of metabolism (e.g., phenylketonuria and maple sugar urine disease), and (3) preterm (LBW) infants who require special supplements or formulas (American Dietetic Association, 1986).

Formula feeding. Commercial formulas offer an alternative to women who cannot or choose not to nurse their infants. They are prepared to approximate the nutritional content of human milk. Most are produced by diluting cow's milk with water and then adding a carbohydrate source such as sucrose or lactose. The butterfat is replaced with vegetable oil, and important vitamins and minerals are added. Although all commercial

ADVANTAGES AND DISADVANTAGES OF BREAST-FEEDING

Advantages to infant

- Offers ideal nourishment; easily digested
- Reduced allergic reactions
- Lower protein and electrolyte load, resulting in a reduced obligatory water loss
- Easily absorbed protein-bound iron
- Protection from immunoglobulin A against viruses and bacteria

Advantage to mother

- Increased energy needs, typically resulting in weight loss
- Increased uterine involution
- Amenorrhea
- Supports maternal-infant bonding

- Convenience
- Low cost

Disadvantages to infant

- Transfer of medications taken by mother
- Inborn errors of metabolism (e.g., phenylketonuria, maple sugar urine disease)
- Possible requirement of special supplements or formulas for preterm (LBW) infants
- Contains low levels of flouride

Disadvantages to mother

- Time constraints with feeding schedules
- Energy drain and fatigue

Developed from the Position of the American Dietetic Association: Promotions of breat-feeding, 1986.

formulas contain iron, some contain more than others, and no clear consensus has been reached concerning its necessity or the possibility of the additional iron increasing the chance for gastrointestinal problems.

A variety of different formulas are available for infants with special needs. Infants who are sensitive to cow's protein or who have lactose intolerance can benefit from lactose-free formulas made with soybean protein. Special formulas that contain a higher proportion of easy-to-digest whey protein and medium-chain triglycerides are available for premature infants. Other formulas have been developed for malabsorption problems and for infants with inborn errors of metabolism.

Transitional stage: introduction of solid foods. After 4 to 6 months of age the child has developed the ability to swallow dilute cereals and pureed foods. In addition, there is an increased ability to digest complex carbohydrates, fats, and protein. Also, the maturing kidneys are better able to handle the higher osmotic loads resulting from the changing diet. Infant cereals are an excellent introduction to solid foods because they can be thinned with formula and are a good source of iron. Commercial baby food is convenient and safe; however, the cost may limit its use. An inexpensive alternative to commercial baby food can be prepared by grinding or straining adult foods.

New foods should be introduced in single ingredient servings, *not* as combination foods such as mixed cereals or stew. Each new food should be given for several days before another food is introduced. This allows for easy indentification of specific food tolerances.

Although these guidelines generally are accepted by health professionals, there is no uniformly accepted opinion among parents on how and when solid foods should be introduced in an infant's diet. The nurse must provide support with the understanding that the views and practices of the individual, family, and physician may vary greatly. Nursing instruction and support must account for the client's needs and opinions while increasing the parents' understanding of the child's unique nutritional needs and how the dietary changes mirror the development of the infant.

Modified adult (toddler period). After 1 year of age only minimal changes from the adult diet are needed. Parents should be encouraged to provide a variety of foods; however, soft foods should be served until the child is able to chew. Parents should be cautioned to serve table food in small pieces to reduce the risk of choking. Hard foods such as raw carrots, frankfurters, peanuts, grapes, and round candies should be avoided (AAP, 1985).

Preschool Period, School-Age Period, and Adolescence

The preschool period is a time when the appetite wanes. The child may go for months without gaining an ounce and be very picky about food. During this period, if the child is getting essential nutrients, it is best to avoid fostering poor eating habits by overanxious bribing or by forcing the child to eat.

The elementary school–aged child should be checked periodically for normal growth and development. Annual height and weight measurements by the school nurse can monitor this progression. During growth spurts nutritional needs may increase, but they can be supplied by a balanced diet. The school-aged child can consume most adult foods. A child's diet should offer variety, support adequate growth and development, maintain ideal body weight, and avoid extremes.

During adolescence the maintenance of proper nutrition is especially challenging. This is an age of rapid growth but also a time when there is a need for independence and autonomy. Convincing adolescents that good nutrition will improve their appearance and raise their energy level may be the only way to enlist their cooperation. For many adolescents the calories provided from snacks is a significant part of the total daily diet. A recognition that snacking behavior can be healthy if the right snacks are provided may help them to maintain a balanced diet.

Assessment of Nutritional Status

Children and adolescents. The community health nurse must be able to screen these young clients and identify those at risk for nutritional problems. Screening tools for the community should be simple and inexpensive and provide easy-to-apply measures that reflect long-term nutritional status (Table 24-3). No single method alone provides a comprehensive measure of a client's status. When available, the combined use of several methods will improve the accuracy of the screening. Examples of nutrition-related problems that can be identified include anemia, obesity, and failure to thrive.

Anthropometrical measures. When height, weight, and age are accurately measured and plotted on standardized growth charts, they offer a sensitive measure of abnormal growth patterns that can indicate nutritional status and hormone function in children (Shils & Young, 1988). Growth rate alone cannot detect disease or good health. The growth charts developed by the National Center for Health Statistics (NCHS) are easy to use and well accepted. Several measurements over time will indicate growth rate. Constant linear growth offers the most important single indicator of a well-nourished child. Shils and Young (1988) suggest that children who fall below the tenth percentile for either weight for age or height (length) for age should have a detailed evaluation. Comparison of a child's height (length) for age, weight for height, and weight for age can offer important clues about a child's nutritional status (Table 24-4).

The NCHS growth charts were developed and standardized on the basis of infants who were typically bottle fed and for whom early introduction to solid foods was common. Healthy, breast-fed infants tend to be leaner and gain weight at a slower rate. Therefore the nurse may see more breast-fed infants at the lower percentiles. This does not indicate any nutritional limitations in breast milk but may be the result of overfeeding the bottle-

TABLE 24-3 Assessment of nutritional status

Measure	Tool used	Results
Anthropometric		
Height/weight for age	Balance beam scale	Serial measures identify normal vs. abnormal growth rates
Head circumference for age	Tape measurement of largest occipital-frontal circumference	Identify undernutrition, disease (e.g., hydrocephalus)
Skin-fold thickness and mid-arm circumference	Lange or Harpenden caliper and tape measure	Percent body fat and muscle mass*
Clinical		
Diet history	Review of eating habits, intake	Identify balanced diet, calorie intake
Physical examination	Visual inspection	Identify obesity/undernutrition, nutritional deficiencies affecting skin, hair, lips, tongue
Laboratory assessment		
Hematocrit or hemoglobin	Blood test	Screen for anemia (iron, folate, B_{12} deficiency)
Total protein/albumin (or retinol-binding protein)	Blood test	Screens for protein status

Adapted from *Pediatric nutrition handbook (2nd ed.)* by the American Academy of Pediatrics, Committee on Nutrition, 1985, Elk Grove Village, IL: Author. Copyright 1985 by the AAP. Modified by permission.
*Most helpful with overnutrition or undernutrition.

TABLE 24-4 Stature, weight, and age as indications of nutritional status

Comparison	Potential interpretation
1. Steady linear growth and weight gain within expected rate	Good long-term nutritional status
2. Very low weight for height	Recent weight loss or slowed weight gain
3. Weight and height low for age	Long-term malnutrition; reflects parents' stature or growth hormone deficiency
4. Excessive weight for height	Obese child (resulting from behavioral, genetic, or systemic disease)

From *Pediatric nutrition in clinical practice* by W.E. Maclean & G.G. Grahm, (1982.) Mendo Park, CA: Addison-Wesley.

fed child (Maclean & Grahm, 1982). Growth charts also are questionable as predictions of protein-calorie malnutrition for LBW infants (< 2.500 kg) (Cooper, Floyd, Ziegler, Kashy, Shinobu, & Heird, 1981).

Clinical appraisal. A review of feeding practices and a physical examination can offer important clues to nutritional status. Visual inspection is useful in identifying obesity and undernutrition. The nurse can use a review of the typical diet of the child to screen for adequate intake and variety in the diet.

With infants and toddlers, questions should focus on feeding schedules, formula preparation, and volume. With the preschool and school-aged child, questions need to target concerns of adequate food sources for vitamins, iron, calcium, protein, and fiber, as well as for other essential nutrients. Emphasis should be placed on developing variety in the diet. The nurse should not expect to produce records that are detailed or accurate enough to identify the dietary content of specific nutrients (e.g., calories and fiber).

Laboratory assessment. Most laboratory tests do not meet the criteria for simplicity, cost, or availability within the community setting. Typically, laboratory measures are used to identify problems of undernutrition such as anemia or protein-calorie malnutrition. The most common mineral deficiency in children is iron deficiency. Both hematocrit and hemoglobin levels can be used to screen for anemia; however, these tests are not specific for malnutrition because not all anemias are the result of poor intake or absorption of iron.

Serum total protein and albumin levels can serve as important assessment tools for underweight children. In evaluating these data, the nurse should recognize that serum protein levels depend on the available supply of both dietary calories and protein.

Early and middle adulthood. A balanced diet and a variety of foods should be encouraged for the adults in today's fast-paced society. Busy lives, fast foods, and stress can place this population at high risk for disease and disability. Health education and promotion activities that emphasize the dietary recommendations of the *Surgeon General's Report on Nutrition and Health* will teach this group how to raise its level of wellness.

Nutritional Concerns of Aging

Nutrition is an important component in maintaining the health, independence, and quality of life of elderly persons (American Dietetic Association, 1987). The community nurse's role includes assessment of individual needs and capabilities and referral to community services when appropriate. These tasks require the nurse to understand the variety of factors that affect the diet, for example, the client's needs as well as physical, social, and economic limitations. The nurse must be able to assess an individual's general nutritional status within a limited data base, and be able to offer practical suggestions that can improve the client's diet.

The elderly represent a heterogeneous group of individuals who have a wide range of health and functional capabilities, social backgrounds, and economic status. Because each individual ages uniquely, persons who are the same chronological age can have significantly different functional abilities and health (Shils & Young, 1988). The nurse should understand the range of changes that are part of the normal aging process and the additional impact of disease (see Chapter 12). This knowledge serves as a basis to judge individual nutritional status and associated health risks.

Physical concerns. Physical concerns encompass both normal aging and chronic disease. Clients need to understand how diet can support medical treatment, which changes are part of the normal aging process, and which symptoms are a result of illness. Physical concerns that affect an individual's nutritional status and health include physical weakness, reduced range of motion, chewing and swallowing problems, loss of sensations, reduced digestive capacity, excretion problems, and food and drug interactions.

Physical changes. Joint stiffness combined with a reduction in muscle mass, motor skills, and vision can limit a person's ability to shop for, transport, prepare, and consume food. The fear of spills in lifting heavy pots and the inability to grasp lids, knives, or stove controls can limit the variety of foods the older adult is able to prepare or enjoy. The nurse can assess limitations of the client's kitchen facilities and recommend modifications. Built-up handles can compensate for a weak grasp, and instruction on how to circumvent limits of strength or mobility can be helpful. Many elderly persons can benefit from enlarged temperature scales on stove dials and from large-print recipes. A review of favorite recipes may lead to arranging for visiting homemaker aides to help with difficult meals by preparing and storing foods in advance.

Chewing and swallowing problems. Teeth that are lost and not replaced or that are replaced with poorly fitting dentures can dramatically reduce the variety and texture of foods the client can consume, for example, the avoidance of raw fruits, vegetables, and meats because of difficulty in chewing. This problem can result in a loss of vitamins, fibers, and other nutrients.

The reduced production of saliva is a normal result of aging and can be further affected by some drugs (e.g., oxybutynin [Ditropan] for incontinence, Donnatal for spastic colon, and diphenoxylate with atropine [Lomotil] for diarrhea). The use of soups, stews, and gravies that are low in fat and salt can help solve the problems of eating when the mouth is dry.

Reduced sensation. The reduction of the sense of smell and taste appears to be a normal part of aging (Cunningham & Brookbank, 1988). This means that foods with stronger flavors (e.g., sweeter and more sour) are preferred. The loss of the sensual pleasure of eating, combined with feelings of isolation and loneliness, can reduce the variety and total intake of food.

Reduced digestive capacity. Age-related reduction of secretions (e.g. hydrochloric acid) by the stomach may reduce the absorption of calcium (American Dietetic Association, 1987). Age-related reduction of digestive enzyme production such as pepsin and lactase can result in malabsorption of proteins and lactose, respectively. Lactose intolerance—the inability to digest large amounts of milk sugar—increases with age. Important sources of calcium, protein, and other nutrients are lost if persons with lactose intolerance are not taught how to include low-lactose milk products in their diet (e. g., aged cheese, yogurt, and Lactaid-treated milk). A decreased ability to digest and absorb fat also can limit food choices. The combination of reduced digestive capacity and a decline in energy needs with a lower metabolic rate (American Dietetic Association, 1987) requires elderly individuals to obtain more nutrients from less food (total calories) or risk obesity.

Excretion problems. Although decreased intestinal motility occurs with aging, the complaint of constipation never should be considered a normal result of aging. Clients should be asked about their use of over-the-counter (OTC) laxatives and their "normal" bowel habits. Factors that can affect chronic constipation include weak intestine muscles, dehydration, low fiber, little exercise, and laxative abuse (Albanese, 1980).

Incontinence, along with a diminished sense of thirst, can be hazardous. Dehydration is one of the most common causes of fluid and electrolyte imbalances in the elderly (Phillips, Phil, Rolls, Ledingham, Forsling, Morton, et al., 1984). This is a concern because the aging kidney has a reduced capacity to concentrate urine (i.e., conserve water). Incontinence may cause an individual to limit intake to avoid embarrassment or inconvenience. The resultant poor hydration and lack of activity also increase the risk of constipation.

Food and drug interactions. Elderly persons are major consumers of drugs, and individuals within this group exhibit a wide range of response to drugs. Side effects from prescription or over-the-counter drugs can alter the intake, absorption, and use of important nutrients (American Dietetic Association, 1987). Effects can include loss of appetite, altered sense of taste and smell, malabsorption, stomach irritation, and nausea. The nurse, physician, pharmacist, and dietitian should review all medications for food and drug interactions on an annual basis.

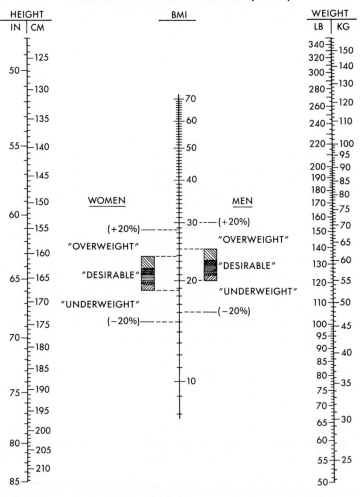

FIG. 24-2 Nomograph for body mass index (kg/m²). *(From "A nomograph method for assessing body weight," by A.E. Thomas, D.A. McKay, and M.B. Cutlap, 1976,* American Journal of Clinical Nutrition, *29, p. 303. Copyright 1976 by American Journal of Clinical Nutrition. Reprinted by permission.)*

Psychosocial concerns. Isolation and depression can affect the client's dietary variety and intake of food (Albanese, 1980). Adjustment to required changes in housing, occupation, and status can place severe stress on individuals, which can result in effects that range from anorexia to overeating. Loss of a mate, friends, or family, forced dependence on others, and financial concerns can alter appetite and affect diet. The enjoyment of food is as much a result of the social setting as the appearance and flavor of the food. The importance of eating as a shared group activity should not be forgotten. For many the social contact provided within group dining, such as congregate meal programs, is the critical element in the development of a healthy appetite.

Food should be recognized as a medium of socialization as well as a biological necessity. The association of food with family, friends, and ethnic identity must be understood in assessing the diet that a client consumes in isolation or one in which favorite foods have been restricted as part of medical treatment.

Economic concerns. Poverty is a common problem for elderly persons. For individuals 85 years and older in the United States, 45% are near or below the poverty level (U.S Senate Special Committee on Aging, 1986). Low income can affect the ability to shop for food (transportation) and limit the availability of adequate refrigeration and food storage facilities. Limited funds to purchase food can reduce variety in the meals and jeopardize nutrition. Thus food stamps can offer an important addition to the available food budget, although the elderly poor do not typically make use of this opportunity.

Nutritional assessment. The tools used to assess the nutritional status of the elderly in the community must be practical and easily obtained, and they should focus on common nutritional risk factors. Easily available measures to assess nutritional risks include weight changes, body mass index, and dietary history. Reichel (1983) believes that accurate body weight offers the single most useful index of an individual's nutritional status. Monthly weight records with the use of an accurate scale can document an individual's progress or risk. It must be understood that weight gains can be the result of many factors: improved appetite and diet, decreased activity, edema, or cheating on a reduction diet. Losses may result from reduced intake because of illness, nausea (possible result of drug side effects), depression, or financial problems. Weight does not measure body composition. A scale cannot be used to determine if weight changes are a result of the gradual loss of lean body mass or the increase of fat tissue that typically occurs with aging (Mohs & Watson, 1986).

Losses in lean body mass, reduction of fat from subcutaneous stores, and the increase of fat around internal organs mean that total body weights and triceps skin-fold measurements are less accurate measures of body fat in elderly persons. The BMI (body mass

---

TABLE 24-5 Evaluating the significance of weight loss

Time interval	Significant weight loss (%)*	Severe weight loss (%)*
1 wk	1.0-2.0	>2.0
1 mo	5.0	>5.0
3 mo	7.5	>7.5
6 mo	10.0	>10.0

From the *Handbook of clinical dietetics* by the American Dietetic Association, 1981, New Haven, CT: Yale University Press. Copyright 1981. Reprinted by permission.

*Percent weight change $= \dfrac{\text{(Usual weight − Actual weight)}}{\text{Usual weight}} \times 100$

index) is one formula that appears to accurately indicate body fat over the life span despite changes in fat distribution and lean body mass (Thomas, McKay, & Cutlap, 1976; Yearick, 1978). It accurately identifies elderly individuals who are overweight or underweight (see Fig. 24-2).

Comparison of the client's weight over time circumvents the problems of individual differences within this diverse population. Significant weight change can be judged as the relationship of weight changes and the usual weight (Table 24-5).

Significant or severe weight loss or gain serves as a signal for a more detailed review of nutritional status (e. g., hemoglobin, hematocrit, and serum albumin levels and diet records).

Diet assessment. Evaluation of a client's ability to plan, shop, prepare, and consume an adequate diet goes beyond a simple recording of a single day's consumption (24-hour recall). Physical, social, and economic factors all must be considered in general assessment of diet. The nurse should consider the following factors:

1. Restrictions in the purchase and preparation of foods (cost, transport, physical capacity, kitchen facilities)
2. Restrictions in food choice because of health (both physician and self-prescribed)
3. Limitations in cooking and food storage
4. Percentage of meals eaten alone
5. Economic status
6. Medications (possible food and drug interactions)
7. Limitations of chewing or swallowing
8. Use of alcohol

Significant weight loss or gain, and diagnosis of diabetes or other nutritionally related disease warrant more detailed diet records and anthropometrical and biochemical data. Consulting dietitians are available within private practice to offer detailed nutritional assessment. Many can offer the use of computer analysis of intake to support dietary intervention.

USE OF THE NURSING PROCESS TO IMPROVE NUTRITIONAL STATUS AND PROMOTE HEALTH

The following case study illustrates how the community health nurse can use the nursing process to improve the health of an elderly client in the community.

Assessment

Mr. Johnston is a 70-year-old white man who recently was discharged from the hospital after being admitted for complaints of prolonged coughing and hoarseness. The client was diagnosed with chronic obstructive pulmonary disease (COPD). He has smoked for more than 50 years. He is a retired laborer, living with his wife. The client enjoys gardening and walking but has limited these activities over the past year because of arthritis. Mr. Johnson has NIDDM, which was diagnosed approximately 15 years ago. He has taken oral hypoglycemics in the past but currently is not using them because of months of negative results in urine sugar tests with Diastix Reagent Strips. The client stated that he has not had any problems with controlling his diabetes; that his negative urine tests were "proof." He indicated that the only problem he has had from diabetes was a small loss of the vision in his left eye. Mr. Johnston noted that he had gained "some weight" over the past year (approximately 18 pounds) but stated that "I have always been a little stocky." The client's current weight is 235 pounds (height, 5 feet 10 inches).

Mr. Johnston has been under treatment for hypertension for the past 5 years, which has been controlled with medication (blood pressure, 157/78). During hospitalization his prescription for chlorthalidone (Hygroton), 50 mg/day, was replaced with triamterene 50 mg/hydrochlorothiazide 25 mg (Dyazide)/day. Other medications included clemastine fumarate (Tavist) three times a day as needed and aspirin for arthritis (up to three tablets (325 mg) every 6 hours.

On his admission Mr. Johnston's blood work-up included the following abnormal results:

	Test result	Normal level
Serum triglycerides	355 mg/dl (high)	40-150 mg/dl
Serum potassium	2.8 mEq/L (low)	3.5-5.5 mEq/L
Serum chloride	92 mEq/L (low)	97-170 mEq/L

The client's blood glucose levels (fasting blood sugar) in milligrams per deciliter were as follows: day 1, 268; day 2, 249; day 3, 238; and day 4, 246. (Normal levels of random blood sugar are 60 to 100 mg/dl.)

Major problems at discharge were (1) chronic obstructive pulmonary disease (COPD), (2) poorly controlled NIDDM, and (3) obesity.

Mr. Johnston's nutritional problems stem from his inability to keep his diabetes under control. He was unable to recognize the severity of his diabetes and failed to stay on his medication regimen and diet. He needs to understand the long-term impact of high blood glucose levels and the limitations of his method of testing for sugar in the urine. A number of factors could be responsible for the consistent false-negative results (e. g., high kidney threshold, impaired vision, ketones, high aspirin use, and out-of-date Diastix).

Mr. Johnston's noncompliance with his diet required assessment of his understanding of (1) the disease process, (2) the relationship between his actions and glucose control, and (3) how these actions affect complication (e. g., vision loss). The client's inability to accurately monitor his glucose levels and diet limited his ability to take responsibility for his treatment. The symptoms of chronic obstructive pulmonary disease contrast directly with those of diabetes and hypertension. For example, breathing difficulties offer immediate limits to daily activities, whereas blood sugar and blood pressure levels are not perceptible.

Mr. Johnston did not appear to view his obesity as a problem. Assessment of his (and his family's) ability and his perceived (and actual) needs will play a pivotal role in treatment. Follow-up visits by a community health nurse for teaching and counseling were scheduled.

Nursing Diagnosis

After an in-depth assessment the following nursing diagnoses were formulated:

1. Knowledge deficit concerning control of diabetes
2. Noncompliance related to knowledge deficit
3. Alteration in nutrition, more than body requirements
4. Potential for vision loss related to uncontrolled diabetes

Planning

1. Instruct client in how to measure glucose levels and test urine for glucose.
2. Counsel the family on the effects of glucose and lipid levels on the body.

RESEARCH HIGHLIGHT

Problem: How can a community health educator effectively provide nutrition information to an elderly population?

Elderly individuals may be placed at nutritional risk as a result of limits in their income, immobility, isolation, and nutritional knowledge. These concerns are compounded if their diet is further restricted for medical reasons. How can a community health nurse circumvent the typical communication barriers and "reach out" to an elderly audience with nutrition information? This highlight describes a format, developed from research, that offers the public health nurse a four-part method for community outreach.

1. *Survey needs:* Elderly audiences reported being interested in learning about nutrition and new methods of food preparation. Respondents felt the lack of transportation, their busy schedules, and cost were barriers to educational activities.

2. *Media selection:* A monthly newspaper distributed free to an elderly audience (pop. 38,000) was selected because it could overcome the barriers of time, transportation, and cost. The print medium was selected over broadcast because it allowed the learner to control the pace of delivery and scheduling of the needed nutrition information.

3. *Development and publication of materials:* The monthly articles consisted of (a) an article addressing a nutrition topic of concern to seniors, (b) easy-to-prepare recipes that allowed readers to apply knowledge gained from the article, and (c) an interview with an elderly peer who tested the recipes.

4. *Evaluation:* The articles were found to develop a substantial readership. Over 68% of those surveyed could recall reading one of the five articles and 25% stated changing dietary habits as a result.

The study demonstrated that a "senior" newspaper that offers nutrition information targeted to seniors can establish a substantial readership and influence reported dietary behaviors. Print media in the form of community newspapers, newsletters, and corporate publications to retired employees could offer effective and inexpensive means to reach an elderly audience.

From "The Response of an Elderly Audience To Nutrition Education Articles in a Newspaper for Seniors" by E.H. Weiss and C.H. Davis, 1985, *Journal of Nutrition Education, 17* (5) pp. 197-202. Copyright 1985 by the *Journal of Nutrition Education.* Reprinted by permission.

3. Teach the family to plan and monitor food intake and, with the dietitian, develop realistic weight goals.
4. Teach the client the interaction between medication and his blood glucose levels.
5. Reduce nocompliance.
6. Counsel the family on the effect of uncontrolled diabetes on the client's vision.

Implementation

1. The client was instructed to monitor blood glucose, the presence of glucose in the urine, and the interaction between his medication and glucose levels. A referral was made to a dietitian to instruct the client in planning meals and monitoring food intake.
2. Teaching and counseling were continued until the client verbalized his understanding of his diabetes and methods of controlling it and noncompliance was reduced.

Evaluation

1. The client verbalized an understanding of the correct way to measure glucose levels and to test urine for glucose.
2. The family verbalized an understanding of the effects of glucose and lipids on the body, as well as the interaction of the client's medication and glucose levels.
3. Planned visits by a dietitian enabled the client and his wife to demonstrate the ability to plan appropriate meals and to monitor food intake.
4. The client verbalized an understanding of the negative effects uncontrolled diabetes would have on his health.
5. The client began losing weight (approximately 1 pound per week). Monthly weight checks and blood pressure checks showed a decrease in both his blood pressure and weight within a 4-month period. He was then given a maintenance diet.

SUMMARY

Nutrition is one of many factors that can affect health. In developed countries (e.g., the United States and Canada) diseases of dietary excess have replaced the problems of nutritional deficiencies. This change is reflected in the number of nutritional guidelines that offer dietary recommendations which reduce the risk of obesity and chronic disease. The general agreement on what is a healthy diet means that the community health nurse can reach a wide range of persons with a common message.

Nutritional needs reflect the client's individual rate of growth and development and the impact of aging and disease. The community health nurse should recognize these differences and identify those at risk through basic screening measures. The nurse also can act as an educator in the area of nutrition. This role can include school-based programs and client-centered activities.

Good nutrition *alone* cannot be expected to alter the course of disease or prevent most diseases; however, it can be an important factor in an individual's health.

CHAPTER HIGHLIGHTS

- Although nutrition alone cannot prevent or alter the course of most diseases, an individual's nutritional status can play a significant role in the treatment and prevention of some diseases.
- In the United States, diseases of dietary excess have replaced problems of nutritional deficiencies.
- There is a general agreement among dietary guidelines as to what constitutes a healthy diet. The surgeon general's recommendations address the areas of fat and cholesterol, weight control, complex carbohydrates and fiber, sodium, alcohol, fluoride, sugars, calcium, and iron.
- Nutritional needs change throughout life to reflect individual rates of growth and development, the impact of aging, and disease.
- The increased nutritional needs during pregnancy are a result of the growth of the fetus and supportive maternal tissue. In addition to increased energy needs, the pregnant woman requires increased amounts of iron, folic acid, and calcium.
- Infant nutrition progresses through the stages of nursing (breast-feeding or formula feeding), transitional stage, and modified adult stage.
- Nutritional concerns of aging include physical changes such as chewing and swallowing

problems, reduced sensation, reduced digestive capacity, excretion and elimination problems, food and drug interactions, psychosocial concerns, and economic concerns.
- The tools used to assess nutrition in the community should be practical, easily available, and focus on common nutritional risk factors.
- A wealth of nutrition resources are available to the community health nurse.

STUDY QUESTIONS

1. Describe the typical adult diet recommended in the *Surgeon General's Report on Nutrition and Health.*
2. Using the nomogram, calculate the body mass index of an adult who is 70 inches tall and weighs 180 pounds.
3. Describe the recommended weight gain during the first trimester of pregnancy and the overall weight gain recommended over 9 months.
4. Identify four nutritional concerns of aging.

REFERENCES

Albanese, A. A. (1980). *Nutrition for the elderly.* New York: Liss.

Alfin-Slater, R. B., Aftergood, L., & Ashley, J. (1986). *Nutrition and motherhood* (2nd ed.). Van Nuys, CA: PM, Inc.

Alpers, D. H., Clouse, R.E., & Stenson, W.F. (1983). *Manual of nutritional therapeutics.* Boston: Little, Brown & Co.

American Academy of Pediatrics, Committee on Nutrition. (1981). Nutrition and lactation. *Pediatrics,* (1986). *68,* 435-443.

American Academy of Pediatrics, Committee on Nutrition. (1985). *Pediatric nutrition handbook* (2nd ed. Elk Grove Village, IL: Author.

American Academy of Pediatrics. (1986). Prudent lifestyle for children: Dietary fat and cholesterol. *Pediatrics, 78,* 521-525.

American Cancer Society. (1984). *Nutrition, common sense and cancer* (Publication No. 2096-LE). New York: Author.

American Diabetes Association. (1987). Nutritional recommendations and principles for individuals with diabetes mellitus. *Diabetes Care,* 10, 126-132.

American Diabetes Association and American Dietetic Association. (1977). A *guide for professionals: The effective application of "exchange lists for meal planning."* Washington, DC/Chicago: Author.

American Dietetic Association. (1981). *Handbook of clinical dietetics.* New Haven, CT: Yale University Press.

American Dietetic Association. (1986). Position of the American Dietetic Association: Promotion of breast feeding. *Journal of the American Dietetic Association, 86,* 1580-1585.

American Dietetic Association. (1987). Position of the American Dietetic Association: Nutrition, aging, and the continuum of health care. *Journal of the American Diabetic Association, 87,* 344-347.

American Heart Association. (1988). Dietary guidelines for healthy American adults. *Circulation, 77,* 721A-724A.

Birch, L. L. (1980). Effects of peer model's food choices and eating behaviors on pre-schoolers food preferences. *Child Development, 51,* 489-496.

Brown, J. E. (1984). Nutrition services for pregnant women, infants, children, and adolescents. *Clinical Nutrition, 3,* 100-108.

Butterworth, C. E., & Tamura, T. (1989). Folic acid safety and toxicity: A brief review. *American Journal of Clinical Nutrition, 50,* 353-358.

Canadian Department of National Health and Welfare. (1982). *Canada's food guide: Handbook* (rev. ed.) Ottawa: Author.

Coates T. J., Jeffery, R. W., & Stinkard, L. A. (1981). Heart-healthy eating and exercise: Introducing and maintaining changes in health behaviors. *American Journal of Public Health, 71,* 15-23.

Coates, T. J., & Thoreson, C. E. (1978). Treating obesity in children and adolescents: A review: *American Journal of Public Health, 68,* 143-151.

Connell, D. B., Turner, R. R., & Mason, E. F. Summary of findings of the school health education evaluation: Health promotion effectiveness, implementation, and costs. *Journal of School Health, 55,* 316-321.

Connor, W. E. (1990). Dietary fiber—Nostrum or critical nutrient? *New England Journal of Medicine, 322,* 193-195.

Cooper, A., Floyd, T., Ziegler, M., Kashy, S., Shinobu, K., & Heird, W. (1981). Nutritional assessment of the low birth weight infant. *Journal of Parenteral and Enteral Nutrition, 5,* 563.

Cunningham, W. R., & Brookbank, J. W. (1988). *Ger-*

ontology: The psychology, biology and sociology of aging. New York: Harper & Row.

Diet, nutrition and cancer. (1982). Washington, DC: National Academy of Sciences/National Research Council.

Edozien J. C., Switzer, B. R., & Bryan, R. B. (1976, July 15). *Medical Evaluation of the Special Supplemental Food Program for Women, Infants, and Children (WIC): Summary and conclusions.* Chapel Hill, NC: University of North Carolina Press.

Ferb, T. E., Glotzer, J., Nester, J. P., & Napior, D. (1980). *The nutrition education and training program: A status report, 1977-1980.* Cambridge, MA: ABT Associates.

Garza, C., & Goldman, A. S. (1985). Effect of maternal nutritional status on lactation performance and infant nutrition. *Perinatology Neonatology, 9,* 11-17.

Gortmaker, S. L., Dietz, W. H., Sobol, A. M., & Wehaler, C. A. (1987). Increasing pediatric obesity in the United States. *American Journal of Diseases of Children, 141,* 535-540.

Hallberg, L. (1982). Iron absorbption and iron deficiency: Human nutrition. *Clinical Nutrition, 36C,* 259-278.

Halberg, L. (1984). Iron. In *Nutrition reviews: Present knowledge in nutrition.* Washington, DC: The Nutrition Foundation.

Harlan, W. R. Hull, A. L., Schmouder, R. L., Landis, J. R., Thompson, F. E., & Larkin, F. A. (1984). Blood pressure and nutrition in adults: The National Health and Nutrition Examination Survey. *American Journal of Epidemiology, 120,* 17-28.

Hoeg, J. M. (1987). Managing the patient with hypercholesterolemia. *Nutrition & the M. D., 13,* 1-3.

Johnson, D. W., & Johnson, R. T. (1985). Nutrition education: A model for effectiveness, a synthesis of research. *Journal of Nutrition Education, 17,* S1-544.

Johnson, P. R., & Roloff, J. S. (1982). Vitamin B_{12} deficiency in infants strictly breast-fed by a mother with latent pernicious anemia. *Journal of Pediatrics, 100,* 917-919.

Karekeck, J. M. (1985). Assessing nutrition status of the elderly. Baltimore: William & Wilkins.

Keys, A., Anderson, J. T., & Grande, F. (1965). Serum cholesterol response to changes in diet. *Metabolism, 14,* 747-787.

Maclean, W.E., & Grahm, G.G. (1982). *Pediatric nutrition in clinical practice.* Menlo Park, CA: Addison-Wesley.

Master, A. M., Lasser, R. P., & Beckman, G. (1960). Tables of average weight and height of Americans aged 65 to 94 years. *Journal of the American Medical Association, 172,* 658-662.

Mohs, M. E., & Watson, R. R. (1986). Nutritional assessment for the elderly. In R. R. Watson (Ed.), *CRC handbook of nutrition in the aged.* Boca Raton, FL: CRC Press.

National Institutes of Health. (1985). Consensus development conference statement: Health implications of obesity. *Annals of Internal Medicine, 103,* 981-1077.

National Research Council. (1989). *Subcommittee on the tenth edition of the RDAs.* Washingtin, DC: National Academy Press.

Olson, C. N., Frangillo, E. A., & Schardt, D.G. (1983). *Final report: An examination of nutrition education practices and materials in elementary schools.* Ithaca, NY: Cornell University.

Phillips, P. A., Phil, D., Rolls, B. J., Ledingham, D.M., Forsling, M.L., Morton, J.J., Crowe, M.J., & Wollner, L. (1984). Reduced thirst after water deprivation in healthy elderly men. *New England Journal of Medicine, 311,* 753-759.

Pregnancy and alcohol warning. (1981). *FDA Consumer, 15,* 2.

Reichel, W. (1983). *Clinical aspects of aging.* Baltimore: Williams & Wilkins.

Roberge, A. G., Sevigny, J., Seoan, N., & Richard, L. (1984). Dietary intake data: Usefulness and limitations. *Progress in Food and Nutrition Science, 8,* 27-42.

Rye, J. A., Hunt, B. N., Nicely, R., & Shannon, B. (1980). The development of a nutrition inservice course for teachers of young children. *Journal of Nutrition Education, 12,* 93-96.

Sarett, H. P., Bain, K. R., & O'Leary, J. C. (1983). Decisions on breastfeeding or formula feeding and trends in infant-feeding practices. *American Journal of Diseases of Children, 137,* 719-725.

Schulette, S. A., & Linkswiler, H. M. (1984). Calcium. In *Nutrition reviews: present knowledge in nutrition.* Washington, DC: The Nutrition Foundation.

Shils, M. E., & Young, V. R. (ed.). (1988). *Modern nutrition in health and disease* (7th ed.). Philadelphia: Lea & Febiger.

Surgeon general's report on nutrition and health. (1987). (Publication No. 88-50210). Washington, DC: U.S. Government Printing Office.

Talmage, H. (1978). Food... *Your choice, levels 1, 2 and 3: Summative evaluation* (Report No. 98). Chicago: University of Illinois at Chicago.

Thomas, A. E., McKay, D. A., & Cutlap, M. B. (1976). A nomograph method for assessing body weight. *American Journal of Clinical Nutrition, 29,* 302-304.

U.S. Department of Agriculture. (1987, April). *Nationwide food consumption survey: Continuing survey of food intake by individuals, low-income women 19-50 years and their children 1-5 years* (1 day Publication No. NFCS, CSF11 86-2). Hyattsville, MD: Author.

U.S. Department of Agriculture and U.S. Department of Health and Human Services. (1985). *Nutrition and your health: Dietary guidelines for Americans* (2nd ed.) (Publication No. Home and Garden Bulletin 232). Washington, DC: U.S. Government Printing Office.

U.S. Public Health Service. (1974, January). *Dietary intake and biochemical findings: Preliminary findings of the First Health and Nutrition Examination Survey, 1971-1972.* Rockville, MD: Author.

U.S. Senate Special Committee on Aging. (1986). *Aging America: Trends and projections* (Publication No. PF337 [1085]. Washington, DC: U.S. Department of Health and Human Services.

Weiss, E. H., & Davis, C. H. (1985). The response of an elderly audience to nutrition education articles in a newspaper for seniors. *Journal of Nutrition Education, 17,* 197-202.

Weiss, E. H., & Kein, C. L. (1987). A synthesis of research on nutrition education at the elementary level. *Journal of School Health, 57,* 8-13.

Whitbourne, S. K. (1985). *The aging body: Physiological changes and psychological consequences.* New York: Springer-Verlag.

Yang, M., & VanItallie, T. B. (1976). Composition of weight loss during short-term weight reduction. *Journal of Clinical Investigation, 58,* 722-730.

Yearich, E. S. (1978). Nutritional status of the elderly: Anthropometric and clinical findings. *Journal of Gerontology, 33,* 657-662.

Environmental Concerns

ARTHUR S. COOKFAIR

This most excellent canopy, the air, look you this brave o'erhanging firmament, this majestical roof fretted with golden fire—why it appears no other thing to me than a foul and pestilent congregation of vapors.

SHAKESPEARE *(HAMLET)*

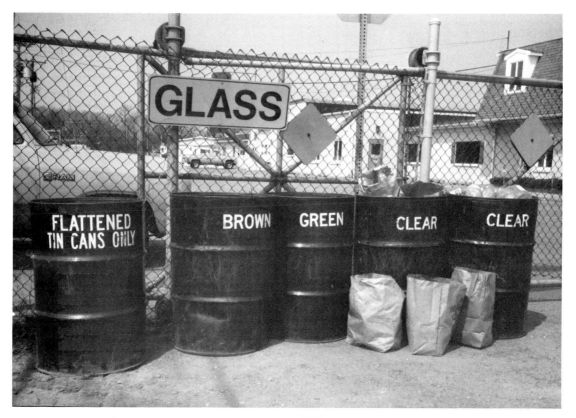

OBJECTIVES

At the conclusion of this chapter the student will be able to:

1. Describe the evolution of environmental issues from a historical perspective
2. Describe the effect of increasing population on the environment
3. Describe the effect of solid waste on the health of the community
4. Describe the problems of hazardous wastes and their harmful effect on the health of the community
5. Describe the hazards of water pollution on the health of the community
6. Describe the effect of noise pollution on the health of the community
7. Describe the problem of air pollution in the community
8. Identify the common sources of radiation hazards in the community
9. Describe appropriate nursing interventions at primary, secondary, and tertiary levels to protect the community from environmental hazards and to rehabilitate the victims of such hazards

KEY TERMS

Air pollution	Open dump
Biomagnification	Pollutant
Chemical wastes	Polychlorinated biphenyls (PCBs)
Environment	Population effect
Formaldehyde	Radioactive wastes
Hazardous wastes	Radon
Incineration	Recycling
Ionizing radiation	Smog
Landfill	Solid waste
Lead poisoning	Water pollution
Noise pollution	

Human concern about the environment and actions to protect it can be traced to the earliest recorded civilizations. The concept of burying human wastes and maintaining a sanitary environment can be found in the Law of Moses (Deuteronomy XXIII:12-13). The Minoan civilization on the island of Crete, as early as 3000 to 1000 BC, disposed of solid wastes by burial in large pits, with layers of earth at intervals.

In a primitive society, on a sparsely populated Earth, the solutions were relatively simple. Nature's purification systems normally could maintain a suitable environment. Water was purified by distillation (evaporation), and the vapors were condensed and returned as rain, cleansing the air as it fell. Ground waters were cleaned by percolation through the soil. Plants and animals died, were decomposed by the action of microorganisms, and eventually returned to the soil to provide nutrients for new life. The elements of this dynamic purification and recycling system maintained a balance. As human population increased and technology advanced, however, nature's purification systems became overloaded. The problem of properly disposing of the products—especially the waste products—of human activity increased in magnitude as well as complexity.

With the advent of industrial societies, not only did the output of human activities increase with population growth (as one might expect), but because of the "progress" of technology, the output per person became greater. The increase in human productivity began to outpace even the dramatic increase in population. To complicate things still further, it has become increasingly apparent that advances in technology are a two-edged sword. On the one hand, useful products of modern technology have resulted in an increase in the standard of living of people throughout the world. On the other hand, that same technology has allowed human beings to use the Earth's resources in the creation of new and sometimes hazardous chemicals.

When the products of human activity enter the environment and affect it adversely, those products are referred to as *pollutants* and we say that the environment has been polluted. Pollution can be defined as an undesirable change in the physical, chemical, or biological characteristics of the air, water, or land that can adversely affect the health, survival, or well-being of human beings or other organisms. The pollution or adverse environmental condition does not have to be one that causes direct physical harm. Excessive or unwanted noise can be considered pollution even though it may cause no physcial injury and the most likely harm will be psychological stress. Similarly, a foul odor can be considered pollution even it its major offense is to the senses.

THE POPULATION EFFECT

It takes little imagination to visualize a correlation between population and the total amount of waste produced by all human activities. The greater the number of people, the greater the amount of waste. Human waste products—biological, chemical, or physical— if present in too great a quantity to be acceptably assimilated by the environment, become pollutants and affect our health or general well-being. As a result, any consideration of environmental issues that may impinge on the health of a community should take into account the effect of population.

World population currently is estimated at a record level of about 5 billion. The population of the United States accounts for about one-twentieth of the total. Both U.S. and world populations are growing but at substantially different rates. Changes in population depend on births, deaths, and migration (immigration and emigration). Numerical changes in total world population occur only as a result of the difference between births and deaths, whereas changes in population of a country (or city or any other unit of population) are influenced by immigration and emigration as people move from place to place.

The average number of babies born (live births), wordwide, is estimated to be about 249 per minute, or about 358,000 per day. Deducting the average number of deaths (100 per minute or 146,000 per day) leaves a net increase in human population of 212,000 persons per day. To illustrate the enormity of such a growth rate, it has been estimated that it takes fewer than 5 days to replace a number of persons equal to all Americans killed in U.S. wars and fewer than 12 months to replace the more than 75 million persons killed in the world's largest disaster—the bubonic plague epidemic of the fourteenth century (Miller, 1986).

As frightening as the *magnitude* of world population growth is, it is further complicated by the fact that the growth is occurring exponentially, or geometrically. The phenomenon of exponential growth can be dramatically illustrated in graphic form, plotting

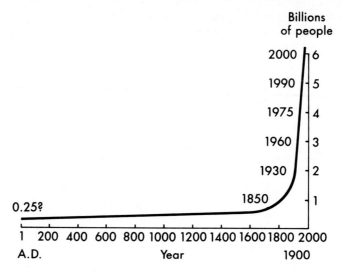

FIG. 25-1 The J-shaped curve of world population growth. *(From* Environmental Science: An Introduction *(p. 3) by G.T. Miller, Jr., 1986, Belmont, CA: Wadsworth. Copyright 1986 by Wadsworth, Inc. Publishing Co. Reprinted by permission.)*

population versus time. The resulting graph is characterized by a distinctive shape that, for obvious reasons, is often referred to as a "J" curve.

The J-shaped curve of human population is shown in Fig. 25-1. From the graph it can be seen that it took about 2 to 5 million years for the population to reach 1 billion but only 80 years to add the second billion; 30 years to add the third billion; 15 years to add the fourth billion, and 12 years to add the fifth billion.

The trends reflected in the *Global 2000 Report** (1980) indicate a virtual certainty that the world population will exceed 6 billion by the year 2000 (assuming no disastrous wars, famine, or pestilence). According to the *Report,* as a result of improved health, life expectancies at birth, for the world population, will increase 11% to 65.5 years. Beyond that, there is considerable doubt and disagreement among demographers as to whether the trend will continue its precipitous climb to environmental disaster or will, for various physical and sociological reasons, level off to a stabilized world population.

The dramatic growth in world population over the last century was due not to a rise in birth rates but rather to a decline in death rates, especially in the less developed countries. The reasons for the decline in death rates include the following (Miller, 1986):

1. An increase in food supplies because of improved agricultural production (partially attributable to the use of chemical pesticides—an environmental two-edged sword)
2. Better food distribution as a result of improved transportation
3. Better nutrition
4. Reduction of diseases associated with crowding—such as tuberculosis—because of better housing
5. Improved personal hygiene, including the use of soap, which reduces the spread of disease
6. Improved sanitation and water supplies, which reduce death rates from plague, cholera, typhus, dysentery, diphtheria, and other fatal diseases

7. Improvements in medical care and public health technology through the use of antibiotics, immunization, and insecticides

Concern for the effect of population growth on the environment usually focuses on the quantity of pollutants produced, that is, the more people, the more pollution. There is, however, another dimension to the environmental effect of people. When the number of persons in a given space, whether it is a city or a planet or a meeting hall, reaches some undefined level of density, the environment becomes less desirable and is referred to in terms such as "crowded" or "congested," which have negative connotations.

A high-population density thus can produce a psychological, if not physiological, stress. In terms of the definitions of pollution and pollutants presented earlier, when population density is high enough, people per se become pollutants.

WASTE DISPOSAL AND DISPERSAL
Solid Waste

The disposal of solid waste probably is the earliest recognized form of environmental problem. Nowhere is the environmental maxim that "everything must go somewhere" more in evidence on a daily basis than in the simple act of carrying out the garbage. When this individual daily ritual is multiplied by the number of persons in a population center, the result can be a logistics problem of staggering proportions. New York City generates 27,750 tons of garbage a day. As staggering as that amount is, it represents but a small fraction of the total commercial, industrial, and domestic waste produced in the United States—estimated at more than 6 billion tons per year.

For regulatory purposes, the U.S. Congress (Resource Conservation and Recovery Act of 1976) has defined *solid waste* as any garbage, refuse, sludge (e.g., from a waste treatment plant), and other discarded material—including solid, liquid, semisolid, or contained gaseous materials resulting from industrial, commercial, mining, and agricultural operations—as well as waste from community activities (Hall, Watson, Davidson, Case, & Bryson, 1986). Within this broad definition, subcategories of hazardous waste and non-hazardous waste also have been defined.

The traditional methods of solid waste disposal include the open dump, the landfill, ocean dumping, and incineration, or some combination of these.

Open dump. The open dump is simply what the name implies, a land area in which garbage and other waste materials are deposited, and little consideration is given to the sanitary conditions of the site. Typically, such dump sites provide a breeding ground for rats, flies, roaches, and other scavengers. The action of such pests as vectors in transmitting communicable disease is well known. Air pollution and water pollution problems associated with open dumps have been common. The Resource Conservation and Recovery Act (1976), which requires that open dumps be closed or upgraded to landfills, prohibits the establishment of new open dumps.

Landfill. The landfill is an improved version of the open dump, in which wastes are covered intermittently with layers of earth to minimize air pollution and accessibility to rats, flies, and other vectors. If care is not taken in the location of a landfill, the potential exists for contamination of ground water and/or surface water because of run-off and leaching. In recent years the term *sanitary landfill* has been applied to landfills that have been located carefully so that the potential for ground water or surface water contamination is minimized and in which the waste typically is spread in thin layers and frequently compacted and covered with a layer of earth. Modern landfills often incorporate systems to prevent ground water contamination and to monitor ground water quality. In the

United States the landfill now is the major method of permanent disposal for nonhazardous wastes. Most of New York City's tremendous daily output of garbage is disposed of in a 3000-acre site—the world's largest landfill—on Staten Island. The Staten Island site, known as Fresh Kills, is not without its problems, however, and its future is uncertain. It rapidly is becoming a symbol of the problem of municipal garbage. It has been estimated that, within a dozen years or so, the piling of wastes at Fresh Kills will result in its becoming the highest point on the eastern seaboard south of Maine. It will rise 500 feet above the New York Harbor, half as high as the Chrysler Building and half again as high as the Statue of Liberty. Similar situations are found in most of the larger landfills around the country. They are becoming saturated.

Ocean dumping. Throughout much of history the oceans have been viewed as the ultimate sink, capable of absorbing an infinite amount of waste. The nations of the world have used the oceans as a disposal site for everything from garbage and sewage to toxic chemicals and radioactive waste. In the early part of this century the ocean dumping of municipal wastes was common in the coastal areas of the United States. In 1933 a U.S. Supreme Court decision, involving New York City, resulted in a prohibition of ocean dumping of municipal waste. However, ocean dumping of other forms of waste continued. The United States took another step forward in 1972 with the passage of the U.S. Ocean Dumping Act. Over the two decades since then, the volume of industrial wastes dumped into U.S. ocean waters has been reduced dramatically. The ocean dumping of sewage sludge (the effluent of sewage treatment plants) continues to increase. In 1973, according to the Environmental Protection Agency (EPA), about 7.9 million tons were dumped into U.S. waters (EPA, 1988).

Recent years have seen an increasing worldwide concern for the potentially harmful effects of indiscriminate ocean dumping. By 1975 some 54 nations, including all the major maritime nations, had agreed to stop the dumping of certain types of chemical, biologcial, and nuclear wastes into the ocean.

Despite the increasing concern and regulation, unacceptably high quantities of slowly degradable and nondegradable plastic products, toxic chemicals, and other potentially harmful substances still find their way to the ocean. The "safe" level, above which pollutants will cause serious harm to the oceanic food chain and to human beings who depend on it, is difficult to determine. It is known that some pollutants, such as polychlorinated biphenyls (PCBs) and certain toxic mercury compounds, can be biologically magnified in marine or fresh water food chains (see Fig. 25-6.) Considerable research into the complexities of ocean systems is necessary before an environmentally sound ocean dumping program will be possible. Nevertheless, future waste management strategies, in the United States and internationally, no doubt will include carefully regulated ocean dumping as one of several waste disposal options.

Incineration. Until recent times the open burning of wastes at home was commonplace. Typically it was carried out in fireplaces, leaf piles, rubbish heaps, and even crude backyard incinerators. Increasing concerns about air pollution have led to the banning of such backyard burning in many areas. The result, of course, has been an increase in the quantity of waste that must be collected and disposed of. The effect varies with location. In 1970 an ordinance banning backyard burning in Sacramento, California, was followed over the next year by a nearly 50% increase in solid waste collected (Tchobanoglous, Theisen, & Eliassen, 1977). Although crude, open burning, whether in the backyard or in an open dump (Fig. 25-2), generally is banned, many metropolitan areas, as well as individual businesses, now use modern, highly efficient incineration techniques as an alternative or as a supplement to landfill disposal. Incineration, used as an adjunct

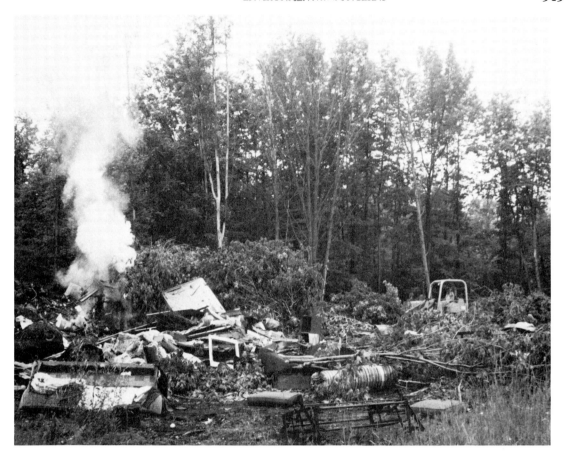

FIG. 25-2 Burning of wastes in an open dump is banned in many communities.

to landfill, can reduce the volume of refuse by 90% or more and, as a result, considerably extend the useful life of a landfill. A modern incinerator is an efficient and a carefully engineered unit designed to maximize the combustion of solid waste while minimizing the emission of pollutants. A modern efficient incinerator, however, requires a high initial investment and is expensive to operate.

The high costs of incineration have led to the development and use of units that use the heat produced from the burning of refuse to generate steam and/or electricty that can be sold to nearby industries or to the local electrical utility (Fig. 25-3). Critics of disposal by incineration have raised questions about environmental hazards associated with the emission of pollutants such as dioxins. Although zero emission of pollutants is not possible, many believe that incineration is the best available technology for disposing of many waste products.

The disposal of waste is further complicated by the difficulty of locating an acceptable site. Whether it is an incinerator or a landfill, "NIMBY" (not in my back yard) is a common community response. No one wants to live near a waste disposal facility, yet everyone needs to dispose of waste.

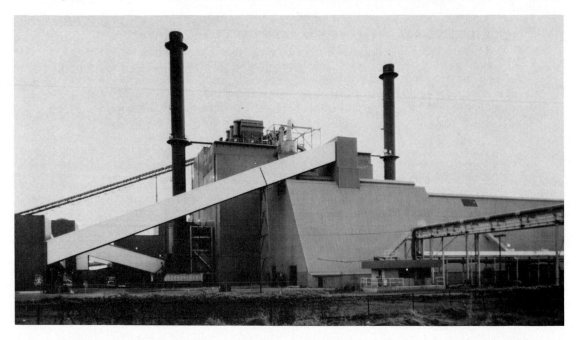

FIG. 25-3 A modern energy from municipal waste facility. This plant has a capacity of more than 600,000 tons of municipal and household waste per year from which a steady supply of steam and electricity is produced.

Recycling. Recycling is an environmental alternative to disposal. Most environmentalists advocate recycling as an environmentally acceptable method of reducing the disposal problem. It is becoming an increasingly attractive alternative as landfills become saturated. Many of the materials that currently are exhausting the capacity of our landfills can be recycled. Among them are paper, textiles, aluminum, glass, scrap iron and steel, rubber, and lubricating oils. A few states have passed mandatory recycling laws that require residents to separate their recyclable materials for collection at the curb, much like regular garbage collection. Thousands of smaller localities have started their own recycling programs. Nine states have enacted "bottle bills" that require purchasers to pay a deposit on cans and bottles, to be refunded to them when the empty container is returned. The distributor then collects them and facilitates recycling. The aluminum industry recycles about 50% of the cans it produces. Recycled aluminum accounts for about a third of the raw material used.

Recycling has another major advantage. In most instances it takes considerably more energy to extract and refine virgin materials than to process recycled materials. For example, the use of recycled aluminum in cans results in a 96% energy savings.

Hazardous Waste: A Product of Modern Technology

As though the sheer volume of waste produced by an affluent and growing U.S. population were not enough of an environmental problem, modern technology has provided a further complication—the production (and ultimately, the disposal) of hazardous wastes.

Radioactive waste. The advent of the nuclear era brought with it the production of nuclear power, nuclear weapons and a new form of medicine, nuclear medicine. All these activities generated radioactive waste that must be processed and safely disposed of and stored. Much of the existing radioactive waste is stored temporarily in deep pools at nuclear plants or in underground tanks. Serious proposals for long-term disposal have included such locations as outer space, underground salt mines, on land beneath the Antarctic ice cap, and in the sediments of the deep ocean floor. As with other hazardous wastes, everyone wants it safely disposed of—somewhere else. Scientists continue to search for the best disposal plan, but the final solution is likely to be as strongly influenced by political as by scientific considerations.

Chemical waste. At the turn of the century the United States was heavily dependent on the importation of chemicals from Germany. The first World War broke that dependency, and a fledgling American chemical industry was spurred into growth. The second growth spurt came with World War II. The postwar period saw the emergence of the United States as a world leader in the manufacture of chemicals and in the creation of new chemicals and new materials. New pesticides, plastics, drugs, synthetic fabrics, coatings, detergents, and a host of other products appeared on the scene and became a part of everyday life. The chemical industry has helped to make possible the highest standard of living the world has known.

That is the good news. The bad news is that with every new pesticide, every new plastic, and every new chemical product comes a potential environmental health hazard from the product itself and from the chemical by-products of its production, from its disposal as waste, and even from the use of the new product itself. By the late 1950s a few voices could be heard raising concerns about the potential environmental pollution from pesticides.

In 1962 Rachel Carson added her voice to the growing concern about our environment. Her book, *Silent Spring,* focused a nation's attention on the environment and, probably more than any other single event, triggered the environmental movement and an environmental awareness that continues to this day. In the years since, "Love Canal" and "Bhopal" have become a part of our vocabulary, and PCBs and methyl mercury have taken their place alongside *Streptobacillus* organisms and the poliomyelitis virus as disease-causing agents.

More than 4 million chemical compounds are known. Of these, it is estimated that more than 60,000 are produced commercially, with about 1000 new compounds being introduced each year (Department of Health, Education and Welfare, 1979).This output of the chemical industry produces the major portion of hazardous wastes. More than 90% of the hazardous wastes produced in the United States come from the chemical, petroleum, and metal-related industries (Miller, 1986).

Since World War II an estimated 6 billion tons of hazardous wastes have been generated in the United States. The improper and often illegal disposal of much of these hazardous wastes has created a series of what many environmentalists refer to as "chemical time bombs"—sites where improperly protected toxic wastes present a very real present or potential health hazard. The EPA has identified nearly 1200 sites as especially hazardous and has placed them on a national priorities list (Fig. 25-4).

Hazardous wastes can become a threat to human health in various ways: direct exposure of persons at or near the disposal site or as a result of accidents during transport to the site; exposure to polluted air resulting from improperly controlled incineration; use of ground water or surface water that has become contaminated by leaching or run-off from waste-disposal sites; and consumption of food contaminated through biological magnification of toxic chemicals (see discussion later in this chapter).

The time interval between the disposal of a chemical in a waste-disposal site and the

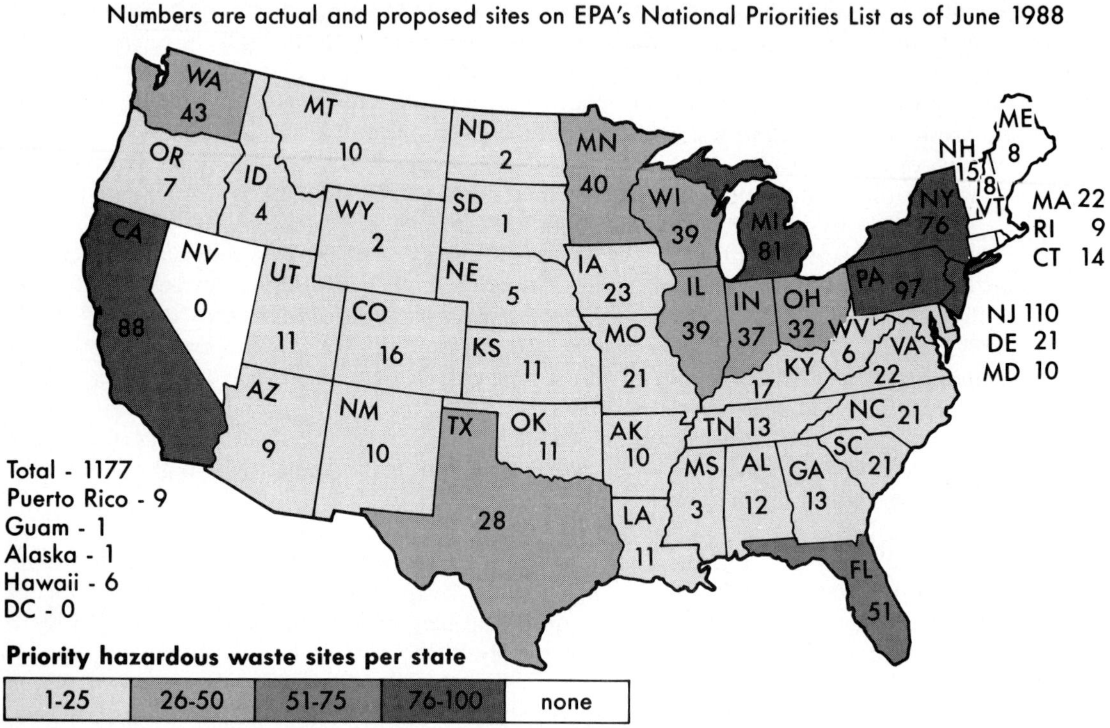

Numbers are actual and proposed sites on EPA's National Priorities List as of June 1988

Total - 1177
Puerto Rico - 9
Guam - 1
Alaska - 1
Hawaii - 6
DC - 0

Priority hazardous waste sites per state

1-25	26-50	51-75	76-100	none

FIG. 25-4 Priority hazardous waste sites per state. Numbers are actual and proposed sited on EPA's national priority list as of June 1988. (*From* National Priority List, Supplementary Lists and Supporting Materials, June 1988, *by the Office of Emergency and Remedial Response (Superfund), 1988, Washington, DC: U.S. Environmental Protection Agency.*)

manifestation of adverse health effects can be divided into three phases (Grisham, 1986):

1. The time required for release across the site boundary
2. The time required for transport through the environment to the site where human exposure occurs
3. The latency period for the manifestation of human health effects

For some chemicals, in some situations, the time period may be extremely brief and may be measured in minutes or hours. In other instances, the time interval may be measured in years or decades—the "chemical time bomb." The following hypothetical "worst case" scenarios illustrate the difference between the two (Grisham, 1986):

1. The driver of a tank truck filled with waste acid arrives at the disposal site and inadvertently drains the acid into a previously dumped cyanide salt mixture, which immediately reacts to form cyanide gas. In a few minutes the gas would be rapidly released into the air; the driver and others in the immediate area then might inhale significant quantities and become immediately, and possibly fatally, ill.
2. A buried drum containing hazardous chemical waste could, over a period of years, rust through, releasing the chemical into the ground, where it would then begin a slow process of migrating through the soil, beyond the disposal site, ultimately

percolating into the ground water. If the chemical were not readily degradable and ground water flow rates were low, the chemical would migrate in the ground water for decades before being pumped out of the ground in drinking water. The latency period between human exposure and manifestation of disease might be extensive, such as for cancer or chronic liver or kidney damage.

The immediate harmful effects of many common chemicals have been long recognized. Arsenic and cyanides are poisonous; strong acids such as sulfuric or hydrochloric acid will burn human tissue, as will strong alkalis, such as sodium hydroxide (lye); ammonia gas will irritate the lungs. Recently, however, there has been a growing concern about the longer range, and sometimes more subtle, effects of many chemicals. Some effects are difficult to detect or to measure, such as mental depression, birth defects, lowering of intelligence, or depressed immunity, which can, in turn, lead to other health effects that are still more difficult to relate to a source.

A chemical health hazard may not be apparent until substantial damage has occurred over a long period of time. In the area of a fishing village on Japan's Minamata Bay, between 1953 and 1960, a strange illness developed and spread among the population. More than 100 persons exhibited symptoms of brain and nerve damage; 19 babies were born with congenital defects; and more than 40 people died. The victims had been eating methyl mercury–contaminated fish from the bay; a plastics manufacturer had been dumping mercury wastes into the bay. Mercury poisoning is now known as Minamata disease and has been diagnosed in other exposed populations.

The health hazards presented by many chemicals are by no means limited to the potential contact resulting from waste disposal. A very real health hazard may be encountered from chemicals contacted in a variety of ways: during the use of a common chemical for the purpose for which it was intended in the home, on the street, and in the workplace or in other environments that are a part of our everyday life. Solvents present in paints and varnishes, pesticide residues on fresh fruits and vegetables, and chemical food additives are but a few of the ways in which we are brought into contact with chemicals—often toxic chemicals—on a daily basis.

Some chemicals are resistant to degradation and will persist and spread throughout the environment until it is virtually impossible to avoid long-term, low-level exposure. The harmful effects of such exposure often are difficult to assess and are controversial even when acute effects from exposure to high concentrations are well known. The saga of PCBs probably is one of the best examples.

PCBs first were manufactured in the United States in 1929. They are a group of toxic, oily, synthetic organic chemical compounds that have been used in the production of plastics, paints, adhesives, hydraulic and heat transfer fluids, dust-control agents on roads, and a host of other industrial uses. Because of their particular electrical properties, they were used extensively as insulating and cooling fluids in electrical transformers and capacitors.

PCBs played a useful role, with little controversy or question about health effects for nearly 40 years. Then, in 1969, they were identified as the causative agent in an outbreak of a disease that afflicted some 1000 persons in southern Japan. The victims exhibited skin discoloration and scaling, severe acne, numbness, neuralgic pains, edema of the eyelids, and marked general weakness. Children born of mothers affected by the PCBs had PCBs in their blood, and some exhibited the same dark pigmentation and eye discharge that had been observed in adult victims. Of 13 recorded births to exposed mothers, 2 were

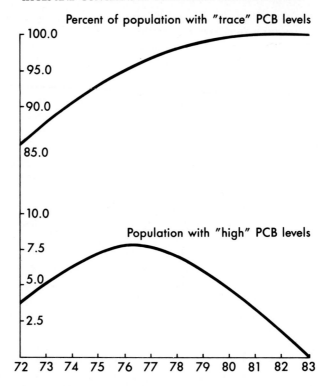

FIG. 25-5 Although nearly everyone now has "trace" levels of PCBs, the percentage of population with "high" levels has gone down. *(From Office of Toxic Substances, 1988, Washington, DC: U.S. Environmental Protection Agency.)*

stillborn and 10 showed the aforementioned symptoms. The victims of what has come to be known as the Yusho disease had eaten food cooked with a rice oil contaminated with PCBs.

In the early 1970s PCBs were found in cow's milk (and subsequently in human milk), many inland and ocean fish, most meats, and in the bodies of human beings. With the Toxic Substances Control Act (TSCA) of 1976, Congress banned the manufacture, processing, and distribution of PCBs except in totally enclosed electrical equipment. Since that time, although the total level of PCBs in food, human beings, and the environment has declined, the actual number of persons with at least trace levels of PCBs has increased. The EPA believes that virtually *all* Americans have PCBs in their bodies (Fig. 25-5).

Despite environmental legislation the story of PCBs is by no means over. The EPA estimates that sealed electrical transformers and capacitors still in use by utility companies contain some 750 million pounds of PCBs. Each year some will be released into the environment from leaking or exploding equipment. More than 250 million pounds have been disposed of in dumps and landfills or have been dispersed, often illegally on roadsides or other areas.

PCBs have been described as the "universal pollutant" (Holum, 1977). They are found in the tissue of marine microorganisms and have migrated upwardly through the food chain to fish and predatory birds, becoming concentrated in the process. Although they are relatively insoluble in water, they are soluble in fats and thus accumulate or are stored

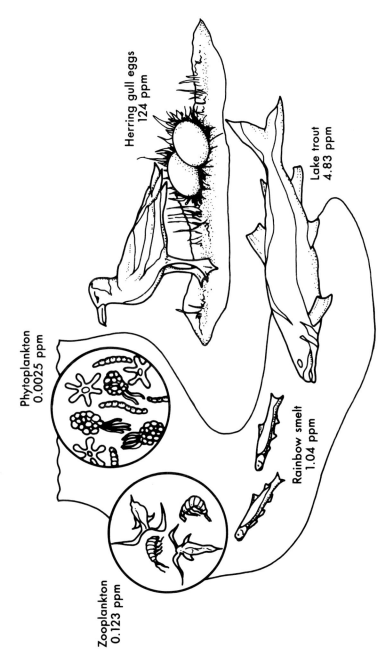

FIG. 25-6 Persistent organic chemicals such as PCBs bioaccumulate and are magnified in the food chain. This diagram shows the degree of concentration in each level of the Great Lakes aquatic food chain for PCBs (in parts per million [ppm]). The highest levels are reached in the eggs of fish-eating birds such as gulls. *(From The Great Lakes, An Environmental Atlas and Resource Book (1987) jointly produced by Environment Canada and the U.S. Environmental Protection Agency, Chicago and Toronto.)*

RESEARCH HIGHLIGHT

The effect of prenatal PCB exposure on visual recognition memory

A sample of 123 white, predominantly middle-class infants (69 males and 54 females) from Grand Rapids, Michigan, was selected for this study. The mothers were screened regarding their fish consumption habits, with 92 being fish eaters and 31 nonfish eaters. The fish eaters had consumed at least 11.8 kg of PCB-contaminated Lake Michigan fish over the 6 previous years. (PCBs accumulate in the body over time, exposing the fetus to risk from PCBs acquired both prior to and during pregnancy). Data on infant feeding patterns were collected at 2, 4, 5, and 7 months, and infants were classified into five categories ranging from exclusively breast-fed to exclusively bottle fed.

At age 7 months, each infant was tested in the laboratory while seated on the mother's lap in front of an observation chamber containing a pivoting stimulus presentation "stage" and administered Fagan's test of visual recognition memory (*Journal of Experimental Child Psychology, 16,* 1973, 424-450.) The test was administered by one of three examiners, who was blind with respect to fish consumption and biological measure of PCB exposure. Each infant was first exposed to a target photo simultaneously in left and right positions. After the infant fixated the target for a total of 20 seconds, the familiar target was paired with a novel target for two 5-second recognition periods, reversing the left-right positions from one period to the next. Visual recognition was defined as the percent of total fixation paid to the novel target for each of the three pairs of targets.

The study suggests a possible relationship between prenatal PCB exposure and deficits in visual recognition memory at 7 months in infants who appeared clinically normal at birth. The authors suggest that further research is needed to determine the potential of the test to predict long-term damage.

From "The Effect of Intrauterine PCB Exposure on Visual Recognition Memory" by S.W. Jacobson, G.G. Fein, J.L. Jacobson, P.M. Schwartz, and J.K. Dowler, 1985, *Child Development, 56,* pp. 853-860. Copyright 1985 by *Child Development.* Reprinted by permission.

in fatty tissue, including human fat tissue. Fish feeding in PCB-contaminated waters often have levels of PCB 1000 to 100,000 times the level of that found in the surrounding water. This "biomagnification" continues upwardly through the food chain (Fig. 25-6). Consumption of Great Lakes coho salmon caught in sport fishing has been noted as a significant source of chronic exposure to PCBs (Cordle, Locke, & Springer, 1982). Consumption of Lake Michigan fish has been correlated with PCB levels in human maternal serum and milk (Schwartz, Jacobson, Fein, Jacobson, & Price, 1983).

The long-term human health effects associated with chronic low-level exposure to chemical pollutants such as PCBs are difficult to assess. Recently, a new multiple-effects model has been proposed that emphasizes subtle behavioral alteration as an early sign of toxicity and as evidence that a particular chemical agent may produce long-term impairment in susceptible persons (Fein, Schwartz, Jacobson, & Jacobson, 1983). In another study (Fein, Jacobson, Jacobson, Schwartz, & Dowler, 1984) it was found that babies born to women who consumed moderate quantities of PCB-contaminated Lake Michigan salmon or trout were smaller than infants in a controlled group.

WATER POLLUTION

Historically, the most serious community health problems associated with water supplies have been waterborne diseases such as typhoid, infectious hepatitis, cholera, and dysentery. In the United States, deaths from these diseases no longer are considered major health problems, but they still are common in many parts of the world. The entry of disease-causing bacteria and viruses into a water supply most commonly occurs through human or animal feces. In the United States and other more developed countries, water-borne diseases are controlled by the purification of sewage in septic tanks or waste treatment plants before being released into the water supply. Although the level of treatment varies depending on the sophistication of the sewage plant, treatment typically includes removal of solids by filtration and sedimentation (primary treatment) and biological processing (secondary treatment). A few sewage plants add a highly sophisticated tertiary treatment stage to remove most of the remaining contaminants. Regardless of how many stages of treatment are employed, the final step is a disinfection process—treating the effluent with chlorine gas before its final discharge.

Measurements of water quality commonly rely on three indicators: (1) the concentration of dissolved oxygen (DO), (2) the biological oxygen demand (BOD), and (3) the fecal coliform bacteria count. Most aquatic animals and plants require oxygen. The DO is the amount of dissolved oxygen gas in a quantity of water at a particular temperature ($20°$C). At that temperature, at normal atmospheric pressure, the maximum concentration of DO is 9 ppm, that is, 9 parts of oxygen per million parts of water.

Organic matter in water is broken down by bacterial action. The amount of DO required for bacterial decomposition is expressed as the BOD as parts per million of DO consumed over a 5-day period at $20°$C and normal atmospheric pressure. When the BOD causes the DO content to fall below 5 ppm, the water is considered to be seriously polluted.

The water quality, for drinking and swimming purposes, is indicated by the number of colonies of fecal coliform bacteria present in a 100-ml sample of water. Water generally is considered safe to drink if it contains fewer than 10 coliforms per liter. In the United States water qualities are mandated by the Clean Water Act (for recreational waters) and the Safe Drinking Act.

Although the sewage treatment and purification may be carried to the point of producing drinkable water, the treated water is not sent directly into the immediate water supply. Instead it generally is discharged into a river, lake, or the water table and once again becomes a part of the natural water supply. When drinking water is taken from some new location, a further purification, which includes chlorination, takes place.

As a result of sewage treatment and drinking water treatment procedures commonly employed in the United States, the incidence of waterborne diseases is low. There is concern, however, about the possible contamination of water supplies with some of the 60,000 commercially produced chemicals. Hundreds of synthetic organic chemicals have been identified in drinking water supplies around the United States. Even the chlorination of drinking water, which purifies the water by killing bacteria, may, at the same time, create another environmental hazard. It has been found that the chlorine reacts with organic compounds present in the water to form chloroform, a chemical known to be toxic in concentrated form (Grisham, 1986).

About half of all Americans rely on ground water as their source of drinking water, the remainder relying on surface water, that is, streams, rivers, lakes, and reservoirs as their source.

NOISE POLLUTION

Noise can be defined as any sound that is unwanted, disagreeable, or harmful to our well-being. It is a physiological or psychological stress. Noise is sound that has become a pollutant.

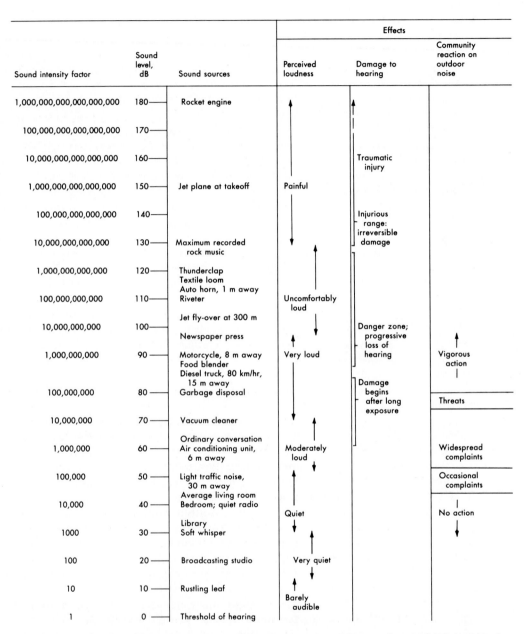

FIG. 25-7 Sound levels and human responses. *(From* Environmental Science *(pp. 536-37) by J. Turk and A Turk, 1988, Philadelphia: Saunders. Copyright 1988 by W.B. Saunders Co. Reprinted by permission.)*

Sound consists of oscillations of atmospheric pressure that are caused by a vibrating object (sound source). It can be characterized or qualified in terms of frequency (pitch), measured in cycles per second or herz (Hz), and in terms of intensity on a scale called a decibel (dB) scale. On the decibel scale the softest sound that can be heard by human beings is given a value of 0 dB. Fig. 25-7 shows the level of intensity (dB) of various common sounds. Because the scale is logarithmic, each 10-dB increase represents a tenfold increase in intensity. Thus a rise in intensity from 10 dB (rustle of leaves) to 40 dB (quiet radio) represents a thousandfold increase.

Noise can be a physiological or a psychological stressor, or both, and can elicit a response ranging from mild irritation to pain or permanent hearing loss. Pain occurs at intensities above approximately 120 dB and hearing loss from prolonged exposure at about 90 dB or above. Hearing loss may occur at lower decibel levels if exposure to the noise is continuous over a very long period of time.

Moderate levels of noise can cause irritability, fatigue, and a reduced ability to cope. Quantifying lower-intensity noise as a psychological stressor is difficult in as much as the response is highly subjective. Cultural, social, and personal differences can affect an individual's perception of sound. What is music to one person may be noise (and thus a stressor) to another.

It is unlikely that, under normal circumstances, noise can be totally eliminated from one's environment. However, much can be done in the community and in the home to minimize or control noise. Noisy machinery often can be replaced by newer, quieter machinery. If this is not possible or practical, ear protection should be used. Traffic noise reaching a home from a busy highway can be lessened by an appropriately placed barrier of trees or shrubs. Noise transmission within a home can be minimized by the use of carpets and draperies and acoustical materials of construction.

AIR POLLUTION

The earliest form of human-induced air pollution probably came into existence when the first human beings learned to start a fire. However, the Earth was sparsely populated, and human ability to affect the quality and composition of the atmosphere was limited. It was not until human beings developed sufficient technology to give birth to the Industrial Revolution that large-scale air pollution from human activities became a problem. The advent of another technological triumph—the internal combustion engine—ushered in the age of the automobile, a new source of air pollution. In the United States, England, and other industrialized nations, laws and regulations limiting the discharge of soot and smoke into the atmosphere came into existence. Although the initial attempts at regulation were of limited effectiveness, they were an indication of a growing concern.

The United States experienced its first major air pollution disaster in 1948, when emissions from steel mills and other industrial facilities became trapped by a combination of topographical and weather factors (temperature inversion) in a stagnant air mass over Donora, Pennsylvania. The heavily polluted air remained stationary for 5 days, resulting in at least 20 deaths and more than 6000 illnesses.

In London, in 1952, an even more deadly air pollution disaster occurred, with the death of some 4000 persons. These and other devastating episodes served to focus attention on the serious nature of air pollution and triggered efforts in the industrialized nations to find a solution.

In the United States a growing concern about the environment throughout the 1960s and specific concern about the health threat from air pollution resulted in the passage of the Clean Air Act of 1970. Under this act the EPA set air-quality standards for those

TABLE 25-1   Health effects of the regulated air pollutants

Criteria pollutants*	Health concerns
	Ozone
Respiratory tract problems such as difficult breathing and reduced lung function. Asthma, eye irritation, nasal congestion, reduced resistance to infection, and possibly premature aging of lung tissue	
Particulate matter	Eye and throat irritation, bronchitis, lung damage, and impaired visibility
Carbon monoxide	Ability of blood to carry oxygen impaired. Cardiovascular, nervous, and pulmonary systems affected
Sulfur dioxide	Respiratory tract problems; permanent harm to lung tissue
Lead	Retardation and brain damage, especially in children
Nitrogen dioxide	Respiratory illness and lung damage
Hazardous air pollutants†	
Asbestos	A variety of lung diseases, particularly lung cancer
Beryllium	Primary lung disease, although also affects liver, spleen, kidneys, and lymph glands
Mercury	Several areas of the brain as well as the kidneys and bowels affected
Vinyl chloride	Lung and liver cancer
Arsenic	Causes cancer
Radionuclides	Causes cancer
Benzene	Leukemia
Coke oven emissions	Respiratory cancer

From EPA: *Environmental Progress and Challenges: EPA's Update* (p. 13) by the Environmental Protection Agency, 1988, Washington, DC: Author.
*Criteria pollutants—those pollutants commonly found throughout the country that pose the greatest overall threat to air quality
†Hazardous air pollutants—those pollutants that can contribute to an increase in mortality or serious illness

common pollutants that posed the greatest overall threat to air quality across the country. Under the Clean Air Act, these pollutants, termed *criteria pollutants,* include ozone, carbon monoxide, airborne particulates, sulfur dioxide, lead, and nitrogen oxides (Table 25-1). Under the Clean Air Act the EPA also is required to set National Emission Standards for Hazardous Pollutants (NESHAPs). Hazardous pollutants are defined as those that can contribute to an increase in mortality or serious illness. Standards have been set for asbestos, beryllium, mercury, vinyl chloride, arsenic, radionuclides, benzene, and coke oven emissions (Table 25-1). Other air pollutants are being analyzed to determine whether they are hazardous and require regulation.

Between 1975 and 1986, federal air pollution control laws in the United States were a major factor in the reduction of the average levels of airborne particulates by 23%, sulfur dioxide by 37%, carbon monoxide by 32%, ozones by 13%, nitrogen dioxide by 14%, and lead by 87%.

As shown by the previous discussion, weather conditions can be critically important in the formation of a smog. Smogs (and fogs) commonly are associated with, or even caused by, an atmospheric condition known as a temperature inversion. The term refers to an "upside down" atmospheric condition. Normally, the atmosphere becomes colder with increasing altitude. In the case of a temperature inversion, a warm air layer forms

TABLE 25-2 Pollutant standards index—health effects information and cautionary statements

PSI	Air quality	Health effects	Warnings
0-50	Good		
51-100	Moderate		
101-200	Unhealthful	Mild aggravation of symptoms in susceptible persons, irritation symptoms in healthy population	Persons with existing heart or respiratory ailments should reduce physical exertion, outdoor activity.
First stage alert			
201-300	Very unhealthful	Significant aggravation of symptoms, decreased exercise tolerance in persons with heart or lung disease, widespread symptoms in healthy population	Elderly persons with existing heart or lung disease should stay indoors, reduce physical activity.
Second stage alert			
301-400	Hazardous	Premature onset of certain diseases, significant aggravation of symptoms, decreased exercise tolerance in healthy persons	Elderly persons with existing heart or lung disease should stay indoors, avoid physical exertion; general population should avoid outdoor activity.
Third stage alert			
401-500	Significant harm	Premature death of ill and elderly; healthy people experience adverse symptoms that affect normal activity	All persons should remain indoors, windows and doors closed; all persons should minimize physical exertion, avoid traffic.

From *Environmental Science* (p. 636) by J. Turk and A. Turk, 1988, Philadelphia: Copyright 1988 by W.B. Saunders Co. Reprinted by permission.

aloft so that the air is colder at ground level. If there is no wind, the air mass is stationary and the warm air layer acts like a lid on the lower atmosphere, sealing in the cooler, lower air and preventing its escape by convection. The pollutants then are trapped near the ground level.

To alert the public to air quality and air pollution conditions, the EPA and other government agencies have developed a pollution standards index (PSI). The index (Table 25-2) uses a scale of 0 to 50 correlated with descriptive terms for air quality, expected health effects, and warnings.

The concentration of air-polluting sources in large cities, such as automobiles, trucks, airplanes, and factories, often in combination with the effect of local topography and weather, can create an extreme air pollution problem referred to as *smog* (derived from the words smoke and fog). Simply stated, smog refers to a situation in which the pollutants are present in such concentrations that visibility is reduced and eye and lung irritation is experienced. Despite the derivation of the word, neither smoke nor fog is a necessary ingredient but either or both may be present. Episodes of smog are a common phenomenon in large cities and highly industrialized areas.

The immediate health effects of smog are generally recognized and have been experienced by millions of city dwellers around the world. It is particularly harmful to elderly persons and to those who suffer from respiratory ailments. The fastest-growing cause of death in New York City in the late 1960s was emphysema. Its incidence rose 500% during that decade. During the same period the incidence of bronchitis rose 200% (Holum, 1977).

RADIATION IN THE ENVIRONMENT

Radiation is energy radiated through matter or space in the form of particles or waves. For purposes of discussion and study, it generally is divided into two types: ionizing and nonionizing radiation.

Nonionizing radiation, which includes such forms of radiant energy as visible light, infrared, ultraviolet, microwaves, and radio waves, involves lower energy, which, as the name implies, does not produce ions. Possibly the most serious health threat from nonionizing radiation is from solar ultraviolet radiation, the principal cause of skin cancer in human beings. It is estimated that between 100,000 and 200,000 new cases of skin cancer occur per year in the United States. Notwithstanding such serious health hazards, public concern about radiation has focused primarily on ionizing radiation.

Ionizing radiation, which includes x-rays, gamma rays, alpha particles, and beta particles, is a high-energy radiation, capable of dislodging electrons from the atoms it hits, to form highly reactive charged particles called ions.

Until Roentgen's discovery of x-rays in 1895, all exposure to ionizing radiation came from natural sources. Scientific and technological developments since then have resulted in a wide variety of human-induced radiation sources based on the application of x-rays and on the development and applications of nuclear energy. However, despite the advent of human-induced radiation sources, the natural background represents the largest source of radiation exposure, about 73% of the total (Mossman, Thomas, & Dritschilo, 1986). Most of the natural background radiation we are exposed to comes from cosmic rays (from outer space), from terrestrial radioactivity (such as in rocks and soil), and from internal sources (from natural radioactive materials present in our air, water, and food). Cosmic rays are estimated to account for about 15% of the total natural background radiation. These radiations are extraterrestrial; that is, they originate in outer space, primarily from galactic sources. Because they must pass through the Earth's atmosphere, their intensity will depend, in part, on altitude. Thus exposure to such radiation would be higher in Denver (altitude, 5000 feet) than in New York City (sea level). Additional cosmic ray exposure, although slight, will occur during air travel; the dose rate from cosmic rays at 35,000 feet is about 100 times higher than at sea level. The risk associated with flying 6000 miles by jet increases by one part in one million the chances of death as a result of cancer caused by cosmic radiation (Table 25-3).

The principal source of natural background radiation is from radon, a radioactive gas formed in rocks and soil. Recently there has been considerable concern over the threat of death from radon-associated lung cancer. Because radon concentration is relatively low in outdoor air and high in indoor air, it is described in the section on indoor pollution.

Man-made radiation sources include medical x-rays or medical applications of radioactive substances, fallout from nuclear weapons testing, emissions from nuclear power plants, and a variety of very low-level sources classified as consumer products, including wrist watches, color television receivers, and smoke detectors.

TABLE 25-3 Risks that increase the chance of death by one part in one million	
Activity	**Cause of death**
Smoking 1.4 cigarettes	Cancer, heart disease
Drinking one-half liter of wine	Cirrhosis of the liver
Spending 1 h in a coal mine	Black lung disease
Spending 3 h in a coal mine	Accident
Living 2 days in New York or Boston	Air pollution
Traveling 6 min by canoe	Accident
Traveling 10 mi by bicycle	Accident
Traveling 300 mi by car	Accident
Flying 1000 mi by jet	Accident
Flying 6000 mi by jet	Cancer caused by cosmic radiation
Living 2 months in Denver on vacation from New York	Cancer caused by cosmic radiation
Living 2 months in average stone or brick building	Cancer caused by natural radioactivity
One chest x-ray taken in a good hospital	Cancer caused by radiation
Living 2 months with a cigarette smoker	Cancer, heart disease
Eating 40 tablespoons of peanut butter	Liver cancer caused by aflatoxin B
Drinking Miami drinking water for 1 year	Cancer caused by chloroform
Drinking 30 12-oz cans of diet soda	Cancer caused by saccharin
Living 5 years at site boundary of a typical nuclear power plant in the open	Cancer caused by radiation
Drinking 1000 24-oz soft drinks from recently banned plastic bottles	Cancer from acrylonitrile monomer
Living 20 years near a polyvinyl chloride plant	Cancer caused by vinyl chloride (1976 standard)
Living 150 years within 20 mi of a nuclear power plant	Cancer caused by radiation
Eating 100 charcoal-broiled steaks	Cancer from benzopyrene
Living within 5 mi of a nuclear reactor for 50 years	Cancer caused by radiation

From "Analyzing the daily risks of life" by R. Wilson, 1979, *Technology Review, 81*(4), p. 45. Copyright 1979 by *Technology Review.* Reprinted by permission.

The largest source of human-induced radiation exposure is from medical and dental x-rays used in the diagnosis and treatment of disease. In the United States it is estimated that more than two thirds of the population receive diagnostic medical examinations, or dental x-rays or both each year. The health effects of high doses of radiation are well known. The largest single source of data is from studies of the survivors of the atomic bombings of Hiroshima and Nagasaki in World War II. At the high levels of exposure involved, a significant number of excess cancers have been documented. There are, however, considerable difficulties in applying the data from such studies to determine health risks from low-level exposures. Mossman et al. (1986) have estimated that fewer than 2% of all cancer deaths may be attributable to ionizing radiation, the greatest portion of which (73%) is from natural background radiation. (See Table 25-3 for a comparison of the risk of death associated with several types of radiation exposure with other environmental or life-style related risks.)

ENVIRONMENTAL DISASTERS

It takes people to make a disaster. The San Andreas fault became a potential disaster site only after San Francisco and other communities were built over it. Similarly, a chemical waste site may become a disaster location only when people move to the site. As the population increases, so does the likelihood of disaster.

Environmental disasters can be natural or human-induced. They may occur with the suddenness of an explosion or the slow pace of toxic chemicals seeping through soil. A contrast in disaster characteristics may be seen in the comparison of two recent human-induced chemical disasters—Love Canal and Bhopal.

Love Canal is probably the most highly publicized chemical waste site disaster to occur in the United States. It began with the dumping of waste chemicals into an abandoned canal nearly a half century ago. Between 1942 and 1952, 21,800 tons of waste chemical's were dumped into the canal. The site was sealed with a clay cap, and for nearly a quarter of a century the hazards buried there seemed all but forgotten as roads, an elementary school, a children's playground, and hundreds of homes were constructed on and around the site. In the mid-1970s, after unusually heavy precipitation, chemical wastes began to surface and to infiltrate into residential basements (New York State Department of Health, 1981). Among the residents there were complaints of unusually high numbers of birth defects, miscarriages, and cancers. The following months and years brought fear, heightened by reports and studies of migrating toxic chemicals and health hazards, fanned by the media, and compounded by a confused societal response. The fear of toxic chemicals, the disruption of lives, the economic instability as the value of homes in the area plummeted, then the mass relocation of hundreds of people, all contributed to what may ultimately be the greatest tragedy of Love Canal—the psychological stress imposed on the victims.

Numerous health studies were undertaken from 1978 to 1984 with varying results and a general lack of coordination. The New York State Department of Health reported a "slight increase" of miscarriages and low birth weight infants associated with one section of the Love Canal neighborhood (New York State Department of Health, 1981). Analysis of blood tests found that residents of some areas, closest to the canal, may face a greater-than-expected risk of liver disease. However, the study also found that none of the individuals with abnormal test results, who subsequently were examined by their physicians, showed any clinical evidence of liver disease. In addition, it was found that the liver functions returned to normal once residents relocated away from the Love Canal neighborhood (Silverman, 1989).

No definitive study has determined the health effects of exposure to chemicals at Love Canal. Those studies that were undertaken have been criticized on various scientific grounds. No deaths appear to be attributable to chemical exposure at Love Canal, and it will take years to determine long-term health effects. Even if the physical health effects to former residents are minimal, the psychological damage still may be great. Those affected will live out their lives in fear of latent chemical effects on them, their children, or their grandchildren.

Other disasters are less subtle in their approach. Late on the evening of Sunday, December 2, 1984, the contents of a chemical storage tank in Bhopal, India, began to rise in temperature, gradually at first. Some time after midnight, driven by a runaway chemical reaction, the tank became dangerously hot and the pressure rose rapidly and uncontrollably. The result was the release of 80,000 pounds of highly volatile, highly toxic methyl isocyanate (MIC) gas. It quickly spread as a foglike cloud over the large densely populated shanty-town neighborhoods near the plant. Many residents died in their beds while others awoke to choking pain and panic. They tried to run from the cloud but were blinded and choked by the gas and died moments later in the streets. The number of dead still is in question. The Indian government estimates the death toll at about 2300, but other estimates range as high as 10,000. The lower number is based on available records from hospitals and burial grounds; the higher estimate is from such data as the number of death shrouds sold in Bhopal in the days that followed. Estimates of those injured range from 10,000 to 200,000, many of them left with permanent respiratory ailments and vision impairment.

M. N. Nagoo, the Madhya Pradesh director of medical services and one of the many physicians who rushed to the disaster site, described the scene in the following words (Lepkowski, 1985, p. 19):

> I tell you, the morning of December 3 was a sight. People running away from Bhopal, volunteers coming in with needed supplies, schoolboys and girls looking after victims, giving them water, tea, bread. I think 70,000 could have died if we hadn't had the right medicines on hand.
>
> Initially 170,000 persons were treated, out of which 11,500 were critically ill and hospitalized. The rest were put in tents or sheds. With the help of volunteer organizations, scouts, students, we organized medical treatment and arranged for water, medicines, and food. There was tremendous cooperation. We have 500 doctors here now, five major hospitals, 22 clinics, and we called 500 more doctors from the outside, plus 200 more nurses and 700 paramedics. Besides the treatment in hospitals, we organized 25 teams of doctors to give treatment in the affected areas.
>
> The state already had enough drugs like cortisone, bronchial dilators, antibiotics, and Lasix (to combat edema). These were the basic ones we used. Then we got a lot of equipment and oxygen from the government of India and neighboring districts. Great Britain, France, and West Germany airlifted respirators and ventilators to us.
>
> We have kept six clinics open around the clock, besides the 35 units already working and the 30-bed hospital we started at the former residence of the police superintendent next to the Union Carbide plant. Seven more clinics have been opened, four of which perform blood and urine tests.

Clinics in Bhopal continue to treat the victims, most of them suffering from lung or eye damage. Among the survivors, possibly thousands are totally or partially blinded.

Love Canal and Bhopal are human-induced disasters, and by hindsight, they may be viewed as tragedies that need not have occurred. Nevertheless, other human-induced disasters will occur, and together with natural disasters, such as floods, tornadoes, earthquakes, and blizzards, they form a part of the environmental health concerns that health professionals can expect to deal with on a short-term, immediate basis as well as on a long-term basis.

POLLUTION IN THE HOME

Because a concerned society has reacted to the need to improve the quality of our environment, factory emissions, toxic wastes, automobile exhaust, and a host of other environmental hazards have been regulated. The quality of the environment we share has been noticeably improved. However, regulatory agencies in the United States are reluctant to intrude into the privacy of citizens' homes in the cause of pollution control.

Even if it were acceptable to regulate the home environment—to set permissible limits on the concentrations of pollutants as is done in occupational settings—it would be next to impossible to monitor and enforce compliance. As a result the health hazards posed by pollution in homes often are in excess of those in the outside environment or

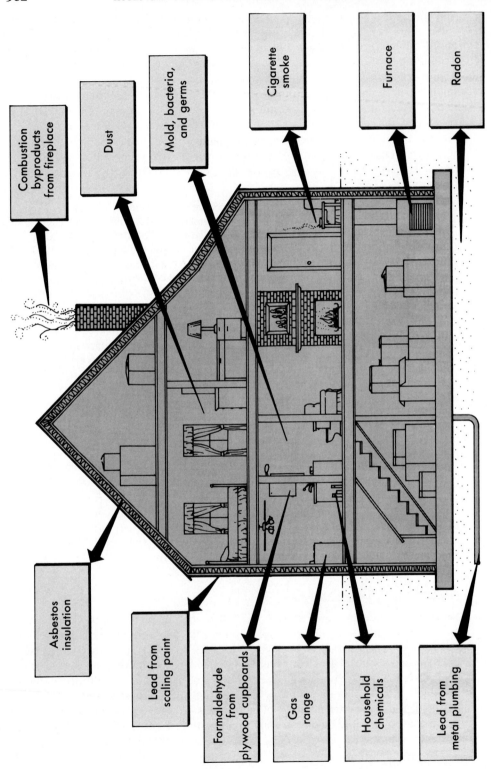

FIG. 25-8 Sources of pollution in the home.

even in industrial settings. The problem is compounded by the fact that most people spend most of their time at home. Fig. 25-8 shows the source of many indoor pollutants.

Some significant indoor air pollutants are included in the following list:

1. *Carbon monoxide* is released by unvented gas stoves, kerosene space heaters, wood stoves, and tobacco smoke. It is a tasteless, colorless, odorless, poisonous gas that can react with hemoglobin in the blood and inhibit the distribution of oxygen by the bloodstream. A smoke-filled room with levels of about 120 ppm of carbon monoxide can cause headaches, dizziness, and a general feeling of dullness. It is known that carbon monoxide can cross the placenta in pregnant women and is believed to be a factor in the lower average birth weight of women who smoke. Approximately 1400 people die annually in the United States from carbon monoxide poisoning, most caused by unvented space heaters.

2. *Asbestos particles* (especially in older homes) are released from fireproofing materials, insulation, ceiling tiles, floor tiles, and other building materials. Asbestos is a generic name for several types of naturally occurring fibrous mineral silicates that were used in industry and construction. All commercial forms have been shown to be carcinogenic to human beings (Leman, Dement, & Wagoner, 1980). Epidemiological studies have focused strongly on exposures in occupational settings. Asbestos insulation, however, has been used in a large number of residences, as well as in public buildings such as schools. Normal aging and deterioration, as well as demolition or remodeling of these structures, will release asbestos fibers into the air and they can be inhaled into the lungs.

3. *Formaldehyde* is a colorless gas, characterized by a strong, pungent odor. It is released in the home environment from particle boards, fiberboards, plywood, and other wood products, as well as from urea-formaldehyde foam insulation. It is strongly suspected as a carcinogen. Exposure to formaldehyde in concentrations in the range of 0.01 to 30 ppm in air has been observed to produce eye, nose, and respiratory tract irritation, headaches, drowsiness, nausea, and diarrhea. An excess of 100 ppm has been characterized as extremely hazardous and possibly fatal. (Committe on Indoor Pollutants, 1981).

4. *Nitrogen oxides* are released indoors from unvented gas stoves and space heaters. At concentrations of 0.05 ppm or higher, not unusual in kitchens where gas is used for cooking, nitrogen dioxide may affect sensory perception and produce eye irritation.

5. *Environmental tobacco smoke* is one of the most familiar indoor pollutants and the major source of indoor airborne particulate matter. In addition to particulates, tobacco smoke contains a variety of other contaminants such as inorganic gases, heavy metals, and various volatile organic compounds, including benzene. It has been well publicized that the person who chooses to smoke greatly increases the risk of the development of heart disease or cancer. Now, however, concern for the health threat of tobacco smoke has been extended to nonsmokers.

The surgeon general has indicated that environmental tobacco smoke—that is, smoke that nonsmokers are exposed to from smokers—poses a risk of lung cancer to the nonsmoker. The EPA states that published risk estimates of lung cancer deaths among such involuntary smokers range from 500 to 5000 per year.

6. *Radon,* which is a colorless, odorless, radioactive gas, is the most serious health threat of the common indoor pollutants. In a survey of 9600 homes in 10 states, the EPA found that 20% are contaminated by potentially health-threatening levels of radon gas. The EPA estimates that radon is responsible for 5000 to 20,000 deaths from lung cancer each year (Table 25-4). According to one estimate (Nero, 1988) hundreds of thousands of Americans are living in houses that have high radon levels, and they receive as large an exposure of radiation yearly as those people living in the vicinity of Chernobyl nuclear

TABLE 25-4 Radon risk evaluation chart				
pCi/l	WL	**Estimated lung cancer deaths due to radon exposure (out of 1000)**	**Comparable exposure levels**	**Comparable risk**
200	1	440-770	1000 times average outdoor level	More than 60 times nonsmoker risk
				4 pack-a-day smoker
100	0.5	270-630	100 times average indoor level	
				2000 chest x-rays per year
40	0.2	120-380		
				2 pack-a-day smoker
20	0.1	60-210	100 times average outdoor level	
				1 pack-a-day smoker
10	0.05	30-120	10 times average indoor level	
				5 times nonsmoker risk
4	0.02	13-50		
				200 chest x-rays per year
2	0.01	7-30	10 times average outdoor level	
				Nonsmoker risk of dying from lung cancer
1	0.005	3-13	Average indoor level	
				20 chest x-rays per year
0.2	0.001	1-3	Average outdoor level	

From Office of Air and Radiation Programs, 1987, Washington, DC: U.S. Environmental Protection Agency.
NOTE: Measurement results are reported in one of two ways: measurement of *radon gas* (pCi/l) or measurement of *radon decay products* (WL).
pCi/l, Picocuries per liter; *WL,* working levels.

power plant did in 1986, when one of its reactors exploded and released radioactive material into the environment.

Radon gas decays to form submicroscopic solid particles called *radon daughters* (actually forms of polonium, a radioactive metal). The solid "daughter" particle, possibly riding piggy-back on a dust particle, can become lodged in the lung and continue to emit radiation. Radon is a natural decay product of uranium and is found in limestone, black shale, and phosphate rock. Most indoor radon comes from rocks and soil around a building and may enter through microscopic cracks and joints in the basement walls.

Testing a home for radon can be fairly simple and relatively inexpensive. Do-it-yourself test kits can be purchased for as little as $10 to $25. Homes with elevated radon levels can be made safe by the use of fairly simple procedures, generally involving ventilation, for a moderate sum, generally about $500 to $1000.

7. *Lead* poisoning has long been recognized as an environmental hazard in the home.

Household water may contain low levels of lead from older plumbing. Probably the most common source is lead-based paint, which, although phased out of use in the 1940s still is prevalent in the painted walls and woodwork of many older homes, especially in low-income urban neighborhoods. Children are particularly vulnerable to lead poisoning from ingestion of chips of scaling paint (see Chapter 9).

NURSING INTERVENTIONS

Community health nurses have as a priority goal the prevention of illness in individuals, families, and groups. An assessment of the stressors in a community that affect the health status of the population must include the environment. The interventions then can be planned that prevent a potential problem from becoming an actual one.

Primary prevention involves anticipating and acting in advance of a health problem. Typically, this includes health education to raise the level of awareness in the community of the potential effect of an environmental stressor.

In a world of increasing concern for environmental hazards, the community health nurse must, when needed, assume the role of environmental risk communicator. The need for such a role was demonstrated when it was found that more than 40% of the persons surveyed in New York State did not know where to go for additional information about indoor radon risks (Boyle & Haltgrave, 1989; Kessler & Levine, 1987). Environmental health education of the individual and the community must stress increased environmental awareness, as well as elimination of unwarranted environmental fears.

Secondary prevention focuses on the detection of existing health problems for the individual, as well as the community level, and responding with early treatment. For individual clients it may include screening and early diagnosis of specific environmental health problems. For example, in communities where asbestos insulation of buildings is common, it may include screening of individual clients for lung cancer and asbestosis and providing treatment as needed. On a community level, secondary prevention might be exemplified by a study to seek out the presence of asbestos insulation in buildings and to initiate remedial action where appropriate.

Tertiary prevention emphasizes rehabilitation and help in the development of an optimal level of functioning. For example, in the case of children suffering from mental retardation or brain damage from lead poisoning, tertiary prevention might involve a special education program to maximize the child's intellectual development. On the community level it might involve an abatement program to "delead" the community.

Application of the Nursing Process

The following case study illustrates the use of the nursing process with a child whose diagnosis was lead poisoning.

Assessment. A community health nurse was referred by a lead-screening clinic to make a home visit on a 3-year-old boy who had been tested for lead levels in his blood. His levels had been abnormally high, and he was considered at high risk for lead poisoning (plumbism), as well as a possible candidate for chelating therapy.

The nurse noted that the house was old, situated in a run-down nieghborhood, and did not seem well maintained. The child lived in a second-floor apartment with his mother, a single parent. The apartment was clean but sparsely furnished. The mother was 18 years old, having given birth to the boy at the age of 15 years. She stated that she received some help from her mother and sister but that she lived alone and maintained her household with some help from social services.

The nursing assessment included a tour of the home. There was a hole in the wall in the boy's bedroom, approximately 1 1/2 feet in diameter. Plaster was falling on the floor. As the nurse watched, the child picked up a small piece and ate it. The mother told him to stop but did not move to halt the behavior. The mother stated that the child was hyperactive and difficult to discipline. Results of a Denver Developmental Screening Test showed him to be within normal developmental stages. However, he did have difficulty sitting still even if bribed with treats and encouraged to cooperate by making a game of the test. A revisit was scheduled for the following week. The mother was asked to sweep up the plaster and call her landlord to fix the wall.

Nursing diagnosis. On the basis of this assessment, the nurse formulated the following nursing diagnosis:

1. Potential for lead poisoning related to unsafe environment
2. Ineffective family coping related to parental knowledge deficit

Planning and implementation. Nursing goals included the following:

1. Arranging for a safe environment for the child
2. Teaching the parent the importance of maintaining a safe environment for the child
3. Teaching the parent appropriate methods of controlling the child's behavior
4. Arranging for follow-up screening to determine the child's lead level

Evaluation. Facilitating the repair of the wall in the child's room became the role of the municipal housing authority. The landlord did not respond to calls from the parent or the nurse. In the meantime the nurse showed the child's mother how to use a plastic paste to repair the wall temporarily.

SUMMARY

This chapter has presented an overview of the environmental factors that can affect the health and well-being of individuals and communities. In recent decades there has been an increasing public awareness of environmental problems. As a result, actions by concerned citizens, as well as legislators, have begun to have a positive effect on pollution. Community health nurses can contribute to the solution of environmental health problems by being well informed and by assuming the role of environmental risk communicator and educator to the individual and the community.

CHAPTER HIGHLIGHTS

- The growth of industry in society created a greater number and variety of waste products in the environment.
- The disposal of solid waste may be accomplished through open dumps, landfills, ocean dumping, or incineration.
- Recyling of wastes offers the advantages of reducing the total amount of waste to be disposed of and preservation of virgin materials.
- Hazardous wastes include radioactive and chemical wastes. Since these wastes are health hazards, proper disposal is critical.
- The latency period between disposal of hazardous waste and the manifestation of adverse health effects may be extremely short, or it may take many years. The effects of many chemicals may be subtle and difficult to detect.
- Water pollution is a serious community health concern because contaminated water

may carry bacteria and viruses associated with diseases such as typhoid, infectious hepatitis, chlorea, and dysentery.

- Excessive noise in the environment can lead to permanent hearing loss, as well as general feelings of stress and fatigue.
- Air pollution is a serious health hazard, especially in large, industrialized cities. Weather conditions also can affect the amount of pollution in the air.
- Environmental accidents may occur quickly or very slowly. They are disasters when they occur in heavily populated areas.
- Pollution in the home is difficult to monitor and regulate. Potential indoor air pollutants include carbon monoxide, asbestos, formaldehyde, nitrogen oxides, tobacco smoke, radon, and lead.

STUDY QUESTIONS

1. Discuss the correlation between population density and pollution in the environment.
2. Describe the difference between open dump and a landfill. List the effect each might have on the health of the people living nearby.
3. Compare the disaster at Love Canal with the disaster at Bhopal.
4. List the negative effects of noise pollution on the health of the individual who experiences it.
5. List the health effects of regulated air pollutants.
6. Describe the adverse health effects from the various forms of radiation.
7. List and describe three indoor pollutants and their effects on the health of the individual.

REFERENCES

Boyle, M. & Holtgrave D. (1989). *Environmental Science and Technology, 23,* 1335-1337.

Committee on Indoor Pollutants. (1981). *Indoor pollutants.* Washington, DC: National Academy Press.

Cordle, F., Locke, R., & Springer, J. (1982). Risk assessment in a federal regulatory agency: An assessment of risk associated with the human consumption of some species of fish contaminated with polychlorinated biphenyls (PCBs). *Environmental Health Perspectives 45,* 171-182.

Department of Health, Education and Welfare. (1979). *Healthy people,* Washington, DC: U.S. Government Printing Office.

Environmental Protection Agency. (1988). *Environmental progress and challenges: EPA's update,* Washington, DC: U.S. Environmental Protection Agency.

Fein, G.G., Schwartz, P.M., Jacobson, S.W., & Jacobson, J.L. (1983). Environmental toxins and behavioral development. *American Psychologist,* 1188-1196.

Fein, G.G., Jacobson, J.L., Jacobson, S.W., Schwartz, P.M., & Dowler, J.K. (1984). *Journal of Pediatrics, 105* (2), 315-320.

The Global 2000 Report to the President. (1980). *Entering the twenty-first century,* (Vol 2, Technical report), Washington DC: U.S. Government Printing Office.

Grisham, J. W., (Ed.) (1986). *Health aspects of the disposal of waste chemicals.* New York: Pergamon.

Hall, R. M. Jr., Watson, T., Davidson, J. J., Case, D. R., Bryson, N. S. (1986). *RCRA hazardous wastes handbook* (7th ed.). Washington DC: Government Institutes.

Hileman, B. (1988, February 8). The Great Lakes cleanup effort, *Chemical & Engineering News,* pp. 22-39.

Holum, J. R. (1977). *Topics and terms in environmental problems,* New York: Wiley.

Jacobson, S. W., Fein, G. G., Jacobson, J. L., Schwartz, P. M., & Dowler, J. K. (1985). The effect of intra-uterine PCB exposure on visual recognition memory. *Child Development, 56,* 853-860.

Kessler, S., & Levine, E. K. (1987). *American Journal of Medical Genetics, 28,* 361-70.

Lemen, R. A., Dement, J. M., & Wagoner, J. K. (1980). Epidemiology of asbestos-related diseases. *Environmental Health Perspectives, 34,* 1-11.

Lepkowski, W. (1985). Bhopal report: People of India struggle toward appropriate response to tragedy. *Chemical & Engineering News, 63*(6), 16-26.

Levine, A. G. (1982). *Love Canal: Science, politics, and people,* Lexington, MA: Heath.

Miller, T. G. (1986). *Environmental science: An introduction,* Belmont, CA.: Wadsworth.

Mossman, K. L., Thomas, D. S., & Dritschilo, A. (1986). Environmental radiation and cancer. *Journal of Environmental Science and Health, 4,* 119-159.

Nero A. V., Jr. (1988). Controlling indoor air pollution. *Scientific American, 258*(5); 42-48.

New York State Department of Health. (1981). *Love Canal special report to the governor and legislature.* Albany, NY: Author.

Schwartz, P. M., Jacobson, S. W., Fein, G., Jacobson, J. L., & Price, H. A. (1983, March). Lake Michigan fish consumption as a source of polychlorinated biphenyls in human cord serum, maternal serum, and milk. *American Journal of Public Health, 73* (3), 293-296.

Silverman, G. B. (1989). Love Canal: A retrospective, *Environmental Reporter, 20*(Pt.2), 835-850.

Tchobanoglous, G., Theisen, H., & Eliassen, R. (1977). *Solid Wastes: Engineering principles and management issues.* New York: McGraw-Hill.

Turk, J. & Turk, A. (1988). *Environmental Science,* Philadelphia: Saunders.

Wadden, R. A., & Scheff, P. A. (1983). *Indoor air pollution: Characterization, prediction and control,* New York: Wiley.

Waldbott, G. L. (1978). *Health effects of environmental pollutants,* St. Louis: Mosby.

Wilson, R. (1979, February). Analyzing the daily risks of life. *Technology Review, 81*(4), 40-46.

Wilson, R., & Crouch, E. A. C. (1988, April 17). Risk assessment and comparisons: An Introduction. *Science, 236,* 267-270.

Substance Abuse

ELIZABETH SHENK

Overall, 70.4 million Americans older than 12 years of age have tried some kind of illicit drug at least once in their lifetime.

(NATIONAL INSTITUTE ON DRUG ABUSE, 1986)

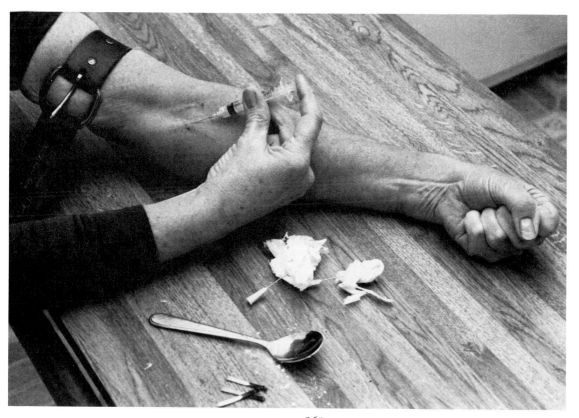

OBJECTIVES

At the conclusion of this chapter the student will be able to:
1. Define the key terms listed
2. Describe the terms *dependence* and *tolerance* as they relate to drug and alcohol use
3. Describe what is meant by enabling behavior
4. Give two reasons that have been proposed to explain the development of chemical dependency
5. Describe four disorders associated with substance abuse and chemical dependency
6. Describe what is meant by the term *drug addiction*
7. Cite at least four populations that are at risk for chemical dependency
8. Discuss the relationship of acquired immunodeficiency syndrome to substance abuse
9. Name at least 10 common substances of abuse
10. Describe aspects of primary, secondary, and tertiary prevention in relation to substance abuse

KEY TERMS

Abstinence	Detoxification
Abuse	Drug abuse
Addiction	Drug addiction
Al-Anon	Habituation
Alcoholics Anonymous	Impairment
Alcoholism	Overdose
Blackout	Substance abuse
Chemical dependency	Tolerance
Cross-tolerance	Withdrawal syndrome
Dependence	

I t is important for the community health nurse to understand substance abuse because of the number of persons it affects. The nurse who works in the community is in a unique position to assist in many different ways in the detection, treatment, and rehabilitation of substance abusers.

ISSUES AND TRENDS IN SUBSTANCE ABUSE

The use of alcohol predates recorded history. Cultures from many parts of the world have used alcoholic beverages to celebrate important events. Alcohol has been consumed as medicine, as a form of magic, and as a part of worship services. In America there have been various legal views on the use of alcohol. In 1642 drunkenness was punishable by a fine. In 1790 a law was passed that gave every soldier a portion of daily liquor. Prohibition, which forbade the production or sale of alcoholic beverages, was enacted in 1919 and repealed in 1933. Even today the use of alcohol is sanctioned by society.

The history of nonmedical drug use goes back thousands of years. As early as 5000

BC the Sumerians referred to a "joy plant" (believed to be the opium poppy plant). Since then, drugs have played a significant role in almost every culture. In the United States the first national awareness of a drug problem occurred in the mid-1860s during the Civil War, when injured and wounded soldiers became addicted to the morphine that was used to relieve pain. In recent years the incidence of drug abuse has risen.

Between 1940 and 1960, drug abuse in the United States was considered to be a ghetto-related phenomenon. As drug use increased, this view was proved untrue. As patients sought drugs from physicians to make them feel better, more and more psychoactive drugs were prescribed. Today Americans classify drug abuse as the number one problem in the United States.

One current trend in substance abuse is the high incidence of acquired immunodeficiency syndrome (AIDS) that occurs with intravenous (IV) drug abuse. The number of persons with AIDS has increased each year, and the reason for the shift in infection source from homosexual white men to a broader group is attributed mainly to IV drug use. Nearly 75% of women with AIDS were infected when either they or their sexual partners used drugs. Because blood-to-blood contact is the most efficient mode of transmission of the human immunodeficiency virus (HIV), sharing a needle is a more certain way of spreading the disease than is sexual contact. In addition, drug abusers do not take the responsibility to protect themselves and others from the spread of the disease as have homosexual men and women.

SCOPE OF THE PROBLEM

Alcoholism is a common health problem that may exacerbate other health disorders. Excessive alcohol consumption can lead to coma or death from acute alcohol poisoning or to numerous other health problems if the drinking continues over a long period of time. (Associated disorders are discussed later in this chapter.)

Estimates are that about 90 million persons use alcohol, and at least 18 million are alcohol abusers or "problem drinkers." In addition, alcoholism affects the functioning of another 30 million friends and relatives of alcohol abusers (Fitzgerald, 1988). Industries lose billions of dollars annually because of alcoholism. This figure includes medical expenses, lost wages, decreased production, motor vehicle accidents, and crime. Nearly half of convicted criminals were found to be under the influence of alcohol when they committed the crime. An alarming number of fatalities from accidents are alcohol related.

It is difficult to estimate the number of persons addicted to drugs. Overall, 70.4 million Americans older than 12 years of age have tried some kind of illicit drug at least once in their lifetime (National Institute on Drug Abuse, 1986), a figure that consitutes about 37% of the population in this age range. The greatest number (33%) have tried marijuana, whereas 10% have experimented with cocaine. The highest rate of use of hallucinogens and inhalants is among young persons.

During the past century a great increase in chemical dependency has occurred among adolescents, women, and elderly persons. In most parts of the world the rate of chemical dependency increases as income increases. The media also influence drug use.

THEORIES OF CAUSATION

Numerous theories have been suggested to explain the causes of chemical dependency. These theories have been divided into the following three main categories:
1. Physiologic
   a. Genetotrophic—related to genetically determined biochemical defect
   b. Endocrinal —caused by dysfunction of the endocrine system

    c. Genetic—30% to 50% risk of alcoholism developing in sons or daughters of alcoholic parents; in 60% of cases alcoholism will develop in identical twins of an alcoholic parent

2. Psychologic
   a. Oral fixation—resulting from lack of a warm, loving relationship with a mother figure during childhood
   b. Behavioral learning theory—association of alcohol ingestion with a positive experience leads to substance abuse

3. Sociocultural or cultural
   a. Cultural—relationship between various groups in society and incidence of alcoholism
   b. Moral—substance abuse as moral fault or sin of the alcohol abuser (Kirk & Bradford, 1987)

Ongoing research continues to determine the causes of substance abuse. No one theory has been found to be all-inclusive. It is apparent, however, that alcohol-addicted persons share common personality characteristics, which include dependency, denial, and delusion. Substance abuse has been found to occur at higher rates in some families. It is likely that the origin of substance abuse is multicausal.

FACTORS THAT PLACE POPULATIONS AT RISK
Poverty

Although the incidence of substance abuse has not been found to be positively correlated with poverty, it is not uncommon to find a greater number of persons addicted to drugs and alcohol among those who live in poverty inasmuch as drug use may result in lost jobs, income, and family. The irresponsibility that usually accompanies chemical dependency makes it difficult for these persons to hold a job and follow through on financial obligations. Thus they become poor.

The impoverished substance abuser poses a special challenge to the community health nurse because of the inadequate resources available to treat those who are without financial resources. The person may want help but may be unable to obtain it. In addition, the impoverished substance abuser may turn to drug dealing or trafficking as a way to escape poverty. It is not uncommon for young persons to earn thousands of dollars a day through drug dealing, which may seem like an easy escape from poverty.

The Homeless. It may be difficult to intervene in treatment of the homeless. Generally the prognosis for this population is poor because of the difficulty in changing patterns of behavior. Detoxification centers, shelters, and other short-term programs that offer medical care, food, and shelter are located in most metropolitan areas. These resources often are inadequate, and long-term provisions for care are not readily available. (Problems of the homeless are discussed in chapter 21).

Culture

A relationship has been found between various groups in society and the use of substances. Jews, Mormons, and Moslems, for instance, have a low rate of alcoholism, whereas the rate among the French is high, and the Soviet Union recently reported a serious problem with alcoholism. Although the reason for this incidence may be in part cultural, experts believe that further study is needed to reach definitive conclusions.

Alcohol abuse among native Americans and native Alaskans is well documented and presents a challenge for the nurse who works with these populations. A major cause of deaths among Indians is directly related to alcohol abuse, including accidents, cirrhosis, suicide, and homicide (Andre, 1979).

In these groups drinking usually is viewed as socially acceptable and may be the focus of get-togethers. There are few sanctions against drunken behavior, and the goal of drinking usually is to get drunk. This outlook almost always leads to problems with alcohol. In addition, drinking is believed to be a way to escape feelings of anger and helplessness, often caused by forced assimilation into modern mainstream society. Even today, Indians who leave the reservation for urban settings often experience long periods of unemployment, which may lead to the use of drugs and alcohol.

To help decrease substance abuse the community health nurse who deals with persons from a different culture needs to be aware of these cultural influences. Involving this population in the planning of effective prevention and treatment programs is essential to positive change.

Youth

A high-risk group for the development of substance abuse is the young. Drug abuse has increased drastically among this group in the United States and other countries. Explanations that have been offered for this increase include the affluence of society and increased leisure time and financial resources as compared with youth of the past.

Drug and alcohol use among adolescents also can serve as a rite of passage from childhood into adulthood. It is associated with the risk-taking and rebellious behavior that often is characteristic of adolescents attempting to determine their own identity. Further, the influence of the peer group usually is stronger than that of the family or church. It has been found that adolescents drink more frequently and more heavily as the extent of drinking among their peers increases.

It also has been found that youth tend to use a variety of mood-altering substances; two substances that are prevalently abused are alcohol and marijuana. Initial experimentation with drinking often takes place within the home with parental approval. As the adolescent becomes older, the drinking takes place outside the home. Although many youths may identify daily drinking as dangerous, they see no harm in getting drunk at a party.

The adolescent who is a substance abuser also may exhibit other problem behaviors, including delinquent behavior, precocious sexual behavior, poor school performance, and a high dropout rate from school. Alcohol-related accidents are common, as are other forms of violence and suicide.

The community health nurse who assists in the treatment of adolescent substance abusers must consider the stability of the family (see the next section in this chapter concerning the family, as well as Chapter 15). Also, identification and treatment of the adolescent can be extremely difficult and expensive. This group generally is treated most effectively in treatment centers equipped with special adolescent services. In addition, it is important to keep in mind normal adolescent developmental tasks and how they affect the problem of substance abuse. Substance abuse can prevent the adolescent from successfully moving through developmental phases.

Family Patterns

Alcoholism and drug abuse have been found to occur more frequently in some families; 50% of all alcohol abusers have an alcohol-addicted parent, grandparent, brother, or sister. Children of alcoholic parents are twice as likely to experience alcohol-related problems as are children of nonalcoholic parents (Fitzgerald, 1988). It also has been found that the children of alcoholic relatives tend to feel a personal immunity to alcoholism because they are certain that they are familiar with the consequences and would never allow themselves to develop such a problem. Family members are affected either directly because of physical, sexual, or emotional abuse or indirectly because of the unpredictability of the alcohol abuser's behavior.

In addition, children and spouses of chemically dependent persons tend to feel a sense of shame and guilt and often exist in isolation from their peer group. They may feel that they have a unique and devastating problem that others are incapable of understanding. Children brought up in a home with alcoholic parents will carry the scars for a lifetime if they do not receive appropriate therapy and help.

Chemical dependency has a disruptive effect on the entire family. Family members often become involved with the alcohol abuser's behavior to the extent that their behaviors become compulsive patterns of dysfunctional reactions that include enabling behavior. Psychiatric treatment of family members or school and behavioral problems of children should alert the nurse to explore the presence of a substance-abuse problem in the family. Chemical dependency must be seen as a family disease, and chemically dependent persons must be treated as part of the family unit if they are to have the best chance to remain abstinent (Captain, 1989).

Jackson (1954) identifies the following seven stages through which the family passes in adjusting to alcoholism or substance abuse:

- Stage 1—Attempts to deny the problem (episodes of excessive drinking are rationalized and not discussed)
- Stage 2—Attempts to eliminate the problem (as the use becomes more of a problem, the spouse may try to control the drinking by throwing out the alcohol or by buying it, and the family becomes more isolated)
- Stage 3—Disorganization of the family (the family equilibrium breaks down, hostility is expressed, children are caught in the middle, and financial and legal problems are common)
- Stage 4—Efforts to reorganize despite the problem (spouse or child assumes a great deal of the alcohol abuser's responsibility and treats the alcoholic as a child
- Stage 5—Attempts to escape the problem (marital separation or divorce may occur, or if the family unit remains intact, the family arranges its life-style around the alcohol abuser)
- Stage 6—Reorganization of part of the family (the spouse and children make a new home without the alcohol abuser, who may threaten or beg to get back into the home)
- Stage 7—Recovery and reorganization of the whole family (if the alcohol abuser maintains sobriety, the family may reunite, but the adjustment may not be easy)

Babies of Addicted Mothers

Women who are addicted to substances during their pregnancies can cause damage to their babies. The number of such infants is increasing; one estimate is that about 10% of newborns suffer from the affects of substance abuse, including the following:

1. The infant is born with an actual addiction and experiences withdrawal symptoms of varying degrees.
2. The infant becomes ill because of the drug's toxic effects.
3. The infant has brain damage or other congenital problems because of the teratogenic characteristics of the drug.

The problems associated with fetal alcohol syndrome have been documented over a long period of time. Women who drink excessively during pregnancy have a higher incidence of infants with birth defects such as mental retardation, growth disorders, and malformed body parts. These women also have a high incidence of spontaneous abortions, stillbirths, and infant deaths. Even moderate drinking can cause birth defects in infants.

The problem of babies of addicted mothers is an area well-suited for intervention from the community health nurse. Not only can education and monitoring during pregnancy prove helpful; the family with an infant suffering from problems caused by addiction will need a great deal of assistance in providing the required care.

One area of need that has been identified to aid this population is the treatment center that can treat the pregnant substance abuser, as well as the mother and baby together after the birth.

Women

The incidence of chemical dependency in women has increased dramatically in the twentieth century. The ratio between alcoholic men and alcoholic women is steadily decreasing. Women also are more likely to be dually addicted or polydrug abusers.

It has been common for society to view chemically dependent women as immoral, whereas the man who is an alcohol abuser is seen as "macho" or "just having fun." The stigma of being a woman substance abuser may increase the denial by all concerned and further handicaps her from obtaining treatment. Studies have found that the family tends to deny the woman's drinking problem longer than does the family of a male, inasmuch as it is difficult for family members to accept that their wife, mother, or daughter has a drinking problem. Because they have been able to conceal their drinking for a longer period of time, women have been known as "closet" drinkers. They also have been protected from facing the consequences of their substance abuse; for example, women are less likely to receive citations for driving while intoxicated (DWI) than are men.

Women also are more likely to go to a family physician for vague complaints and receive a prescription for a mood-altering drug such as diazepam (Valium) or chlordiazepoxide (Librium). These drugs often are combined with alcohol consumption, which leads to polyaddictions and cross-tolerance.

The Elderly

The problem of substance abuse in elderly persons is receiving more attention as the true nature of the problem is coming to light. Estimates are that perhaps 5% to 10% of persons older than 60 years of age are alcohol or drug abusers. These problems often develop as a result of stress, loss, depression, and other negative aspects of aging. Alcohol is the substance most abused by the elderly, followed by prescribed mood-altering drugs. (Caroselli-Karinja, 1985).

Older persons who began to have drinking problems early in life may exhibit signs of late stages of alcoholism, including liver cirrhosis, polyneuropathy, malnutrition, alcohol-related dementia, Wernicke-Korsakoff syndrome, and cerebellar degeneration. The progression seen in long-term chronic alcohol abusers covers a period of 20 to 40 years, whereas deterioration in persons who begin drinking heavily in later years is relatively rapid.

Chemical dependency in the elderly often goes undetected and untreated. The effects of the abuse may be explained as a sign of senility or chronic brain syndrome or as a natural consequence of growing older. Also, society may view substance abuse in the elderly as untreatable or may believe that the elderly deserve this "pleasure" in life. The community health nurse can be invaluable in detecting chemical dependency in an elderly person with a history of malnutrition, falls, depression, or other alcohol-related physical disabilities.

Nurses

Nurses have been found to be at high risk for the development of substance abuse and chemical dependency. Although it is difficult to estimate precisely the incidence in nurses, the American Nurses' Assocation (ANA) estimates that between 6% to 8% of nurses have a substance abuse problem (ANA, 1984). Identification of these nurses may be extremely difficult inasmuch as they often resist treatment because of the stigma. Traditionally, nurses have been believed to be immune from such problems or to know better and society may view nurses who abuse alcohol with disdain. In addition, affected nurses may fear legal or licensing reprisals, which may prevent them from seeking help.

Nurses are at risk for chemical dependency for a number of reasons. The work is viewed as stressful and demanding with few positive rewards (Green, 1989). Nurses may feel they have little control over their own working situations. They also have ready access to many mood-altering drugs, especially narcotics (the drugs most abused by nurses). Often, however, substance abuse in a nurse begins with legal prescriptions for drugs. The nurse continues to obtain a supply of drugs from legal sources for as long as possible and begins to divert drugs only when the addiction worsens. Some nurses have been found to come from dysfunctional families and may enter nursing to feel good about who they are. Because of this co-dependent behavior, they are at increased risk of developing substance abuse themselves (Zerwelch & Michaels, 1989).

One study of 100 nurses showed that those who abuse drugs often are high achievers (Bissell & Haberman, 1984). Most were in the top third of their class, held demanding and responsible jobs, were highly respected for excellent work habits that continued after substance use became heavy, and were ambitious and achievement oriented, often working on advanced degrees.

The community health nurse should be aware of the possibility of chemical dependency in colleagues. Some signs of substance abuse in nurses include excessive absenteeism and tardiness, excessive medication errors, illogical charting, isolating themselves at work, poor judgment and mistakes, appearing at work early and staying late, and signs of drug withdrawal. As the chemical dependency worsens, so will the job performance. Behavior that interferes with job performance should be documented.

Just as the general public, nurses tend to turn their backs on chemically dependent colleagues. They may enable them by covering up for them, ignore them for fear of getting involved, or refuse to admit the possibility of an alcohol or drug problem. However, the worst thing that a nurse can do regarding a chemically dependent colleague is to do nothing.

Most states have now established peer-assistance programs that offer assistance to the impaired nurse. These programs usually are linked with a state board of nursing or a professional organization, or both.

COMMON SUBSTANCES OF ABUSE
Alcohol

Alcohol is a central nervous depressant. The so-called stimulating effect of alcohol occurs because the first areas affected are the higher centers of the brain that control judgment

TABLE 26-1 Effects of varying blood alcohol levels	
Level (mg)	**Effect**
50-75 (0.05-0.075%)	Pleasant, relaxed state, mild sedation, loosening of inhibitions
100-200 (0.1-0.2%)	Overt signs of intoxication: loosening of the tongue, clumsiness, beginning emotional changes
200-400 (0.2-0.45%)	Severe intoxication: difficulty speaking, stumbling, emotional lability
400-500 (0.4-0.5%)	Stupor, coma
>500 (0.5%)	Usually fatal

and self-control. As alcohol intake increases, other areas of the brain also are affected. Unconsciousness may occur, respirations may slow, and death may result.

Alcohol does not require digestion and is absorbed in both the stomach and the intestine. An empty stomach increases absorption. After ingestion, small amounts of alcohol are lost through breathing and in the urine, but 90% of alcohol is broken down by the liver. The active ingredient in alcoholic beverages is ethyl alcohol, or ethanol. A 12-ounce bottle of beer, a 4-ounce glass of wine, and 1 1/2 ounces of "hard liquor" contain similar amounts of alcohol.

Alcohol has a diuretic effect. Increased amounts of electrolytes, including potassium, magnesium, and zinc, may be excreted in the urine of a heavy drinker. Prolonged use of alcohol has a toxic effect on the mucosa of the intestine, which results in decreased absorption of thiamine, folic acid, and vitamin B_{12}.

Alcohol is not converted to glycogen, and it provides the body with calories but no minerals or vitamins. One ounce of alcohol provides 200 kcal, but these are "empty calories." This accounts for malnourishment in many alcohol abusers who maintain near-normal body weight.

Blood alcohol levels depend on the amount of alcohol ingested and the size of the individual. Most states designate blood alcohol serum levels of 100 mg/100 ml (0.10%) as the legal limit for driving a motor vehicle. Higher blood alcohol levels have increasingly more side effects (Table 26-1).

Stimulants

Stimulants are natural and synthetic drugs that have a strong stimulating effect on the central nervous systems and are accompanied by a feeling of alertness and self-confidence. When stimulants reach the brain, they cause the neuron transmitters to fire off messages too quickly. Other results include dilation of the pupils, increases in pulse and blood pressures, reduction of fatigue, reduction of appetite, and an increase in concentration. When the feeling of alertness wears off, however, the person experiences fatigue and depression, as well as a feeling of lethargy and anxiety. Drugs included in this category are amphetamines, cocaine, caffeine, and nicotine (Fitzgerald, 1988). These drugs will be discussed separately.

Stimulants have the potential to produce tolerance, but usually they do not cause symptoms of physical withdrawal. Psychological dependence is common. Side effects of stimulant use include restlessness, dizziness, insomnia, headaches, diarrhea, constipation, and lack of appetite. Persons who ingest a large amount of stimulants over a period of time may experience extreme agitation and anxiety. Death may occur as a result of a cerebral hemorrhage or heart attack. Collapse from exhaustion during the use of stimulants can occur. Withdrawal can lead to profound depression and suicide.

Amphetamines

Amphetamines are synthetic psychoactive drugs that are available in capsule or tablet form. Current belief is that amphetamines increase the release of norepinephrine. The resulting stimulation increases alertness, concentration, learning ability, and attention span. Medical uses of amphetamines include the treatment of narcolepsy, obesity, fatigue, and depression. Methylphenidate (Ritalin), an amphetamine-like drug, often is used to treat children who are hyperactive. Commonly used amphetamines and their brand names are dextroamphetamine (Dexedrine), metamphetamine (Methidrine), and amphetamine (Benzedrine). Street names include pep pills, dexies, bennies, ups, speed, crystal, meth, and whites.

Cocaine

Cocaine (gold dust or champagne of drugs) has been called the recreational drug of the 1980s. Estimates are that there are 5000 new cocaine users daily and that as many as 8 million persons use cocaine more than once a month. As many as 1.6 million persons are addicted to cocaine (Fitzgerald, 1988). It is a psychoactive drug that comes from the leaves of the South American coca bush. It was first used by the members of early South American tribes, and its use was encouraged by the Spaniards, who found that the natives worked longer and harder and needed less food when they used cocaine.

At one time cocaine was used as an ingredient in many products, including syrups, nasal sprays, cigarettes, liquors, and cola beverages. It also was recommended, at one time, as a treatment for alcoholism. In 1914, the nonmedical use of cocaine was prohibited. It is used medically as an anesthetic of choice for some procedures of the nose and throat and as a part of Brompton's mixture, which is administered for pain control in patients with cancer.

Cocaine is similar to the neurotransmitter norepinephrine. It mimics norepinephrine's action in carrying neuron impulses between cells. With the use of cocaine the brain cuts back on its own production of norepinephrine; when the cocaine "high" wears off, the supply of norepinephrine is depleted, which leads to the cocaine "crash." Continuous use of cocaine can result in a more permanent depletion of the neurotransmitter, which produces a parkinsonian-type syndrome.

Cocaine is ingested by sniffing, smoking, or injection. Cocaine also may be "free-based" (a process of heating the drug to separate it from impurities). When free-based cocaine is injected, it produces a high that is more intense and short-lived than when cocaine is smoked.

A newer form of cocaine that is now readily available in most locations is called "crack," a mixture of cocaine and common baking soda and water. It gets its name from the sound it makes as it is used. It is less expensive than other forms of cocaine and is considered highly addicting (Fitzgerald, 1988). Other street names for cocaine include blow, coke, dust, flake, nose candy, rock, snow, super-blow, toot, and white.

Chronic sniffing of cocaine can destroy the nasal tissues. Smoking it can cause lesions in the lungs. Tolerance and psychological dependence can develop, and an overdose can cause convulsions, respiratory paralysis, and death. A cocaine psychosis has been reported that is characterized by a loss of pleasure and orientation, by hallucinations, and by insomnia. Abrupt withdrawal from cocaine does not lead to physical withdrawal.

Caffeine

Caffeine is the most accepted and most used psychoactive substance in the United States. Many beverages, medications, and other products contain caffeine. It has been used as an additive in carbonated beverages since the early 1900s. Because of its availability and widespread use, most persons do not view caffeine as a drug.

In its pure state, caffeine is a white powder or consists of white, needle-shaped crystals. It stimulates the central nervous system (CNS), the digestive system, and the kidneys. Body metabolism is increased, and blood pressure is raised. Large doses of caffeine cause tachycardia, headaches, nervousness, insomnia, and stomach distress. Physical dependence occurs with a regular intake of 350 mg for an adult (a cup of brewed coffee contains 75 to 155 mg). Withdrawal symptoms are severe headache, irritability, and fatigue.

Nicotine

Nicotine is one of the most widely abused drugs today. It is far easier to become addicted to cigarettes than to alcohol or to other drugs. Smoking also is physically damaging. It has been linked to heart and blood vessel disease, chronic bronchitis, emphysema, and cancer.

The tobacco plant belongs to the genus *Nicotiana*, a member of the nightshade family. Evidence has been found that tobacco use occurred as early as 200 AD. Tobacco is ingested by chewing or inhaling. The nicotine in tobacco acts as a stimulant to the CNS and also acts as an appetite depressant. Withdrawal symptoms include a decrease in heart rate, weight gain, impairment of psychomotor performance, nervousness and anxiety, headaches, fatigue, and insomnia.

Barbiturates

Barbiturates are synthetic drugs that are classified as sedative-hypnotic agents. They are derived from barbituric acid and are used medically to treat high blood pressure, epilepsy, and insomnia and to sedate patients before and during surgery.

Barbiturates are swallowed (capsule or elixir form), used as a suppository, or injected. Drugs of this class were first synthesized in the early 1900s. Street names of barbiturates include yellow jacket (pentobarbital), red devil (secobarbital) phennie (phenobarbital), blue heaven or blue devil (amobarbital), barbs, downs or downers, rainbows, blues, and goof balls.

Barbiturates cause depression of the CNS, including slowing of physical and mental reflexes. Continued use of these drugs can cause physical and psychological dependence, as well as tolerance. Barbiturates produce a feeling of well-being, euphoria, and relief from anxiety. Side effects include difficulty in breathing, lethargy, nausea, and dizziness. Alcohol and other CNS depressants potentiate the effects of barbiturates. Withdrawal symptoms include irritability, restlessness, anxiety, and sleep disturbances. In severe form, withdrawals may cause convulsions and delirium.

Tranquilizers

Drugs classified as tranquilizers generally are referred to as major and minor tranquilizers. The major tranquilizers include drugs used to treat psychiatric illlnesses and generally are not abused.

Minor tranquilizers are psychoactive drugs that are taken to reduce anxiety. First developed in 1950, they are commonly prescribed and are available in capsule, tablet, and liquid forms. Common types of tranquilizers are those found in the benzodiazepine family and include chlordiazepoxide (Librium), diazepam (Valium), oxazepam (Serax), lorazepam (Ativan), and clorazepate (Tranxene). It is estimated that more than 65 million prescriptions are written yearly for Valium, 75% by physicians who are not psychiatrists (Fitzgerald, 1988).

Hallucinogens

Hallucinogens are drugs—both natural and synthetic—that affect the mind and produce changes in perception and thinking. Included in this category are phencyclidine (PCP), lysergic acid diethylamide (LSD), mescaline, psilocybin, and 3,4-methylenedioxyamphetamine (MDA). Hallucinogens are found in the streets in a wide range of forms, including powder, peyote buttons, mushrooms, capsules, and tablets. LSD may be found on blotter paper, chips, and sheets of paper, including tattoos or stamplike pictures of cartoon figures. Hallucinogens usually are taken orally, although MDA may be sniffed or injected. These drugs sometimes are placed on sugar cubes or mixed in other food. PCP may be sprinkled on marijuana and smoked. When it is combined with marijuana, it is called *sheba*. PCP may be injected or snorted. Some common street names for hallucinogens are listed in Table 26-2.

Most of the effects of hallucinogens are psychological, although nausea and vomiting are common reactions. These drugs act as stimulants at first and produce depressed appetite, dilated pupils, and increases in body temperature and heart and respiration rates. Hallucinogens have a profound psychological effect that often is described as a process of amplication, with the drug acting as a catalyst. These processes are called "trips." A person's attempts to resist the effects of the drug seem to increase the chances of a negative experience, or a "bad trip." These negative experiences are characterized by tremendous confusion, unpleasant sensory images, and extreme panic. With large doses of PCP there may be respiratory or cardiac arrest. Flashbacks may occur with the use of hallucinogens; that is, the user reexperiences the effects of the drug without having taken it again.

Narcotics

Narcotics are drugs that are derived from the opium poppy or are produced synthetically. In the nineteenth century tincture of opium was called God's own medicine (GOM). In general, narcotics lower the perception of pain. Narcotics include heroin, morphine, opium, codeine, meperidine, and methadone. Narcotics are injected, sniffed, smoked, or taken by mouth. Street names for heroin include H, horse, junk, hard stuff, smack, and scag.

TABLE 26-2   Common street names of hallucinogens

Drug	Street name
LSD	Acid, barrels, blotter, domes, microdots, purple haze, windowpane
Mescaline	Buttons, cactus, mesc, mescal buttons
MDA	Love drug, mellow drug of America
Psilocybin	Magic mushroom, shroom
PCP	Angel dust, animal tranquilizer, crystal, dust, hog, embalming fluid, KJ killer, peace pill, synthetic marijuana

Effects of narcotics include shallow breathing; reduced hunger, thirst, and sexual drive; and drowsiness. The user may experience euphoria, lethargy, heaviness of the limbs, and apathy. Overdose of narcotics can cause coma, convulsions, respiratory arrest, and death. If narcotics are injected, there is a risk of hepatitis or AIDS and other infections such as septicemia. With narcotics, tolerance and physical and psychological addiction develop. Withdrawal may be painful and requires medical supervision. Clonidine (Catapres) often is used for detoxification. Symptoms of withdrawal include nausea, cramps, chills, sweating, restlessness, and runny nose.

Cannabis

Cannabis, or marijuana, comes from the Indian hemp plant (*Cannabis sativa*). It can grow wild; it also is fairly easily cultivated. It grows throughout the world, and its use has been recorded as long ago as 2700 BC. It usually is smoked as a cigarette (joint or reefer) or in a pipe or "bong." Slang terms for marijuana include dope, grass, herb, joint, pot, reefer, roach, smoke, snuff, and weed. Marijuana has been used for medical and nonmedical uses for more than 3000 years. Its popularity as a street drug began in the nineteenth century, and it is commonly abused today. Hashish or hash is more concentrated than marijuana and produces more intense symptoms. The primary psychoactive agent of marijuana is tetrahydrocannabinol (THC) (Fitzgerald, 1988). In low doses it acts as a mild sedative. In higher doses it has properties similar to the hallucinogens.

Marijuana's role in reducing eye pressure in glaucoma and in controlling side effects of chemotherapy is being evaluated. Physical effects of marijuana include drying of the eyes and mouth, increase in appetite, reddening of the eyes, and impairment of short-term memory. It raises the heart rate and blood pressure while lowering the body temperature and producing loss of coordination and possible confusion. Research shows that marijuana may affect chromosome division and cause birth defects. Persons who smoke marijuana have been found to have a lowered resistance to infection. Also, the tar content of marijuana cigarettes is 7% to 20% that of regular cigarettes, leading to respiratory problems (Fitzgerald, 1988). Marijuana is fat-soluble and may be stored in the body for as long as several months.

Psychological effects of marijuana include an altering by perception by the senses. The user has a sense of well-being and intoxication, although depression and panic may occur. Marijuana is psychologically addictive and anxiety reactions may occur.

Deliriants

Deliriants are any chemicals that give off fumes or vapors that, when inhaled, produce symptoms similar to intoxication. They may be called inhalants. The fumes or vapors from inhalants are sniffed through the nose, or the vapors are put into a bag or captured in a balloon to increase the concentration of the inhaled fumes.

The history of the use of inhalants is traced back to ancient Greece. Sniffing of commerical products and solvents was first documented in the 1950s. Deliriants or inhalants have a psychoactive or mood-altering effect when the vapors are inhaled and sniffed. Most fall into one of three categories: solvents, aerosol sprays, or anesthetics. Solvents include commercial products such as glue, gasoline, kerosene, lighter fluid, "white out," and nail polish remover. Aerosol products include hair sprays, deodorant, insecticides, and cookware sprays. Anesthetics that are used recreationally include ether, chloroform, and nitrous oxide. Amyl nitrate and butyl nitrate, drugs used for treatment of cardiac disease, also are abused; these are called whippets.

Almost all inhalants are CNS depressants that slow the user's heart rate, brain activity, and breathing. Other effects include slurred speech, blurred vision, inflamed mucous membranes, light-headedness, ringing in the ears, watering eyes, loss of coordination, and excessive nasal secretions. With high doses, the user may lose consciousness or have seizures. The effects are immediate and usually last 20 to 45 minutes.

The prolonged use of inhalants may lead to liver, kidney, blood and bone marrow damage. The sniffing of toluene, found in gasoline and commerical cleaners, has been linked to irreversible brain damage, which can manifest as forgetfulness, inability to think clearly, depression, irritability, hostility, and paranoia. Use of large amounts of aerosols or solvents can cause death as a result of cardiac arrest after arrhythmias. Death from inhalants usually is caused by suffocation because of the displacement of oxygen in the lungs. Sniffing of inhalants from a bag or balloon increases the risk of suffocation.

CHEMICAL DEPENDENCY

Alcoholism and drug addiction are commonly referred to as chemical dependency. Most modern definitions of dependence concerning drug addiction and alcoholism consist of two parts—physical and psychological dependence. Physical dependence refers to a physiological state in which the continuous and prolonged consumption of a drug or alcohol leads to the user's adaption to its presence. Tolerance then develops. If the use of alcohol or drug use stops, withdrawal symptoms occur. Psychological dependence refers to the craving for a drug or alcohol.

The terms *habituation* and *addiction* also have been used to define the nature and extent of drug use. Drug habituation includes repeated use of a drug to a point to which psychological dependence occurs. Drug addiction includes craving, psychological dependence, and physical dependence.

Dual Diagnosis

Chemical dependency is a primary illness; however, chemically dependent persons often have other psychological problems, such as depression or anxiety. Many problems disappear when drinking and drug use cease. It is important to diagnose and treat chemical dependency before other psychological problems are investigated.

Psychiatric and psychological symptoms may, however, make recognition of an addiction problem more difficult. Determining the correct diagnosis is a task for an expert in chemical dependency and psychiatry or psychology. Persons with a dual diagnosis may be more difficult to treat and may require treatment with medication such as antidepressants.

USE OF THE NURSING PROCESS
Assessment

It is important to collect both subjective and objective data about the patient suffering from alcoholism. Subjective data include the person's normal using or drinking pattern, as well as the date and time of the last drink or use of drugs. The specific drink or drug used and the quantity used is important. Table 26-3 shows a chemical use history form that may be helpful in determining a drinking or drug-using pattern.

Any past history of tremors, hallucinations, delusions, or delirium tremens (DTs) should be assessed. Past periods of abstinence, normal diet patterns, the presence of problems (e.g., legal, occupational, or family) and any family history of chemical dependency are evaluated. The occurrence of blackouts is considered diagnostic. It is important for the community health nurse to remember that the defense mechanism of denial will be present in both the substance abuser and the family in untreated chemical dependency.

Classification	Drug name	Date of last use	Amount	Frequency	Length of use	Usual amount	Method of use
Barbiturates							
Tranquilizers							
Alcohol							
Marijuana							
Opium							
Heroin							
Narcotics							
Cocaine							
Stimulants							
Hallucinogens							
Inhalants							
PCP (dust)							
Amphetamines							
Caffeine							
Hash/hash oil							
Analgesics							
Others							

TABLE 26-3 Chemical use history

The information gained from the affected person may not always be accurate, and it is helpful to validate it with families or significant others.

Objective data that can be important include an abnormal response to preoperative medication, anesthesia, or sedatives. The existence of tremor, morning nausea, or skin conditions should be assessed, as well as mental functioning, general behavior, and the relationship of weight to height. The occurrence of tachycardia, hypertension, neuropathies, and petechiae is significant. The presence of ascites and a positive result of a blood alcohol, urine alcohol, or drug screen should alert the community health nurse to take an in-depth history. Another objective sign in the IV drug abuser is track marks. If the person has been injecting into the veins, needle marks or small scabs may be present on the hands, forearms, or instep. The abuser may attempt to hide sites of injection and use the veins of the penis or the conjunctival vessel of the eyelid.

Diagnosis

A diagnosis of psychoactive substance dependence, including alcoholism, is based on the specific criteria presented here (Kirk & Bradford, 1987).

1. At least three of the following signs:
   a. Substance often taken in larger amounts or over a longer period than intended
   b. Persistent desire for the substance or one or more unsuccessful efforts to cut down or control substance use
   c. A great deal of time spent in activities necessary to get the substance, taking the substance, or recovering from its effects
   d. Frequent intoxication or withdrawal symptoms when the individual is expected to fulfill a major role obligation at work, school, or home
   e. Important social, occupational, or recreational activities given up or reduced because of substance use
   f. Continued substance use despite knowledge of having a persistent or recurrent social, psychological, or physical problem caused by or exacerbated by the use of the substance
   g. Marked tolerance: need for markedly increased amounts of the substance to achieve intoxication or the desired effect
   h. Characteristic withdrawal symptoms
   i. Substance often taken to relieve or avoid withdrawal symptoms
2. Persistence of some symptoms of the disturbance for at least 1 month or repeated occurrences over a longer period of time

Diagnostic tests. Routine blood tests often reveal abnormalities that are directly related to alcoholism. These include elevated liver enzymes, hypoglycemia, and abnormal blood protein levels. Magnesium levels may be decreased. It is not uncommon to find anemia and other evidence of poor nutrition in alcoholic patients.

One diagnostic test used to detect drug abuse is the urine or blood drug screen. The amount of time after use that drugs can be detected in the urine varies from a very short time for alcohol and cocaine to a long time for benzodiazepines and cannabis. It is possible to have a minimally positive drug test result for cannabis because of a long period of "passive inhalation" from close contact with someone smoking and exhaling marijuana fumes. Urine testing usually is not used to detect alcohol because it is metabolized very rapidly. Alcohol blood levels are much more accurate. The breathalyzer test is used by law enforcement agencies to determine alcohol levels in the blood.

Nursing diagnoses. Nursing diagnoses by the community health nurse for the person with substance abuse depend on the condition and nursing assessment of the person. They may include the following:

1. Activity intolerance
2. Anxiety
3. Coping, ineffective individual and family
4. Denial, ineffective
5. Fear
6. Fluid volume, excess or deficit
7. Health maintenance, altered
8. Home maintenance management, impaired
9. Incontinence
10. Infection, potential for

11. Injury, potential for
12. Knowledge deficit
13. Mobility, impaired physical
14. Noncompliance
15. Nutrition, altered: less than body requirements
16. Self-care deficit
17. Self-esteem, disturbance in
18. Sensory-perceptual alteration
19. Social interaction, impaired
20. Spiritual distress
21. Thought processes, altered
22. Violence, potential for

Implementation

Primary prevention. Prevention of chemical dependency is a complex issue, partly because of the almost unlimited financial resources of the illicit drug industry, as well as its power. Primary prevention attempts to prevent alcohol and drug problems before they begin. Legal efforts have been made to restrict the sale of alcohol to minors and to institute heavier penalties for driving while intoxicated and for drug trafficking. The federal government also has scheduled drugs according to their addictiveness. Unfortunately, many of these efforts have not been highly successful. Other efforts have been aimed at monitoring the influence of mass media on attitudes and behaviors.

The key to prevention is in part education. This includes teaching fairly young children about the dangers of alcohol use and abuse. Many elementary schools now start these programs as early as the first or second grade. In addition, working with children can increase their self-esteem so that they may be better able to avoid peer pressure to drink or use drugs as they become older. This is similar to strategies that promote prevention by improving an individual's ability to deal with the environment without drug use. These include problem solving, assertiveness, stress management, parenting, and values clarification. The goal in part is to help individuals improve interpersonal relationships, communication, and self-esteem.

Another attempt to educate persons involves families and employers of alcohol and drug abusers. They are taught that alcoholism is a disease that needs treatment. Alcohol abusers usually are surrounded by persons who enable their substance use and abuse, for example, the spouse who calls the employer to say that the drunk or hung-over mate is sick with the flu. Without this enabling behavior, which includes making many excuses for the affected person, the substance abuser might seek help sooner.

Community health nurses are in an excellent position to implement substance-specific primary prevention for clients and families. All the settings in which community health nurses work offer opportunities to introduce the subject of substance abuse in day-to-day health care and teaching. These settings include schools and occupational and clinic sites.

Secondary prevention. Prompt diagnosis and treatment can be important in assisting alcoholic abusers to once again become productive members of society. More and more programs are being developed to detect substance abusers; some are occupational programs or employee-assistance programs. These programs generally accept the assumptions that the most clear-cut mechanism for defining problems related to drug use is the immediate supervisor's awareness of impaired performance on the job and that chemical dependency is accepted as a medical problem. Generally, disciplinary procedures are suspended while the person receives treatment.

Tertiary prevention

Planned confrontation (intervention). Some still believe that it is only when the alcohol abuser desires and seeks help that treatment can be effective. Unfortuantely, often by the time an alcohol-dependent person realizes the need for help, much has been lost. Recently, a process called intervention has been used to assist the alcohol abuser in asking for help. Interventions are planned confrontations by individuals who care about the addicted person. They present facts or data about specific and descriptive events. The tone of the intervention should be nonjudgmental. The goal of the intervention is to have the alcohol abuser see and accept reality so that the need for help is realized. It is best to have immediate help available (Johnson, 1987).

Nursing care. Care for the alcohol- or drug-addicted client in the acute phase involves detoxification efforts to prevent acute withdrawal. Detoxification is undertaken in a controlled setting or under supervision of the physician or nurse. The person is closely watched and treated for complications as needed.

Medications. Medications used in the initial period of detoxification include chlordiazepoxide (Librium) or a similar drug. The drug is used in decreasing doses for its sedating and anticonvulsant effect during detoxification. The dosage can be as great as 50 mg every 3 hours in the first 24 hours. Anticonvulsant therapy may include phenytoin (Dilantin) and magnesium sulfate. The anticonvulsant agent may be continued longer if the person has a history of seizures.

Specific medications may differ from setting to setting. In some, alcohol or paraldehyde is used in the detoxification process. Whatever medication is used, it is important to realize that alcohol and drug abusers may require large doses of medication to safely withdraw from the substance.

Another medication that may be used in the treatment of alcohol abuse is disulfiram (Antabuse), which blocks the enzymatic action needed to metabolize alcohol. If the person drinks, the drug will cause symptoms of nausea, vomiting, palpitations, and general sick feelings. Antabuse is used voluntarily by the person as a help in maintaining sobriety. It is important for the community health nurse who deals with the person on an Antabuse regimen to realize what effects will occur if he or she drinks while taking this drug.

Methadone maintenance. One approach to the treatment of narcotics addiction is the methadone maintenance program. Methadone is a synthetic drug, and the average daily dose is much less expensive than is heroin or morphine. The drug is given legally as a part of a rehabilitation program. Methadone itself is addictive. Because methadone is easily available through legal channels, some experts believe that it is essentially the same as taking maintenance doses of other drugs such as insulin. Other persons disagree, however, because they believe that the use of methadone encourages addiction and replaces one drug with another.

Nutrition therapy. Many alcohol-addicted persons enter treatment with a history of poor nutrition. They may have received most of their calories from alcohol or have no appetite for food. As the condition of the alcohol abuser improves, the appetite usually improves also. The emphasis is on three well-balanced meals a day, with free access to snacks. Many clients find that they crave sugar in this period. If the alcohol-dependent person has problems with cirrhosis of the liver, dietary modifications may be needed. In cases of DTs, intravenous or nasogastric feedings may be necessary. In the acute withdrawal period, vitamin supplements including thiamine, are almost always used.

Associated disorders of alcohol withdrawal. When alcohol is not available to a person in whom a physiological dependence has developed, withdrawal symptoms occur. These symptoms range from mild tremors to severe agitation and hallucinations. The type

TABLE 26-4	Disorders associated with alcohol abuse
Body system	**Disorder**
Hepatic	Hepatitis, cirrhosis, fatty liver
Gastrointestinal	Cancer of the mouth and esophagus, irritation of the stomach or pancreas, difficulty in absorbing food
Neurological	Organic brain disease with confusion, Wernicke-Korsakoff syndrome, disorders of peripheral nerves (neuropathies)
Cardiovascular	Enlarged heart, high blood pressure, increased cholesterol levels, low blood sugar, anemia, coronary artery disease, congestive heart failure, arrhythmias
Musculoskeletal	Disorders of muscles (myopathies), trauma, gout
Immunological	Increased susceptibility to infection
Skin	Abscesses, rashes
Psychological	Depression, anxiety, passive-aggressive personality, antisocial personalities, food addictions (bulimia or anorexia nervosa)

and seriousness of the symptoms depend on several factors. Alcohol abusers at high risk include older persons, persons with a previous history of delirium tremens, persons with nutritional problems, and persons with other illnesses. Symptoms of alcohol withdrawal includes diaphoresis, tachycardia, elevated blood pressure, tremors, nausea and/or vomiting, anorexia, restlessness, hallucinations, and convulsions.

The tremors associated with alcohol withdrawal usually are seen 6 to 48 hours after the last drink. They may persist from 3 to 5 days. The hands are involved first, but the tremors may become generalized, with involvement of the feet, tongue, and trunk. Seizures may occur from 12 to 24 hours after the last drink. Usually these are grand mal seizures and are not preceded by an aura.

Delirium tremens (DTs) is an acute complication of alcohol withdrawal that interferes with brain metabolism. The rate of death can be as high as 15%, even with treatment. Signs that indicate Delirium tremens (DTs) may occur include tremors, increased activity, confusion and disorientation, fear, and an elevated temperature. DTs often occur suddenly, 3 to 4 days after the last drink. The condition lasts from 2 days to a week but at times can last as long as 4 weeks.

Other disorders that occur with substance abuse include those found in Table 26-4.

Addicted persons who inject drugs are at risk for diseases such as hepatitis and AIDS. Often, they share needles and equipment or reuse them without sterilization between periods of use. They also demonstrate resistance to more responsible use because of blackouts or the character traits that accompany the disease.

Education. Educating the alcohol-addicted person about the disease is very important. Education includes teaching about the disease concept, medical aspects of the disease and accompanying complications, the need for continued abstinence, and signs and symptoms of relapse. The importance of aftercare, including Alcoholics Anonymous (AA), of being honest with physicians and dentists, and of learning how to express feelings in a more positive way are stressed. This area is one in which the community health nurse can be extremely helpful and effective in assisting the person and family in recovery issues. It also is important to educate the person about what drugs to avoid, as well as about products that contain alcohol, such as mouthwash, cough syrup, and aftershave lotion.

Rehabilitation. The treatment objective for substance abuse is to assist persons to completely stop using the substance and to understand that they can never take one drink or mood-altering drug without the danger of relapse. Alcohol- and drug-addicted persons who are not currently using their substance of choice are not considered cured, only recovering. Treatment may take place in an inpatient setting or in an outpatient clinic. There is more and more emphasis on treatment in the outpatient setting. This emphasis has occurred partly because of financial concerns of insurance companies but also because few studies have demonstrated a significant difference between inpatient and outpatient treatment. Further, outpatient treatment allows the person to remain in a familiar setting.

Group therapy often is used. Its goal is to enable the person to see the relationship between the abused substance and the negative consequences that have resulted. Positive reinforcement, caring, emotional support, and encouragement also are very important. The group can point out negative behaviors and defense mechanisms and offer possible solutions to its members' problems.

Many recovering alcoholics attend AA meetings or a similar 12-step group. These groups serve self-acknowledged substance abusers whose goal is to stay sober and help other substance abusers gain sobriety. AA groups meet regularly in most communities. Some groups are listed in the local telephone book or in a local directory of meetings. A telephone call to AA will bring help in the form of a returned call or a visit from an AA member to the alcohol-addicted person who desires help.

THE 12 STEPS OF ALCOHOLICS ANONYMOUS

1. We admitted we were powerless over alcohol—that our lives had become unmanageable.
2. Came to believe that a power greater than ourselves could restore us to sanity.
3. Made a decision to turn our will and our lives over to the care of God as we understood Him.
4. Made a searching and fearless moral inventory of ourselves.
5. Admitted to God, to ourselves, and to another human being the exact nature of our wrongs.
6. Were entirely ready to have God remove all these defects of character.
7. Humbly asked Him to remove our shortcomings.
8. Made a list of all persons we had harmed, and became willing to make amends to them all.
9. Made direct amends to such people whenever possible, except when to do so would injure them or others.
10. Continued to take personal inventory and when we were wrong promptly admitted it.
11. Sought through prayer and meditation to improve our conscious contact with God as we understood Him, praying only for knowledge of His will for us and the power to carry it out.
12. Having had a spiritual awakening as a result of these steps, we tried to carry this message to alcoholics, and to practice these principles in all our affairs.

The Twelve Steps are reprinted with permission of Alcoholics Anonymous World Services Inc. Permission to reprint the Twelve Steps does not mean that AA has reviewed or approved the content of this publication, not that AA agrees with the views expressed herein. AA is a program of recovery from alcoholism. Use of the Twelve Steps in connection with programs and activities which are not patterned after AA but which address other problems does not imply otherwise.

AA and other similar programs are founded on 12 steps (see box on p. 588) that assist the alcohol abuser to admit his or her powerlessness over alcohol and other drugs. Other groups that have been formed as a result of the success of AA include Al-Anon, Families Anonymous, and Overeaters Anonymous.

Peer assistance programs for nurses. Over the last decade many states have developed programs to assist nurses who are impaired by either alcohol or drug use. Before the start of peer assistance programs the nurse often would be fired or be free to move to another facility where the abuse could continue.

Peer assistance programs have several goals: (1) to assist the impaired nurse to receive treatment, (2) to protect the public from the untreated nurse, (3) to help the recovering nurse reenter nursing in a systematic, planned, and safe way, and (4) to assist in monitoring the continued recovery of the nurse for a period of time. The reentry of the nurse may include a restriction on passing narcotics or other drugs for a designated period (ANA, 1984; Green, 1989).

These programs are based on one nurse helping another nurse. Most volunteers in these programs are recovering nurses or nurses who work in the area of chemical dependency or psychiatric nursing.

Evaluation

Evaluation of clients with chemical dependency involves input from the clients themselves, as well as from family members or significant others, employers, or teachers. Questions to consider include whether the affected persons are staying sober and abstinent and whether they are able to function in society with minimal anxiety. Their medical condition should be under fairly good control, and they should demonstrate positive coping mechanisms. Sleeping patterns, nutritional status, and self-concept all should show improvement. Lastly, the community health nurse needs to assess the entire family system, to ensure that all members are moving toward recovery.

SUMMARY

Chemical dependency or substance abuse is a problem of large dimension. Without proper intervention and treatment the person who is chemically dependent will wreak havoc on self, others, and the community in general. Chemical dependency is a medical disease that can be treated in a variety of settings by skilled professionals. To be most effective, treatment must take place within the context of the family or support systems.

Substances that are abused are many and varied. Some, such as cocaine, are illegal whereas others are available by prescription. Alcohol continues to be highly abused, even by teenagers. Chemical dependency has been on the increase in adolescents, women, and elderly persons.

Community health nurses are in an excellent position to assist in the prevention of substance abuse by providing primary, secondary, and tertiary intervention. The nurse's primary prevention activities include education; secondary prevention includes identification and assessment, as well as assisting with treatment; and tertiary prevention aspects includes assisting with rehabilitation.

 ### CHAPTER HIGHLIGHTS

- The community health nurse frequently sees the problem of substance abuse in the community.
- Alcoholism and drug addiction are commonly referred to as chemical dependency.

- Dependency may be psychological and physical and is defined as the need to continue the use of drugs and/or alcohol to prevent withdrawal.
- Efforts to prevent chemical dependency have included legal and educational efforts.
- Persons with chemical dependency also may suffer from a psychiatric diagnosis (called dual diagnosis).
- At least 18 million persons are considered "problem drinkers" in the United States today.
- There is a genetic component to the development of chemical dependency.
- Alcohol provides the body with "empty calories" and heavy drinking can cause damage to many body systems, especially the liver.
- Denial and delusion commonly are seen in persons with untreated chemical dependency.
- Substance abusers may require large doses of medications to prevent withdrawal symptoms during detoxification.
- Many of the problems found in alcoholism may be due to nutritional problems.
- The so-called stimulating effects of alcohol occur because the first areas of the brain affected are the higher centers that regulate self-control and judgment.
- Alcoholics Anonymous, or a related 12-step group, has been found to be highly effective in treatment because it helps the person accept his or her powerlessness over drugs or alcohol.
- The basic types of drugs that are abused are stimulants, depressants, hallucinogens, narcotics, cannabis, and deliriants.
- Caffeine is the most accepted and most widely used psychoactive drug in the United States.
- Drug addiction includes craving, psychological dependence, and physical dependence.
- Drug-addicted persons who inject drugs are at increased risk for the development of AIDS and hepatitis.
- Nurses are at increased risk for the development of alcoholism and chemical dependency.

STUDY QUESTIONS

1. What role does denial play in the disease of chemical dependency?
2. Explain the following terms and cite differences among them: dependency, addiction, psychological tolerance, physical tolerance, and cross-tolerance?
3. How can the community health nurse assist with primary, secondary, and tertiary prevention?
4. How can a 12-step program benefit the substance abuser?

REFERENCES

Adams, F. (1988). Drug dependency in hospital patients, *American Journal of Nursing, 88*, 477-481.

Alcoholics Anonymous. (1976). New York: Alcoholics World Services.

Alice, M. Two reports, one disease. *American Journal of Nursing, 88*, 660-661

American Nurses' Association. (1984). *Addiction and psychological dysfunction in nursing: The profes-sion's response to the problem.* Kansas City, MO: Author.

Andre, J. (1979). *The epidemiology of alcoholism among American indians and Alaskan natives.* Albuquerque: Indian Health Service.

Beattie, M. (1987). *Co-dependent no more.* Minneapolis: Hazeldon Foundation.

Bissell, L., & Haberman, P. (1984). *Alcoholism in the professions.* New York: Oxford University Press.

Captain, C. (1989). Family recovery from alcoholism: Mediating family factors. *Nursing Clinics of North America, 24,* 55-68.

Caroselli-Karinja, M. (1985). Drug abuse and the elderly. *Journal of Psychosocial Nursing and Mental Health Services, 23,* 25-30.

Cermak, T. (1986). *Diagnosing and treating co-dependence.* Minneapolis: Johnson Institute.

DaDalt, R. (1986). Changing patterns of drug diversion. *American Journal of Nursing, 86,* 792-794.

DiCicco-Bloom, B., Space, S., & Zahaurek, R.P. (1986). The homebound alcoholic. *American Journal of Nursing, 86,* 167-169.

Edens, K., et al. (1987). *How to use intervention in your profession.* Minneapolis: Johnson Institute.

Estes, N.J., & Heinemann, M.E. (1986). *Alcoholism: development, consequences, and interventions* (3rd ed.). St. Louis: Mosby.

Fitzgerald, K. (1988). *Alcoholism: The genetic inheritance.* New York: Doubleday.

Flood, M. (1989). Addictive eating disorders. *Nursing Clinics of North America, 24,* 45-54.

Gay, G. (1982). Clinical management of acute and chronic cocaine poisoning. *Annals of Emergency Medicine, 11,* 77.

Green, P. (1989). The chemically dependent nurse. *Nursing Clinics of North America, 24,* 81-94.

Haack, M., & Hughes, T. (1988). *Impairment in nursing: Clinical perspectives and program development.* New York: Springer.

Huffman, A. (1987). Body and behavioral experiences in recovery from alcoholism. *Rehabilitation Nursing, 12,* 188-192.

Hughes, T. (1989). Models and perspectives of addiction: Implications for treatment. *Nursing Clinics of North America, 24,* 1-12.

Hutchinson, S. (1986). Chemically dependent nurses: The trajectory toward self-annihilation. *Nursing Research, 35,* 196-201.

Jack, L. (1989). Use of milieu as a problem-solving strategy in addiction treatment. *Nursing Clinics of North America, 24,* 69-80.

Jackson, J. (1954). The adjustment of the family to the crises of alcoholism. *Quarterly Journal of Studies in Alcoholism, 15,* 526-586.

Johnson, V. *I'll quit tommorrow.* New York: Harper & Row.

Johnson, V. *Intervention.* Minneapolis: Johnson Institute.

Kelley, R. (1987). The path to addiction and recovery. *American Journal of Nursing, 87,* 176-177.

Kirk, E., & Bradford, L. (1987). Effects of alcohol on the CNS: Implications for the neuroscience nurse. *Journal of Neuroscience Nursing, 19,* 316-335.

Long, B.C., & Phipps, W.J. (1988). *Medical-surgical nursing: A nursing process approach* (2nd ed.). St. Louis: Mosby.

Malice. Two reports, one disease. *American Journal of Nursing, 88,* 660-661.

Matteson, M., & McConnell, E. (1988). *Gerontological nursing: Concepts and practice.* Philadelphia: Saunders.

Mosby's medical & nursing dictionary, (2nd ed.). (1986). St. Louis: Mosby.

National Institute on Drug Abuse. (1986). Rockville, MD: Author.

Nuckols, C., & Greeson, J. (1989). Cocaine addiction: Assessment and intervention. *Nursing Clinics of North America, 24,* 33-44.

Powell, A., & Minick, M. (1988). Alcohol withdrawal syndrome. *American Journal of Nursing, 88,* 312-315.

Sullivan, E., Bissell, L., & Williams, E. (1988). *Chemical dependency in nursing: The deadly diversion.* Menlo Park, CA: Addison-Wesley.

Tweed, S. (1989). Identifying the alcoholic client. *Nursing Clinics of North America, 24,* 13-32.

Vandegaer, F. Cocaine—The deadliest addiction. (1989). *Nursing 89, 19,* 72-74.

Which nurse is likely to become chemically dependent? (1988). *American Journal of Nursing, 88,* 791-794.

Williams, E. (1989). Strategies for intervention. *Nursing Clinics of North America, 24,* 95-108.

Zerwekh, J., & Michaels, B. (1989). Co-dependency: Assessment and recovery. *Nursing Clinics of North America, 24,* 109-120.

Legal and Ethical Issues

CORINNE T. STUART

Value turnover is now faster than ever before in history. While in the past a man growing up in society could expect that its public value system would remain largely unchanged in his lifetime, no such assumption is warranted today, except perhaps in the most isolated of pre-technological communities.

ALVIN TOFFLER, 1970

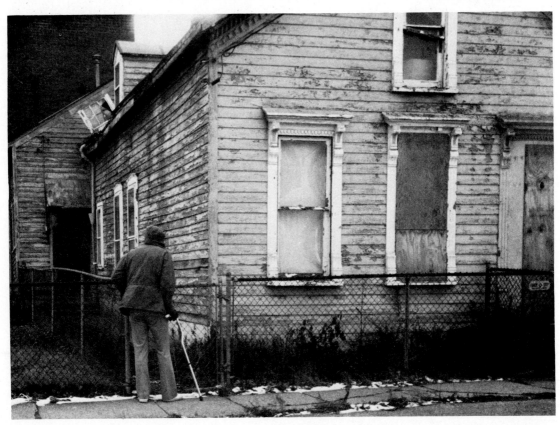

OBJECTIVES

At the conclusion of this chapter the student will be able to:

1. Define the key terms listed
2. Identify three types of law as they relate to community health nursing practice
3. Identify those diseases that, according to communicable disease control centers, are reportable by law
4. Apply the ethical principle of informed consent as it relates to immunization protocol, as well as other community health procedures
5. Identify a situation in which the community health nurse can be held liable for neligence and malpractice
6. Identify steps in the process of ethical analysis according to Leah Curtin's model
7. Apply the decision-making process of ethical analysis to a clinical situation
8. Identify the ethical principles and ethical theory implied in case examples

KEY TERMS

Abuse
Autonomy
Beneficence
Case law
Common law
Confidentiality
Constitutional law
Deontological (formalist) theory
Ethical dilemma
Ethics
Fidelity
Fundamental human rights
Informed consent

Judicial law
Justice
Legal rights
Legislation
Negligence
Nonmaleficence
Regulation
Special rights
Teleological (consequentialist) theory
Truth telling
Utilitarianism
Values
Values clarification

Health care in the community is far from new. A quiet revolution, however, has occurred. Changes are due to the high cost of institutional care, changes in federal regulations regarding hospital stays, the advent of advanced technology adaptive for use in the home, and the growth of supportive community services. These factors allow certain treatments to take place at home that previously were reserved only for the "sacred" halls of the hospital.

As discussed in Chapters 18 and 19, many persons with chronic disease, terminal illness, paralysis, and disabilities of old age remain in their own homes. Community health agencies provide nursing care and a variety of therapies such as physical, occupational, respiratory, speech, and counseling. Help with household chores, Meals on Wheels, and a host of other services also are available. Complex care in the home that could not have been considered previously now is possible for clients ranging in age from the newborn to the elderly. With specific instruction individuals have learned to perform complicated procedures. Fortunately, some equipment has become simpler and easier to handle, thus enabling the client and/or care giver to perform the required task to maintain the client at home.

LEGAL ISSUES
Types of Laws

Three types of laws affect community health nursing practice. The first is constitutional law, which is mandated by federal and state constitutions. The community health nurse (CHN) refers to this type of law for answers to questions in selected practice situations, for example, state requirements for quarantine or isolation of persons with a communicable disease. The state may actively intervene to protect the health, safety, and welfare of its citizens.

The second type of law is called legislation and regulation. This type is mandated by state, local, or federal legislative branches of government. The CHN, regardless of employment category—official or private voluntary agency—is subject to legislation and regulations. An example of this type of law is the CHN's compliance with Medicare (federal law) or Medicaid (state enforced) legislation and regulations to enable the private agency that provides home health care to receive financial reimbursement. Other examples are given throughout this chapter.

Common law is the third type of law that affects community health nursing. Common law derives from previous decisions made by a court (legal precedent). It is influenced by justice, fairness, and tradition. Subsequent court decisions are often based on common law (Northrop & Kelly, 1987).

CHNs must be technically competent and well versed in the nursing process. It is also prudent to be aware of the laws affecting community health nursing practice.

The CHN is vulnerable to malpractice lawsuits: "Professional negligence or malpractice is defined as an act or failure to act when a duty is owed to another that was not reasonable and that leads to injuries compensable by law" (Northrop, 1988, p. 121). The CHN works independently, as compared with the hospital employed nurse. To facilitate early assessment and care of clients discharged from the hospital to home care service, the CHN may have to function on the basis of verbal orders for a brief period of time. These medical orders must be carefully evaluated by the CHN before actual implementation. Written orders signed by the referring physician must become a part of the client's record as soon as possible. Agencies should have specific policies regarding this matter.

Any change in the client's condition must be verbally communicated to the attending physician. Documentation of the specific changes and contact with the physician must be noted on the client's record. If the CHN questions the safety of the client's remaining in the home either because of the client's incompetence or worsening medical status, options need be considered for protective action to be taken. Again, it is the responsibility of the home health care agency to formulate policies that help direct the individual action of the CHN under its employ. Standing orders, sometimes known as medical directives or protocols set by the agency, serve to assist the CHN. To properly evaluate such orders the CHN must be familiar with and abide by such documents as the state Nurse Practice Act and state regulations, as well as the standards of community health nursing practice.

The following case* illustrates how careful home health care agencies must be in providing personnel with the desired degree of skill necessary for client care.

*From "Case in point: Roach v. Kelly health care (742 p. 2d 1190— or)[11] (Home health care and legal issues) by A.D. Tammelleo (Ed.) in *The Regan Report on Nursing Law* (Vol. 28, No., 7), December 1987, Providence, RI: Medica Press. Copyright 1987 by Medica Press, Inc. Reprinted with the express permission of A.D. Tammelleo, J.D. and Medica Press, Inc.

ISSUE: As the DRG systems are causing patients to be discharged quicker and sicker than ever before, there is a concomitant increase in the need for vital home health care services. This has led to an overwhelming demand for home health care services which are in some cases provided by Voluntary Nurses Associations, (VNA) and in other cases by private Home Health Care (HHC) agencies. This interesting Oregon case illustrates how careful Home Health Care agencies must be in providing personnel with the requisite degree of skill and training necessary for each patient.

CASE FACTS: In October, 1983, Edna Tuson, an 87-year-old widow, lived at home by herself in Portland, Oregon. Early that month, Mrs. Blaufus, her daughter, noticed signs of forgetfulness and confusion in Edna Tuson. Mrs. Blaufus arranged for the Visiting Nurses Association (VNA) to provide home nursing visits several times a week to ensure that her mother was taking her medication and that her blood pressure would be monitored. On two occasions in early November, Edna Tuson fell at home and was unable to get up until a visitor discovered her. On November 17, a VNA nurse found Mrs. Tuson obviously confused and showing signs of a stroke, which was later confirmed by a physician. Mrs. Blaufus arranged for Kelly Health Care, Inc. and Kelly Services, Inc. to provide twenty-four hour live-in care for her mother. As was its normal custom in such cases, Kelly used Certified Nursing Assistants (CNAs) rather than Home Health Aides (HHAs) to provide the care. CNAs receive sixty hours of training, with an emphasis on caring for patients in an institutional setting under the direct supervision of a nurse. HHAs receive an additional sixty hours training, with emphasis on home care, including attention to home safety. Kelly employees began living with Mrs. Tuson at the end of November, 1983. Her condition deteriorated gradually. She became less aware of her surroundings and less able to care for herself. She also developed bedsores. One sore on her coccyx did not heal. On January 5, 1984, Kelly's nursing supervisor, Nurse Gray, visited Mrs. Tuson in her home. Nurse Gray's visit was partly to determine Mrs. Tuson's competency for a conservatorship proceeding and partly to conduct a regular supervisory inspection. Nurse Gray discovered that the sore on the coccyx was worse. Mrs. Blaufus took her mother to a physician, who changed the treatment for the sores by instructing the CNA on duty to turn Mrs. Tuson every two hours. The CNA believed that the doctor intended that the patient be turned throughout the night as well as during the day. She turned Mrs. Tuson every two hours until 6:30 a.m. the following morning. The aide went to sleep shortly after 6:30 a.m. the following morning and did not awaken until approximately 11:30 a.m., and found Mrs. Tuson on the floor with her face against a baseboard heater, severly burned. Mrs. Tuson was hospitalized for more than two weeks and then stayed in a nursing home until her death from other causes in July, 1984. The personal representative of Mrs. Tuson's estate brought an action for personal injuries against Kelly Health Care, Inc., Kelly Services, Inc. and Nurse Charlotte Gray. The Circuit Court, Multnomah County, entered Judgement against the plaintiff. The plaintiff appealed.

COURT OPINION: The Court of Appeals of Oregon reversed the Judgement of the Lower Court in part and affirmed the Judgement of the Lower Court in part. The Court held that a jury could reasonably find that Certified Nursing Assistants were attempting to provide care that they were not qualified to provide. The Court further found that the Trial Court should have instructed the jury on the agency's violation of regulations as negligence per se. The Court also found that there was insufficient evidence to justify submitting the case to a jury on the issue of Nurse Gray's personal negligence, thus affirming that portion of the Lower Court's decision which entered Summary Judgement for Nurse Gray.

LEGAL LESSON: Under Oregon law, a Home Health Agency must be licensed, if it is primarily engaged in providing skilled nursing services and at least one of several other services, including Home Health Aide Service. The Court found that Kelly was licensed at the time it provided care for the patient. The Court held that a CNA is not qualified to provide home health aide services which require a HHA. The Court rejected Kelly's contention that an HHA was not necessary because Kelly was providing only "personal care," not Home Health Care and that "personal care" services are exempt from licensing. The Court recognized that applicable law exempts from the definition of "Home Health Agency" those personal care services that do not pertain to curative, rehabilititative or preventative aspects of nursing. However, the Court further rejected Kelly's claims that its employees simply assisted the patient with personal and household tasks and provided companionship as a substitute for family members. The Court found that a jury could conclude that the CNAs provided total care for a woman who could no longer think clearly or meet her basic needs. That care, a jury could find, included at least curative and preventative aspects of nursing.

Needless to say, a responsibility and an obligation exist to provide necessary care to any client who is discharged from the hospital to home and who requires further medical supervision. Hospital discharge planners have been guided by legal requirements, as well as moral obligation, for many years. Although there is no federal mandate, most states have legislation that requires a written plan of care, with appropriate agency contact and physician referral for those clients in need of home care. If this is lacking, the hospital can be charged with abandonment and allegations of negligent discharge.

Professional Expectations and Standards

Community health nursing, as defined by the American Nurses' Association (ANA), is a synthesis of nursing practice and public health practice applied to the promotion and preservation of the health of its populace. This practice is general, comprehensive, and continuing. It is not limited to a particular age or diagnostic group. Activities involve health promotion, health maintenance, and prevention of disease for the population as a whole, as well as to individuals, families, or groups (ANA, 1986).

It is imperative that the CHN be knowledgeable regarding the Standards of Community Health Nursing Practice as set by their professional nursing organization, the ANA. These standards and the "reasonable person" rule are presented in Chapter 3.

In any lawsuit the party accused of negligence, the defendant, is held accountable to the standards of practice of the particular specialty. The person filing the complaint or claim on the basis of substantive law is known as the plaintiff. Substantive law may be classified as civil, administrative, or criminal law (Northrop & Kelly, 1987).

Actually there have been few negligence cases involving CHNs, either in the private or public health care arena; however, this is likely to change as a result of the tremendous growth of home health care agencies. The following case* serves as an illustration.

A PHN received a telephone call from a private medical doctor (PMD) requesting TB services for a patient. Two different versions of what the conversation was came out at trial. The PMD said he discussed the patient's condition with the PHN and told the PHN that the patient had a positive sputum culture and that he had not treated anyone with TB for several years, so was unfamiliar with the drugs. He testified that he asked the nurse to put the patient on the health department's protocol and treat her and that he informed the patient that she was now under the care of the health department for the TB. The PMD denied prescribing any drugs for the patient.

The PHN, on the other hand, relayed to the court that she and the PMD discussed available treatment of TB; that the PMD ordered a standard combination of ethambutol, isoniazid, and vitamin B-6 for the patient; and that the PMD asked her to deliver the drugs to the patient on the following Monday.

In order to facilitate the patient beginning the treatment as soon as possible, the PHN went to her supervisor, a part-time health department physician, for his signature on the

*From *Legal issues in nursing* (p. 202) by C.E. Northrop and M.E. Kelly, 1987, St. Louis: Mosby. Copyright 1987 by The C.V. Mosby Co. Reprinted by permission.

prescriptions. She marked the prescriptions per telephone order of PMD, noting the PMD's name. The health department physician signed the forms, and the PHN made the home visit later that day.

During the home visit the PHN testified she warned the patient that the drugs could affect her kidneys and that the patient should watch her urine for a red coloring. The PHN learned during the home visit that the patient had cataracts. The remainder of the conversation with the patient was disputed. The PHN testified that she checked the patient's vision with a 10-foot eye chart and recorded the readings as 10/100 in the right eye; 10/50 in the left eye.

The patient, supported by testimony from her sister who was present during the initial home visit, stated that the PHN told her she had forgotten the eye chart and to check the patient's vision she asked the patient to identify certain objects in the room. The patient testified that the PHN told her to watch the whites of her eyes and to notify her physician if they turned yellow. Interestingly, the eye chart the PHN said she used did not have a 10/100 line. The PHN further testified that she told the patient to watch for any decreased visual acuity.

The patient took the medications prescribed for one month. At the end of the month another PHN made a home visit, delivering another month's supply of drugs. The PHN testified she checked the patient's vision. It was undisputed that during the home visits made in the following 2 months the patient's vision was not checked. The patient suffered rapid loss of vision during these 4 months. Uncontradicted expert testimony was presented at trial stating that if vision checks had been performed, the patient's loss of vision could have been detected, the ethambutol would have been stopped, and vision loss possibly could have been reversed.

In the fifth month of taking the drugs the patient saw the PMD for a regular checkup. She informed the PMD of her vision problems; however, it was disputed by the PMD to what extent the patient had informed him about the extent of the loss. Another month went by until the patient went to see the ophthalmologist, who immediately referred her to a neurologist who admitted her to the hospital, saw the ethambutol, and immediately concluded that it was the cause of her vision loss.

On procedural grounds the court remanded this case for a new trial. However, the court made several points which the trial court was to follow. The court determined that there was evidence in the record from which a jury could find, in pertinent part, that the:

1. PHN was negligent in failing to properly inform the patient of side effects of the drugs and to check the vision
2. PMD was negligent in failing to assess the patient's condition; that the PMD was still the patient's physician, not the health department
3. Health department was negligent for the PHN's negligent conduct; that the health department physician who was her supervisor may be liable but only for his own failure to properly supervise the PHN

Public Health Law

The public health nurse (PHN) and the CHN are employed in the public sector, primarily in local, state, or federal agencies or in the private sector. The CHN working for a private health agency must be as aware of the public health laws as the nurse employed by a public agency even though she or he may not be as directly affected by them.

The enforcement of public health laws to protect the public's health is primarily the responsibility of the individual, the state, or the province. Laws vary from state to state. PHNs working in any public health agency must be aware of the public health legislation in that state. They must work within the limitations of their written job description and must know the policies and correct procedures of practice for which they are held accountable.

Cynthia Northrop (1987), a registered nurse and an attorney, reports three areas in which public health nursing case law is prevalent: communicable disease control, hereditary diseases and other conditions, the environment, sanitation, and housing.

The federal government created the Public Health Service (PHS) and the Centers for Disease Control (CDC). It is required by law that all states and territories of the United States report the occurrence of certain diseases on a weekly, monthly, and annual basis. Diseases that require official mandatory notification are acquired immunodeficiency syndrome (AIDS), chickenpox, measles (rubella), mumps, aseptic meningitis, gonorrhea, hepatitis, salmonellosis, syphilis, shigellosis, and tuberculosis (CDC, 1982).

The problem of AIDS (see Chapter 22) has been named the number one priority of the Public Health Service (1985). The legal issues pertaining to AIDS include the problem of confidentiality, transmission of the disease, and the issue of mandated screening. The guidelines developed by CDC are comparable to standards that can be used in malpractice cases and other litigation (Northrop & Kelly, 1987).

Some states require the reporting of additional diseases to their public health departments. CHNs must be familiar with the state laws under which they practice. Accurate reporting and detailed records must be kept. Communicable disease legislation affords the state the right to investigate the disease, to enter the premises, the inspect the individual, to order physical examinations and diagnostic tests, and, if necessary, to quarantine persons. Actual reporting is required of physicians, hospitals, and laboratories. Frequently it is the PHN who serves as the case finder. The PHN must then inform the public health physician and the PHN supervisor of these findings. If the PHN is negligent or fails to meet this legal responsibility, the PHN could be held liable and subject to civil proceedings. Depending on the court's decision and the state board of licensure, the PHN faces a fine or a license suspension or revocation.

The importance of confidentiality is uppermost. Because of the legal requirement of reporting, state legislatures have allowed for an acceptable breach of confidentiality and have even granted civil immunity from suit for good faith reporting (Illinois Annotated Statutes, 1985). Yet the necessary data such as name, address, sex, age, race, and suspected or confirmed disease must remain confidential within the confines of the health department and not be made available for public scrutiny (Maryland Health, 1982).

As yet no cases have been cited against a PHN for breach of confidentiality or for failure to report a communicable disease. It is the PHN who most frequently intervenes with protective measures to prevent the spread of disease and to provide corrective treatment for the individual and family affected by the disease. This places the additional responsibility of legal obligations on the nurse (Northrop & Kelly, 1987).

Concerns of Community Health Nurses

Abuse. The enforcement of public health laws and local, state, and federal regulations fall under the scope of concern of the CHN. In respect to case law (interpretation of law through completed cases that serve as precedents), usually is involved in cases of child abuse or termination of parental rights (Northrop & Kelly, 1987).

Child abuse includes emotional as well as physical abuse. It ranges from violent physical attacks that cause severe injury to passive neglect that may manifest in malnutrition or other problems. Sexual abuse ranges from fondling to rape. In 1974 Congress passed the Child Abuse Prevention and Treatment Act (Misener, 1986). One of the provisions of this act required states to enact mandatory reporting legislation in order to be eligible to receive grant funds. All 50 states have passed laws that mandate reporting of child maltreatment. Underreporting occurs mainly because of the reluctance of health care providers to get involved in family matters. Any nurse who suspects that a child has been abused must report the case to the proper authorities. Failure to report such cases could lead to further injury or even to the death of the child. The CHN could be subject to criminal punishment. It is incumbent upon the nurse to know the local and state laws governing the definition and reporting of child abuse. State statutes provide protection from civil suit for anyone reporting child abuse (Lancaster & Kerschner, 1988).

The abuse of elders by a spouse, other family members, or care giver in the home has become more evident in recent years. Often the CHN who renders care and supervision in the home is the person who detects evidence of such abuse. When inadequate food, clothing, shelter, and physical care to meet safety needs, as well as overt physical and psychological assault is suspected or clearly indicated, the CHN must intervene as early as possible. Aside from any official reporting required by law to protective agencies or to community mental health or social work services, the CHN, supported by the health agency (employer), must be influential in seeking to provide protective living arrangements. The CHN is subject to be called upon for testimony in a court of law and must act responsibly in this role.

Immunization. Mandatory state requirements of immunization programs to prevent communicable diseases have been under attack in recent years because of serious adverse reactions sometimes caused by the vaccine for pertussis. There always has been the opportunity for clients to reject state-required immunization if it conflicts with religious beliefs. The vast majority of parents, however, agree to the immunization process for their children as a prevention strategy. The question of informed consent must be raised. Are the risk factors presented to the parents? Is this the responsibility of the physician, the CHN, or the person who administers the vaccine? One state passed laws designating the collection of data regarding the adverse reaction to the pertussis vaccine for the purpose of developing guidelines for circumstances under which the vaccine should be delayed or not given at all. This clarification helped to identify categories of recipients who were more vulnerable than the general population to major adverse reactions. Consent procedures were designed, published, and distributed to all physicians and concerned health care providers (Maryland Health, 1985b). Under this specific legislation the CHN is considered a health care provider and consequently is held legally accountable. Therefore, in response to the previously asked questions, the CHN does have the duty to inform parents, to take a careful history to determine cause for any possible exception for administering the pertussis vaccine, to provide adequate information regarding the nature of an adverse reaction, and to realize the importance of immediate reporting to the appropriate authority. Fig. 27-1 shows an example of a consent form that provides the necessary information.

The law specifically addresses the importance of record-keeping responsibilities. Complete information pertaining to the vaccine, date, manufacturer, lot number, and other identifying information on the vaccine used must be kept in the child's health record. The signature and title of the health care provider, most frequently the PHN, must be given, and accurate reporting of any adverse reaction to the vaccine is essential (Maryland Health, 1985a).

Lawsuits concerning issues of negligence, product liability, and informed consent for state-mandated treatments have involved PHNs. The PHN has been the defendant, the witness, or the party who gave the medication, immunization, and/or treatment that brought the case to trial.

Professional liability insurance. The question of malpractice insurance for the CHN

IMPORTANT INFORMATION ABOUT DIPHTHERIA, TETANUS, AND PERTUSSIS AND DTP, Dt, AND Td VACCINES

Please read this carefully

WHAT IS DIPHTHERIA?

Diptheria is a very serious disease which can affect people in different ways. It can cause an infection in the nose and throat which can interfere with breathing. It can also cause an infection of the skin. Sometimes it causes heart failure or paralysis. About 1 person out of every 10 who get diptheria dies of it.

WHAT IS TETANUS?

Tetanus, or lockjaw, results when wounds are infected with tetanus bacteria, which are often found in dirt. The bacteria in the wound make a poison which causes the muscles of the body to go into spasm. In the United States, four out of every 10 persons who get tetanus die of it.

WHAT IS PERTUSSIS?

Pertussis, or whooping cough, causes severe spells of coughing which can interfere with eating, drinking, and breathing. In the United States, approximately 70 percent of reported pertussis cases occur in children younger than 5 years. Pertussis is a more serious disease in young children and more than half of the children less than 1 year of age reported to have pertussis are hospitalized. In recent years, over 2,000 cases of pertussis have been reported each year in the United States. Complications occur in a substantial proportion of reported cases. Pneumonia occurs in one of every four children with pertussis. For every 1,000 reported pertussis cases, 22 develop convulsions and/or have more severe problems of the brain. In recent years, an average of nine deaths due to pertussis occurred annually.

Before vaccines were developed, these three diseases were all very common and caused a large number of deaths each year in the United States. If children are not immunized, the risk of getting these diseases will go back up again.

DTP, DT, AND Td VACCINES:

Immunization with DTP vaccine is the best way to prevent these diseases. DTP vaccine is actually three vaccines combined into one shot

to make it easier to get protection. Advisory committees of the United States Public Health Service and the American Academy of Pediatrics recommend DTP vaccine be used in children up to their seventh birthday. The vaccine is given by injection starting early in infancy. At least three shots are needed to provide initial protection. Young children should get three doses in the first year of life and a fourth dose at about 15 months of age. A booster shot is important for children who are about to enter school and should be given between their fourth and seventh birthdays. The vaccine is very effective at preventing tetanus—over 95 percent of those who get the vaccine are protected if the recommended number of shots is given. Although the diptheria and pertussis parts of the vaccine are not quite as effective, they still prevent most children from getting disease and they make the disease milder for those who do get it. Because pertussis is not very common or severe in older children, those 7 years of age or older should take a form of the vaccine that has a lower concentration of the diptheria part. This vaccine which contains no pertussis part and a lower concentration of the diptheria part is called Td vaccine. Boosters with the Td vaccine should be received every 10 years throughout life.

DEFERRAL OF DTP IMMUNIZATION:

Children who have had a serious reaction to previous DTP shots should not receive additional pertussis vaccine (see WARNING). A preparation called DT vaccine is available for them which does not contain the pertussis part. Also, children who have previously had a convulsion or are suspected to have a problem of the nervous system should not receive DTP vaccine until a full medical evaluation has been made.

POSSIBLE SIDE EFFECTS FROM THE VACCINE:

With DTP vaccine, most children will have a slight fever and be irritable within 2 days after getting the shot. One-half of children develop some soreness and swelling in the area where the shot was given. More serious side effects can occur.

(Please read other side)

A temperature of 105°F or greater may follow 1 out of 330 DTP shots. Continuous crying lasting 3 or more hours may occur after 1 in every 100 shots and unusual, high-pitched crying may occur after 1 in every 900 shots. Convulsions or episodes of limpness and paleness may each occur after 1 in every 1,750 shots. Rarely, about once in every 110,000 shots, other more severe problems of the brain may occur, and permanent brain damage may occur about once in every 310,000 shots. Side effects from DT or Td vaccine are not common and usually consist only of soreness and slight fever. As with any drug or vaccine, there is a rare possibility that allergic or more serious reactions or even death could occur.

Although some people have questioned whether DTP shots might cause Sudden Infant Death Syndrome (SIDS), the majority of evidence indicates that DTP shots do not cause SIDS.

PERSONAL OR FAMILY HISTORY OF CONVULSIONS:

Children who have had a convulsion and children who have a brother, sister, or parent who has ever had a convulsion are more likely to have a convulsion after receiving DTP vaccine. The advisory committees recommend that because of the overall risk of pertussis disease and the fact that the risk of convulsions is still very low: (1) children with a personal history of a convulsion and whose nervous system problem is stable may receive DTP vaccine; and (2) children with a family history of convulsions should receive DTP vaccine. However, you should tell the person who is to give the immunization about such a history and discuss the possibility of using an anti-fever medicine.

PREGNANCY:

Babies born under unsanitary conditions to unimmunized women have a risk of developing tetanus during the newborn period (neonatal tetanus). Neonatal tetanus can be prevented by immunization of adult women. Women who have not received Td earlier and who are thought to be at risk of delivering their babies under unsanitary conditions should be immunized during pregnancy.

Td vaccine is not known to cause special problems for pregnant women or thier unborn babies. Doctors usually do not recommend giving any drugs or vaccines to pregnant women unless there is a specific need. Pregnant women who need Td vaccine should receive it, preferably during the second and/or third trimesters.

WARNINGS—SOME PERSONS SHOULD NOT TAKE THESE VACCINES WITHOUT CHECKING WITH A DOCTOR:

- Anyone who is sick right now with something more serious than a cold.
- Anyone who has had a convulsion or is suspected to have a problem of the nervous system.
- Anyone who has had a serious reaction to DTP, DT, or Td shots before, such as: an allergic reaction to any vaccine component; a temperature of 105°F or greater; an episode of limpness and paleness; prolonged continuous crying; an unusual, high-pitched cry; or a convulsion or other more severe problem of the brian.
- Anyone taking a drug or undergoing a treatment that lowers the body's resistance to infection, such as: cortisone, prednisone, certain anticancer drugs, or irradiation.
- Anyone who has had a serious reaction to a product containing thimerosal, a mercurial antiseptic.

QUESTIONS:

If you have any questions about diphtheria, tetanus, or pertussis or DTP, DT, or Td immunization, please ask us now or call your doctor or health department before you sign this form.

REACTIONS:

If the person who received the vaccine develops a temperature of 105°F or greater, continuous crying lasting 3 or more hours, an unusual high-pitched cry, a convulsion, an episode of limpness and paleness, or a severe problem of the brain, the person should be seen promptly by a doctor.

If the person who received the vaccine gets sick and visits a doctor, hospital, or clinic in the 4 weeks after immunization, please report it to:

Continued.

FIG. 27-1 Example of a consent form providing information about the benefits and risks associated with the diphtheria-pertussis-tetanus (DPT), diphtheria-tetanus (DT), and tetanus and diphtheria (Td) vaccines. (*From Immunization: A Handbook for Schools by the University of the State of New York, 1982, Albany, NY: State Education Department. Copyright 1982 by the University of the State of New York. Reprinted by permission.*)

PLEASE KEEP THIS PART OF THE INFORMATION SHEET FOR YOUR RECORDS

I have read or have had explained to me the information on this form about diptheria, tetanus, and pertussis and DTP, DT and Td vaccine. I have had a chance to ask questions which were answered to my satisfaction. I believe I understand the benefits and risks of the DTP, DT, and Td vaccine and request that the vaccine checked below be given to me or to the person named below for whom I am authorized to make this request.

Vaccine to be given ☐ DTP ☐ DT ☐ Td

INFORMATION ABOUT PERSON TO RECEIVE VACCINE (Please Print)			
Last Name	First Name	Mi	Birthdate	Age
Address			
City	County	State	Zip
x Signature of person to receive vaccine or person authorized to make the request.			Date

FOR CLINIC USE
Clinic ident.
Date Vaccinated
Manuf. and Lot No.
Site of injection

FOR DATA PROCESSING USE ONLY (OPTIONAL)

VACCINE HISTORY: PLACE CHECK ☐ IN BOX IF HISTORY PREVIOUSLY SUBMITTED

DTP:	m/d/yr	m/d/yr	m/d/yr	MEASLES:	m/d/yr	MUMPS:	m/d/yr
POLIO:	m/d/yr	m/d/yr	m/d/yr	RUBELLA:	m/d/yr	HAEMOPHILUS b:	m/d/yr

FIG. 27-1, cont'd For legend see p. 601.

is debatable. Many lawyers believe it not only unnecessary but undesirable for nurses to buy malpractice insurance. If the nurse is known to have this form of insurance, the prosecuting attorney may sue for higher financial damages. Contrary to this viewpoint, professional nursing organizations believe it is in the nurse's best interest to carry this protection. It would seem imperative that certain nursing specialists such as the nurse midwife and the nurse anesthetist have this protection. It may be equally important for CHNs to carry their own malpractice insurance, in addition to that provided by their employers. This action serves as a statement that they can no longer rely on others to protect their legal interests but instead will assume this responsibility. Ultimately it is the individual nurse's choice.

ETHICAL ISSUES

Nurses always have been concerned about professional ethics and moral choices. One cannot consider ethics without commenting on the nature of values. "Values may be considered to be a set of beliefs and attitudes for which logical reasons can be given. Values are significant in that they influence perceptions, guide our actions, and have consequences" (Aroskar & Davis, 1983, p. 199). Each of these values has an ordered priority that may or may not be subject to change over time. The CHN brings personal values to the field of practice. These values may conflict with those values of the client and/or families with whom the CHN is interacting. Thus the nurse must make a conscious effort to explore the values and covert motivations that direct each person's behavior. Values clarification is a process of discovery that "attempts to bring to conscious awareness the values and underlying motivations that guide one's action" (Steel & Harmon, 1983, p.13). This clarification process does not indicate the right or wrong of alternative actions, but it does provide some assurance that the course of action chosen by the person is consistent and in accordance with his or her beliefs and values.

The respect for values that differ from one's own requires understanding, tolerance, and a high degree of acceptance. When personal values interfere with the attainment of desired objectives in the prevention of disease or the maintenance of health, the CHN may be instrumental in assisting the client and family in the examination of their values. At no time should the CHN force his or her own values on the client. Appreciation by both parties—health care provider and client—of the other's values would serve to establish common ground upon which to build a more positive relationship. This mutual respect more easily facilitates the nursing process and the achievement of client-centered objectives.

Ethics itself has been defined as principles and rules that dictate personal conduct in a given situation (Davis & Aroskar, 1978). Ethical conflicts that arise in nursing practice situations usually are caused by a conflict between moral values (Fry, 1985). Discussions of ethical solutions to problems concern what is "good" and what is "bad." The concepts of "right," and "wrong," and "obligation" are integral to this concern.

The ANA (1985) developed a code to provide a framework for the consideration of nursing responsibilities and obligations. It considers the special rights of nurses on the basis of the relationship of nursing to society in providing an essential service to the sick and to populations at risk. Nursing responsibility is based on the fundamental principle of respect for persons and their inherent dignity and worth. This respect is basic to moral principles such as autonomy (self-determination), beneficence (doing good), nonmaleficence (avoiding harm), fidelity (keeping promises), truth telling, and justice (treating people fairly). The following specific items in the code relate to these principles (ANA, 1986, p. 3):

- Providing nursing services with respect for the human dignity of all who require nursing service, regardless of social or economic status, personal attributes, or the nature of their health problems
- Safeguarding client rights to privacy and confidentiality
- Safeguarding the well-being and safety of the individual, group, and community clients and of the public, recognizing that in limited instances responsibility for the public's health and safety may temporarily take priority over individual autonomy
- Assuming responsibility and accountability for nursing judgements and actions
- Seeking consultation, accepting responsibilities, and delegating nursing activities to others, based on the criteria of informed judgement, individual competence, and qualifications
- Participating in the profession's efforts to protect the public from misinformation and misrepresentation
- Working with others to promote community and national effort to ensure the availability and accessibility of high-quality health services for all people

Responsibility carries with it the corresponding right or authority to fulfill one's responsibilities as a professional person. Of particular concern to nurses are *fundamental human rights, legal rights, and special rights.* A right is that to which a person has a just claim. Fundamental human rights are claims recognized by law that are legally enforceable. These include rights protected by the Constitution of the United States. Every U.S. citizen has the right to bring suit, civil or criminal, seeking damages or other legal relief. The *Patient's Bill of Rights* lists basic human rights, as well as a number of legal rights of clients, whether or not the health care agency supports this document. CHNs must alert their clients to these rights and be supportive to the point of advocacy.

The Nurse Practice Act gives nurses certain legal privileges but also defines the limits of practice in each specific state. The nurse is held accountable by law to specific standards of practice in the particular specialty.

Some would argue that nurses have no special rights. According to the Ethics Committee of the ANA, however, special rights and/or privileges of the professional nurse are those that arise out of the nurse-client relationship. For example, nurses are not required to participate in care that would violate the bounds of acceptable practice or the nurse's own deeply held religious or moral beliefs. Nor are nurses morally required to place themselves at serious personal risk. Therefore in such situations the nurse must provide for adequate coverage and/or appropriate referral to maintain nursing care: otherwise the nurse could be charged with abandonment. Standards of nursing care designed for specialty areas of practice also afford nurses special rights to ensure safe client environments. The right of the CHN for client advocacy takes on a new dimension for decision making and implementation that often includes political action (ANA, 1986a).

Theories of Ethics

Nursing ethics is concerned with the nurse's legal, ethical, and professional obligations in practice. Of the many theories of ethics, only two major ones are briefly addressed here.

Teleological (consequentialist) theory. This theory states that the rightness or wrongness of an action is determined by the results of that action or by its consequences. It implies that one ought to do that which is conducive to one's goals. In other words, the end justifies the means.

The most common teleological theory, utilitarianism, is often thought of as the greatest-happiness principle, or the greatest good for the greatest number of people (Curtin & Flaherty, 1982).

Deontological (formalist) theory. A second theory, known as deontology, or formalism, was developed by Immanuel Kant, an eighteenth-century philosopher. According to this philosophy, the rightness or wrongness of an action is based on the nature of the action or the motives behind the action, but not on the results or consequences of the action. The rightness of the action is based on principles and action and on a respect for one's moral duty (Curtin & Flaherty, 1982).

Ethical Problems in Community Health Nursing

Empirical research in nursing and ethics has almost exclusively focused on nurses in the hospital setting. Consequently, little is known about the ethical problems confronting CHNs. This lack, however, does not imply a paucity of ethical problems in the home or community, as demonstrated in the following excerpt*:

> This is the first study to focus primarily on ethical problems in community/public health nursing. Little is known about the ethical problems confronting nurses in community settings as empirical research in nursing and ethics has focused almost exclusively on nurses in hospital settings. While most nurses are employed in hospital and other institutional settings, the majority of patients and clients are elsewhere in the health care system. For example, patients with more complex nursing needs are returning home as hospital stays become shorter. Findings of the study have implications for nursing practice, education, administration, research, health agency policy, and public policy.
>
> Questionnaires were sent to over one thousand staff nurses providing direct patient care and employed in community/public health nursing agencies (primarily public health nursing and hospital-based home care agencies) in Minnesota. Three hundred nineteen responses are being used for data analysis which is not yet completed. Sixty-seven percent of the respondents have baccalaureate degrees with fifty-seven percent having a major in nursing. The majority of patient care caseloads are characterized by clients over the age of 65 with long-term chronic illness. About fifteen percent of the caseloads were identified primarily as maternal/child health.
>
> Respondents identified ethical problems as a spectrum of situations ranging from situations where difficult choices are required to those where duties and obligations conflict. They were given a list of thirty-six items depicting ethical situations and asked whether they experienced the identified situation in their practice and to indicate the severity of the situation as an ethical problem. The *ten most frequently experienced ethical situations* (with ties for 1st and 7th places) were:
>
> > 1A. Client's incompetence to make or participate in major decisions about care/treatment,
> > 1B. inadequate care of client by self or family,
> > 2. limited reimbursement for needed client care,
> > 3. medical orders such as *Do Not Resuscitate*,
> > 4. disagreement with physician about treatment decisions,
> > 5. disagreement with client about treatment decisions,
> > 6. disagreement with client's family/close friends about treatment decisions,
> > 7A. withdrawal or stopping of treatment,
> > 7B. misuse/abuse of medication by client or family,
> > 8. request from client to be allowed to die,
> > 9. confidentiality of client information, and
> > 10. inadequate information for client or family to make decisions about care/treatment.
>
> The *ten leading ethical problems by degree of severity* (with a tie for 10th place) were:
>
> > 1. abuse of client's rights,

*From *Epidemiology of Ethical Problems in Community Public Health Nursing in Minnesota* by M. Aroskar, January 1988, unpublished manuscript, University of Minnesota, Biomedical Ethics Center. Reprinted by permission.

   2. lack of administrative support for establishing and maintaining a working environ-
      ment which enhances quality patient care,
   3. inadequate care of client by self or family,
   4. termination of client care by agency due to lack of reimbursement,
   5. coercion of nursing staff by administration,
   6. limited reimbursement for needed client care,
   7. questionable competency of other (not nurses) health professionals,
   8. lack of collegial support for establishing and maintaining a working environment
      which enhances quality patient care,
   9. coercion of client by family,
 10A. research protocols which jeopardize client rights, and
 10B. inadequate information for client or family to make decisions about treatment.

The *ten most severe ethical problems encountered in practice by more than half of the
respondents* were:

   1. inadequate care of client by self or family,
   2. client's incompetence to make or participate in major decisions about care/treat-
      ment,
   3. limited reimbursement for needed client care,
   4. disagreement with physician about treatment decisions,
   5. disagreement with client about treatment decisions,
   6. disagreement with client's family/close friends about treatment decisions,
   7. misuse/abuse of medications by client or family,
   8. questionable competency of other (not nurses) health professionals,
   9. inadequate information for client or family to make decisions about care/treatment,
      and
  10. coercion of client by family.

Respondents were also asked to identify and describe the most significant ethical problem
which they encountered in their practice, their response to it, and what mechanisms they
thought would be useful to deal with ethical problems in their practice. This data is being
analyzed. The descriptive data that is available from the study has implications for education
in undergraduate, graduate, and continuing education nursing programs. The data could be
used for review of existing agency policy, possible development of new agency policy, and to
influence public policy.

Ethical Dilemmas

An ethical dilemma involves the problem of trying to make the right choice between two
or more equally undesirable alternatives (Curtin & Flaherty, 1982). Knowledge of the
two theories discussed earlier can be helpful in the resolution of an ethical dilemma.
However, what constitutes an ethical dilemma for the CHN? Every problem is not necessarily of an ethical nature, nor is every ethical problem a dilemma.

   Models for ethical analysis. The following excerpt* offers an excellent model for
the analysis of an ethical dilemma:

   1. Gather as much information as possible about the situation (Assess).
      a. Background information
      b. Data base
      c. Relevant information

*From *Nursing Ethics: Theories and Pragmatics* (p. 61) by L. Curtin and M. J. Flaherty, 1982, Bowie, MD: Brady.
Copyright 1982 by Robert J. Brady Co. Reprinted by permission.

2. Identify the ethical problem. State exactly what the dilemma is.
3. Identify all of the persons who may have a part in making the decision in terms of:
   a. Scope of authority
   b. Rights
   c. Responsibilities
   d. Duties
   e. Ability to implement any given action
4. Identify the courses of action—the possible courses of action you could take. Project as accurately as you can the consequences of taking a given course of action.
5. Develop and apply an ethical ideal. This involves the deontological approach—looking at the principles behind the various potential courses of action—[and] the teleological approach—looking at the consequences that may result from the action.
6. Reach a resolution. The option that upholds the highest principles and achieves the best consequences is selected.

One must be aware that the social expectations and legal requirements may influence one's decision; however these are extrinsic to the analysis and should not be confused with right and wrong. Societal expectations and the law are not necessarily right or wrong.

Another framework that may help in attempting to resolve ethical dilemmas is the bioethics approach, which identifies six principles that can serve as guidelines in decision making when the nurse deals with ethical dilemmas (Brent, 1986, p. 615):

1. Autonomy—the right to make one's own decisions
2. Nonmaleficence—the intention to do no wrong
3. Beneficence—the principle of attempting to do things to benefit others
4. Justice—the distribution, as fairly as possible, of benefits and burdens
5. Veracity—the intention to tell the truth
6. Confidentiality—the social contract guaranteeing another's privacy

After resolution, action must take place. It is hoped that the individual will be consciously aware of the ethical theories and principles involved in this decision-making process and will rely on careful reflection and, academic acknowledgment of the theory and ethical principles applied.

The following analysis of this case study is based on Curtin and Flaherty's model (p. 609) for ethical analysis and decision making.

Step No. 1. Background information regarding the case has been gathered.

Step No. 2. The ethical problem is the decision to be made by the VA HBHC program regarding the acceptance of this case for continued nursing care and supervision in a home in which provision of adequate care by the client and care giver is highly questionable.

It is equally undesirable to keep the client in the hospital against his wishes. He is considered medically stable and eligible for discharge to his home. The high cost of hospitalization is unwarranted, providing he can receive adequate medical supervision at home.

Step No. 3. Identification of those parties involved in the decision, according to the scope of authority, rights, responsibilities, and ability to implement recommended action, are the following: the staff of the HBHC program, the physician, CHNs, social worker, nutrition consultant, physical therapist, the referral party from the hospital inpatient unit, and those individuals important in the situation: the client, Mr. T, and his care giver, Mr. J.

Step No. 4. Identification of possible courses of action and projection of possible consequences of such action are included in the following list:

Proposed options	Possible consequences
1. Keep Mr. T in the hospital (Mr. T wishes to return home)	a. Mr. T unhappiness and possible noncompliance b. High cost to the hospital, question of justification c. Assurance of adequate medical care d. Discontinuation of Mr. J's care giver responsibilities
2. Transfer Mr. T to a skilled nursing facility	a. Mr. T's unhappiness b. Possible noncompliance c. Financial costs d. Assurance of adequate nursing care e. Discontinuation of Mr. J's care giver responsibilities
3. Return Mr. T to home with more frequent visits by the CHN plus additional support services to client and care giver, such as Meals on Wheels, home health aide	a. Mr. T's happiness b. Higher incentive to follow medical regimen c. Mr. T and Mr. J daily receipt of needed assistance in complying with treatment plan d. Additional expense, but less than hospital or nursing home e. Longer duration between hospitalizations

Step No. 5. The ethical ideal is applied on the basis of the principles (deontological approach) behind the potential courses of action and consideration of the consequences (teleological theory) that may result from the action.

The ethical principles most evident are those of autonomy/self-determination versus paternalism; the client desires to return home whereas some of the health professionals believe he should not. Should not this client's autonomy be respected? Should not Mr. T have the right to determine where he wishes to live, in his own home, despite the fact that the health care team believes it is in the best interest of the patient (paternalistic viewpoint) to receive inpatient care provided by the VA hospital or care in a local skilled nursing facility?

The principles of beneficence—doing good—versus nonmaleficence—prevention of harm—also come into play. Option Nos. 1 and 2 may be viewed by the medical director of the HBHC program as the most desirable choices, that by not returning Mr. T to his home, harm (due to inadequate care) will be prevented from occurring, that is, nonmaleficence. This far outweighs the beneficent act of allowing him to return home, beneficent as viewed from the client's perspective that good has been done for his happiness.

In contrast, in option No. 3 the beneficence principle is enacted by the action to engage additional support systems to maintain Mr. T in his home. This takes precedence over the possible danger of harm being done by the client's return home because steps have been taken to lessen this probability.

According to the utilitarian viewpoint, one must calculate the consequences that result from certain actions taken and then ask how much value and how much disvalue would result in the lives of all affected parties. One then is morally obliged to choose the action that maximizes intrinsic value for all affected (Beauchamp & Childress, 1983).

Step No. 6. In terms of reaching a resolution, Robert Veach (1981) makes the following point: It is wrong to view any health professional as a primary decision-maker for patients and to maintain an image of any health care professional as existing in an exclusive, isolated patient-professional relationship (p. 19).

The client, if competent, should be the primary decision maker. Often the physician,

CASE STUDY: INADEQUATE CARE OF PATIENT BY SELF AND CARE GIVER

Mr. T is a frail but competent 63-year-old black man who is five foot eight inches, weighs 92 pounds, and resides at home with his friend and care giver, Mr. J. Mr. J is in his sixties and seems fairly reliable. Mr. T has never been married and has no living relatives. He has limited physical ability as a result of chronic obstructive pulmonary disease (COPD). He has neuropathy of his lower extremities, degenerative joint disease, and peripheral vascular disease. He has a cataract and corneal opacity of the left eye, with evidence of glaucoma. He is malnourished because of poor caloric intake. He is wheelchair bound and needs support standing and transferring from wheelchair to bed and bathroom.

His ability to function in activities of daily living is restricted because of shortness of breath on exertion, as well as severe impairment of his vision. He is able to dress and feed himself. He has no permanent teeth, has refused to use dentures, and consequently is on a soft-diet regimen with supplementary feedings of ensure, a high caloric nutritional liquid.

The two men live on the first floor of a home in need of repair. It is not always clean or free from litter. Mr. T is a veteran of World War II and receives home visits for nursing supervision from the Veterans Administration (VA) hospital-based home care program (HBHC). The medical director of the program is a physician who visits the client periodically. Mr. T takes a large number of prescribed medications that require correct administration. He receives respiratory therapy through the use of a intermittent positive pressure breathing (IPPB) machine and oral inhalation therapy (Vanceril).

The other recommended breathing exercises and postural draining positions are performed reluctantly, if at all. The care giver has been taught and supervised by the nurse regarding his participation in this treatment; however, his insistence on and consistency in the performance of these treatments for Mr. T is doubtful.

The CHN visits weekly and pours the medication for a full week in a special container that identifies the days and times the medicine is to be given. Mr. J then assumes the responsibility for giving the medicine to Mr. T. On occasion the CHN may find a pill or two that was not given; however, the caretaker usually is dependable in this area.

Mr. J prepares the meals. Although the CHN has repeatedly instructed both client and caregiver on the importance of eating a nourishing diet, preferably small amounts of food four to six times a day, it becomes apparent on questioning the client that Mr. T's daily intake usually is limited to two meals a day with Ensure as a supplement. Financial problems are not the issue because there is a sufficient pension and all medications and treatment equipment are provided by the VA hospital.

Mr. T has required hospitalization from time to time because of an exacerbation of his COPD or because of his cachectic state. His last hospitalization required intensive respiratory care. After stabilization, the recommendation for discharge to home with oxygen when necessary was made with the stipulation that his condition would be followed up by the HBHC program.

---

the nurse, the client, and the family each has a different goal. It is important that those who are confronted with ethical problems and/or dilemmas work as a team in the decision-making process (Cody, 1986).

Mr. T's life span certainly is limited because of his poor prognosis, and the health care team chose option No. 3 as the most logical decision: to return Mr. T to his home with continued nursing and medical supervision plus additional support systems for both client and care giver. This resolution upholds the principle of autonomy over paternalism. Respect for the client's rights and desire to go home is honored above the need to have a more rigidly controlled treatment environment such as the hospital or nursing home.

The opportunity for greater benefits for Mr. T in permitting his discharge to the home seems to outweigh the probability of harm being done to him. This demonstrates beneficence over nonmaleficence.

According to the utilitarian viewpoint option No. 3 allows for the greatest happiness for the greatest number of persons.

This case is but one example. Questions of confidentiality, truth telling, do-not-resuscitate (DNR) orders, informed consent, and discontinuation of tube feedings are but a few of the many ethical problems confronting CHNs (Aroskar, 1988). The client's competence, questions of safety, and a diagnosis of terminal illness also have significant bearing in the analysis of any ethical problem.

Because community health agencies provide service to frail elderly clients, CHNs should be familiar with the Older Americans Act. This basic legislation relates to the elderly and places special emphasis on the older person's right to choose living arrangements, medical care, and life-style. Of course, these premises may conflict with the reality of the highly dependent elderly person's condition. In dealing with persons of reduced competency, the principle of autonomy and free choice becomes idle rhetoric (Streib, 1983). How can free choice be honored when incompetent persons may endanger their own lives as well as the lives and safety of others? When society must assume the economic costs, how can one demand free choice?

These questions cannot be easily answered. They do serve as a stimulus and help us to recognize the need for study and investigative search.

SUMMARY

Community health nurses must be continually alert to the legal and ethical issues that concern their practice. As the number of clients receiving nursing care in the home increases, so does the likelihood that the nurse will be involved in cases involving negligence or malpractice. To provide safe and prudent care, the nurse must be familiar with local, state, and federal laws, his or her state's Nurse Practice Act, and the ANA Standards for Community Health Nursing Practice.

Ethical issues that affect the community health nurse only recently have begun to be studied. Ethical problems include abuse of clients' rights, inadequate care of clients, disagreements with physicians, clients, and families over treatment, and termination of client care.

CHAPTER HIGHLIGHTS

- Because of the great number of technological advances in home health care in recent years, the community health nurse who practices independently often is placed in a vulnerable position. Although until now the number of lawsuits has been few in community health nursing, the number is likely to increase.
- The three types of law that affect community health nursing practice are constitutional law, legislation and regulation, and judicial and common law.
- Community health nurses must be familiar with the Standards of Community Health Nursing Practice as established by the ANA. They are obliged to practice within the

confines of these standards, as well as within the scope of practice set by the state legislature in which they are licensed.

- Public health law is prevalent in the areas of communicable disease control, hereditary disease, and environment, sanitation, and housing. Federal law requires that the occurrence of certain communicable diseases be reported to the Centers for Disease Control.
- Community health nurses often become involved in cases involving child abuse. All cases of suspected child abuse must be reported to the proper authorities.
- The community health nurse often has the duty to provide informed consent to clients. One common situation for the community health nurse is that of informing parents about the possible risks associated with routine childhood immunizations.
- The community health nurse must make the decision concerning whether to carry his or her own professional liability insurance.
- Ethics has been defined as principles and rules that dictate one's conduct in a given situation. The ANA *Code for Nurses with Interpretive Statements* provides a framework of ethical conduct for the nurse.
- Nurses should be familiar with the moral and ethical principles of autonomy, beneficence, nonmaleficence, fidelity, truth telling, and justice.
- Two major theories of ethics that may guide nursing practice are the teleological (consequentialist) theory and the deontological (formalist) theory.
- Although many ethical problems exist in the home and community settings, most research on ethics in nursing has focused on the hospital setting. Therefore less is known about the ethical problems unique to community health nursing.
- An ethical dilemma exists when an individual must make a choice between two or more equally undesirable alternatives. Curtin and Flaherty's model for ethical analysis can be used to resolve an ethical dilemma.

STUDY QUESTIONS

1. Describe three types of laws that relate to community health nursing practice.
2. List specific information parents should be given regarding adverse reactions that may occur as a result of some immunization protocols.
3. Compare the teleological or consequentialist theory to the deontological or nonconsequentialist theory.
4. Apply the Curtin and Flaherty's model to the following case study.

Mr. B. is a 70-year old man who lives alone in a sparsely furnished, one-room house. It has no hot water and is heated by a space heater. The house is dirty, and Mr. B. insists on his need to keep two German shepherd dogs on the premises for his protection. He has lived in the house for 5 years and is accustomed to the lifestyle. The CHN is visiting to assess his needs related to diabetes mellitus, recent blindness, and his inability to inject or measure needed daily insulin. To maintain Mr. B. in the home it will be necessary, she determines, to visit daily to administer the insulin, and place a home health aide in the house to assist with activities of daily living. Visits and placement of the aide are complicated by the fact that the dogs are very territorial, and access to the home is impossible if Mr. B. is sleeping. There is no phone so he cannot be reached before a visit. An alternative option is nursing home placement. A decision must be reached. Mr. B. does not wish to leave his home.

REFERENCES

American Nurses' Association. (1985a, April). *Issues in professional nursing practice: Vol. 4. Ethical dilemmas in nursing practice* (NP-68D 1.5M). Kansas City, MO: Author.

American Nurses' Association, Report of Committee on Ethics. (1985b, June). *Ethical dilemmas confronting nurses* (C-165 2M). Kansas City, MO: Author.

American Nurses' Association. (1985c, July). *The code for nurses with interpretive statements* (G-56-12M). Kansas City, MO: Author.

American Nurses' Association, Report of Committee on Ethics. (A-86). *Enhancing quality of care through understanding nurses' responsibilities and rights.* Kansas City, MO: Chairperson M. Aroskar.

American Nurses' Association Council of Community Health Nurses. (1986). *Standards of community health practice,* CH-2 10M4, p. 3, Kansas City, MO: Author.

American Nurses' Association. (1986b, April). *Standards of community health nursing practice* (ANA Council of Community Health Nurses, CH-2 10M). Kansas City, MO: Author.

Aroskar, M. (1988, January). *Epidemiology of ethical problems in community/public health nursing in Minnesota* (Study Report). Unpublished manuscript, University of Minnesota, Biomedical Ethics Center.

Beauchamp, T., & Childress, J. (1983). *Principles of biomedical ethics* (2nd ed.). New York: Oxford University Press.

Brent, N. J. (1986). Legal and ethical issues in family and community health nursing. In B. B. Logan & C. E. Dawkins (Eds.), *Family-centered nursing in the community* (pp. 613-634). Menlo Park, CA: Addison-Wesley.

Centers for Disease Control. (1982). 42 U.S.C., 236, 289c-4, 247d, 436a.

Cody, M. (1986). Withholding treatment: Is it ethical? *Journal of Gerontological Nursing, 12*(3), 24-26.

Conrad, P. (1987). The noncompliant patient in search of autonomy. *Hastings Center Report, 17*(4), 15-17.

Curtin, L., & Flaherty, M. J. (1982). *Nursing ethics: Theories and pragmatics.* Bowie, MD: Robert J Brady Co.

Davis, A. J., & Aroskar, M. (1983). *Ethical dilemmas and nursing practice,* (2nd ed.). New York: Appleton-Century-Crofts.

Davis, A. J., & Aroskar, M. (1978). *Ethical dilemmas and nursing practice.* New York: Appleton-Century-Crofts.

Fry, S. T. (1985). Values and health. In B. W. Spradley (Ed.), *Community health nursing concepts and practice* (2nd ed.) (pp. 106-128). Boston: Little Brown & Co.

Illinois Annotated Statutes. (1985). Ch. 126, 21 (Smith-Hurd Suppl).

Jameton, A. (1984). *Nursing practices: The ethical issues.* Englewood Cliffs, NJ: Prentice-Hall.

Lancaster, J., & Kerschner, D. (1988). Violence and human abuse. In M. Stanhope & J. Lancaster (Eds.),

Community health nursing: Process and practice for promoting health (2nd ed.) (pp. 663-681). St. Louis: Mosby.

Lynn, J. L. (1986). *By no extraordinary means the choice to forgo life-sustaining food and water.* Bloomington: Indiana University Press.

Maryland Health—General Code Annotation. (1982), No. 18-205 (e), (f), and (h) and 18-322 (b) (1982) (confidential tuberculosis registry).

Maryland Health—General Code Annotation. (1985a). No. 18-330 (Suppl.).

Maryland Health—General Code Annotation. (1985b). No. 18-332 (Suppl.).

Misener, T. R. (1986, July). Toward a nursing definition of child maltreatment using serious vignettes. *Advances in Nursing Science, 8*(4), 1-14.

Northrop, C. E. (1988). Governmental, political, and legal influences on the practice of community health nursing. In M. Stanhope & J. Lancaster (Eds.), *Community health nursing: Process and practice for promoting health* (2nd ed.) (pp. 109-126). St. Louis: Mosby.

Northrop, C. E., & Kelly M. E. (1987). *Legal issues in nursing.* St. Louis: Mosby.

Public Health Service. (1985, August). *Facts about AIDS.* Washington, DC: U.S. Department of Health and Human Services.

Steel, S. M., & Harmon, M. V. (1983). *Values clarification in nursing* (2nd ed.). East Norwalk, CT: Appleton-Century-Crofts.

Streib, G. F. (1983). The frail elderly: Research dilemmas and research opportunities. *The Gerontologist, 23*(1), 40-44.

Tammelleo, D. (Ed.) (1987, December). Case in point: Roach v. Kelly health care (742 P. 2d 1190—OR) (Home Health Care and Legal Issues) In *The Reagan Report on Nursing Law* (Vol. 28, No. 7). Providence, RI: Medica Press.

Toffler, A. (1970) *Future Shock.* New York: Random House, Inc.

University of the State of New York, State Education Department. (1982). *Immunization: A handbook for schools* (2nd ed.). Albany, NY: Author.

Veatch, R. (1981). Nursing ethics, physician ethics, and medical ethics. *Law, Medicine and Health Care, 9,* 19.

Veatch, R., & Fry, S. (1987). *Case studies in nursing ethics.* Philadelphia: Lippincott.

Voell, P. (1988, August 9). Health care at home on rise. *The Buffalo News,* section D, p. 1.

Professional Issues: The Future of Community Health Nursing

CAROL BATRA

The power of forming any correct opinion as to the result must entirely depend upon an enquiry into all the conditions in which the patient lives.... Minute enquiries into conditions enable us to know that in such a district will be the excess of mortality, that is, the person will die who ought not to have died before old age.

FLORENCE NIGHTINGALE

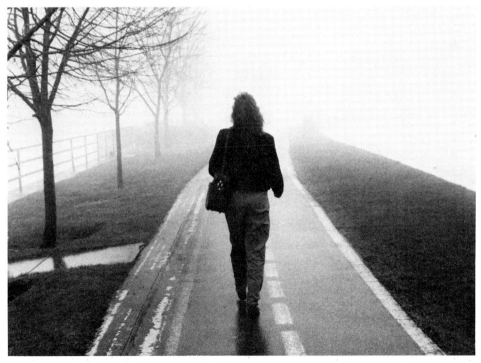

OBJECTIVES

At the conclusion of this chapter the student will be able to:

1. Define the key terms listed
2. Describe community health nursing professional issues from the perspective of the metaparadigm of nursing
3. Describe the ambiguities in terminology relevant to the client in community health nursing
4. Recognize ethical issues in environmental hazards for the community health nursing role
5. Predict health policy issues of the future
6. Discuss the problems of quality, access, and cost in relation to the health care system and federal legislation
7. Contrast meanings, models, and paradigms of health
8. Identify issues in the development of community health nursing theory and in each of the phases of the nursing process
9. Describe actions needed in community health nursing as a result of future trends in the health care delivery system and in consumers and nursing

KEY TERMS

Access to care	Health behavior paradigms
Adaptive model of health	Leadership
Clinical model of health	Metaparadigm of nursing
Community as client	Nursing center
Community health nursing diagnosis	Nursing entrepreneurship
Community health nursing theory	Person
Consumer trends	Political action
Cost of care	Quality of care
Critical competencies	Role performance model of health
Environment	Theory development
Eudaemonistic model of health	Third-party reimbursement

T he professional issues that present a challenge to community health nursing have been raised throughout the previous chapters in relation to the specific topics under discussion. In this chapter these issues are discussed from the perspective of the metaparadigm of nursing. The metaparadigm of any discipline reflects its members' identification of the discipline's own unique and specific areas of interest. It is therefore the collective philosophy, orientation, or world view adopted by the members of the particular discipline (Firlit, 1990).

THE METAPARADIGM OF NURSING

Most disciplines have a single global metaparadigm. Considerable agreement now exists that the metaparadigm of nursing includes the four key concepts of person, environment, health, and nursing (Fawcett, 1984). The concept of person will be addressed by a discussion of the different definitions for the "client" in community health nursing. The

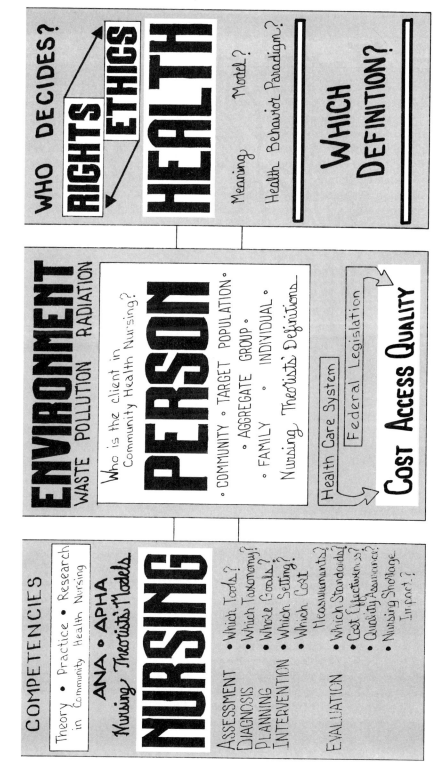

FIG. 28-1 Professional issues affecting community health nursing within the metaparadigm of nursing.

environment concept will be used to examine the natural environment issues discussed in Chapter 25, along with the issues of cost, access, and quality of the total health care system. The concept of health will be devoted to the issues of who determines health and who has the right to health. The concept of nursing itself will encompass an examination of the issues pertaining to each phase of the nursing process—assessment, diagnosis, planning, intervention, and evaluation—relevant to community health nursing. Fig. 28-1 demonstrates the professional issues that affect community health nursing from the perspective or structure of the metaparadigm of nursing.

After a discussion of the professional issues, the chapter concludes with a look at possible directions and the future of community health nursing and a discussion of trends in the health of the overall population, from acute to chronic illness and the changes in the health care system, which have increased the importance of discharge planning and quality assurance. The need for the community health nurse to act as a leader, to effect planned change, and to become involved politically will show the challenging role for nurses who choose a career in the field of community health nursing.

Person

Definition of community as the client. The focus and recipient of nursing care is known as the "client." In community health nursing the precise definition of this term is unclear, often abstract, and multidimensional. Throughout the text and particularly in Chapter 3, the Betty Neuman health care system model definition of client is offered as the focus of client care in the community and the basis for nursing assessment, nursing diagnosis, and nursing interventions.

Chapters 9 through 12 suggest that the client in community health nursing is the individual and possibly the family. Similarly Chapters 16 through 19 and 21, 22 and 23 emphasize the individual as client for discharge planning; home health care; and high-technology, chronic illness, and high-risk aggregates; communicable diseases; and the developmentally disabled.

Chapters 13 through 15 portray the family as the client for community health nursing. Functional and dysfunctional families are included here, along with families from different cultures.

Chapter 6 states that the group is the client in community health nursing. Community development groups support client advocacy; for example, the Gray Panthers group educates the elderly in their rights for rent control. Support or self-help groups use peer cohesiveness for behavior control, for coping with stress, or for personal growth. Educational groups provide information on preventive health.

In Chapter 4 wellness and health promotion models are presented from the perspectives of the individual and the family as the client. The multilevel approaches toward community health (MATCH) model specifies target populations of individuals, organizations, and governments. Individuals as clients are influenced to reduce personal risk factors. Organizations are influenced through policies and practices to reduce environmental risk factors for disease. Governments are influenced through public action and legislation to reduce environmental risk factors for disease.

Occupational health nursing, as presented in Chapter 20, is similar to the MATCH model's concept of client in its health care and safety concerns of the adult working population in the working environment. Chapter 26, in describing environmental issues, further suggests that these three target populations of the MATCH model are the client for community health nursing.

Effie Hanchett (1988) views community as client as a continuum of conceptions: an aggregate, a system, or a field. Each concept represents a more integrated, holistic view of the community. Hanchett points out that few nursing theorists deal directly with the community. Many of their models have been extended to be applied to the family as client (Clements & Roberts, 1983).

Hanchett extends the nursing theories of Dorothea Orem, Callista Roy, Imogene King, and Martha Rogers* and applies them to the community as client. She sees Orem's theory of self-care deficit as compatible with the concept of community as aggregate. In the industrialized world, Orem's self-care requisites are managed by the community as a system or group. Roy's model of the person as an adaptive system can be applied to the community as an adaptive system. Then the functions of the community would be viewed as community behaviors in response to stimuli. From King's framework the focus for defining the community as a system would be the interaction of the personal, interpersonal, and social systems. Within Rogers' world view of human-environmental field process, descriptions of community-environmental patterns, such as motion or conscious partic-ipation in change, would be the focus of concern. Selection of a particular nursing the-oretical framework would influence the structure of the assessment of the community as client, as well as the diagnoses and focus of the nursing interventions. (See Table 1-3 for a list of selected nursing theorists who have influenced the development of community health nursing.)

Barbara Spradley (1990) uses three criteria for identifying the types of community in community health practice:

1. Geography: Geographical boundaries, as in a census tract or a county
2. Common interest, as in a group of migrant workers or an industrial site and its neighborhood
3. Health problem or community of solution, as in air pollution or teen drug abuse

Spradley further differentiates the client labels in community health nursing historically:

1. Individual: District nursing (1860-1900) focused on the sick poor
2. Family: Public health nursing (1900-1970) focused on the needy public
3. Population: Community health nursing (1970-present) focused on the total com-munity

What exactly is meant by the term "community"? What are the definitive character-istics of the recipients of community health nursing practice? Do individuals, families, groups, and communities have the same needs and goals? Still other related terms used to describe community health nursing clients are aggregates, target populations, and systems. What are the dimensions of communities? Current definitions of community health nursing practice seem to assume that these questions have been answered. There is a great need for clarification of whether the community is (1) the setting or the context of the individual's existence, (2) the setting or context of nursing interventions, or (3) the primary client (Hamilton, 1983).

Ethical issues in defining the client. Who shall be the priority recipients of com-munity health nursing practice? Who shall have access to care? Who shall pay for the care? What should be the level of care?

All these questions pertain to the person concept of the metaparadigm. The nature of the clients needing community health nursing care with increasing frequency now

---

*See Marriner-Tomey (1989) for definitions of health by nursing theorists mentioned in this chapter.

include clients with acquired immunodeficiency syndrome (AIDS), the elderly and chronically ill and their care givers, the acutely ill who require high-tech home health care, and the high-risk populations of substance abusers and the homeless. Who determines which of these challenging populations will be the client for the community health nurse?

Environment

Environmental health issues. Chapter 25 raises many issues about environmental health and its influence on community health nursing. Assessing clients' environments for all the various pollution possibilities (solid and hazardous wastes; water, air, and noise pollutions; and radiation hazards) raises the ethical issue of truth telling or whistle blowing when problems are identified. Clients' environments and possible corresponding health problems can include family homes (e.g., radon gas), schools (e.g., asbestos insulation), businesses, industries, and other occupational health settings, as well as health care settings (e.g., radiation, communicable disease, hospital-acquired disease, and treatment hazards).

Even teaching clients about environmental hazards raises similar ethical concerns for the community health nurse. As the public becomes increasingly knowledgeable about human-created pollution and environmental hazards, the community health nurse will face even greater questions and dilemmas, perhaps, than those faced by the nurse in the hospital setting.

Health care system: cost, access, and quality issues. What happens in community health nursing practice is totally controlled by what is happening in the total health care system and particularly what is happening politically and economically at the national, state, and county governmental levels.

A 1987 study by the American College of Healthcare Executives addressed the issues that affect national health policy for the 1990s (Wesbury, 1988). The number-one policy issue that was named most critical by the 1600-member panel of experts was the aging of America. In addition to an increased need for health care services, the growing numbers of elderly persons also means that this group will have far more influence on who will be elected to public office. The American Association of Retired Persons (AARP) is a politically aggressive group that will continue to grow in influence.

The second most critical issue involved governmental payment decisions. The third issue was the implications of AIDS. They felt that by 1995 there would be a cure for AIDS.

This study revealed that health care executives believed nurses should be most concerned with quality of care and the issue of minimal access to care. Quality of care will become better defined and better measured in terms of clinical outcomes. Although quality usually is assessed by peer review, commercial insurance plans will produce more demands for quality care. The computer will be used more frequently for quality assessment and for evaluating effectiveness of care and client outcomes, as well as for cost-management structures. The malpractice scene will continue to be debated regarding the excessively high costs versus the poor quality care offered by only a minority of providers. How much money can be or should be awarded for the results of poor quality care? What controls should there be for abuse of financial compensation through lawsuits?

Access to care will continue to be a major problem. National health insurance is not expected to be in place in the 1990s, particularly with the federal government's current struggle to lower the national deficit. Approximately 15% of the U.S. population does not have health insurance, and an even larger percentage has inadequate coverage. Consequently, those with coverage will have no difficulty finding care whereas those without coverage will find it increasingly difficult to obtain access to care. Without any national programs forecast for indigent care, local solutions will become imperative. In reality, however, what will happen is that the federal health care agenda will be driven by the deficit and by concerns about Medicare. The panel of health care executives also predicts that hospitals will continue to close, particularly the small hospitals, as a result of fewer admissions and a continually decreasing length of stay.

The panelists believed that there will be continued development of alternative delivery systems, with eventually an equal number of health maintenance organizations (HMOs) and preferred provider organizations (PPOs). Health care reimbursement methods will continue to be based on a diagnosis-related group (DRG) prospective payment system. The issue here will be whether the hospital or the physician should receive the payment or whether the government should move toward a combined DRG payment, with hospital and physician payment. The greatest likelihood would be that a third-party administrator would receive the check to be allocated appropriately to the physician and to the hospital. This study predicted that physician fee-for-service would be replaced by a capitation system for family care providers, with a fee schedule for specialists. This group also predicted that nurses or other provider groups would have few chances of creating new fee-for-service programs. They believed the government was moving away from fee-for-service in favor of capitation-type payment programs. Medicare beneficiaries will be paying more, and employees can expect to pay more for their care. State and local governments will have to pick up the increasing costs of indigent care.

Federal legislation: cost, access, and quality issues. Harrington (1988), Gould (1989), and Pera and Gould (1989) report that the quality of home health services delivered by some agencies is substandard, and yet the regulation of home health care quality is underdeveloped. The home care sector of the health care industry has the least amount of external monitoring. The Medicare home health care certification program was enacted to try to deal with this issue in the Omnibus Budget Reconciliation Act of 1987 (P.L. 100-203) in December 1987. However, the implementation of this Act has still a long way to go in terms of specific standards and policies.

Medicare will pay for home health services for those with short-term rehabilitation needs. The federal Health Omnibus Program Extension of 1988 increased the availability of home health care for persons with AIDS through block grants to states. These funds are very limited, however, and reserved for chronic conditions; after specified times the individual must pay for continued services. Compounding these two issues is the fact that the demand for home health services is escalating because of the increase in chronic conditions, the increase in life span, and the prospective payment system for hospitals, which gives them greater incentives to discharge patients as early as possible. An editorial in the *AARP Bulletin* (January 1990) indicated that "more than 800,000 errors a year" were identified in the treatment of Medicare cases and that elderly clients are being discharged from hospitals "quicker and sicker."

The Medicare Catastrophic Coverage Act of 1988 was meant to expand Medicare coverage. The new law, in effect as of January 1, 1989, provided for unlimited hospital and hospice coverage after deductible fees were met, as well as for increased coverage from 100 to 150 days a year for acute care in a skilled nursing home. By January 1, 1990, coverage for home health services was increased from 3 weeks per year to 38 consecutive days per year and for an indefinite period of home care for 6 or fewer days per week. Prescription drug expenses after a $600 annual deductible would be paid for by Medicare at a 50% rate in 1991, 60% in 1992, and 80% in 1993 (Demkovich, 1988).

This apparent progress in catastrophic coverage came to a halt when Congress repealed the program in November 1989, only 16 months after this landmark legislation was signed into law. Unlimited hospital coverage; expanded home health, hospice, and skilled nursing care; and expanded prescription drug coverage were all withdrawn (Carlson, 1990). The result was a return to limited home health care benefits for those with chronic health problems.

A study by Phillips, Scattergood, Fisher, & Baglioni (1988) raised the suspicion that nonpublic home health agencies were providing reimbursable care, leaving the nonreimbursable care to public agencies. Proprietary agencies proliferated in the early 1980s when they were able to be certified as Medicare providers without having state licensure. Hospital-based home health agencies also entered the picture in the early 1980s. These providers have continued to expand as the effects of the prospective payment system decreased the need for hospital beds. Hospitals saw the opportunity of entering the home care market as a means of financial gain. Not surprisingly, with the proliferation of agencies, federal costs of Medicare reimbursement have been escalating. The denials of home care claims started to increase, and home care services began to be determined by carefully labeled terminology and limited services.

Patricia Moccia (1989) predicts trends of ever-quickening decline of acute care "empires" as a result of changing population demographics. She sees a resultant shift of service needs to out-of-hospital technology and procedures, leading to a continued oversupply of hospital beds. She sees increased public scrutiny of health care policies and an increased demand for quality standards. Last, it is disturbing to note that she forecasts an increasingly sick citizenry in the United States, with rapidly deteriorating public health. As is shown in Chapters 2, 8, and 27, access, quality, and cost historically are the three big issues that stand out in every dimension of the health care of the public.

Health

Meaning of health. Health is a concept with many different interpretations. There is consensus that health is a quality to be attained and preserved; however, there is no clear agreement on exactly what this state of health is. Nevertheless it is imperative that this important concept be specified to establish public health policy at local, regional, state, and national levels.

Chapter 4 explores various definitions of health from the World Health Organization, Halpert Dunn, Don Ardell (high-level wellness), Rene Dubos, and Ivan Illich. Nursing theorists' definitions of health also are reviewed from the perspectives of Betty Neuman, Margaret Newman, Rosemary Parse, and Nola Pender. Wellness models such as Irwin M. Rosenstock's health belief model, Dorothea Orem's self-care theory, and Barbara Blattner's holistic nursing approach to wellness are contrasted. Chapter 4 concluded that the focus of community health nurses should be on *Health* services, not *Illness* services. Such a focus would cut health care costs.

Models of health. Judith Smith (1985) tried to clarify the meaning and level of health that are deemed desirable for a community in order to determine measureable goals for delivering health care. She asked the following questions: (1) What are the goals to be achieved by health care? (2) What is a sufficient extent of improvement of health care? (3) What is the level of health to which the care is to raise the individual or the community? Smith categorized all the concepts of health that have been proposed into four models, ranging from a state of minimal health to one of the maximal condition of general well-being. She labeled these models as clinical, role performance, adaptive, and eudaemonistic (1983; 1985). Figure 28-2 shows how each one deals with a continuum of states from health to illness (Smith, 1983).

The clinical model of the view of health as the absence of disease is most allied to the focus of medical practice. That is, health is achieved when the signs and symptoms

HEALTH-ILLNESS CONTINUUM

	HEALTH	ILLNESS
Clinical model	Absence of signs or symptoms	Conspicuous presence of signs or symptoms
Role-performance model	Maximum expected performance	Total failure in performance
Adaptive model	Flexible adaptation to environment	Total failure in self-corrective response
Eudaimonistic model	Exuberant well-being	Enervation, languishing debility

FIG. 28-2 Smith's four models of health. *(From* The idea of health: implications for the nursing professional (p. 32) *by J. A. Smith, 1983, New York, Teachers College Press. Reprinted by permission.)*

of disease are eradicated. In public health science this view is comparable to the epidemiological approach toward health (Chapter 7). Few nursing theorists have such a biomedical view of health. Only Joyce Travelbee (1971) partially used this narrow perspective in defining "objective" health as "the absence of discernible disease, disability, or defect," which is determined by the outward effects of illness on the individual. Ida Jean Orlando (1961) and Ernestine Wiedenbach (1964) alluded to a state of distress and "need-for-help," which may fall under the clinical model.

The role-performance model adds the dimension that healthy individuals must fulfill a role in society. Hildegard Peplau (1952) viewed health from this perspective, stating that health implies "forward movement of human processes in the direction of creative, constructive, productive, personal and community living."

The adaptive model views health as the effective functioning of adaptive systems. It implies that people have the capacity to adjust to changing circumstances through growth, expansion, and creativity. All the nurse theorists who advocate a systems approach, such as Imogene King (1971), Myra Levine (1974), Dorothy Johnson (1980), Betty Neuman (1982), and Sr. Callista Roy (1984) would be included in the adaptive model of health.

Smith's fourth model is the eudaimonistic conception of health, wherein health includes qualities such as self-actualization, fulfillment, and loving. The views of nurse theorists such as Florence Nightingale (1860), Martha Rogers (1970), Margaret Newman (1979), Rosemary Parse (1981), and Joyce Fitzpatrick (1983) are most closely allied to Smith's last model of health.

Smith (1985) reinforces the nature of the continuum and overlapping features of these models in asking the following question. If resources for public health are limited, how should adequate minimal health be defined? If we cannot specify positive tests for minimal levels, can we determine what should be adequate or necessary conditions for

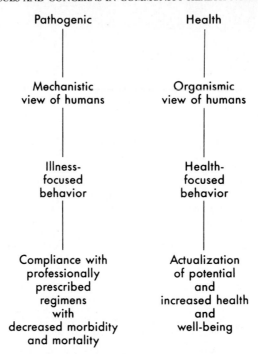

FIG. 28-3 Two major paradigms of health concepts. *(From "Health behavior: evolution of two paradigms" by S. C. Laffrey, C. J. Loveland-Cherry, and S. J. Winkler, June 1986, Public Health Nursing, 3(2) pp. 92-100. Copyright 1986 by Public Health Nursing. Reprinted by permission of Blackwell Scientific Publications, Inc.)*

health? Smith points out that historically public health agencies have aimed to maintain health by implementing programs that can be controlled by the public without the need for the individual's cooperation. The traditional Nightingale concerns still are pertinent: sanitation of water and streets, waste disposal, food inspection, physical environment, and atmosphere regulation. Controlling these conditions has provided an indirect minimum standard of adequate health, preventing the rise and spread of disease. This control has made possible the achievement of health as interpreted by Smith's first three models. Implementation of public health policy on the basis of Smith's fourth (eudaemonistic) model of health would require the development of opportunities in cultural, educational, and recreational activities for the achievement of community health.

Health behavior paradigms. Laffrey, Loveland-Cherry, and Winkler (1986) noted that health behavior can vary in definition from (1) use of health care services, (2) compliance with medically prescribed regimens, (3) routine activities of life such as eating and sleeping, and (4) actions taken to prevent illness to (5) actions taken to achieve a higher level of well-being. They described health behavior from the evolution of two major paradigms in the literature (Fig. 28-2). Health behavior is defined according to the individual's perception of the key concepts: person, environment, and health. There are two major views of these concepts: the pathogenic or disease paradigm whereby health is freedom from disease and the health paradigm wherein health is a subjective human phenomenon and involves the entire life situation of the individual. These views demonstrate how the general shift today in public health nursing science is toward the health paradigm, whereas earlier literature focused exclusively on the disease paradigm. Laffrey et al. hope that disease prevention can be incorporated as one factor in health promotion, the latter being of a much broader scope than is disease prevention. This issue is especially important in terms of the nursing profession's increased emphasis on health behavior and the stated goal of health promotion.

Rights to health and to health care. An issue related to the definition of health is that of who has the right to health and health care. The extent and nature of public care for individual health continue to be a controversial issue. Are all persons entitled to equal health care? If resources are inadequate for the demand, who will interpret the measurement of health? Who will determine the fair allocation of health care? Smith supports the concept of equal access to health care if only a minimal adequate amount of health care is available rather than unlimited services.

Jean Goeppinger (1984) added to the complexity of this issue by indicating that many individuals and communities do not choose to participate actively in health care matters. In such cases a specification of health standards can be difficult to implement. Furthermore the United States has been concerned historically with the individual, not the collective. How then can any public body determine what will be the level of health for a collective, a community? This situation would be contrary to our much-protected belief in free choice.

Mary Ann Ruffing-Rahal (1987) has shown the differences between resident-identified and provider-identified community priorities (Table 28-1). The fact that the residents prioritized two issues not mentioned by providers (environmental concerns and crime prevention) points out how crucial it is to have a common understanding of the definition of health in a particular community. Measures to reflect sensitivity to this issue of client

TABLE 28-1 Comparison of resident-identified versus provider-identified community priorities

Category	Resident priority			Provider priority		
	Rank	No.	%	Rank	No.	%
Environmental concerns*	1	39	13.6	—	—	—
Alcohol and substance abuse	2	36	12.5	4	24	8.4
Crime prevention*	3	26	9.0	—	—	—
Teen pregnancy	4	20	7.0	2	28	9.8
Primary health care/preventive services	5	15	5.2	3	28	9.8
Nutrition	6	15	5.2	7	16	5.6
Cardiovascular diseases	7	15	5.2	5	21	7.3
Senior services	8	14	4.9	1	30	10.5
Financial resources	9	14	4.9	9	13	4.5
Emotional/mental health	10	12	4.2	8	15	5.2
Child health†	—	—	—	6	20	7.0
Accident prevention/auto safety†	—	—	—	10	12	4.2
Other		81	28.2		80	27.9
TOTAL		287	100.0		287	100.0

From "Resident/Provider Contrasts in Community Health Priorities" by M.A. Ruffing-Rahal, 1987, *Public Health Nursing, 4(4),* p. 242. Copyright 1987 by Blackwell Scientific Publications, Inc. Modified by permission.

*Priority cited only by residents.
†Priority cited only by providers.

input for defining health for a specific community are crucial to plan for health care services that will be effectively used by that community's citizenry.

Nursing: Community Health Nursing Issues

The fourth key concept in the metaparadigm of nursing is nursing itself. In this area there is an abundance of professional issues that affect community health nursing. These issues are examined from the perspective of nursing theory and research and then according to each of the phases of the nursing process in terms of community health nursing.

Theory development and research. Chapter 1 outlines the contributions of nursing theory to community health nursing. There continues to be, however, a lack of conceptual clarity and of theory development regarding community health nursing. Hamilton and Bush (1988) provide a framework for analyzing theory for use in community health nursing (Fig. 28-3). They suggest that there may be four routes to developing community health nursing theory:

1. The sum of two distinctly different types of theory (i.e., public health and generic nursing)
2. The transformation of theory from a nonnursing discipline into community health nursing theory
3. Generic nursing theory transformed into community health nursing theory
4. Theory derived from a unique community health nursing perspective

They further elaborate on issues to be answered, depending on which of these aforementioned approaches would be most acceptable:

1. Should there be greater emphasis on joint research with disciplines outside of nursing to stimulate research and theories that can be applied to community health nursing practice?
2. How much community health nursing practice is generic nursing, and how much, or what part, is uniquely community health nursing?
3. Should research and theory parallel those in such fields as anthropology, epidemiology, community medicine, or sociology, or do nurses need to develop separate research and theory based on their unique contributions to community health?

Historical research concerning the work of Nightingale, Lillian Wald, and others provide much insight into community health nursing practice over time. Qualitative research methods would be helpful to differentiate the experiences of generic and community health nurses and to identify the experiences of community health clients. Patterns of practice and structures for practice would be examined in terms of their corresponding responses to the political, social, economic, and legal environments. Questions that would be helpful to understand the process of community health nursing include the following:

1. Whom do community health nurses assess: the individual, family, group, or community?
2. What do community health nurses assess?
3. What nursing diagnoses do community health nurses use?
4. What types of nursing interventions do community health nurses use in practice?
5. How do interventions differ with differences in client focus?
6. How is community health nursing evaluated?

In terms of education of community health nurses, a number of issues arise that may throw some light on community health nursing theory development:

Emerging Theory Specifically for Community Health Nursing

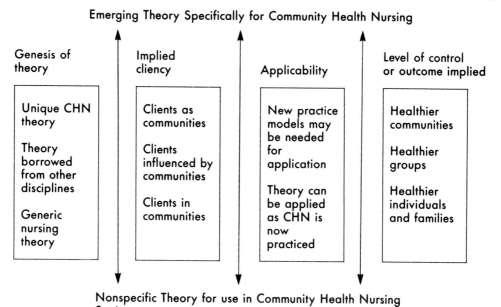

FIG. 28-4 Framework for analyzing theory for use in community health nursing. *(From "Theory development in community health nursing: issues and recommendations" by P. A. Hamilton and H. A. Bush, Summer 1988, Scholarly Inquiry for Nursing Practice 2(2) pp. 145-160. Copyright 1988 by Scholarly Inquiry for Nursing Practice, published by Springer Publishing Company, Inc., New York 10012. Reprinted by permission.)*

1. What are the unique concepts of community health nursing taught by nursing educators?
2. How is community health nursing taught in educational programs: as a discrete content area or "integrated" throughout the curriculum?
3. What is the relative emphasis in nursing education programs between community health nursing and other areas of nursing or generic nursing?
4. Should community health nurses be prepared at the level of:
   BSN (Bachelor of Science in Nursing), or
   MSN (Master of Science in Nursing, with a major in Community Health Nursing), or
   MPH (Master of Public Health, not a nursing degree at the graduate level, but with a BSN as prior preparation).
5. What clinical settings should be used for teaching community health nursing?

One report (Jones, Davis, and Davis, 1987) examined the results of an exhaustive study on these very issues and concluded with nine recommendations. Among these were that the baccalaureate program needs to develop not only basic nursing skills but also nursing theory and practice skills involved in public health nursing. The study was conducted by representatives of official health agencies and baccalaureate nursing programs. The box lists the critical competencies for public health nurses according to topic areas agreed upon by the agency staff and faculty.

Nursing assessment. The previously listed research questions for understanding community health nursing suggest that there may be a wide variety of areas that are considered appropriate and necessary for assessment in community health nursing.

Chapter 3 provides a community assessment guide based on categories and terminology from Betty Neuman's health care systems model. Chapter 4 presents areas of assessment in terms of the components of wellness. Chapter 5 suggests that an educational assessment must be performed for health teaching in the community. Chapter 7 describes epidemiological methods of collecting data, and Chapter 8 provides guidelines for a needs assessment for quality assurance. Chapter 13 offers a variety of tools for a family assessment, and Chapter 14 provides detailed guidance for conducting a cultural assessment of a family. Through the use of the structure of Neuman's framework to describe the characteristics of dysfunctional families, Chapter 15 demonstrates an easily used tool to assess these families. Chapter 17 identifies all the components necessary to perform an assessment for discharge planning.

It can be concluded from this wealth of available assessment tools that the instrument to be selected depends upon the client with whom the community health nurse is concerned at any point in time. In addition, many more assessment guides exist that are compatible with the particular nursing theory or model adopted by the community health nurse in practice. Another area necessitating the use of tools for client assessment requirement is that of satisfying the reimbursing agency's requirement to justify the need for the provided care. Instruments for needs assessment must evaluate the functional capacity of the client, the need for nursing and other health care requirements to meet the client's needs and to assist with functional incapacities, and the resources available to meet those requirements. The issue is clearly one of how organized data collection can be conducted in community health nursing, with an endless assortment of structures for that data collection to take place.

Nursing diagnosis. With the lack of clarity in terms of nursing assessment in community health nursing, it follows that nursing diagnosis in community health nursing is equally undeveloped. Patti Hamilton (1983) provided an extensive analysis of community nursing diagnoses, pointing out that nursing diagnoses typically are generated from assessments of the individual but that they need to reflect the community. She believes that classifications of community nursing diagnoses will evolve in the future. Now research needs to be undertaken first on what communities are like and on what ways nurses enter into association with communities. Furthermore, ascertaining the scope of effectiveness of nurses with communities as clients is necessary for the development of community nursing diagnoses.

Throughout the text examples of nursing diagnoses relevant to the community are suggested. Those in Chapter 3 are given within the Neuman's framework for one community with low-level wellness and another with high-level wellness. Any of the other nursing theorists' frameworks possibly could have produced different nursing diagnoses or different language in the nursing diagnoses.

Chapter 5 points out that one of the 72 nursing diagnostic categories is that of knowledge deficit related to managing a health problem. The knowledge deficit category can be used extensively as a basis for all the health teaching conducted by community health nurses. Chapter 10 provides selected nursing diagnoses from the North American Nursing Diagnosis Association (NANDA)– approved nursing diagnostic categories for the school-aged child, and Chapter 12 does the same for the older adult.

In a critique of the concept of community health diagnosis (Marjorie Muecke, 1984) proposes the following steps to identify the community of concern:

1. Identification of the community's health risk
2. Specification of the characteristics of the community and its environment that are etiologically associated with the risks
3. Specification of the health indicators that verify the risk

Phyllis Andrews (1990) identifies criteria that set community nursing diagnoses apart from individual or family nursing diagnoses:

1. The diagnosis is generated from assessments, not only of the state of individuals but also of the state of the community as a physical, sociocultural, experiential entity.
2. Relational statements imply intervention not by providing direct client services—although these may be the ultimate result—but by instituting some change in the present community.
3. The implied direct client is the community; the indirect client is the individual.

For example, passing a state law prohibiting smoking in public places may be the result of a community diagnosis of increased number of respiratory diseases related to air pollution. The total community is the direct client targeted for the intervention, whereas the individual is the indirect client.

The lack of an existing and nationally recognized categorization of the reasons for a visit by a community health nurse points out the lack of a common understanding of community nursing diagnosis. Valid and reliable systems for classifying home visits in terms of the presenting problem(s) potentially amenable to the interventions of community health nurses would group clients in an organized and retrievable fashion to facilitate evaluations of interventions and client outcomes. Measures of case mix and severity of illness are necessary to judge the intensity of needed nursing care. The combination of these measures might lead to the development of DRGs for home health practice.

Nursing goals. Jean Goeppinger (1984) examines the principal issues of community health nursing from the perspective of the following questions:

1. What are the goals of community health nursing practice?
2. What are the target systems that community health nurses intend to change?
3. What roles are particularly appropriate for community nurses?
4. In what settings do community health nurses practice?

A variety of position statements articulated the goals of community health nursing practice in the year 1980. The American Nurse's Association Division on Community Health Nursing published *A Conceptual Model for Community Health Nursing.* The Public Health Nursing Section of the American Public Health Association published *Definition and Role of Public Health Nursing in the Delivery of Health Care.* These statements provided such divergent positions that a question arises: should the goals be eclectic, extensive, and inclusive or focused, restrictive, and exclusive?

Nursing intervention. Settings for community health nursing practice lead to a question of whether community health nursing is setting-specific. Is it community-oriented simply because of its site or is it community-oriented because it emphasizes the collective need?

Two newer and related developments in nursing community settings are the nursing center concept and nurses in private practice or nursing entrepreneurship. Nursing centers may be referred to as community nursing organizations, nurse-managed centers, nursing clinics, or community nursing centers (American Nurses' Association, 1987). These centers give clients direct access to professional nursing services that are holistic and client-centered and that are reimbursable at a reasonable fee level. These may be freestanding businesses, or they may be affiliated with universities or other service agencies. The relationship of the nursing center to the other agencies that offer community health nursing services is an interesting issue.

The development of private practice in nursing, a new organizational model for nursing services, has led to increased motivation for the acquisition of third-party reimbursement for nursing services. The American Nurses' Foundation (1988) conducted a study on the characteristics, organizational arrangements, and reimbursement policies of nurses in private practice. Nursing centers may be one such setting for nursing entrepreneurs. This movement may provide one means of responding to the competitiveness for limited resources and the pressures for new methods of care delivery. On the other hand, this movement contradicts the findings of the health care executives' study mentioned earlier, whereby they predicted that nurses would have few chances of creating new fee-for-service programs. Issues continue to be raised concerning the sources of financing for nursing care, the mechanisms for paying nurses, and the systems of organizing and delivering nursing care.

A related nursing intervention issue is that of the measurement of costs of community health nursing in the home health care setting. Christine Kovner (1989) categorizes alternatives into four models: per visit, acuity of care, hourly, and by diagnosis. She recommends a time-based approach adjusted for differential use of supplies.

Evaluation of nursing care. Measurement of the outcome of community health nursing leads to a variety of questions and issues:

1. What are the consequences of organizing care around reimbursement guidelines rather than in terms of a theory-based approach?
2. What level of focus of community health nursing is most cost effective: individuals, families, groups, or communities?
3. What are the effects of changes in referral patterns, level of illness of clients referred, intensity of services required, and quality of services delivered?
4. What measures of client outcomes in terms of behavioral or functional changes can be used to evaluate the interventions of community health nurses?
5. What are the effects of different management procedures for various types of clients?
6. What is the effect of various management structures and types of agencies on the way home care is delivered?
7. What are the relationships among client assessment, care plans, and client outcomes?

Beverly Flynn and Dixie Ray (1987) contrast several quality assessment criteria or measurement strategies for a quality assurance program, categorizing them according to environmental, structure, process, or outcome measures. They point out a major problem with existing criteria: that different agencies use different classification schemes for their client populations, thereby reducing the possibilities of sharing methods or comparing services across agencies. Classifications may be by diseases or problem categories. Multiple problem populations present even greater difficulties. Very few of the existing criteria have established either reliability or validity. Chapter 8 provides a variety of quality assurance models, methods, and programs and a long list of issues that require creative responses.

A final and crucial issue that faces the nursing profession and the outcomes of client care is that of the critical nurse shortage existing in the 1990s which is expected to grow worse. The Secretary's Commission on Nursing (Department of Health and Human Services, 1988) was established to develop recommendations on the problems related to the recruitment and retention of nurses. Its final report, which was published in December 1988 and produced 16 recommendations and 81 directed strategies, addressed the following issues:

1. Utilization of nursing resources
2. Nurse compensation
3. Health care financing
4. Nurse decision making
5. Development of nursing resources
6. Maintenance of nursing resources

The Commission warns that the health of this nation will be at risk if these recommendations are not implemented. Briefly, it advocates adequate staffing levels and innovative staffing patterns, with the use of automated information systems in health care delivery organizations. Methods for costing, budgeting, reporting, and tracking nursing resource utilization should occur collaboratively by health care delivery organizations, nursing associations, and government and private health insurers. Compensation of registered nurses should be increased by a one-time adjustment that targets geographical, institutional, and career differences. Innovative compensation options should expand pay ranges for experience, performance, education, and demonstrated leadership. The government should reimburse at levels sufficient to allow health care organizations to recruit and retain nurses necessary for adequate client care.

Greater representation and active participation of the nursing profession in decision-making activities should be fostered within health care policy-making, regulatory, and accreditation bodies. Employers of nurses should ensure active nurse participation in the governance, administration, and management of their organizations. Employers of nurses, as well as the medical profession, should recognize the appropriate decision-making authority of nurses in relationship to other health care professionals. Close cooperation and mutual respect between nursing and medicine is essential.

Financial and nonfinancial barriers to the acquisition of nursing education should be minimized and the promotion of positive and accurate images of nursing fostered. Research and demonstrations concerning health care financing and nursing practice, nurse supply and demand, and health care cost and quality should be sponsored.

The Commission further stated that the nursing shortage that is well publicized in hospitals and nursing homes (in 1988 137,000 registered nurse vacancies were reported) also is being experienced in the home care sector. Urban agencies and agencies without hospital affiliation reported having the most severe nurse-recruitment problems. The ambulatory care sector had the greatest shortage of nurse practitioners, nurse managers, and clinical nurse specialists. The Commission emphasized that the current shortage of registered nurses is primarily a result of increased demand as opposed to decreased supply. This situation is consistent with the decrease in hospital stays and the resultant increased need for out-of-hospital nursing care. If the recommendations from the Secretary's Commission on Nursing are acted upon, the future opportunities for nursing, particularly community health nursing, are exciting and optimistic.

THE FUTURE OF COMMUNITY HEALTH NURSING
Future Trends

Colleen Conway-Welch (1990) discussed the view of the immediate future (5 to 15 years) as proposed by the 1986 National Commission on Nursing Implementation Project. The major forces for shaping the role of nursing in the health care environment are considered to be the following:

1. Shifting payment systems
2. Increased proportion of the aged population
3. Increased competition among health care providers
4. Increased complexity of client needs and severity of client conditions
5. Government intervention in cost containment

Trends in the health care delivery system. The health care delivery system will continue to be driven by a business orientation and profit motive, which will be fueled by government intervention to contain costs. The result will be changes in structure and delivery. This business orientation will demand more precise justification of costs and substantive data on the results of intervention. The emphasis will be on productivity, making the need for the monitoring of quality even more crucial. This trend will necessitate the development of data on the cost/benefit outcomes of nursing care.

The shifting payment system and the explosion of technology will cause client populations to make a shift away from acute care hospitals. Multi-tiered care systems and the problems of dealing with uncompensated care may increase. To lower the costs of long-term care, services for the management of chronic illness and the need for home care services will increase dramatically (Conway-Welch, 1990).

Consumer trends. The profile of the consumer of health care will shift to an increasing proportion of elderly persons, with escalating needs for uncompensated care. The greater numbers of immigrant populations will require larger numbers of nurses who speak a second language and have an understanding of ethnic diversity.

Although self-care and wellness services will increase, consumers may not take advantage of these services. Rather they will continue to use the health care system for illness care. Futurists predict that consumers will develop a more responsive health care system.

With the increasing frequency of decision making by clients, families, and health care providers in terms of extending life through procedures and equipment, the quality of life will be a main concern. Thus ethical issues will be an increasing concern (Conway-Welch, 1990).

Nurses and nursing. Because the government's role in health care is expected to continue, nurses must learn to be adept at influencing public policy. Nursing organizations will have to be involved in the public arena in order to influence policy. The public arena may be the workplace, the community, the state legislature, or Congress.

The changing settings of health care delivery will necessitate a larger number of nurses to practice outside the hospital setting. At the same time advanced preparation will be needed to manage the increasingly complex needs of clients in the acute care setting.

It is expected that there will be a shortage of nurses prepared at the baccalaureate level and an oversupply of nurses with associate degrees to meet evolving needs for more highly educated nurses. It is critical that planned change include the shifting of one educational system to another. The future nurse's practice will be based on a greater use of research and scientific data. This trend, which will result from the explosion of technology, further supports the need for educational remapping.

Because of the changes in ways that health care will be delivered, it is expected that nurses will provide services in a greater diversity of settings, consistent with the business orientation of health care services. Contractual agreements, private practice, professional collaboration, consultation, and other nursing entrepreneurial endeavors will be multiplying (Conway-Welch, 1990).

Political action. Debbie Ward (1989) discusses the impact on public health nursing of the 1988 Institute of Medicine Committee for the Study of the Future of Public Health. This study demonstrated the importance of national attention and collective action in its sample list of problems:

1. Immediate crises: acquired immunodeficiency syndrome (AIDS), health care for the indigent
2. Enduring problems: injuries, teen pregnancy, high blood pressure, smoking, substance abuse
3. Looming problems: hazardous waste, Alzheimer's disease (i.e., long-term care)

Ward pointed out that the Committee advocates political involvement and action by nurses, especially in the community health nursing arena.

Nurses can and should develop and continually cultivate relationships with legislators and other public officials. They can contact legislators through organized lobbying by nursing groups. If an agency does not have a legislative liaison, the nurse can volunteer for the job. If there already is such a position, the nurse should talk to that person and volunteer as an interested nurse. In individual written and personal contacts with local, state, and federal legislators, the nurse always should be identified as a nurse. The nurse also can offer services as a resource on nursing and health issues to the mayor, school board, or housing authority.

The community health nurse should learn, understand, and practice good community relations and citizen participation techniques and speak to organizations such as the Rotary Club, church, Parent-Teacher Association, and other groups on the real work of community health nursing. Agencies can print a brochure outlining the educational and background capabilities of community health nurses. Each nurse should have a business card and should present one to all clients. Every client should be informed about what a community health nurse can do. Forming and supporting citizens' advisory groups will lend support to agencies and programs.

Community health nurses should build and cultivate relationships with professional and citizen groups interested in health issues, social services, and environmental protection. They can bring business people to adult day-care facilities, shelters, or schools for tours and special events, with media coverage, demonstrating the worth of nursing to the cost-driven care system. They can join in efforts to analyze and assign value to community health nursing and to translate community health nursing into comprehensible terms like hours and dollars.

Community health nurses can and should build and cultivate strong public, street-level community relationships. They can carry out long- and short-term community projects such as lead screening and health fairs, join with neighborhood organizations, and use neighborhood resources, such as grocery stores, as sites for public health education and outreach (Committee for the Study of the Future of Public Health, 1988; Ward, 1989).

Leadership and change. Timothy Porter-O'Grady (1990) has called for clear lead-

CRITICAL COMPETENCIES FOR PUBLIC/COMMUNITY HEALTH

Key topical areas

Epidemiology
Aggregates, cultural patterns, populations at risk
Wellness and disease prevention
Continuity of care
Interagency/interdisciplinary collaboration for prevention and health care needs

Important topics

Case finding and case management
Ability to operate autonomously or as a team member
Family and community assessment
History-taking
Consumerism
Communicable disease control, mental hygiene, nutrition, ethics

Graduate topics

Political process
Community assessment
The environment
Agency management and health administration
Health planning
Statistics and research

From *Public Health Nursing: Education and Practice,* by D.C. Jones, J.A. Davis, and M.C. Davis, 1987, Washington, DC: U.S. Government Printing Office. Modified by permission.

ership for establishing new organizational systems for the delivery of nursing care. He states that nursing practice must be defined in concrete terms so that it can be measured. Nursing's contribution to the profits of the organization must be clearly identified. This means that the value of nursing service must be defined in terms of costs and revenues. Nurses must be able to convince the consumer that health care needs can best be met by the range and quality of services of nurses.

Pamela Maraldo (1990) has reinforced these dictates in suggesting that nurses, as professionals, must muster nursing's resources in areas that will have the greatest impact on the most people. Nursing must move in the directions of the greatest strategic leverage and invest resources that will yield the greatest power for nursing. Maraldo sees the new role of nurses—as case managers and in private practice arrangements—as a strategy for increasing the prestige of nursing in the public's eye. A logical route for nurses in practice is to assume the authority and responsibility for making decisions about client care. Working for financial independence in the reimbursement of nursing care in and out of the hospital and across settings is an important ingredient in achieving this increased leverage for nursing. Again, political involvement is crucial to providing leadership for changes in community health nursing.

SUMMARY

Although the field of community health nursing is full of opportunities in a wide variety of settings, many challenges are ahead, which will require leadership and nurses with commitment to become involved in much more than direct client care. Given the breadth of clients targeted and client needs in community health nursing, decisions concerning where to place financial and professional energies will have to be made.

The lack of standardization in cost analysis, in assessment tools, and in nursing diagnosis taxonomies across agencies makes it difficult to collect information that would be useful in reaching decisions concerning priorities. Community health nurses need a broad educational background and professional expertise to provide nursing care to community health clients, as well as to deal with the demands and complexities of the health care system. Political involvement is vital for understanding community health nursing and for providing the leadership necessary for the nurse to be an advocate for the client in community health nursing.

CHAPTER HIGHLIGHTS

- The term *client* in community health nursing has many different interpretations, such as individual, family, group, community, and target population.
- With increasing consumer understanding of environmental hazards, the community health nurse will face many ethical dilemmas in reporting and teaching about identified hazards.
- Cost, access, and quality of health care will become an increasing problem, with aging population trends and government roles in financing health care.
- Health has many meanings, each of which determines different public health policies and client goals.
- The unique focus and critical content of community health nursing theory, research, and education need to be clarified.
- Organized data collection for the field of community health nursing is difficult because of the large number of assessment tools, each focused on or restricted to a particular client, setting, or purpose.
- Community health nursing diagnosis is undeveloped as a basis for the classification of health care needs of the community client.
- National nursing organizations have developed divergent goals for community health nursing practice.
- Community health nursing practice may be specific to a setting or to a specifically defined client group.
- Nursing centers and nursing entrepreneurship—newer developments for offering nursing care directly to the client—are significant motivators for third-party reimbursement for nursing.
- Quality assurance measures in community health nursing lack consistency in classification systems, thus limiting comparisons across agencies or for cost-effectiveness.
- The Secretary's Commission on Nursing recommended immediate steps to address the nursing shortage.
- The future of community health nursing will evolve to a greater business orientation, dealing with more ethical issues in care, increased involvement and expertise in political action, and ultimately more power in influencing health care for clients.

STUDY QUESTIONS

1. How does the definition of client in community health nursing influence interventions by the nurse? Give an example.

2. How does the definition of health in the community influence the goals agreed upon by the client and the community health nurse? Use an example to demonstrate your explanation.

3. How are the issues of cost, access, and quality of care affecting the health of the increasing population of elderly persons?

4. Describe an environmental hazard the community health nurse will have to deal with and the ethical issues that may be experienced by the nurse.

5. Why is it going to be necessary for the community health nurse of the future to become very politically active?

REFERENCES

American Nurses Association. (1987).*The nursing center: Concept and design.* Kansas City, MO: Author.

American Nurse's Foundaton. (1988).*Nurses in private practice: Characteristics, organizational arrangements and reimbursement policy.* Kansas City, MO: Author.

Andrews, P. B. (1990). Nursing diagnosis. In P. J. Christesen & J. W. Kenney (Eds.). *Nursing process: Application of theories, frameworks, and models* (3rd ed.). St. Louis: Mosby.

Carlson, E. (1990, January). A family affair: Millions are unable to get insurance. *AARP Bulletin,* p. 1.

Clements, I. W. & Roberts, F. B. (Eds.). (1983). *Family health: A theoretical approach to nursing care.* New York: Wiley.

Committee for the Study of the Future of Public Health, Institute of Medicine: (1988). *The future of public health,* Washington, DC: National Academy Press.

Conway-Welch, C. (1990). Emerging models of postbaccalaureate nursing education. In J. C. McCloskey & H. K., Grace (Eds.). (1990). *Current issues in nursing,* (3rd ed.). pp. 137-144. St. Louis: Mosby.

Demkovich, L. (1988, Autumn). Special report on medicare. *AARP News Bulletin.*

Department of Health and Human Services. (1988). *Secretary's Commission on Nursing: Final report,* Washington, DC: U.S. Government Printing Office.

Fawcett, J. (1984). *Analysis and evaluation of conceptual models of nursing.* Philadelphia: Davis.

Firlit, S. L. (1990). Nursing theory and nursing practice: Do they connect? In J. C. McCloskey and H. K. Grace, (Eds.). *Current issues in nursing,*(3rd ed.). pp. 4-11. St. Louis: Mosby.

Flynn, B. C. and Ray, D. W. (1987). Current perspectives in quality assurance and community health nursing. *Journal of Community Health Nursing, 4*(4),187.

Goeppinger, J. (1984). Primary health care: An answer to the dilemmas of community nursing. *Public Health Nursing, 1*(3),129-140.

Gould, E. J. (1989). Home care nursing: Professional and political issues. *Journal of the New York State Nursing Association, 20*(1):4-7.

Hamilton, P. A. (1981). *Health and Consumerism,* St. Louis: Mosby.

Hamilton, P. A. (1983). Community nursing diagnosis. *Advances in Nursing Science, 5*(3),21-36.

Hamilton, P. A. and Bush, H. A. (1988). Theory development in community health nursing: Issues and recommendations. *Scholarly Inquiry for Nursing Practice, 2*(2),145-160.

Hanchett, E. S. (1988). *Nursing frameworks and community as client.* East Norwalk, CT: Appleton & Lange.

Harrington, C. (1988). Quality, access, and costs: Public policy and home health care, *Nursing Outlook, 36*(4),164-166.

Jones, D. C., Davis, J. A., and Davis, M.C. (1987). *Public health nursing: Education and practice,* Washington, DC: Department of Health and Human Services.

Kovner, C. (1989). Public health nursing costs in home care. *Public Health Nursing, 6*(1),3-7.

Laffrey, S. C., Loveland-Cherry, C. J. & Winkler, S. J. (1986). Health behavior: Evolution of two paradigms. *Public Health Nursing, 3*(2),92-100.

Maraldo, P. J. (1990). The aftermath of DRGs: The politics of transformation. In J. McCloskey and H. K. Grace, (Eds.). *Current issues in nursing* (3rd ed.). pp. 387-392. St. Louis: Mosby.

Marriner-Tomey, A. *Nursing theorists and their work* (2nd ed.). St. Louis: Mosby.

Moccia, P. (1989). Shaping a human agenda for the nineties: Trends that demand our attention as managed care prevails. *Nursing & Health Care, 10*(1),14-17.

Muecke, M. A. (1984), Community health diagnosis in nursing, *Public Health Nursing, 1*(1),23-25.

Neuman, B. (1982). The Neuman systems model: Application to nursing education and practice. East Norwalk, CT: Appleton Century Crofts.

Nightingale, F. (1969). *Notes on nursing: What it is and what it is not.* New York: Dover. (original work published in 1860)

Pera, M. K. & Gould, E. J. (1989). Home care nursing: Integration of politics and nursing, *Holistic Nursing Practice, 3*(2),9-17.

Phillips E. K., Scattergood, D. M., Fisher, M. E. & Baglioni, A. J. (1988). Public home health: Settling in after DRGs? *Nursing Economics, 6*(10),31.

Porter-O'Grady T. (1990). Decentralization of nursing practice. In J. C. McCloskey & H. K. Grace, (Eds.). *Current issues in nursing*, (3rd ed.). pp. 310-315. St. Louis: Mosby.

Ruffing-Rahal M. A. (1987). Resident/provider contrasts in community health priorities. *Public Health Nursing, 4*(4),242-246.

Smith, J. A. (1983). *The idea of health: Implications for the nursing professional*, New York: Columbia University Teachers College Press.

Smith, J. B. (1985). Levels of public health. *Public Health Nursing, 2*(3),138-144.

Spradley, B. W. (1990). *Community health nursing: Concepts and practice* (3rd ed.). Glenview, IL: Scott, Foresman & Co.

Ward, D. (1987). Public health nursing and the future of public health. *Public Health Nursing, 6*(4),163-168.

Wesbury S. A. (1988). The future of health care: Changes and choices. *Nursing Economics, 6*(2),59-62.

Glossary

A

Abstinence: Total voluntary avoidance of a substance or an activity.

Abuse: Any type of physical or emotional maltreatment of another individual, ranging from violent attacks to passive neglect.

Accelerating change: Quickening of the pace of change in society.

Access to care: The availability of health care, particularly for individuals unable to pay for it.

Accountability: To be answerable to someone for something.

Accreditation: A voluntary system by which agencies are recognized as having met predetermined standards of the accrediting body.

Acquired Immune Deficiency Syndrome (AIDS): A disease caused by a virus that effects cell-mediated immunity. It has a long incubation period, follows a protracted and debilitating course, is manifested by various opportunistic infections, and is always fatal at this time.

Active immunity: A long-term resistance to disease brought about naturally by infection or artificially by innoculations of the agent itself in killed or modified form.

Activities of daily living: Actions such as bathing, dressing, and toileting that are normally performed on a daily basis.

Activity theory: Theory of aging stating that most older adults maintain a high level of activity to promote well-being and satisfaction. The amount of activity is influenced by previous life-style.

Adaptive model: A model that views health as the effective functioning of adaptive systems.

Addiction: Compulsive, uncontrollable physical or psychological dependence on a substance or habit.

Adjourning: The fifth and final stage of group development, in which the group terminates its task and comes to some kind of closure.

Admission criteria: Factors to be considered when evaluating a client's suitability for receiving high-technology care in the home.

Adolescence: The period of life between the ages of 13 and 20 years. In western societies adolescence may be prolonged.

Adult day care: Services designed to meet the unique needs of older adults who live in the community but cannot function completely autonomously and may need some supervision. Services include socialization and health promotion.

Affective domain: One of three domains concerning learning behaviors; deals with expression of feelings, interests, attitudes, values, and appreciation.

Agent: A factor, inanimate or animate, whose presence or lack of presence may lead to disease, disability, or death.

Aggregate: Collection of individuals who share similar characteristics or experience common factors.

Aging: The process of growing older.

AIDS: Abbreviation for acquired immune deficiency syndrome.

AIDS related complex: A subclinical form of AIDS.

Air pollution: Concentration of dust, soot, and other particles in the atmosphere that may increase the incidence of illness.

Al-Anon: Support group for family members of alcoholics or other substance abusers.

Alcohol: A central nervous system depressant consumed in liquid form that may impair one's judgment, cause unconsciousness, and damage the liver if consumed in excess.

Alcoholics Anonymous: Self-help groups of recovering alcoholics whose goal is to stay sober.

Alcoholism: The excessive use of alcohol to the point of addiction.

Altered coping mechanisms: Lack of ability to problem solve in a positive way. May result in acts of subjugation and aggression as a manifestation of anger and frustration by prisoners in a jail.

Alzheimer's disease: A progressive dementia of unknown etiology characterized by confusion, memory failure, disorientation, and inability to carry out purposeful movements. The course may take a few months to seven years to progress to a complete loss of functioning.

American Nurses Association (ANA): The national professional association of registered nurses in the United States.

American Association of Occupational Health Nurses (AAOHN): Association formed by nurses practicing in occupational health, to improve nursing services and offer opportunities for nurses interested in this area of practice.

American Association of Retired Persons (AARP): Organization providing information and various benefits to persons over 50 years of age.

Analytical study: Epidemiological study conducted by formulating and testing a hypothesis.

Anthropometric measures: Measurement of growth by comparison of height, weight, and age to standardized growth charts.

Antibody: A protein found mostly in serum that is formed in response to exposure to a specific antigen.

Antigen: Substance that stimulates the formation of an antibody.

Antitoxin: Antibody formed in response to a toxin.

Apgar score: A system of scoring an infant's condition on five factors 1 minute and again at 5 minutes after birth. The maximum score is 10. Those with low scores (less than 4) need immediate attention to survive.

Apnea monitoring: Use of a device that monitors the client's (usually an infant) breathing and sounds an alarm if breathing stops.

Artificial immunity: Immunity acquired by inoculation of the agent in killed or modified form.

Assessment: A systematic collection of data that assists one in identifying the needs, preferences, and abilities of a client.

Association: A relationship between two factors or events which demonstrate that they occur more frequently together than one would expect by chance alone.

Asthma: A respiratory disorder characterized by paroxysmal dyspnea and wheezing due to constriction of the bronchi.

Autism: A developmental disability characterized by abnormal emotional, social, and language development. The autistic child may engage in repetitive and ritualistic behavior and appears to be unable to progress beyond a fixed developmental stage.

Autocratic leadership: Leadership style in which decisions are made by the leader, with little or no input from the group members.

Autonomy: The quality of being self-governing, including the right to make one's own decisions.

Autonomy vs. shame and doubt: Stage of development during the toddler period described by Erikson as one when the toddler wishes to gain control of the world.

B

Bacillus: A genus of aerobic, gram-positive, spore-producing bacteria.

Basic structure: In Neuman's model, all the variables that keep the individual or community functioning as a unit, as well as its unique characteristics.

Beliefs: Statements that one holds to be true, but which may or may not be based on empirical evidence.

Beneficence: The quality or state of being, doing, or producing good.

Biological hazards: Infection-producing organisms found in the environment, such as bacteria, viruses, molds, fungi, and parasites.

Biomagnification: The concentration of pollutants upwardly through the food chain.

Blended family: Family resulting when two adults who were part of previous families join together to form a new family.

Blindness: The inability to see. Children who are blind from birth will experience greater developmental delays than those who lose their sight later in childhood.

Body Mass Index: Expression of the relationship between a person's height and weight.

Breastfeeding: The sucking of milk by an infant from the mother's breast.

C

Calcium: A mineral found in dairy foods and green leafy vegetables, necessary for the formation of healthy teeth and bone mass.

Calorie: The amount of energy needed to raise the temperature of one gram of water $1°$ C, used to measure the energy value of food.

Candidiasis: Infection caused by a species of Candida, usually Candida Albicans, characterized by pruritius, a white exudate, peeling, and easy bleeding.

Carrier: A person who harbors and can pass on a specific disease or infectious agent but who does not present with symptoms of the disease.

Case Control Study: A retrospective study that identifies a group of persons with a disease or disability and a group of similar persons without the disease or disability. The two groups are compared to determine what possible factor(s) might account for the difference in incidence of disease.

Case law: Law based on court or jury decisions.

Causality: The relationship between two events in which one precedes the other and the direction of influence and nature of effect are predictable and reproducible.

Cerebral palsy: A motor function disorder affecting movement and muscle coordination caused by a nonprogressive brain defect or lesion present at birth or shortly after.

Certification: Recognition of a nurse in a speciality practice attesting to his/her expertise in the speciality field as shown by the meeting of predetermined requirements.

Chain of transmission: A complicated mode of transmission involving a causative agent, a host, and an environment.

Chemical dependency: Addiction to drugs and/or alcohol.

Chemical hazards: Chemical agents found in the environment or workplace that may have adverse effects on health.

Chemical wastes: Byproducts created by the manufacture of chemicals; these include hazardous and nonhazardous substances.

Cholesterol: Fatty substance found in foods of animal origin that is associated with a high risk of cardiovascular disease.

Chronic illness: Illness or disease that is permanent, leaves a residual disability, causes a nonreversible pathological condition, and requires long-term rehabilitation or supervision.

Chronic low self esteem: NANDA-approved nursing diagnosis of long-standing self-evaluation/feelings about self or self-capabilities.

Chronicity: Ongoing disease process that may require intervention to maintain the highest level of wellness possible or restore the highest level of functioning.

Client: The recipient of care; may be an individual, family, or a group.

Client eligibility: Client and care giver factors to assess when determining whether an individual can be admitted to a home care program.

Client teaching: Imparting of information to a client.

Clinical model: Health is viewed as the absence of disease.

Cognitive domain: One of three domains concerning learning behaviors; deals with intellectual ability.

Cohort: A group of persons who share a common characteristic.

Cohort study: Study of a group of persons over time (a specified period) who share a common characteristic.

Common law: Law based on principles such as precedent, justice, fairness, and respect for individuals.

Communication: The giving or receiving of information or messages.

Community: A practice setting, a target of service, or a small group within a larger population.

Community as client: The entire community as the focus and recipient of nursing care.

Community assessment: The process of describing a community, its patterns of morbidity and mortality, and identifying patterns of disease or potential health problems in the community.

Community development group: Groups that come together to support advocacy.

Community health nurse: A nurse who works to promote and preserve the health of populations, and who utilizes a holistic approach to care for the health of individuals in the community.

Community health nursing: A synthesis of nursing theory and public health practice applied to promoting and preserving the health of populations. Health promotion, health maintenance, health education and continuity of care are utilized in an holistic approach to the management of the health care of individuals.

Community health nursing diagnosis: Nursing diagnosis that is generated from the state of the community and for whom the direct target of intervention is the community itself.

Community Health Nursing Theory: Nursing theory applicable to community health nursing; it may be adapted from generic nursing theory, or derived from a unique community health nursing perspective.

Comparison group: Any group compared to a group being studied; a control group.

Complex carbohydrates: Carbohydrates containing a large number of glucose molecules, such as those found in cereals and whole grain foods; starches.

Compliance: Cooperation and participation in the prescribed therapeutic regimen by the client.

Concurrent audit: Quality assurance audit performed by comparing the chart with predetermined criteria during the episode of care.

Confidentiality: The social or legal contract guaranteeing another's privacy.

Conflict: Disagreement within a group.

Confounding variable: A factor that causes change in the frequency of disease and also varies systematically with a third causal factor being studied.

Congenital anomaly: An abnormal condition present at birth.

Constitutional law: Law based on federal and state constitutions.

Continuing care: The process of activities between and among patients and providers to coordinate ongoing care.

Continuity of care: Personalized, continuous care that begins at the point of entry into the health care system and continues until the health related problems and needs are resolved by means of interpersonal, interdisciplinary communication with the focus on the patient and his family.

Continuity theory: Theory of aging stating that many adults maintain lifestyles like those they had in young adulthood.

Continuum of care: An integrated, client-oriented system of care composed of both services and integrating mechanisms that guides and tracks clients over time through a comprehensive array of health, mental health, and social services spanning all levels of intensity of care.

Correctional institution: Facility for incarceration of individuals convicted of a crime; includes minimum, medium, and maximum levels of security.

Cost containment: Achieving a given objective with an awareness of and a responsibility to keeping the overall costs of services at an appropriate manageable level.

Crisis: An upset in a steady state.

Criteria: Measurable statements that reflect the intent of a standard.

Cross-sectional study: A study that determines the presence or absence of causal factors of disease or disability for each member of a population at a single point in time.

Cross tolerance: Use of one substance increases the user's tolerance for similar substances.

Culture: A distinctive way of life that characterizes an ethnic group and which is passed down from generation to generation; learned patterns of behavior.

Cultural assessment: Systematic appraisal of a client's cultural beliefs, values, and attitudes.

Cultural diversity: Differences in values, beliefs, and attitudes among people of different cultures.

Culture-bound: The belief that one's culture is the only "correct" view of the world and the expectation that others conform to this view.

Cystic fibrosis: An inherited disorder of the exocrine glands causing abnormally thick secretions of mucus, elevation of sweat electrolytes, increased organic and enzymatic constituents of saliva, and overactivity of the autonomic nervous system beginning in infancy. The glands most affected are those in the pancreas and respiratory system. Treatment is directed at preventing respiratory infections. There is no cure but the advent of effective antibiotics has prolonged the life span.

Cytomegalovirus (CMV): A member of a group of large species-specific herpes type viruses with a wide variety of disease effects; it may cause serious illness in newborns and individuals with depressed immunity.

D

Day care: Care of infants and children while parents are occupied with work or school.

Day Care Center: A state licensed facility where children ranging from infancy through school-age are cared for while the parents are working, or otherwise unable to care for their children.

Death of permanence: Lack of stability in relationships and material possessions caused by a rapidly changing society.

Defining characteristics: Signs and symptoms identified to describe various states of health.

Deinstitutionalization: The practice of discharging mental patients from institutions to halfway houses and group homes or, in some instances, to the streets.

Dementia: A condition of deteriorated mentality.

Democratic leadership: Leadership style in which decisions are made jointly by the group leader and its members.

Denial/Appeals: Refusal of third-party payers to provide reimbursement for services and the process of requesting reconsideration.

Dental caries: Progressive decay or destruction of a tooth.

Denver Developmental Screening Test: Test for evaluating the motor, social, and language skills of children 1 month to 6 years of age.

Deotological (formalist) theory: Theory of ethics stating that the rightness or wrongness of an action is determined by the nature of the action or motives behind it, not the results.

Dependence: Physical or psychological state in which the continuous and prolonged consumption of a substance leads to the user's adaptation to its presence.

Depressant: A substance that slows the functioning of a body system.

Depression: A state of feeling sad.

Descriptive survey: Collection and analysis of existing information, which may lead to formulation of hypotheses and further study.

Detoxification: Withdrawal of an addicting substance under controlled conditions to minimize side effects.

Developmental disability: A chronic disability due to emotional or physical impairments that manifests itself before adulthood and interferes with a person's ability to function normally in society.

Developmental model: The belief that developmentally disabled individuals are not ill and development is a lifetime priority.

Diagnosis-related groups (DRG): Classification of medical conditions into 23 major diagnostic categories and 470 diagnostic groups, which are used to determine the payment reimbursable by Medicare and other third-party payors.

Diagnostic category: Classification used to describe various states of health that the nurse can treat.

Diet: The foods eaten by an individual, with regard to nutritional qualities, composition, and effects on health.

Dietition: Individual trained in nutrition who assists clients in improving nutritional status.

Direct transmission: Transmission of a disease that occurs when an agent directly affects a host through an accessible portal of entry.

Disability insurance: Financial assistance given to individuals in some states, who have documentation from a physician that they cannot work due to a disability.

Discharge planning: Assessment of needs and arrangement or coordinating of services for patients and clients as they move through the health care system.

Disease prevention: Activities that prevent or contain the spread of disease.

Disengagement: Pattern in which rigid, impermeable boundaries separate members of a family.

Disengagement theory: Theory that older adults and society undergo a mutual withdrawal that is an inevitable part of the aging process.

District nursing: The beginnings of public health nursing, as established in England.

Down's syndrome: Developmental disorder resulting from the presence of an extra chromosome on the twenty-first pair causing distinct physical characteristics and mental retardation.

Drug abuse: Use of drugs for nontherapeutic reasons.

Drug addiction: Physical or psychological dependence on a drug.

Dysfunctional family: Family that experiences a severe level of anxiety and responds to a crisis by perceiving it as an overwhelming burden.

E

Ecomap: A schematic drawing showing interactions between a family and other systems in the community.

Education for All Handicapped Children Act: Public Law 94-142, mandating that a "free and appropriate education" be available for all children, regardless of disability.

Educational group: Group formed for the purpose of providing information and education.

Educational need: Need that can be satisfied by a learning experience.

Educational Resource Centers: Regional facilities offering education in various areas of occupational safety and health.

Ego: That aspect of a personality that defines the person's identity to the self; the conscious organized mediator between a person and reality.

ELISA test: A laboratory technique for detecting specific antigens or antibodies, commonly used in the diagnosis of AIDS.

Enabling: Behavior by one person that encourages another to continue acting in a dysfunctional manner by shielding that person from the consequences of the dysfunctional behavior.

Enculturation: The raising of children within a family to conform to the requirements of the social group in which they were born.

Endemic: The habitual presence of a disease or infectious agent in a defined geographical area or population.

Enmeshment: Family pattern in which sharing among members is extreme and intense and where individuality and independence are viewed negatively.

Environment: The combination of all factors that influence the health of a person.

Environmental sensitivity: The process of becoming aware of the effects of the environment on health and working to improve the quality of the environment to raise the level of health in a community.

Epidemic: An outbreak of disease that is sudden and widespread across many localities, regions, or populations.

Epidemiology: Science concerned with the various factors and conditions that determine the occurrence and distribution of health disease, defect, disability, and death among groups of individuals.

Epidemiological process: The phases of epidemiological investigation, starting with descriptive study and progressing to analytical study and experimentation.

Epidemiologic triangle: The relationship between an agent, host, and environment necessary for disease to occur. Elimination of any one of these may eliminate the occurrence of disease.

Ergonomics: The study of humans at work to understand the complex relationships among people, physical and psychological aspects of the work environment (such as facilities, equipment, and tools), job demands, and work methods.

Ethical dilemma: The problem of choosing between two or more equally undesirable alternatives.

Ethics: The study of principles and rules that guide one's conduct.

Ethnicity: Affiliation with a value system and with people who share that system.

Ethnocentrism: The tendency to judge others on the basis of one's own cultural beliefs.

Etiological and contributing factors: Those physiological, situational, and maturational factors that can cause a health problem or influence its development.

Eudaemonistic conception of health: View of health that includes qualities such as self-actualization, fulfillment, and loving.

Examination stage: Developmental stage described by Robert Havinghurst as occuring during later maturity.

Existentialism: A chiefly twentieth century philosophy that is centered upon the analysis of existence and of the way humans finds themselves existing in the world, that regards human existence as not describable or understandable in scientific terms. It stresses responsibility and freedom of choice in the individual.

Extended family: Several generations of a family living together.

Extrafamily stressors: Influences on a family from political, social, and cultural issues.

Extrinsic motivation: Forces outside the individual that cause one to act; rewards or punishments.

F

Factor: Cause or variable that may produce an effect.

Family: A group of people, including at least one adult, who are related to each other by blood or social contract.

Family day care: Care for up to six children in a neighborhood home.

Family developmental tasks: Responsibilities connected with each particular stage of family life.

Family life cycle: Period beginning with formation of a family and ending with its dissolution.

Family violence: Any act by one family member toward another that causes pain or injury, including physical, emotional, and sexual abuse.

Fidelity: Ethical principle related to keeping promises.

Flexible line of defense: In Neuman's model, a protective buffer for preventing stressors from breaking through the solid line of defense.

Fluoride: A mineral, which when incorporated into the tooth structure, helps to prevent tooth decay.

Folk healers: Individuals believed by some cultural groups to have the ability to cure illness.

Formaldehyde: A colorless gas often found in homes and suspected to be a carcinogen.

Forming: The initial stage of group development, in which members assemble and begin to assume a sense of common identity.

Fragile elderly: Those older adults who require extended long-term care.

Frontier Nursing Service: An organization founded in 1925 by Mary Breckenridge in Lexington, Kentucky, to provide health care to rural families. It is still in existence today.

Fundamental human rights: Claims recognized by law that are legally enforceable.

G

Gamma globulin: Passive immunizing agents obtained from pooled human plasma.

Generativity vs. Stagnation: Erickson's developmental task of middle adulthood, in which the individual is concerned with achieving major life goals.

Genogram: An assessment tool resembling a family tree which may be used to depict a family's structure.

Glaucoma: Eye disease characterized by increased intraocular pressure, which can cause progressive loss of sight if untreated.

Goal: An aim or end toward which intervention is directed.

Group: An open system composed of three or more people held together by a common interest or bond.

Growth and development: General rates of physical growth and cognitive development provide milestones from which the infant and child are assessed.

H

Habituation: Repeated use of a drug to the point at which psychological dependence occurs.

Hazard: The probability that a substance will produce harm under specific conditions.

Hazardous wastes: Substances that can threaten health if people are exposed to them.

Health: Optimal system stability, that is the best possible state for an individual, group, or community at any given time.

Health behavior contract: A formal, written agreement designed to systematically change a client's behavior to improve health.

Health behavior paradigms: Models to explain clients' health behavior, including the health paradigm and the disease paradigm.

Health Belief Model: Rosenstock's theoretical model stating that an individual's decision to perform a health action is determined by perceptions of susceptibility to an illness, severity of the illness, and personal threat of the illness.

Health care delivery system: An organized interrelated system that provides health care to a population.

Health education: Program directed to the general public that attempts to improve and maintain the health of a community.

Health Maintenance Organization (HMO): A prepaid health cooperative with an emphasis on health maintenance and illness prevention. Members prepay their medical fees and all health care is provided by the HMO.

Health promotion: Activities designed to improve one's health and prevent disease; a component of primary prevention.

Hearing loss: The inability to hear, which may range from very mild to profound (total). If present at birth, hearing loss will cause delays in language acquisition and learning.

Hepatitis: Communicable disease caused by a virus and spread by the fecal-oral route, causing inflammation of the liver.

Herd immunity: The resistance of a group or community to invasion and spread of an infectious agent.

Herpes simplex: Infection caused by a herpes simplex virus that produces small, transient, irritating, and sometimes painful fluid-filled blisters on the skin and mucous membranes.

Hiatal hernia: Herniation of the stomach through the esophagous.

High-level wellness: A concept of optimal health that emphasizes the integration of mind, body, and environment.

High risk aggregate: A collection of individuals who share similar characteristics or experience common factors that place them at risk for death, disease, or disability.

High tech care: Use of advanced equipment in the provision of nursing care, including infusion therapy, phototherapy, apnea monitoring, and ventilator therapy.

High touch care: Those elements of care that are the results of therapeutic relationships among the client, nurse, and other care givers.

Holistic approach: Approach to nursing emphasizing the interrelationship of the body, mind, spirit, and environment in maintaining a wellness state.

Holistic health: An approach emphasizing the mind-body connection in health and illness.

Home health agency: Agency or organization providing skilled nursing and related services for clients in their homes.

Home health aide: Paraprofessional who assists with a client's personal care in the home.

Home health care: The provision of health care and health related services to persons in their place of residence; skilled nursing care. Direct care provided by the "laying on of hands", or by teaching or demonstration. It may also include assessment and observation of a client who is medically unstable.

Homeless Person's Survival Act: Act passed by the U.S. Congress in 1986 that made homeless persons eligible to receive food stamps, SSI, Medicaid, AFDC, or VA benefits and to be included in the Job Training Partnership Act.

Homeless population: Those people whose primary nighttime residence is a public or private shelter, emergency lodging, park, car, or abandoned building.

Hopelessness: NANDA-approved nursing diagnosis of "a subjective state in which an individual sees limited or no alternatives or personal choices available and is unable to mobilize energy on own behalf."

Hospice: Treatment for terminally ill clients, with emphasis on palliative rather than restorative care. The goal is to keep the client at home, pain free and symptom free.

Host: A person or animal susceptible to disease or disability.

Human Immunodeficiency Virus (HIV): A retrovirus that is transmitted directly through body fluids; it is the virus that causes AIDS.

Hypothesis: A supposition provisionally adopted to explain an event and guide investigation.

I

Imaging: A mental picture of something not actually present.

Immunity: The condition of being able to resist a specific disease or disability.

Immunization: Administration of a living modified agent, a suspension of killed organisms or an inactivated toxin to protect susceptible individuals from infectious disease.

Immuno suppressive chemotherapy: The administration of drugs which depress the functioning of the immune system, whether intentionally or unintentionally.

Immunoglobulin: A protein that behaves like an antibody or is formed in response to an antigen.

Impairment: Any disorder in structure or function resulting from anatomic, physiologic, or psychologic abnormalities that interfere with normal activities.

Incidence: The frequency of newly occurring cases of a disease in a specified population during a given time period.

Incineration: The burning of waste products to dispose of them.

Incubation period: The time interval between contact with an infectious agent and appearance of the first sign or symptom of a disease.

Indigent: Lacking in resources to reimburse providers for health care.

Indirect transmission: Transfer of disease via a vehicle (food or water), vector (insect), or through the air.

Individual roles: Specialist roles within a group that serve members' own needs rather than those of the group as a whole.

Industrial hygiene: The environmental science of identifying and evaluating physical, chemical, and biological hazards in the workplace and devising ways to control or eliminate them.

Ineffective family coping: NANDA-approved nursing diagnosis defined as "the state in which a family demonstrated destructive behavior in response to an inability to manage internal or external stressors due to inadequate resources."

Infant: An individual from birth to 1 year of age.

Infant mortality: The statistical rate of infant death during the first year after live birth.

Informed consent: A client agreement to comply with treatment after receiving sufficient information about the procedure(s), inherent risks, and acceptable alternatives.

Infusion therapy: Administration of medications, fluids, or nutrition via the intravenous route.

In-home care: Care for a child in his or her own home by a relative, friend, or other babysitter.

Initiative vs. guilt: Stage of development experienced by preschoolers. According to Erikson, this stage is characterized by conflict between a desire for independence and dependence on the parents.

Inner harmony: A component of wellness focusing on relaxation and stress reduction.

Instrumental activities of daily living: Activities such as shopping and housekeeping that must be performed in order to live independently.

Integrity vs. anxiety and dispair: Erikson's stage of development experienced by older adults, in which one's life and accomplishments are evaluated.

Integument: An enveloping layer of skin.

Interfamily stressors: Factors that influence a family as it interacts with other systems in the environment, such as schools or health care facilities.

Intermediate care facility: A residential facility that allows developmentally disabled individuals with medical problems to live in the community and also obtain treatment necessary for their physical needs.

Intimacy vs. isolation: Erikson's stage of development experienced by young adults, characterized by the need to establish an intimate relationship in order to achieve a sense of well-being.

Intrafamily stressors: Conflicts within the family itself.

Intrinsic motivation: Forces within the individual that cause one to act, including values, beliefs, attitudes, unmet needs, and emotions.

Ionizing radiation: High-energy radiation, including x-rays, gamma rays, alpha particles, and beta particles.

Iron: A mineral necessary to prevent anemia, fatigue, and impaired wound healing.

J

Judicial law: Law based on court or jury decisions.

Justice: The distribution, as fairly as possible, of benefits and burdens; treating people fairly.

K

Kaposi's sarcoma: A malignant neoplasm often associated with AIDS.

Kin network family: Nuclear families or unmarried members who live in close proximity and work together to exchange goods and services.

Knowledge deficit: State in which the individual experiences a deficiency in cognitive knowledge or psychomotor skills that alter health maintenance.

L

L'Arche: Communities for the mentally retarded based on the attitudes of interdependence and mutual value.

Laisséz-faire leadership: Leadership style in which group members are given little direction and are free to make their own decisions.

Landfill: Area where solid wastes are stored and covered intermittently with layers of earth.

Latchkey child: A child who takes care of him- or herself in the absence of the parent.

Later maturity: The period of life from age 65 until death.

Lead poisoning: Toxic condition caused by ingestion of lead through lead based paint or water. If prolonged, it may result in hyperactivity or mental retardation.

Leadership: A process used to move a group toward achieving a goal.

Learning: Process of acquiring new knowledge, skills, or attitudes that are synthesized to produce behavior change in the individual.

Learning disability: A group of disorders affecting the acquisition and use of speaking, listening, reading, writing, reasoning, or mathematical abilities.

Least restrictive environment: A setting most like that inhabited by people without disabilities; to be used for education of developmentally disabled children.

Legionnaires' disease: An acute bacterial pneumonia caused by infection by *Legionella pneumophila* and characterized by influenza-like symptoms.

Legislation and regulation: Law mandated by state, local, or federal legislative branches of government.

Levels of care: Classification of health care service levels by the kind of care given, number of people served, and the people providing the care. The levels include acute, subacute, skilled, custodial, and chronic.

Licensure: A legal process assuring the public that an individual has met minimum requirements.

Lifestyle Assessment Questionnaire: A tool that allows clients to objectively assess their health behaviors.

Lines of resistance: In Neuman's model, the internal factors that help a client defend against a stressor.

Logotherapy: A theory of psychotherapy described by Victor Frankl which focuses the individual on the unique meaning of life by striving to find a concrete reason for existence.

Long-term care: The provision of care on a recurring or continuing basis to persons with chronic physical or mental disorders.

Low birth weight: Infant whose weight at birth is less than 2500 g, regardless of gestational age.

Lymphoma: Neoplasm of the lymphoid tissue.

M

Maintenance roles: Behaviors within a group that are an attempt to keep the group working together harmoniously.

Maturational crisis: Transitional period that occurs across the life cycle, requiring acquisition of new sets of behavior and psychological growth.

Medical regimen: Therapeutic measures prescribed for clients by physicians and directed toward management or cure of illness or disease.

Medical self-care: Actions taken to monitor one's own health, such as monitoring diet and exercise or performing breast self-examination.

Medicaid: Federal health insurance program for poor individuals and families.

Medicaid certified agency: An agency that qualifies and meets the standards of the state government in regards to reimbursement by Medicaid.

Medicare: Federal health insurance progam for individuals age 65 and older or some younger, disabled individuals.

Medicare certified agency: An agency that qualifies and meets the standards of the federal government in regards to reimbursement by Medicare.

Melting-pot approach: Belief that cultural diversity recedes as groups adopt traits from the dominant culture.

Menarche: The onset of menstruation.

Menopause: Cessation of menses.

Mental retardation: Subaverage intellectual functioning existing concurrently with deficits in adaptive behavior, as shown by an IQ of less than 70 and inability to perform the skills needed for personal independence and social responsibility.

Metacommunication: Nonverbal communication; body language.

Metaparadigm of nursing: The specific and unique philosophy of nursing, including the concepts of person, environment, health, and nursing.

Midlife crisis: Feeling of dissonance sometimes experienced in middle age if earlier developmental tasks have not been completed.

Molestation: The making of annoying sexual advances with injurious effect.

Moral: Of or relating to principles of right or wrong in behavior.

Morbidity: The relative incidence of disease.

Mortality: The relative incidence of death.

Motivation: That which stimulates one toward action or inaction.

Motivational theory: Identifies major "satisfiers" and "dissatisfiers" that affect group productivity.

Multiple risk factors: A web of interacting events that place certain aggregates at risk.

Multiple sclerosis (MS): An inflammatory disease of the central nervous system, causing degeneration of the myelin sheath, and resulting in neurologic dysfunction with periods of exacerbation and recovery.

N

National Institute of Occupational Safety and Health (NIOSH): Branch of the U.S. Public Health Service whose responsibilities include investigating workplace illness and accidents as well as the presence of workplace hazards.

Natural history of disease: Stages in the process of development and progression of a disease without intervention by humans.

Natural immunity: Immunity caused by acquisition of antibodies as the result of a previous infection or existing from birth.

Negligence: Failure to act in a reasonably prudent manner, resulting in harm.

Neuman's definition of nursing: A unique profession that is concerned with the variables affecting an individual's response to stress.

Nightingale, Florence: The founder of modern nursing.

Noise pollution: Sound that is unwanted, annoying or harmful; excessive noise exposure can cause permanent hearing loss.

Noncompliance: Client refusal or inability to comply with the treatment plan.

Nonmalfeasance: The intention to do no wrong.

Normalization: The concept of treating disabled individuals in the same manner as all others; giving them the same options and opportunities in everyday life.

Norming: Third stage of group development in which rules for participation are established and members begin to feel more relaxed.

Nuclear family: Family consisting of a husband, wife, and one or more children.

Nuclear family dyad: Adult couple without children, or whose children have grown and left home.

Nurse: An individual concerned with the diagnosis and treatment of human responses to actual or potential health problems. The nurse's role is to keep the client system stable through accuracy in the assessment of effects and possible effects of environmental stressors and in assisting client adjustments required for an optimal wellness level.

Nursing center: Community center giving the client direct access to professional nursing care that is holistic and client-centered.

Nursing process: A systematic approach to nursing, consisting of five components: assessment, diagnosis, planning, implementation, and evaluation.

Nursing Theory: A systematic body of knowledge that attempts to define the role of the nurse and guides nursing practice.

Nutrition: The science that studies the effects of foods eaten on one's health.

Nutritional assessment: Use of various methods and tools to evaluate an individual's intake of food and nutrients.

O

Obesity: Body weight significantly greater than that recommended for an individual's height.

Objective: Statement of intended outcomes or results to be achieved by the client.

Occupational health: The health of the worker and its effect on his or her ability to function in the workplace.

Occupational health history: Collection of information about a client's past and current employment, to identify actual or potential health hazards in the work setting.

Occupational health nursing: The application of nursing principles to help workers achieve and maintain the highest level of wellness throughout their lives. This specialized practice is devoted to health promotion in the occupational environment based on prevention of illness and injury.

Occupational illness: Abnormal condition or disorder, other than one resulting from an occupational injury, caused by exposure to environmental factors associated with employment.

Occupational injury: Any injury such as a cut, fracture, sprain, amputation, etc. which results from a work accident or exposure in the work environment.

Occupational Safety and Health Act (OSHA): Government act passed in 1970 to ensure healthful and safe working conditions.

Occupational Safety and Health Administration (OSHA): Agency created by the OSHAct that works to improve health and safety in the workplace by educating workers and establishing standards and regulations.

Official agency: Agency operated by the government.

Omnibus Budget Reconciliation Act: Legislation passed in 1982 which cut funding for many domestic programs and reduced the allowable income for families to qualify for Aid to Families With Dependent Children.

Open dump: A land area where solid wastes are deposited, with little regard for sanitary conditions.

Opportunistic infections: Infection or disease caused by normally nonpathogenic bacteria and viruses when the environment is suitable, (i.e., when the host's resistance is compromised).

Outcome: Results of care that is rendered.

Overdose: High dose of a drug that may be life-threatening; emergency care is often required.

P

Palliative: Serving to relieve without curing.

Palliative care: Care given to moderate the pain and discomfort caused by a disease that is terminal.

Paraprofessional: A trained aide who assists a professional nurse.

Parenting: The process of raising children and passing on one's values, attitudes, and beliefs.

Passive immunity: A resistance to disease brought about artificially by inoculation of specific protective antibodies (hyperimmune) or serum (immune serum globulin) which is of short duration. Natural passive immunity is passed from mother to child through the placental barrier in the last trimester of pregnancy or through breastfeeding.

Pathogenicity: The ability to produce clinically apparent illness.

Performing: Fourth stage in group development, in which group members function as a unit to complete the task at hand.

Period of communicability: Time period during which a communicable disease can be transmitted from an infected person.

Phototherapy: Treatment of jaundice caused by excess bilirubin by exposure to intense fluorescent light.

Physical fitness: The ability to carry out daily tasks with alertness and vigor, without undue fatique, and with enough energy reserve to meet emergencies or to enjoy leisure time pursuits.

Physical hazards: Factors in the workplace that contribute to occurrence of injury such as equipment, lighting, noise, and temperature.

Place: In epidemiology, a location where a disease is more likely to occur.

Plague: Contagious disease caused by a bacillus that has historically been prevalent in crowded and unsanitary conditions and appears to be transmitted by rodents to fleas to humans. It spread rapidly through Europe in the fourteenth century.

Play: Any spontaneous or organized activity that provides enjoyment, entertainment, amusement, or diversion. It may be structured or unstructured, and allows children to express feelings, develop cognitive and motor skills, and socialize.

Pneumocystis carinii: A protozoan that is a causative agent of plasma cell pneumonia.

Political action: The process of becoming involved in community relations and with government officials to bring about change.

Pollutant: Any unwanted substance that enters the environment and affects it adversely.

Polychlorinated biphenyls (PCBs): Toxic chemical compounds that were used in industry and have been found in many humans, animals, and food sources, causing a variety of health effects.

Population effect: As the population increases, so does the amount of waste produced.

Power: The ability to influence and/or control others.

PRECEDE Model: Health education planning model that identifies factors in one's environment that motivate an individual to exhibit certain health behaviors.

Prematurity: The state of an infant born any time prior to the thirty-seventh week of gestation regardless of birth weight.

Preoperational stage: Piaget's stage of development experienced by preschoolers, characterized by the development of representational thought and the ability to solve simple problems.

Presbycusis: Loss of hearing due to aging, including a lessened ability to understand speech.

Presbyopia: Changes in vision due to aging, including a loss of ability of the lens to accomodate to near and far vision.

Preschool or Nursery School: A facility which may or may not be state licensed, where children aged 3 years to 5 years attend full- or half-day school that prepares them for kindergarten.

Preschooler: Child 3 to 4 years of age.

Prevalence: The number of existing cases of a disease or occurrences of an event at a particular point in time.

Prevention: The act of stopping or interrupting the progression of disease.

Primary prevention: Actions taken to prevent the occurrence of disease.

Private sector: The component of the health care delivery system financed by private funds and comprising physicians in private practice, private hospitals, and outpatient services.

Process: A series of activities used to deliver care.

Program evaluation: Systematic process of collecting information to determine the worth of a set of activities designed to produce a certain outcome.

Proprietary agency: A privately owned, profit making organization defined under section 501 of the Internal Revenue Code as ineligible for tax exemption.

Prospective Payment System: Payment for medical conditions is predetermined according to the diagnosis-related group (DRG).

Prospective study: Study that starts with a group (a cohort) all considered to be free of a given disease but who vary in exposure to a factor suspected of causing the disease.

Provider: A person or agency providing health care services to clients.

Psychological hazards: Factors in the workplace that affect the worker's response to the work environment, often resulting in stress, fatigue, or depression.

Psychomotor domain: One of three domains covering learning behaviors; deals with skills known as motor skills.

Psychotropic drugs: Drugs that affect the recipient's behavior and perception.

Puberty: The condition of becoming able to reproduce sexually, marked by maturing of sexual organs and development of secondary sex characteristics.

Public health: The health of the community, with particular regard to areas such as the water supply, waste disposal, air pollution, and food safety.

Public Health Nursing: A field of nursing that synthesizes the body of knowledge from the public health sciences and professional nursing theory for the purpose of improving health in the entire community.

Public Law 94-142: The Education for All Handicapped Children Act, mandating that all disabled infants and children are entitled to a "free and appropriate" education.

Public sector: The component of the health care delivery system financed by taxes and comprising federal, state, and local health departments.

Q

Quality: Conformance to standards leading to a degree of excellence.

Quality assurance: A planned systematic process of evaluating care according to predetermined standards and criteria; followed by taking appropriate corrective actions to ensure excellence.

R

Race: Specific physical and structural characteristics that are transmitted genetically and distinguish one human type from another.

Radioactive wastes: Waste products that are hazardous and decompose over time, spreading into the environment if not disposed of properly.

Radon: A colorless, odorless, inert radioactive gas which may be found in the home. It is a decay product of radium.

Rate: Ratio of cases of disease or deaths to the total population in a given time period.

Ratio: The relationship between two numbers expressed as a fraction; the value obtained by dividing the numerator of a fraction by the denominator.

Readiness to learn: The state of being both willing and able to make use of instruction.

Reality orientation: Nursing intervention designed to assist a cognitively impaired individual in maintaining awareness of the environment.

Recycling: Methods of reusing waste materials, reducing the total amount of waste and conserving resources.

Referral: A mechanism for communication, coordination, and collaboration between and among health care settings and disciplines, to ensure continuity of care.

Regression: A retreat or movement backwards; a return to an earlier, more primitive form of behavior.

Reimbursement: Payment for services by a third party (i.e., someone other than the recipient, such as private insurance, Medicare, or Medicaid).

Relationships: In a group, the bonds between its members.

Research process: The systematic use of scientific process to find answers to questions. Research may be descriptive or analytical. It is always objective.

Reservoir: Living organisms or inanimate objects that harbor an infectious agent.

Reservoir of infection: A continuous source of infectious disease.

Resistance: The inherent capacity of a human being to resist untoward circumstances (such as disease, malnutrition or toxic agents).

Restorative health care: Health services provided to help clients regain a maximum level of health and independence following a debilitating illness or injury.

Retrospective study: A study that looks back for a relationship between one condition occurring in the present and another that occurred in the past, such as comparing people diagnosed as having a disease to those who do not (controls).

Retrospective audit: Comparison of the client's chart with predetermined criteria after the episode of care has been completed.

Retrovirus: A single piece of RNA surrounded by a protein coat. Instead of flowing from DNA to RNA it reverses the process and makes itself into a piece of DNA. It then infects the nucleus of the cell. HIV is a retrovirus.

Risk: Exposure to a situation which may result in an injury, illness, or other loss.

Risk management: A program designed to eliminate or control health care situations having the potential of injury, danger, or liability to clients.

Role performance model: View of health stating that healthy individuals must fulfill a role in society.

Rubeola: Acute, contagious viral infection causing fever, rash, upper respiratory symptoms; lay term, measles.

S

Salmonella: Gram-negative bacilli which produce fever, acute gastroenteritis, bacterimia and localized infection. The mode of transmission is water- or food-borne.

Sandwich generation: Middle-aged adults who are raising their own children and caring for aging parents at the same time.

Saturated fats: Fats whose molecular structure contains the maximum possible number of hydrogen atoms. They are often linked with an increased incidence of cardiovascular disease.

Scapegoating: Blaming one family member for the problems confronting the family. It is usually an unconscious process.

School nursing: Provision of nursing services, including health promotion and disease prevention, to children and adolescents within the school setting.

Scoliosis: An abnormal, S-shaped curve of the spine.

Screening: Identification of unrecognized disease or disability by mass examination of entire populations or high risk groups.

Seasonal: Occurring periodically at certain times of the year.

Secondary prevention: Actions taken to detect and treat disease in early stages.

Self-care: The practice of activities that individuals initiate and perform on their own behalf in maintaining life, health, and well-being.

Self-efficacy model: A useful tool for bringing about desired behavioral changes in a specific area of lifestyle by considering the individual's belief that he or she can perform a specific behavior and that performing the behavior will cause a change in health status.

Self transcendence: Focusing on others as a way to find purpose and meaning in life.

Senecense: The state of being old; the process of being old.

Sensorimotor period: Piaget's stage of development experienced from birth to 2 years of age, in which the infant explores the environment through the five senses.

Seroconversion: The appearance of specific antibodies in blood serum that has previously been free of them.

Shared leadership: Group situation in which two individuals share the leadership responsibilities.

Significant other: Person considered by an individual to be special, this person may be directly responsible for patient care in the home.

Single parent family: Family consisting of one parent living with one or more children.

Situational cisis: Crisis resulting from unexpected changes, causing disequilibrium in the individual or family.

Skilled services: Services that require the knowledge and skills of a professional to perform or teach.

Smog: Air pollution present in concentrations high enough to reduce visibility and cause irritation in the eyes and lungs.

Social vulnerability index: A tool that could be used to determine those populations in greatest need of health services. It takes into account the factors of social pathology, economic well-being, education, access to health care, and health status.

Socialization: The process of learning the social requirements of one's cultural group.

Sodium: An element contained in salt and necessary in small amounts for the body to maintain a proper fluid balance.

Solid waste: Any garbage, refuse, sludge or other discarded material resulting from industrial, commercial, mining, and agricultural operations or from community activities.

Special rights: Rights accorded to the nurse that arise out of the nurse/client relationship.

Spermatogenesis: The production of male gametes, including meiosis and transformation of the four resulting spermatids into protozoa.

Spiritual nursing: Intervention in which the nurse assists the client to relate positively to his or her deepest inner self and allows the expression of concerns and fears about death and other aspects of the essence of life.

Spirituality: A component of health related to the core of existence, sensitivity or attachment to religious values relating to the belief system of the individual.

Stereotype: The belief that all members of a cultural group behave in the same way.

Standard: A broad statement of the agreed upon level of excellence.

St. Vincent de Paul: Founder of the Sisters of Charity in the early seventeenth century.

Storming: Second stage of group development in which members bargain for position within the group and conflicts arise.

Stressors: In Neuman's model, environmental forces that may altar system stability.

Substance abuse: Use of drugs or substances for reasons other than to achieve a therapeutic effect.

Support group: Group in which members assist each other in meeting a common need. Also called self-help group.

Surveillance: The process of monitoring incidence and prevalence of communicable diseases through accurate record keeping and data collection, to assist health professsionals to monitor dangerous outbreaks of disease. It can also facilitate effective health planning to intervene and control the spread of communicable disease.

Systemic mycosis: A chronic, malignant neoplasm of the skin which is caused by a fungus.

T

Task roles: Behaviors within a group that contribute to completion of the group's task.

Teaching: A process that facilitates learning. It includes activities that are a deliberate action which help the student learn. Health teaching is an act in which a client is assisted to become an active member of the health team and to reach an optimal level of health.

Teaching/learning process: Process in which knowledge, attitudes, and skills are imparted to and integrated by the learner.

Teaching situation: The environment in which teaching will take place. It includes the physical, interpersonal, and external environment.

Team conference: Interdisciplinary case conference where all disciplines involved in a patient's care meet to evaluate and revise the plan of care.

Teleological (consequentialist) theory: Theory of ethics stating that the rightness or wrongness of an action is determined by its results or consequences.

Teratogenic effects: Incomplete or improper fetal development caused by external substances.

Tertiary prevention: Actions taken to limit the spread of disease or disability, improve health, and/or maintain stability.

Therapeutic or medical play: Play activities where children can dress up as health care staff and can act out medical procedures such as giving "shots" to dolls, giving "anesthesia" to teddy bears, and so on. This helps children learn about and prepare for experiences with the health care system.

Third party reimbursement: Payment by a third party insurer for any claims made by a health care provider for health care services rendered to the insured consumer.

Time: In epidemiology, data is collected regarding when a disease occurs, to discover trends in health and disease.

Tinea capitus (ringworm): A contagious fungal disease transmitted by direct contact.

Toddler: A child between 1 and 2 years of age.

Tolerance: The need to use larger doses of a drug to achieve the desired effect.

Toxicology: Study of the adverse effect of certain agents on the biological system.

Toxin: A poisonous substance usually produced by the invading microorganism.

Toxoid: A toxin that has been treated to alleviate toxic properties but retain its antigenic quality, usually to stimulate antibody production.

Trajectory: A curve or surface that passes through a given set of points or intersects a given set of curves or surfaces at a constant angle.

Trajectory of chronic illness: The course, or predictable path, of an illness over time.

Trust vs. mistrust: Erikson's stage of development experienced in infancy, when the infant develops a bond with parents and/or other caretakers.

Tuberculosis: Communicable disease caused by droplet infection which causes fever, fatigue, weight loss, coughing, chest pain, hemoptysis, and hoarseness.

Turner's syndrome: A congenital syndrome, in females, caused by the absence of one of the two X chromosomes.

U

Uniform Needs Assessment Instrument: Assessment tool, currently in development, that was mandated by the Omnibus Budget Reconciliation Act of 1986, and can be used to evaluate a client's need for continuation of services.

Universal precautions: Use of protective barriers, such as gloves, masks, and protective eyewear to protect mucous membranes from exposure to blood and body substances. Fundamental to this concept is the practice of treating all patients as if they are infected with a blood-borne disease and taking appropriate protective measures.

Utilitarianism: The greatest-happiness principle, or the greatest good for the greatest number of people.

Utilization review: A set of activities directed toward reviewing care for its appropriateness for a specific client.

V

Vaccine: Substance developed and administered to produce active immunizations.

Values: Views and beliefs that guide one's behavior.

Values clarification: The process of understanding one's own values and how they guide behavior.

Variable: Any attribute, phenomenon or event that can have different values.

Varicella: Viral infection causing fever, rash, and malaise, also known as chicken pox.

Vector: Any carrier, particularly one that transports an infectious agent.

Vehicle: An inanimate substance that transports an infectious agent to a susceptible host (e.g., food, water).

Vendors: Distributors of durable medical equipment in the home.

Ventilator care: Use of a mechanical device to assist with breathing in cases of pulmonary failure.

Veracity: The intention to tell the truth.

Virulence: The power of a microorganism to produce disease.

Visiting Nurse's Association (VNA): Private, nonprofit agencies originally founded to provide health care and education to the poor, funded by charitable contributions and fees based on clients' ability to pay.

W

Wald, Lillian: A public health nurse who founded the Henry Street Settlement in New York City and worked to improve the health of the city's poor residents.

Water pollution: Presence of disease-causing bacteria and viruses in the water supply, often through human or animal feces, or through the dumping of solid wastes in the water supply.

Web of causation: An interrelationship of multiple factors that contribute to disease or disability.

Well-being: An individual's perceived condition of existence, pleasure, and kinds of happiness.

Wellness: A dynamic, fluctuating state of being, encompassing physical, psychological, and spiritual health.

Western blot test: A laboratory blood test to detect the presence of antibodies to specific antigens.

Wheel model: Epidemiologic model of human-environment interactions that are necessary for disease to occur.

Wholism: According to Neuman, relationships and processes arising from wholeness, dynamic freedom, and creativity in adjusting to stress in the internal and the external environment.

Withdrawal syndrome: The unpleasant and sometimes life-threatening physiologic changes that occur when some drugs are withdrawn after prolonged, regular use.

Workman's Compensation: Laws requiring employers to be financially responsible for wages lost as a result of occupational illness or injury.

Z

Zoonosis: Disease of animals that is transmissible to humans, (e.g. rabies).

Index

A

A Patient's Bill of Rights, 99
A Plan for Implementation of the Standards of Nursing Practice, 171
AA; *see* Alcoholics Anonymous
AAIN; *see* American Association of Industrial Nurses
AAOHN; *see* American Association of Occupational Health Nurses
AARP; *see* American Association of Retired Persons
Abdellah, Faye, influence of, on development of community health nursing, 17*t*
Abuse
  child, 194, 598-599, 611
    assessing young children for, 198
    developmentally disabled and, 502
    of primary and secondary school age children, 217, 219
    in school-age childen, 232
  drug; *see* Drug abuse
  elder, 599
  substance; *see* Substance abuse
Accidents
  death in middle-aged adults due to, 248
  death rates in young and middle-aged adults from, 240*t*
  environmental, 560-561, 566
  involving children from birth to five years, 192-193
  involving primary and secondary school age children, 215
  motor vehicle
    deaths of young adults due to, 236, 238
    involving young children, 193
  non-motor vehicle, involving young children, 192-193
  prevention of
    parent education in, 195
    in young children, 192-193
  school nurse's role in prevention of, in school-aged children, 226-227
Accountability, professional, 162
Accreditation, 162-163
Acculturation, definition of, 302
ACLF; *see* Adult congregate living facilities
Acne, 231
Acquired immune deficiency syndrome
  children with, right to education for, 501

Acquired immune deficiency syndrome—cont'd
  diagnosis of, 479
  early stages of, 478-479
  family with, 480
  history of, 474-475
  incidence and prevalence of, 474, 475*t*
  intravenous drug abuse and, 571
  legal issues pertaining to, 598
  nutritional needs in, 479
  pathology of, 479
  period of communicability of, 478
  transmission of, 475-476, 478, 483
Activities of daily living, 373
  hopeful experiences maximized by, 341
  instrumental, 373
Activity theory of aging, 261
Acuity, visual, in school-aged children, 230
Acute myocardial infarction, death rates in young and middle-aged adults from, 239*t*
Addiction, drug, 582
Adjourning, by groups, 126-127
ADL; *see* Activities of daily living
Adolescence
  definition of, 209, 232
  late, definition of, 209
Adolescents
  assessing nutritional status of, 526-528
  cognitive development of, 214
  developmentally disabled, 496
  diet for, 526
  female, increased calcium intake by, 520
  height and weight of, 213
  major causes of mortality and illness in, 215-221
  personality development in, 214
  physical growth and development of, 213
  social behavior development of, 226*t*
  substance abuse by, 573
Adulthood
  early and middle, nutrition in, 528
  young, comparison of models of developmental theories of, 237*t*

Adult(s)
  congregate living facilities for, 269
  height and weight chart for, 242t
  in later maturity; see Older adults
  obesity in, criteria for, 515
  reduction of cholesterol levels in, 514
  young and middle-aged, 235-252; see also Middle-aged
      adults; Young adults
Advocacy
  client, by community health nurse, 604
  definition of, 132
Age of Enlightenment, nursing and medicine influenced by,
      5t, 19
Agent, disease caused by, 146
  communicable, 466
Aggregates
  definition of, 450
  high-risk, 450-461
  at risk, 461; see also High-risk aggregates
Aging
  activity theory of, 261
  developmental tasks of, 257-261, 271
  normal physical changes during, 256-257
  nutritional concerns of, 528-532, 535-536
  process of, 256-257
  psychosocial theories of, 261, 271
AIDS; see Acquired immune deficiency syndrome
Air, pollution of, 555-558, 567
Alcohol, 570
  abuse of, 577
      by native Americans, 572-573
      by older adults, 575
      by school-aged children, 220-221
      statistics on, 590
      by youth, 573
  consumption of, recommendations regarding, 518
  dependence on, by school-aged children, 227
  effects of varying levels of, 576t
  withdrawal from, disorders associated with, 586-587
Alcoholic, nursing assessment of, 582-583
Alcoholics Anonymous, 588, 590
Alcoholism, 571; see also Alcohol, abuse of
  diagnosis of, 584
  in dysfunctional families, 323-324
Alzheimer's disease, 266, 413-414
American Association of Industrial Nurses, 424
American Association of Occupational Health Nurses, 424
American Association of Retired Persons, 269
American College of Surgeons' Hospital Standardized Pro-
      gram, 158
American Hospital Association, 22
American Medical Association, 22
American Nurses' Association
  model of quality assurance developed by, 182
  purpose and function of, 13t
  quality assurance model developed by, 159, 170-175

American Nurses' Association—cont'd
  standards of quality assurance developed by, 179
American Public Health Association, 159
American Red Cross, 11
  purpose and function of, 13t
American Red Cross Nursing Service, 11
Amitriptyline, 503
Amphetamines, abuse of, 578
ANA; see American Nurses' Association
Analytical studies, 152-153
Anemia
  iron deficiency, 193
  pernicious, in older adults, 266
Angina pectoris, death rates in young and middle-aged adults
      from, 239t
Antabuse; see Disulfiram
Anthropometric measures, nutritional status assessed using,
      526-527
Antibiotics
  gonorrhea treated with, 472
  initiation of, in supervised setting, 392
  type one and type two, 392
Antiquity, influence of, on nursing and medicine, 4, 5t, 6-7
APHA; see American Public Health Association
Apnea monitoring, home, 401-402
Army Nurse Corps, 11, 14
Army school of nursing, 13
Arsenic, health affected by, 556t
Arterial disease, chronic occlusive, 265
Asbestos
  diseases caused by exposure to, 431t
  health affected by, 556t
  home pollution caused by, 563
Assessment, definition of, 39
Assessment instrument, for discharge planning, 375, 377-
      378, 380
Atabrine; see Quinacrine
Ativan; see Lorazepam
Attention-deficit disorders, 493
Attraction power, definition of, 129
Audiovisual materials, evaluation of, 116
Audit
  health care, 175
  nursing, evaluation of health care by, 159
Autism, 492-493
Autonomy, client, 603, 607, 608
AZT; see Zidovudine

B

Bandura, self-efficacy model developed by, 73-74
Barbiturates, abuse of, 579
Barton, Clara, contributions of, to nursing profession,
      10-11
Basic core, in Neuman's health care systems model, 41
Basic structure, in Neuman's health care systems model, 41
  immunity and, 465

Behavior
  drug-related, in young people, 222
  drunken, 573
  dysfunctional, in families, 344
  health
    definitions of, 622
    paradigms of, 622-623
  modification of, in developmentally disabled, 502-503
Beneficence, 603, 607, 608, 610
Benzene, health affected by, 556*t*
Benztropine mesylate, 503
Beryllium, health affected by, 556*t*
Bhopal, India, chemical exposure at, 560-561
Bills of mortality, 140
Binocularity, children with, 230
Biofeedback, inner harmony achieved using, 90
Biological oxygen demand, 553
Birth control, effect of, on family structure, 278
Birth rate, 150
  calculation of, 152
Birth weight, low, higher risk for mortality and morbidity
    associated with, 450
Black Death, 139-140
  influence of, on nursing and medicine, 8
Blended family, 278
Blindness in children, 494
Blood circulation, understanding, 5*t*
Blue Cross, 29
Blue Shield, 29
Blue Shield of Northern California, wellness movement
    and, 67
BMI; *see* Body mass index
BOD; *see* Biological oxygen demand
Body language, family communication and, 281
Body mass index, 515
  nutritional status of older adults assessed by, 531-532
Book of Surgery, 4, 6
Boys, height and weight measurements for, 210*t*
Breckinridge, Mary, establishment of Frontier Nursing Ser-
    vice by, 15
Brothers and Sisters of Mercy, 9
Bubonic plague
  historical evolution of epidemiology and, 139-140
  nursing and medicine influenced by, 8

C

Cadet Nurse Corps, 14
Caffeine, 590
  effects of, 579
Calcium
  increased intake of, 520
  increased requirements for, during pregnancy, 522
Calcium disodium edetate, lead poisoning treated with, 194
Calda de la Mollera, 312*t*
Calendar, care-giver, in high-tech home care, 389-390
Canada, health care delivery system in, 34

Cancer
  children with, 217
  young adults with, 242
Candidiasis, 479
Cannabis, abuse of, 581
Car seats for young children, 193
Carbohydrates, complex; *see* Complex carbohydrates
Carbon disulfide, diseases caused by exposure to, 431*t*
Carbon monoxide
  health affected by, 556*t*
  home pollution caused by, 563
Carcinoma, terminal, case study about client with, 415
Cardiovascular system
  in older adults
    changes in, 257
    physical assessment of, 262*t*
  in older adults, physical assessment of, 265
Care-giver, high-tech home care, calendars kept by,
    389-390
Case study, 153
Case-control study, 153
Case-specific rate, 150
  calculation of, 152
Catepres; *see* Clonidine
Causality, 141, 144-146
Causation
  chains of, 144, 146
  web of, 144-146
CDC; *see* Centers for Disease Control
Centers for Disease Control, 25, 598, 611
Cerebral palsy, 489-491
  types of, 490
Certification, 162, 182
  comparison of, with licensure, 163*t*
CHAMPUS; *see* Civilian Health and Medical Programs of Uni-
    formed Services
Chelation therapy, lead poisoning treated by, in young chil-
    dren, 194
Chemical dependency, 582; *see also* Substance abuse
  causes of, 571-572
  clients with, evaluation of, 589
  diagnosis of, 584
  effect of, on families, 574
  incidence of, in women, 575
  nursing diagnoses for, 584-585
  in older adults, 575-576
  prevention of, 585-586
  statistics on, 571
  types of, 589
  work affected by, 576
Chemicals
  diseases caused by exposure to, 431*t*
  hazardous, 547-552
    in workplace, 429, 431-432
  teratogenic effects of, 431
Chest, assessment of, in school-aged children, 229

Chewing, problems with, nutrition in older adults affected
    by, 529
Child abuse, 194, 598-599
    assessing young children for, 198
    in primary and secondary school age children, 217, 219
    in school-aged children, 232
Child Abuse Prevention and Treatment Act, 598
Child neglect, 194
Child-rearing
    by black American families, 315-316
    cultural variations in, 307-308
    by Eastern Asian families, 310
    by Hispanic American families, 312-313
    by native American families, 314
Children; see also Adolescents; Primary-school children
    abuse of; see Child abuse
    with AIDS, 480
        right to education for, 501
    assessing nutritional status of, 526-528
    from birth to five years, 187-205
        health problems of, 192-194
    blind, 494
    chronic illness involving, 411
    deaths and death rates in, 216t
    developmentally disabled, 495-496
        interaction of community health nurse with,
            488-489
    with Down's syndrome, 491
    dying, parents role with, 416
    fat intake by, 514
    female, height and weight measurements for, 211t
    latchkey, 199, 219
    male, height and weight measurements for, 210t
    mentally handicapped, education of, 488-489, 506
    moral and spiritual development of, 214-215
    primary and secondary school age, 208-233
    primary-school; see Primary-school children
    school-aged; see School-aged children
    with sensory disorders, 494-495
    sick, day-care centers for, 203-204
    signs of maturation in, 213
    with special needs, day care for, 204
    weight reduction program for, 516
    young, physical growth and development of, 188
China, health care delivery system in, 34
Chlamydia, 471t
Chlorazepate, 580
Chlordiazepoxide, 575
Chlorination, 553
Chlorpromazine, 503
Cholesterol, fats and, reduction of, 513-515
Chromium/chromates, diseases caused by exposure
    to, 431t
Chronic illness
    across the life span, 411-414
    definition of, 409-410, 417

Chronic illness—cont'd
    effects of, on personality development, 410-411, 417
    financial assistance for, 416-417
    home health care and, current issues in, 416-417
    home health care for, 409-418
    incidence of, 409, 417
    involving primary and secondary school age children,
        215, 217
    in older adults, 409
    trajectory of, 414, 416, 417
Chronic obstructive pulmonary disease, death rates in
        young and middle-aged adults from, 240t
Chronic occlusive heart disease, 265
Chronicity, definitions of, 409-410
Cirrhosis, death rates in young and middle-aged adults
        from, 241t
Civilian Health and Medical Programs of Uniformed Ser-
        vices, home health care financed by, 356
Clean Air Act of 1970, 555-556
Clean Water Act, 553
Client
    community as, definitions of, 616-617, 633
    conceptual view of, 17
    continuing care needs of, criteria for, 369-370
    cultural assessment of, 304-308
    dying, 414, 416
    ethical issues in defining, 617-618
    ethnic group affiliation of, 304
    health beliefs and practices of, assessment of, 306
    racial background of, 304
    satisfaction of, quality of health care assessed by, 176
    values and beliefs of, assessment of, 304-305
Client system boundaries, 39
Client teaching, 119; see also Health teaching
    definition of, 100
    implementation of plan for, 116
Client-nurse contract, 111. 112t
Coal and Mine Safety Act of 1969, 425
Cocaine, 221
    abuse of, 578
Code for Nurses with Interpretative Statements, 603-
        604, 611
Coercive power, definition of, 129
Cognitive learning theories, 100
Cohabiting couple, retired, 278
Coke oven emmissions, health affected by, 556t
Communicability, period of, associated with AIDS, 478
Communication, 319
    with black Americans, 315
    care-giver and client, in high-tech home care, 389-390
    with different ethnic groups, 307
    with Eastern Asians, 310
    with Hispanic Americans, 312
    with native Americans, 314
Communication theory, for families coping with problems,
        281-282, 297

Community
   clarification of, 617
   as client, definitions of, 616-617, 633
   definitions of, 39, 58
   developmentally disabled persons in, 486-506
   functions of, formation of groups for, 124-125
   groups in, community health nurses and, 122-136
   health and wellness in, 65-94
   health of
      interrelationship of health of family and, 294-296, 297
      multilevel approaches toward, 77, 93
   health teaching in, 96-120
   high-risk aggregates in, 450-461
   L'Arche, 504
   nursing assessment of, Neuman's approach to, 40-41
   nutrition in, 512-536
   perception of, 38, 58
   relationship between occupational health and, 436
   rights of developmentally disabled to be part of, 504
   types of, 617
Community health agencies, accreditation of, 163
Community health nurse
   care provided by, evaluation of, 628-629
   client advocacy by, 604
   client assessment and teaching by, for high-tech home
      health care, 390
   concerns of, 598-603
   critical competencies for, 632
   in day-care center, 197-204
   discharge planning by, evaluation of, 374
   health teaching by, 105
   involvement of, with quality assurance, 178-180, 181
   on-call support provided by, in home health care, 386
   political actions of, 631
   responsibilities of, related to immunizations, 599, 611
   role of
      with adolescent substance abusers, 573
      with children from birth to five years, 196-204
      in delivery of high-tech care, 384-385, 406
      with developmentally disabled, 488-489, 505
      with environmental health problems, 565-566
      with high-risk aggregates, 462
      in program development for high-tech home health
         care, 387
   in schools, 221-233, 232, 233
      historical perspective of, 221-223
   vulnerability of, to malpractice lawsuits, 594-596,
      599, 603
   young children in the community and, 196-197
Community health nursing
   application of epidemiological concepts to, 153
   definition of, 18-19, 38, 58, 596
   education and, 119
   ethical dilemmas for, 606-610, 611
   focus of, 97, 98
   future of, 630-633

Community health nursing—cont'd
   historical overview of, 3-19
   issues and concerns in, 509-633
   issues in nursing affecting, 624-629
   measuring costs of, 628
   nursing assessment in, 624-625
   nursing diagnoses relevant to, 626
   nursing goals in, 627
   nursing theory and, 16-17
   organized data collection in, 626, 633
   professional expectations and standards for, 596-597
   professional issues in, 614-634
   quality assurance in, 156-182, 633
   settings for, 627-628, 633
   standards of, 18
   theory development and research in, 624-625
   third-party reimbursement for, 628
   types of laws affecting, 594-596, 610
Community of concern, 626-627
Community of interest, 39
Complex carbohydrates, fiber and, increased consumption
   of, 516-517
Compliance, client, health teaching and, 117, 119
Comprehensive Health Services amendment of 1966, 23
Conceptual framework, definition of, 282
Confidentiality, 598, 607
Congentin; see Benztropine mesylate
Congestive heart failure, 265
Constipation, older adults affected by, 529
Consumerism, health care delivery impacted by, 161-162
Continuity of care; see also Discharge planning
   care plan for, 374-375
   components for providing, 374-375
   definition of, 370
   following discharge, changes in health care delivery sys-
      tem affecting, 371
   qualifications for person planning, 380
   referral systems for, 369, 369-370, 375, 380
Continuity theory of aging, 261
Contract
   client-nurse, developing, 111-113
   health behavior, 74
Coping
   ineffective, nursing care plans for dysfunctional families
      with, 337-342
   strategies for, 90
Coronary heart disease, alcohol intake and, 518
Correctional institutions
   risk for morbidity and mortality in, 453-456
   standards for nursing care in, 455-456
Cost containment, health care, 31, 33-34
Council for National Defense, 14
Crack, 221, 578
Crisis, definition of, 280
Crisis theory, for families coping with problems, 280-
   281, 296

Criteria mapping, case management and, 177

Cross-sectional study, 152

Cross-tolerance, drug, 325, 327

Crusades, influence of, on nursing and medicine, 5*t*, 8

Cultural groups
  in United States and Canada, 319
  value orientations among, 305*t*

Cultural healers, 309

Culture
  assessment of, 303-308, 319
    guide for, 317
  definition of, 302, 318
  developing sensitivity to, 300-301
  family as bearer of, 299-319

Culture-bound, definition of, 300

Curanderos, 311

Cystic fibrosis, case study of child with, 412

Cytomegalovirus, 479

D

Dark Ages, influence of, on nursing and medicine, 5*t*, 7

Data collection
  methods of, 154
  types of, 148-151

Day-care
  adult, 269
  children from birth to five years in, 198-199
    interactions with peers and parents by, 201
    stressors on, 202
  for children with special needs, 204
  family, definition of, 199
  nursing intervention in, 202-204
  types of, 199

Day-care center
  community health nurse and, 197-204
  definition of, 199
  policies and procedures of, 199-201
  prevention of infection in, 202-203
  for sick children, 203-204
  staff-to-child ratio in, 199-200

dB; *see* Decibel scale

DDST; *see* Denver Developmental Screening Test

Death of permanence, health needs of young and middle-aged adults affected by, 235

Death rate(s)
  in children, 216*t*
  crude, 150
    calculation of, 152
  worldwide decline in, 542-543

Death rate(s), age-specified, 150
  calculation of, 152

Death(s); *see also* Mortality
  causes of, in children, 216*t*
  from drug-related causes, 238, 241*t*
  major causes of, in young and middle-aged adults, 252
  risk of, from radiation exposure, 559*t*

Decibel scale, 555

Deinstitutionalization, 458, 462, 487, 506

Delano, Jane, contributions of, to nursing profession, 11

Deliriants, abuse of, 581-582

Delirium tremens, 587

Denver Developmental Screening Test, 195

Department of Health and Human Services, 25

Dependence, definition of, 582

Depression, in older adults, 261, 263
  nutrition affected by, 531

Detoxification, 590
  clonidine used for, 581
  medications used during, 586

Developmental model, needs of developmentally disabled met using, 488, 495, 506

Developmentally disabled
  attitudes toward, shifts in, 486-488, 505
  behavior modification in, rights concerning, 502-503
  care and treatment of, legal and ethical views involving, 500-505, 506
  case study on, 498-500
  community and, 486-506
  education of, 500-501
  least restrictive environment for, 494
  living arrangements for, 488, 495
  marriage by, 496-497
  rehabilitation of, primary objective of government in, 495
  rights of
    to be part of a community, 504
    to choose, 503
    to leisure and retirement, 502
    to marry and have children, 502
    to normalization, 505
    to reach full potential, 503-504
    to sexual expression, 501
  role of community health nurse with, 488-489
  sexual activity of, 496-497

Dexedrine; *see* Dextroamphetamine

Dextroamphetamine, 503

Diabetes mellitus
  death rates in young and middle-aged adults from, 240*t*
  fiber intake in, 517
  middle-aged adults with, 249
  noninsulin dependent, weight management for, 513-514, 516
  older adults with, 266
  weight reduction program and, 516

Diabetics
  alcohol consumption by, 518
  sugar intake by, 520

Diagnosis, nursing; *see* Nursing diagnosis(es)

Diagnosis-related groups, 23
  health care costs and, 34

Diazepam, 575

Diazepoxide, detoxification with, 586

Diet; *see also* Nutrition
  adolescent, 526
  of black American culture, 316
  cultural variations in, 308
  of Eastern Asian cultures, 311
  healthy, 535
    recommendations for, 512-521
  of Hispanic American culture, 313
  infant, stages of, 523-526, 535
  of native American culture, 314
  in older adult, assessment of, 532
  for preschool children, 526
  for school-aged children, 526
  for toddlers, 526
Dietary goals, 66, 87
Digestion, changes in, nutrition in older adults affected
    by, 529
Dilemmas, ethical
  definition of, 606
  models for analysis of, 606-610, 611
Diphtheria, 469*t*
Diphtheria/pertussis/tetanus, immunization against, 472
Disability
  developmental, definitions of, 489, 505-506
  learning, 493-494
Disabled, developmentally; *see* Developmentally disabled
Disasters, environmental, 560-561, 566
Discharge plan
  for high-tech home health care, 401
  simple versus complex, 380
Discharge planner, 379-380
Discharge planning, 368-380; *see also* Continuity of care
  for continuity of care, recent changes affecting, 371
  critical information required for, 375
  definitions of, 370, 380
  evaluation of, 374
  guidelines for, 372
  historical perspective on, 369-370
  legislation affecting, 370-371
  primary nurse and, 379-380
    case studies for, 376-377
  process of, 371-374, 380
  roles in, 378-380
Disease(s)
  affecting young and middle-aged adults, 252
  cardiovascular, middle-aged adults affected by, 248
  caused by chemical exposure, 431*t*
  cerebrovascular, death rates in young and middle-aged
    adults from, 240*t*
  communicable, 464-483
    common, 469*t*-471*t*
    in day-care centers, 202-203
    definition of, 468
    epidemiological triad for, 465-466, 483
    legislation regarding, 598
    prevention of, 468, 472, 483

Disease(s)—cont'd
  communicable—cont'd
    reportable by law, 598
    screening for, 472, 483
    surveillance of incidence of, 467-468, 482
    transmission of, 465-467
  frequency of, measures of, 151
  incidence of, 149
  infectious
    exposure of health workers to, 432-433
    middle-aged adults affected by, 248
  native Americans' concept of, 313
  natural history of, 141
  prevention of, definition of, 70
  primary prevention of, 141
  related to occupation, difficulties in determination
    of, 443
  secondary prevention of, 141
  skin, occupational illness and, 426-427
  tertiary prevention of, 141
  waterborne, 552-553
Disengagement, 333-334, 345
Disengagement theory of aging, 261
Disorders, sensory, children with, 494-495
District Nursing Service, 10
Disulfiram, during detoxification, 586
DO; *see* Oxygen, dissolved
Donabedian, Avedis, quality of health care impacted by, 159,
    164-165
"do-not resuscitate" orders, in high-tech home health
    care, 398
Down's syndrome, 491-492
DRGs; *see* Diagnosis-related groups
Drug abuse, 570-571
  deaths from, 238, 241*t*
  in school-aged children, 220-221
  by youth, 573
Drug abuser, nursing assessment of, 582-583
Drug Enforcement Agency, 25
Drugs; *see also* Medications
  abuse of; *see* Drug abuse
  addiction to, 571, 582, 590
  antipsychotic, for developmentally disabled, 503
  behavior related to use of, by school-aged children, 222
  dependence on, by school-aged children, 227
  interaction of, with food consumed by older adults, 529
  nonmedical use of, 570-571; *see also* Drug abuse
  psychostimulant, for developmentally disabled, 503
  psychotropic, for developmentally disabled, 502-503
DTs; *see* Delirium tremens
Dumping; *see also* Waste dumps
  ocean, 544
Dunn, Halpert, wellness movement and, 68
Durant, Jean Henri, International Red Cross founded by, 10
Dutch East India Company, organized health care provided
    by, 22

Dysfunction
  cues of, 333
  in families; *see* Family(ies), dysfunctional
  sexual, middle-aged adults affected by, 250

E

Early and Periodic Screening, Diagnosis and Treatment Program, 196
ECM; *see* Erythema chronicum migrans
Ecological study, 153
Ecomap, family health assessed using, 286-287, 297
Education
  client; *see also* Client teaching; Health teaching
    about apnea monitoring, 401-402
    about home infusion therapy, 401
    about substance abuse, 585
    about ventilator therapy, 403-404
  client and family, in providing continuity of care, 375
  community health nursing and, 119
  parent, about health promotion in young children, 195
  rights to, for developmentally disabled, 500-501
  of substance abuser, 587
Education for all handicapped children act, 488-489, 506
Educational resource centers, 446
Educational resource centers, education in occupational health care provided by, 424
Elavil; *see* Amitriptyline
Elderly, the; *see* Older adults
ELISA; *see* Enzyme-linked immunosorbent assay
Emergency treatment, in day-care center, 200-201
Emissions, seminal, in puberty, 213
Empacho, 312*t*
Enabling, 334, 345
Enculturation, definition of, 302
Endocrine system, in older adults, physical assessment of, 262*t*, 266
End-result idea, development of, 158
Enmeshment, 333, 345
Entrepreneurship, nursing, 627, 628, 633
Environment
  for communicable disease, 466
  concept of, in nursing, 618-620
  concerns about, 540-566
  conducive to learning, 109
  crowded, 543
  disasters and, 560-561, 566
  effect of population growth on, 541-543
  hazards in, community health nursing and, 633
  hazards in, wellness affected by, 94
  home, pollution in, 561-565
  least restrictive, for developmentally disabled, 494
  in Neuman's health care systems model, 40
  radiation in, 558-559
  sensitivity to, wellness and, 91
Enzyme-linked immunosorbent assay, HIV identified by, 479
Epidemics, influence of, on nursing and medicine, 5*t*, 8

Epidemiological triad for communicable disease, 465-466, 483
Epidemiological triangle, 146
Epidemiology, 138-154
  application of, to community health nursing, 153
  concepts in, 141-148
  definition of, 154
  historical evolution of, 139-141
EPSDT; *see* Early and Periodic Screening, Diagnosis and Treatment Program
ERCs; *see* Educational resource centers
Ergonomics, workplace, 429
Erythema chronicum migrans, 473
Erythema infectiosum, 469*t*
Ethical dilemmas, models for analysis of, 606-610, 611
Ethics
  definition of, 603, 611
  deontological theory of, 604-605
  nursing practice guided by, 604-605, 611
  teleological theory of, 604
Ethnic groups, health beliefs and practices of, 306
Ethnicity, definition of, 302
Ethnocentrism, definition of, 300
Ethylene oxide, diseases caused by exposure to, 431*t*
"Evaluating the Quality of Medical Care," 159
Evaluation
  definition of, 40, 167
  formative, 167
    guidelines for, 169
  summative, 168
    guidelines for, 169
  supervisory, quality of health care and, 176
Examination stage, in older adults, 260
Excretion, problems with, nutrition in older adults affected by, 529
Exercise
  aerobic, 85, 93
  isokinetic, 86
  isometric, 86
  isotonic, 86
  wellness affected by, 93
  yoga and stretching, 86
Exercise programs, wellness, counseling clients about, 86
Experimental study, 154
Expert power, definition of, 129
Expression, sexual, right of developmentally disabled to, 501
Extended family, 277
Extrafamily stressors, 326*t*, 335

F

Family of orientation, 277
Family(ies)
  with AIDS, 480
  assessment of, 279-280
    conceptual frameworks for, 282-283

Family(ies)—cont'd
  as bearer of culture, 299-319
  blended, 278
  communication in, and coping with problems, 281-282
  coping patterns of, 280-282
  culturally diverse, 308-316
  definition of, 277, 296
    by Neuman's health care systems model, 295-296
  developmental tasks for, 282
    associated with life cycle, 283t
  dysfunctional, 321-345
    case study applying nursing process to, 342-343
    characteristics of, 322-325, 326t
    developmental variables associated with, 326t, 334
    goal setting in, 336-337
    NANDA classification of, 323, 345
    nursing assessment of, 325-335
    nursing care of, 336
    nursing concerns about, 324-325
    nursing diagnoses for, 335-336
    nursing intervention with, 336-337
    physiological variables associated with, 325, 326t, 327, 330-331
    psychological variables associated with, 326t, 331-333
    sociocultural variables associated with, 326t, 333-334
    spiritual variables associated with, 326t, 333
  of Eastern Asian origin, 309-311
  extended, 277
  functional, 279-280
    characteristics of, 296
  health of
    assessment of, 279-280
    Neuman's health care systems model and, 283-284
    tools for assessment of, 284-292
  ineffective coping by, nursing care plans fo, 337-342
  interrelationship of health of, and health of community, 294-296, 297
  kin network, 277-278
  life cycle of, 282, 283t
  members of, cultural variations in attitudes towards, 308
  nuclear, 277, 296
  nursing care of, nursing process applied to, 284-294
  occupational health nursing and, 434
  pattern of substance abuse in, 573-574
  problems in, coping with, 280-282
  role of
    in black American culture, 315
    in Eastern Asian cultures, 310
    in Hispanic American culture, 312-313
    in native American culture, 314
  roles within, 278-279, 296
    coping with problems and, 281
  same sex, 278
  single-parent, 277
  stressors affecting, 326t, 334-335, 345

Family(ies)—cont'd
  structure of
    in dysfunctional families, 322-324
    evolving, 278
  three-generation, 277
  types of, 277-278
  as unit of service, 275-297
  unity of, 280
  unmarried couple/child, 278
  unmarried parent/child, 278
  violent, profile of, 328t-331t
  wellness in, and wellness in community, 274
Farr, William, impact of, on epidemiology, 140
Fats, cholesterol and, reduction of, 513-515
Females
  incidence of chemical dependency in, 575
  increased calcium intake by, 520
  postmenopausal, iron overload in, 520-521
Fertility rate, 150
  calculation of, 152
Fetal alcohol syndrome, 518, 575
Fetus, development of, maternal nutrition and, 522, 523
Fiber, dietary, 516-517
Fidelity, 603
Fifth disease, 469t
Flashbacks, 580
Flesch formula, 116
Flexible line of defense, in Neuman's health care systems model, 41
  immunity and, 465
  strengthening of, 342
  weakening of, 335
Flexible line of defense in Neuman's health care systems model, 40
Flexner report, quality of health care affected by, 158
Fliedner, Theodur, influence of, on nursing and medicine, 8
Fluoride, recommendations for, 519
FNS; see Frontier nursing service
Fog formula, 116
Folic acid, increased requirements for, during pregnancy, 522
Folk healers, 311
Food and Drug Administration, 25
Food groups, basic, 87
Foods
  drug interactions with, nutrition in older adults affected by, 529
  fiber-rich, 516, 517
  high in complex carbohydrates, 517
  high-sodium, 518
  iron-rich, 520
  rich in folic acid, 522
  solid, introduced to infants, 525
Formaldehyde, home pollution caused by, 563
Formula feeding, 524-525
Formulas, epidemiological, commonly used, 149-150, 152

Framingham study, 68
Free-basing, 578
Frontier Nursing Service, 15-16
Fry formula, 116
Fundamental human rights, 604
Furazolidone, *Giardia lamblia* treated with, 202
Furoxone; *see* Furazolidone

G

Galen, influence of, on nursing and medicine, 5*t*, 7
Gasoline, diseases caused by exposure to, 431*t*
Gastric secretions, reduced, nutrition in older adults affected by, 529
Gastrointestinal system, in older adults, physical assessment of, 262*t*, 265
Gaunt, John, impact of, on epidemiology, 140
Genitourinary system, in older adults, physical assessment of, 262*t*, 265
Genogram, family health assessed using, 286, 297
Giardia lamblia, in day-care centers, 202
Giardiasis, in day-care centers, 202
Giftedness, spirit of, in L'Arche communities, 504
Girls, height and weight measurements for, 211*t*
Glaucoma, middle-aged adults affected by, 250
Goal setting, realistic, in dysfunctional families, 336-337
God's own medicine, 580
GOM; *see* God's own medicine
Gonorrhea, 471*t*
    antibiotics used to treat, 472
Goodrich, Annie Warburton, army school of nursing and, 13
Greece, ancient, influence of, on nursing and medicine, 5*t*, 7
Grey Nuns of the Sacred Heart, contributions of, to nursing profession, 9-10
Group(s)
    characteristics of, 125, 136
    community development, 132
    conflict within, 130, 136
    definition of, 123-124, 136
    development of, stages of, 125-127, 136
    eductional, 133-134
    forming, 125-126
    functions of, 124, 136
    individual roles in, 127, 128
    leader of, 128-129
    leadership of, effective, 128-129, 136
    roles within, 127-128, 136
    self-help, 132-133
    small, initiating, 135
    socioeconomical specialist role in, 127
    support, 132-133
    task roles within, 127
    types of, 132-134, 135

H

Habituation, drug, 582

Haldol; *see* Haloperidol
Hallucinogens, abuse of, 580
Haloperidol, 503
Hand, foot, and mouth disease, in day-care centers, 203
Hand washing, proper, in day-care centers, 203
Handicapped, mentally; *see also* Developmentally disabled
    attitudes towards, 486-488
    dying and, 498
    sexuality in, 501
Harmony, inner, wellness and, 88-91
Harvey, William, influence of, on nursing and medicine, 5*t*, 8
Hazards
    environmental, community health nursing and, 633
    occupational, experienced by hospital employees, 435
    workplace
        biological, 432-433
        categories of, 428-434, 446
        chemical, 429, 431-432
        ergonomic, 429
        physical, 428-429
        psychological, 433-434
Healers, cultural, 309
Health
    activities to promote, in children, 194-196
    adaptive model of, 621
    chemical hazards to, 547-552
    clinical model of, 620-621
    in community, 65-94
    definition of, 38-39, 70, 620
        black American, 315
        Eastern Asian, 309
        Hispanic American, 311
        native American, 313
        in Neuman's health care systems model, 40, 58
    effect of air pollutants on, 556*t*
    environmental, 618, 633
    eudaimonistic model of, 621-622
    family
        Neuman's health care systems model and, 283-284
        tools for assessment of, 284-292
    family, assessment of, 279-280
    hazardous wastes as threat to, 547-552, 566
    holistic, definition of, 70
    of homeless, 458, 459*t*
    models of, 620-622
    occupational, 446
        emphasis of, 434
        government involvement in, 424-425, 446
        maintenance of, 427-428
        programs for, 443, 445-446, 447
        relationship between community and, 436
    problems with; *see* Health problems
    promotion of; *see* Health promotion
    rights to, 623-624
    role-performance model of, 621

Health—cont'd
  and safety, in day-care center, 200
  teaching client about; *see* Client teaching; Health teaching
  third wave of, 67
  in workplace
    attitudes about, 428
    maintenance of, 427-428
Health behavior contract, 74
Health belief model, 102-103, 120
  for wellness, 71-72
Health belief model for wellness, 93
Health care
  access to, 618-619
  alternative delivery systems for, 619
  changes in, 593-594
  consumer demands and needs for, 161
  continuing; *see also* Continuity of care
    criteria for, 369-370
  continuity of; *see* Continuity of care
  continuum of, 369
  cost crisis in, wellness movement and, 67
  cost of, 35
    containment of, 31, 33-34
    quality assurance and, 160-161
    wellness movement and, 93
  cost-effective, 370
  in day-care center, 200-201
  delivery of; *see* Health care delivery system
    at home; *see* Home health care
  federal legislation affecting, 619-620
  financing, 29-30, 618-620
  financing of, 35
  forces shaping role of nursing in, 630
  home; *see* Home health care
  increased cost of, theories about, 33-34
  legal issues in, 594-603
  level of, 370
  managed, definition of, 397
  quality assurance in, 164-175
  quality of, 618
    costs and, 160-161
    federal government involvement in, 25
    methods of assessing, 175-177
    sentinel approach to, 177
  quality of, trajectory method for evaluating, 177
  rights to, 623-624
  in 1990's, issues affecting, 618-619
  services for, competition in, 161
Health care delivery system(s), 21-35
  changes in, nursing leadership in, 631-632
  components of, 25-29, 35
  evaluation of, 30-34
  evolution of role of federal government in, 23-24
  federal government involvement in, 25
  federal legislation affecting, 24-25*t*
  historical perspective on, 22-25

Health care delivery system(s)—cont'd
  impact of prospective payment system on, 162
  influence of technology on, 163
  involvement of black ministers in, 315
  issues involving, 618-619
  Neuman's model of, 40-44, 58
    prevention of illness in school-aged children using, 223-232
  in other countries, 34
  primary skilled services in, 355
  private sector of, 28-29, 35
  public and private sectors of, 2
  public sector of, 25-28
  secondary services in, 355
  state governments involvement in, 25, 28
  trends in, 630
Health care practices
  of black Americans, 315
  of Eastern Asians, 309
  health beliefs of ethnic groups and, 306
  implications of value orientations for, 305*t*
  of native Americans, 313-314
  religious influences on, 306-307
Health care worker
  occupational health hazards experienced by, 435, 446
  universal precautions taken by, 433
Health departments
  development of, 22
  local, 28, 35
  state, 25, 28, 35
Health education; *see also* Client teaching; Health teaching
  assessment of, 106-108
  definition of, 70
  planning models for, 102-103
  for young adults, 244
Health history, occupational, 438-442, 443, 446-447
Health insurance
  payment of high-tech home health care by, 396, 397
  private, home health care financed by, 356
Health insurance, independent, 30
Health Maintenance Act of 1973, 23, 24*t*
Health Maintenance Organizations, 29-30
  payment for high-tech home health care by, 397
Health Omnibus Program Extension of 1988, 619
Health problems
  associated with water supplies, 552-553
  environmental, role of community health nurse with, 565-566
Health promotion
  American Hospital Association's policy statement on, 66-67
  definition of, 70
  in schools, 223-232
  in senior citizen center, 266-269
  in young adults, 244
  in young children, use of play in, 194-195

Health Services Administration, 25
Health teaching; *see also* Client teaching
  in community, 96-120
  community health nurse as source for, 105
  definition of, 119
  goals of, 103
  in groups, advantages of, 134
  historical background on, 97-89
  legal issues in, 99
  as part of discharge planning, 373-374, 380
Healthy People, 67
Hearing
  assessment of, in school-aged children, 230-231
  loss of
    in children, 494-495
    occupational, 428
  in older adults
    changes in, 257, 258t
    physical assessment of, 263, 265
Heart
  chronic occlusive disease of, 265
  diseases of, death rates in young and middle-aged adults
      from, 239t
Heart failure, congestive, 265
Heart rate
  maximum, 86
  target, 85-86
Hebrews, influence of, on nursing and medicine, 6
Height and weight
  nutritional status of children indicated by, 526, 527t
  of primary-school children, 209, 212
  in school-aged children, 227-228
Height and weight chart
  for adults, 242t
  for boys, 210t
  for girls, 211t
Hematological system, in older adults, physical assessment
      of, 262t, 266
Henderson, Virginia, influence of, on development of com-
      munity health nursing, 17t
Hepatitis, viral, 472-473
Hepatitis A, 472-473
Hepatitis B, 432-433, 473
  young adults affected by, 242
Heptavax B, contraction of Hepatitis B prevented by,
      473
Herd immunity, 148
Hernia, hiatal, middle-aged adults affected by, 249
Heroin, 580
Herpes, 471t
Herpes simplex, 479
Herz, 555
Hettler, William, wellness movement and, 69
High-Level Wellness, 68
High-Level Wellness: An Alternative to Doctors, Drugs and
      Disease, 68

High-technology home health care
  assessment of client eligibility for, 388-396
  clinical laboratory services associated with, 388
  communication abilities of client and care-giver associ-
      ated with, 389-390
  denial of, appeal process for, 398-399
  discharge from, appeal for, 399-400
  drug therapy restrictions in, 392
  legal issues involving, 397-399, 401, 406
  payment for, 396-397, 406
  planning for use of, 386-404
  program development support for, 387
  service area logistics for, 388
  services associated with, 384, 406
  team members associated with, 384-386, 406
High-touch care, 383-384
  integration of, with high-tech home health care, 406
Hill-Burton Act of 1946, 23, 24t
Hill-Burton Act of 1946 quality of health care affected by,
      158-159
Hippocrates, influence of, on nursing and medicine, 5t, 7
History
  chemical use, 582-583
  health, occupational, 438-442, 443, 446-447
  nursing, discharge planning using, 373
HIV; *see* Human immunodeficiency virus
HMOs; *see* Health maintenance organizations
Home, pollution in, 561-565, 567
Home care coordinator, role of, in discharge planning,
      378-379
Home health aide
  home health care provided by, 352
  role of, in delivery of high-tech care, 386
Home health care
  accreditation of, 163
  advanced technology in, 383-406; *see also* High-tech-
      nology home health care
  for chronically ill, 409-418
  for chronically ill, current issues in, 416-417
  clients requiring, 350-351, 366
  definition of, 350, 366
  financing of, 355-356, 366
  future trends in, 365-366
  high-technology; *see* High-technology home health care
  hospital-based agencies providing, 354-355
  influence of Florence Nightingale on, 10
  logistical aspects of, 356-357, 365
  Medicare payments for, 619
  nursing assessment for client receiving, 365
  nursing shortage in, 629
  private agencies providing, 353-354, 354
  professionals involved in providing, 351-352, 366
  proprietary agencies providing, 354
  quality of, 159-160
  trends in, 619-620
  types of agencies providing, 352-355, 366

Home health care—cont'd
    Visiting Nurse Association and, 353
Home visit, cultural assessment during, 304
Homebound, definition of, 355
Homeless, the
    definition of, 457
    demographical characteristics of, 457-458, 462
    health problems experienced by, 458, 459t
    numbers of, in major cities, 457t, 458
    nursing diagnoses for, 460
    substance abuse by, 572
Homeless Person's Survival Act, 458, 460
Homelessness
    causes of, 458
    solutions for, 460
Homicide
    among adolescents, 232
    death rates in young and middle-aged adults from, 241t
    involving primary and secondary school age children, 217
Homicide, and middle-aged adults, 248
Hopelessness
    cues for identifying, 332
    ineffective family coping related to, nursing care plan for, 341-342
Hospice
    concept of, 414, 416, 417
    home health care provided by, 355, 366
Hospital and Diagnostic Services Act of 1957, Canadian, 34
Hospitals, private, 28
Host, for communicable disease, 466
Human immunodeficiency virus, 475, 478-479, 483
    children with, 217
    intravenous drug abuse and, 571
Human immunodeficiency virus, death rates in young and middle-aged adults from, 241t
Humanists, influence of, on nursing and medicine, 5t, 8
Humor, inner harmony achieved using, 91
Hygiene, dental, for young children, 193-194
Hypertrophy, prostatic, in older adult males, 265
Hypnosis, inner harmony achieved using, 90
Hz; *see* Herz

I

ICFs; *see* Intermediate care facilities
Identity, developing sense of, in adolescence, 214
Identity diffusion, 214
Illness
    causes of, according to native Americans, 313
    chronic; *see* Chronic illness
    common causes of
        in middle-aged adults, 248-250
        in young adults, 242
    in family members, influence of family structure on, 322
    occupational; *see* Occupational illness
Illness-wellness continuum, Travis', 68
Imagery, inner harmony achieved using, 90

Imipramine, 503
Immune globulin, hepatitis A treated with, 472
Immunity, 148, 464-465, 482-483
    changes in, in older adult, 257
    changes in, in older adults, 260t
    dynamics of, demonstrated by Neuman's health systems model, 465-483
Immunizations
    informed consent about, 599, 611
    of normal infants, 225t
    primary prevention of communicable disease by, 472, 483
    of school-aged children, 224-226
    for young adults, 244
Immunoblot, HIV identified by, 479
Immunological system, in older adults, physical assessment of, 262t
Implementation, definition of, 39
Incidence rate, 149
    calculation of, 152
Incineration, 544-545
Incontinence, older adults affected by, 529
Individuation, definition of, 488
Infant mortality rate, 149
    calculation of, 152
Infants
    of addicted mothers, 574-575
    chronic illness affecting, 411
    cognitive development of, 188-189
    developmentally disabled, 495-496
    feeding recommendations for, 514
    formula feeding, 524-525
    growth and development of, 205
    immunization of, recommended schedule for, 225t
    iron needs of, 521
    low birth weight, maternal prepregnancy weight and, 522
    nutritional requirements for, 523-526
    at risk, 450-452
    stages of diet for, 523-526, 535
Infections
    opportunistic, associated with AIDS, 479, 483
    prevention of, in day-care centers, 202
    reservoirs of, 146
    transmission of, 146, 148
Influenza, death rates in young and middle-aged adults from, 240t
Informed consent
    in high-home health care, 398
    related to immunizations, 599, 611
Infusion therapy, home, diagnosis appropriate for, 400
Ingestion, exposure to chemical agents by, 431-432
Inhalants, abuse of, 581-582
Inhalation, exposure to chemical agents by, 431
Injury
    back, in workplace, 428
    work-related; *see* Occupational injury

INS; *see* Intravenous nursing society
Institutionalization, of older adults, 254
Instrumental activities of daily living, 373
Insurance
  health; *see* Health insurance
  independent, 30
  malpractice, 599, 603, 611
  private
    home health care financed by, 356
    payment for high-tech home health care by, 396, 397
  professional liability, 599, 603, 611
Interfamily stressors, 326*t*, 335
Intermediate care facilities for developmentally disabled, 488
International Red Cross, 10-11
Intimacy, crisis of, in young adults, 236
Intrafamily stressors, 326*t*, 335
Intravenous Nursing Society, 396
Investigation, field, 153
Iron, requirements for, 520-521
  during pregnancy, 521-522
Iron supplements, side effects of, 522
Isolation, nutrition of older adults affected by, 531

J

Jenner, Edward, influence of, on nursing and medicine, 8
Johnson, Dorothy, influence of, on development of community health nursing, 17*t*
Joint Commission on Accreditation of Healthcare Organizations, 162-163
    quality assurance model developed by, 165-167
  quality of health care affected by, 158
Joint Commission on the Accreditation of Hospitals, 22
  quality of health care affected by, 158, 159
Justice, 603, 607

K

Kaposi's sarcoma, 479
Kidneys, changes in, in older adult, 257
Kin network family, 277-278
Knowledge deficit, nursing diagnosis of, 110-111, 120
Knowles, John, wellness movement and, 66
Korean War, influence of, on nursing, 14

L

La Raza, 311
Laboratory services, associated with high-tech home health care, 388
Lactaid, 522
Lactose, intolerance to, 522
Landfill, 543-544
Language, barriers in, 307
L'Arches community, 504
Latchkey children, 199

Laws
  common, 594
  community health nursing practice affected by, 594-596, 610
  constitutional, 594
  public health, 597-598, 611
  workmen's compensation, 425
Lawsuits, malpractice, vulnerability of community health nurse to, 594-596, 599, 603
LBW; *see* Infants, low birth weight
LDL; *see* Low-density lipoprotein
Lead
  health affected by, 556*t*
  home pollution caused by, 564-565
  poisoning with, case study on, 565-566
Leader, group, 128-129
Leadership
  autocratic, 130, 131*t*
  democratic, 130, 131*t*
  group
    effective, 128-129, 136
    shared, 129, 136
  laissez-faire, 130, 131
  styles of, 130-131, 136
Learner in community health practice, 108
Learning, 120
  ability for, 108
    by older adults, 254
  affective, 101-102
    teaching methods associated with, 115*t*
  client, motivation and, 108-109
  cognitive, 100-101
    teaching methods associated with, 115*t*
  conditions of, 104*t*
  definition of, 99-100, 119
  domains and levels of, teaching methods and, 115*t*
  environment conducive to, 109
  mental retardation and, 504
  psychomotor, 102
    teaching methods associated with, 115*t*
  readiness for, 108
  types of, 100-103, 119
Learning disabilities, 493-494
Learning objectives, preparation of, 111
Learning theories, 119
  cognitive, 100
  definition of, 100
Least restrictive environment for developmentally disabled, 494
Legislation
  communicable disease, 598
  community health nursing affected by, 594
  federal, health care affected by, 619-620
Legitimate power, definition of, 129
Leininger, Madeline, influence of, on development of community health nursing, 17*t*

Leukemia
  death rates in young and middle-aged adults from, 239*t*-240*t*
  lymphatic, in older adults, 266
Librium; *see* Chlordiazepoxide
Licensure, 162, 182
  comparison of, with certification, 163*t*
Life, right to, for developmentally disabled, 500
Life expectancy, 256
Lines of resistance, in Neuman's health care systems model
  immunity and, 465
  weakening of, 335
Lines of resistance in Neuman's health care systems model, 40
Liver disease, death rates in young and middle-aged adults from, 241*t*
Logotherapy, 250-251, 252
Lorazepam, 580
Love Canal, chemical exposure at, 560
Low-density lipoprotein, 514
LSD; *see* Lysergic acid diethylamide
Lyme disease, 473-474
Lymph nodes, enlarged, in school-aged children, 228-229
Lymphatic system, in older adults, physical assessment of, 262*t*, 266
Lysergic acid diethylamide, 580

M

Mal de ojo, 312*t*
Males, adult, iron overload in, 520-521
Malpractice insurance, 599, 603, 611
Malpractice lawsuits, vulnerability of community health nurse to, 594-596, 599, 603
Managed care, definition of, 397
Marijuana, abuse of, 581
Marine Hospital, 23, 35
Marriage, developmentally disabled and, 496-497
MASH; *see* Mobile army surgical hospital
MATCH model, 77, 93
Material safety data sheets, 425
Maternal mortality rate, 150
Maturational crisis, definition of, 280
Maturity, later, definition of, 254
MDA; *see* 3,4-methylenedioxyamphetamine
Measles/mumps/rubella, immunization against, 472
Medicaid, 23, 24*t*, 29
  home health care financed by, 356
  payment for high-tech home health care by, 397
Medical Care Act of 1966, Canadian, 34
Medical unit, self-contained and transportable, establishment of, during Vietnam War, 14
Medicare, 23, 24*t*, 29
  home health care financed by, 355, 619
  payment for high-tech home health care by, 396-397
Medicare Catastrophic Coverage Act of 1988, 23, 619-620

Medications; *see also* Drugs
  administration of, by nonmedical personnel in intermediate-care facility, 502
  antidepressant, for developmentally disabled, 503
  establishing dosage schedules for, 394-395
  planning for storage of, in high-tech home health care setting, 392, 394
  seizure, for developmentally disabled, 502-503
  use of
    in day-care center, 201
    during detoxification, 586
Meditation, inner harmony achieved using, 90
Mellaril, 503
Melting-pot, 302-303
Menarche, in girls, 213
Menopause, 247
Mental discipline learning theories, 100
Mental health
  in older adults, assessment of, 262*t*
  in school-aged children, 220-221, 227
Mental retardation, 492, 503-504; *see also* Developmentally disabled
  attitudes towards, 486-488
Mercury, health affected by, 556*t*
Mescaline, 580
Mesothelioma, due to asbestos exposure, 431
Metaparadigm, definition of, 614
Metaparadigm of nursing, 614-629
Methadone, 586
3,4-methylenedioxyamphetamine, 580
Methylphenidate, 503
MHR; *see* Heart rate, maximum
Microwaves, effects of, on health, 429
Middle Ages, influence of, on nursing and medicine, 5*t*, 7-8
Middle-aged adults
  chronic illness involving, 411-413
  common causes of illness in, 248-250
  developmental tasks for, 247-248
  major causes of mortality in, 248
  midlife crisis in, 250
  spiritual development of, 250-251
Midlife crisis, 250
Minamata disease, 549
Minister, black, as member of health team, 315
Missionaries of Charity, 16
Mobile army surgical hospital, establishment of, during World War II, 14
Model Standards: A Guide for Community Preventive Health Services, 172
Molestation, sexual, involving school-aged children, 219
Morbidity, 149
Morphine, use of, in high-tech home health care, 392
Mortality; *see also* Death(s)
  bills of, 140
  infant, 450-451
    nursing prevention of, 452

Mortality; *see also* Death(s)—cont'd
  major causes of, in young and middle-aged adults, 236, 237, 239t-241t, 252
Mortality rate, 150
  calculation of, 152
  definition of, 149
Mother D'Youville, contributions of, to nursing profession, 9-10
Mother Teresa, 16
Mothers, addicted, babies born to, 575-575
Motivation, 120
  client learning affected by, 108-109
  of group members, 131-132
Motivation maintenance theory, 131-132, 136
Motivators, 132
Moulder, B., occupational health nursing impacted by, 423
MSDs; *see* Material safety data sheets
Multiple sclerosis, case study on adult with, 413
Mumps, 469t
Muscles
  changes in, in older adult, 256
  growth of, in adolescents, 213
Musculoskeletal system in older adults
  changes in, 259t
  physical assessment of, 262t, 265
MUST; *see* Medical unit, self-contained and transportable

N

NAHC; *see* National Association for Home Care
Narcan, administration of, in high-tech home health care, 393-394
Narcotics, abuse of, 580-581
National Association for Home Care, 350
National Coalition for the Homeless, 460
National Emission Standards for Hazardous Pollutants, 556
National Health Planning and Resources Act of 1974, 23, 25t
National Institute for Occupational Health and Safety, 424, 425
National Institutes of Health, 25
National League for Nursing, purpose and function of, 13t
National League for Nursing Education, purpose and function of, 13t
National League of Nurses, 12
National Organization for Public Health Nursing, 11-12
National Organization of Public Health Nurses, purpose and function of, 13t
National Student Nurses' Association, purpose and function of, 13t
Native americans, alcohol abuse by, 572-573
Natural history, 141
Navane; *see* Thiothixene
Needs assessment, 167
  guidelines for, 168

Negligence, 596-597
Neonatal mortality rate, 150
Neoplasms, malignant
  death rates in young and middle-aged adults from, 239t-240t
  middle-aged adults affected by, 248
  young adults affected by, 238, 239t-240t
Nephritis, death rates in young and middle-aged adults from, 241t
Nephrosis, death rates in young and middle-aged adults from, 241t
Nephrotic syndrome, death rates in young and middle-aged adults from, 241t
Nervous system
  changes in, in older adults, 256-257, 260t
  peripheral, effect of cumulative trauma on, 429
NESHAPs. *see* National Emission Standards for Hazardous Pollutants
Neuman, Betty, influence of, on development of community health nursing, 17
Neuman community-client assessment guide, 59-61
Neuman's health care systems model, 40-44, 58
  application of
    to immunity, 465
    to prevention of illness in school-aged children, 223-232
  definition of family by, 295-296
  interaction between health of family members and family's wellness shown by, 283-284
  interrelationship of family health and community health shown by, 295-296
  nursing assessment/intervention involving young adults based on, 243
Neurological system, physical assessment of, in older adults, 262t, 266
Nicotine, effects of, 579
Nightingale, Florence
  influence of, on development of community health nursing, 17
  use of epidemiological model by, 140
Nightingale, Florence, contributions of, to nursing profession, 10, 19
Nightingale School of Nursing, 22
Nineteenth century, influence of, on nursing and medicine, 6
NIOSH. *see* National Institute for Occupational Health and Safety
Nitrogen dioxide, health affected by, 556t
Nitrogen oxide, home pollution caused by, 563
Nocturnal emission in puberty, 213
NOHPN. *see* National Organization for Public Health Nursing
Noise
  definition of, 553
  in workplace, hearing loss related to, 428
Noise pollution, 553-555, 567

Noncompliance, 120
    client teaching and, 117
    in high-tech home health care, 398-399, 401
Nonmalefeasance, 603, 607, 608, 610
Normal line of defense in Neuman's health care systems
        model, 40, 41
    immunity and, 465
    strengthening of, 342
    weakening of, 335
Normalization
    definition of, 488
    rights of, developmentally disabled to, 505
Norming in groups, 126
Nuclear family, 277, 296
Nuclear family dyad, 277
Nurse Practice Act, 604
Nurse Training Act of 1964, 23, 24*t*
Nursery school, definition of, 199
Nurse(s)
    chemical dependency by, 576-577
    community involvement by, 631
    home health, safety tips for, 357
    home health care planning by, 351
    occupational health; *see* Occupational health nurse
    political involvement by, 631
    primary, discharge planning and, 376-377, 379-380
    prison, role of, 454
    public health; *see* Public health nurses
    recruitment and retention of, 629
    responsibilities and obligations of, 603-604
    rights of, 604
    role of
        conceptual view of, 17*t*
        in home health care, 351, 355, 366
    school, developmentally disabled children and, 489
    shortage of, 629
    substance abuse by, 576
        assistance programs for, 589
    as wellness advocates, 93
Nursing
    community health; *see* Community health nursing
    entrepreneurship in, 627, 628, 633
    ethical issues in, 603-610
    issues in, related to community health nursing, 624-629
    metaparadigm of, 614-629
    nutrition provided to infants by, 524-525
    occupational health, 422-447, 446
        definition of, 434
        history of, 423-426
        Wilkinson windmill model of, 436
    private practice in, 627, 628
    public health, definition of, 18; *see also* Community health
            nursing
    theories of ethics guiding, 604-605, 611
Nursing assessment, cultural, 303-308, 319
    guide for, 317

Nursing audit, evaluation of health care by, 159
Nursing care
    home; *see* Home health care
    spiritual, for older adults, 270-271
    standards for, in correctional institutions, 455-456
Nursing centers, 627-628, 633
Nursing diagnosis(es), 292
    definition of, 40, 110
Nursing diagnosis(es), community, 626-627, 633
Nursing history, discharge planning using, 373
Nursing interventions, 58, 292
    in day-care, for children from birth to five years, 202-204
Nursing model, holistic, 79-80, 93
Nursing organizations in United States, 13*t*
Nursing practice, development of standards for, 159
Nursing process, 58
    applied to high-tech home health care, 404-405
    applied to low-income urban community, 44-52
    applied to suburban community, 53-57
    for chronically ill client, 416
    in community, 37-58
    components of, 39-40
    Neuman's views on, 58
    in occupational setting, 443
        case study on, 444-445
    to provide culturally appropriate care, 316-318
    stages of group development parallel to, 125-127, 136
    teaching/learning process and, 105-119, 120
Nursing theory, community health nursing and, 16-17, 19
Nutrition; *see also* Diet
    assessing status of, 526-528
    changes in, throughout life, 521-532, 535
    in community, 512-536
    during detoxification, 586
    factors affecting, in older adults, 528-532, 535-536
    infant, provided by nursing, 524-525
    maternal, fetal development affected by, 522, 523
    need for, in AIDS, 479
    during pregnancy, 521-523
    total parenteral
        in home health care setting, 395
        medicare coverage of, 396-397
    wellness and, 86-88
Nutritionists
    home health care provided by, 352
    role of, in delivery of high-tech care, 386

O

Obesity
    adult, criteria for defining, 515
    prepregnancy, 522-523
    young adults affected by, 242
Objective(s), learning, preparation of, 111
OBRA; *see* Omnibus Budget Reconciliation Act
Observation, direct, quality of health care assessed by,
        175-176

Occupational health nurses, roles and functions of, 434-446
Occupational illness, 434
  definition of, 426, 446
  difficulties in diagnosis of, 443, 447
  impact of, 427
  manifestations of, 426-427
  statistics on, 426
Occupational injury, 434
  definition of, 426, 446
  impact of, 427
  statistics on, 426
Occupational Safety and Health Act, 23, 24t, 424, 443
Occupational Safety and Health Administration, 23, 424-425
Occupational therapists, home health care provided by, 352
Ocean dumping, 544
OHN; *see* Occupational health nurse
Older adults, 253-271
  abuse of, 599
  assessment of diet of, 532
  assessment of nutritional status of, 531-532
  chronic illness affecting, 409, 413-414
  common health problems of, 261-266
  community resources for, 269
  developmentally disabled, 497-498
  disability in, prevention of, 258t-260t
  fragile, 270
  improving nutritional status of, case study on, 532-535
  increase in, discharge planning for continuity of care affected by, 371
  normal cognitive changes affecting, 257
  nursing diagnoses related to, 267
  nutritional concerns of, 528-532, 535-536
  physical assessment and health history of, systems approach to, 262t
  physical needs of, senior citizen centers and, 268
  psychological problems in, 261, 263
  psychosocial needs of, senior citizen centers and, 266-267
  senior citizen center for, 266-269
  spiritual nursing care for, 270-271
  substance abuse by, 575-576
Older Americans Act, 610
Omnibus Budget Reconciliation Act of 1987, 23, 25t, 375, 619
Opiates, administration of, in high-tech home health care, 393-394
Orem, Dorothea, influence of, on development of community health nursing, 17t
OSHA; *see* Occupational Safety and Health Administration
OSHAct; *see* Occupational Safety and Health Act
Osteoporosis, 265
  relationship between dietary calcium and, 520
Oxazepam, 580

Oxygen, dissolved, in water, 553
Ozone, health affected by, 556t

P

Parenteral therapy
  guidelines for determining therapeutic response to, 391
  home, client with history of substance abuse and, 395-396
  initiation of, in high-tech home care, 391
Parenting; *see* Child-rearing
Parents Anonymous, 340
Parkinson's disease, 266
Passenger vehicle safety, 193
Paternalism, 608
Patient's Bill of Rights, 604
PCBs; *see* Polychlorinated biphenyl
PCP; *see* Phencyclidine; *Pneumocystis carinii* pneumomia
Peer review, quality of health care and, 176
Pentamidine, aerolized, AIDS treated with, 479
Peplau, Hildegard, influence of, on development of community health nursing, 17t
Performing by groups, 126
Periodontal disease, young adults affected by, 242
Peripheral nervous system, effect of cumulative trauma on, 429
Peripheral venous access, 391
Person, concept of, in nursing, 616-618
Personality development
  in adolescents, 214
  Erikson's stages of, effect of chronic illness on, 410-411, 417
Pharmacist, role of, in delivery of high-tech care, 385
Phencyclidine, 580
Phenytoin, during detoxification, 586
Phototherapy, home, 402
  criteria for, 403
PHS; *see* Public Health Service
Physical dependency, 325
Physical examination, of school-aged children, 228
Physical fitness, 85-86
Physical therapists, home health care provided by, 351
Physicans, home health care planning by, 351
Physicians, 28
  on-call support provided by, in home health care, 386
  role of, in delivery of high-tech care, 385
Pilocarpine eye drops, 250
Pitch, 555
P.L. 94-103, 489, 490, 491, 505-506
P.L. 94-142, 488-489, 491, 495, 506
P.L. 98-527, 489, 490, 491, 500
Plague
  human, in United States, 467-468
  influence of, on nursing and medicine, 8
Planning, definition of, 39
Plaque, dental, 519

Play, 190-191, 205
structured, 191
supervision of activities of, 192
therapeutic, in young children, 195
types of, 191
use of, in health promotion for young children, 194-195
Plumbism in young children, 194
Pneumocystis carinii pneumonia, 474, 479
Pneumonia, death rates in young and middle-aged adults from, 240*t*
Poisoning
lead
case study on, 565-566
in young children, 194
mercury, 549
Poliomyelitis, 469*t*
Pollutants, types of, 556
Pollution
air, 555-558, 567
effect of population growth on, 543
in homes, 561-565, 567
noise, 553-555
water, 552-553, 566-567
Pollution standards index, 557
Polychlorinated biphenyl, 549-552
ocean dumping of, 544
Population
high-density, 543
world, growth in, 541, 542
Poverty
older adults affected by, 531
substance abuse associated with, 572
Power
coercive, definition of, 129
expert, definition of, 129
Power, social, 129, 136
PPD; *see* Purified protein derivative
PPS; *see* Prospective payment system
Preadolescence, definition of, 209
PRECEDE model, 102-103, 120
Pregnancy
consumption of alcohol during, 518
increased calcium intake during, 520, 522
increased need for folic acid during, 522
iron requirements during, 521-522
nutritional needs during, 521-523, 535
screening for nutritional risks during, 522-523
substance abuse during, 574-575
teen-age, 220
weight gain and energy needs during, 521
Prematurity, higher risk for mortality and morbidity associated with, 451
Presbycusis, 257, 258*t*
Presbyopia, 258*t*
Preschool program, definition of, 199

Preschoolers
cognitive development of, 189-190
developmental screening of, 195-196
diet for, 526
health screening of, 196
Prevalence rate, 149
calculation of, 152
Primary prevention, 58
of chemical dependency, 585
of communicable disease, 472m 483
in correctional institutions, 456
of disability in older adults, 258*t*-260*t*
of disease, 141
in epidemiology, 141
of homelessness, 460
for ineffective family coping related to family violence, 338-339
for ineffective family coping related to hopelessness, 341
for ineffective family coping related to substance abuse, 337
of infant mortality, 452
involving school-aged children, 224-227
involving young adults, 244
involving young children in day-care centers, 202-203
in Neuman's health care systems model, 40, 44, 224
Primary-school children
cognitive development of, 214
major causes of mortality and illness in, 215-221
personality development of, 214
physical growth and development of, 209-213
social behavior development of, 226*t*
vital signs in, 212
Prisoners
demographic characteristics of, 453-454
high risk for mortality and morbidity among, 453-456
Professional review organizations, 162
Program, definition of, 167
Proprietary health care agencies
home health care provided by, 354, 366
quality assurance and, 161
PROs; *see* Professional review organizations
Prospective payment system
effect of, on continuity of care, 371
health care delivery system affected by, 162
for home health agencies, 365
PSI; *see* Pollution standards index
Psilocybin, 580
Psychological dependency, 325
Puberty, 209, 213, 232
Public health law, 597-598, 611
Public health nurses
critical competencies for, 632
responsibility of, to report communicable diseases, 598
Public health nursing, 18, 19; *see also* Community health nursing

Public Health Service, 598
Purified protein derivative, 472

Q

Quality, emphasis on, in health care field, 163-164
Quality assurance
  American Nurses' Association model for, 159, 170-175, 182
  American Nurses' Association standard for, 179
  in community health nursing, 156-182, 633
  definition of, 157, 181
  future of, 180-181
  goal of, 157
  historical perspectives of, 158-160
  involvement of community health nurse with, 178-180, 181
  Joint Commission model of, 165-167
  methods for assessing, 175-177
  models of, 165-175
  nursing's impact on, 159
  program evaluation model for, 167-170
  research and, 180
  roles in, 178-180
  societal forces influencing development of, 160-163
Quality Patient Care Scale, 159
QUALPACS; *see* Quality Patient Care Scale
Queen Victoria, contributions of, to nursing profession, 10
Quinacrine, *Giardia lamblia* treated with, 202

R

Radiation
  definition of, 558
  environmental, 558-559
  exposure to, in workplace, 428-429
  ionizing and nonionizing, 429
Radionuclides, health affected by, 556*t*
Radon, 558
  home pollution caused by, 563-564
Ramazzini, B., occupational health nursing influenced by, 423
Rates
  calculation of, 152
  epidemiological, 149
Readability, formulas to measure, 116
Reality orientation, 270
Record-keeping, responsibility for, 599
Recycling, 546, 566
Red Cross
  American, 11
    purpose and function of, 13*t*
  International, 10-11
Referrals for continuity of care, 375, 380
  historical perspective on, 369
Rehabilitation, substance abuser, 588
Relative numbers, 149-150
Relative risk, 150

Relative risk—cont'd
  calculation of, 152
Relaxation, progressive, 90
Religion, health beliefs and practice influenced by, 306-307
Rennaisance, nursing and medicine influenced by, 5*t*, 8
Reorganized American Nurses' Association, purpose and function of, 13*t*
Research
  epidemiological, methods used in, 151-153
  quality assurance and, 180
Resources, informational, related to need for health education, 107*t*
Respiratory system, in older adults
  changes in, 257
  physical assessment of, 262*t*, 265
Respite care for older adults, 269
Retardation, mental, 492, 503-504; *see also* Developmentally disabled
  attitudes towards, 486-488
Retirement, 261
Reward power, definition of, 129
Rheumatic fever, death rates in young and middle-aged adults from, 239*t*
Rheumatic heart disease, death rates in young and middle-aged adults from, 239*t*
Rickettsia, Rocky Mountain Spotted Fever caused by, 467
Right, definition of, 604
Right to life, for developmentally disabled, 500
Ringworm, 471*t*
Risk management, 177-178
Ritalin; *see* Methylphenidate
Rocky Mountain Spotted Fever, *Rickettsia* as cause of, 467
Rogers, Martha, development of community health nursing influenced by, 17*t*
Rome, nursing and medicine influenced by, 5*t*, 7
Rosenstock, health belief model developed by, 71-72
Rubella, 469*t*
Rubeola, 470*t*

S

Safe Drinking Act, 553
Safety
  in correctional institutions, 454
  emphasis on, for children, 205
  guidelines for, for health care workers, 433
  health and, in day-care center, 200
  occupational
    government involvement in, 424-425, 446
    programs for, 443, 445-446, 447
Salmonella, transmission of, 466
Sandwich generation, 247, 251
Scabies, 469*t*
Scapegoating, 334, 345
Scarlet fever, 470*t*
Schemes, development of, in infants and toddlers, 188

School nurse, involvement of, with developmentally disabled children, 489
School-age years, definition of, 209, 232
School-aged children. *see also* Adolescents; Primary-school children
  chronically ill, nursing diagnoses related to, 218
  diet for, 526
  height and weight of, assessment of, 227-228
  major causes of mortality and illness in, 215-219, 232
  mental health of, 220-221
  mentally or physically impaired, tertiary prevention for, 231-232
  physiological measurements of, 228-229
  social behavior development of, 226*t*
Schools
  community health nurse in, 221-233
  health promotion in, 223-232
Scoliosis in school-aged children, 231
Screening
  for communicable diseases, 472, 483
  preschooler, 195-196, 205
Seat belts, 193
Secondary prevention, 58
  of communicable disease, 472, 483
  in correctional institutions, 456
  of disability in older adults, 258*t*-260*t*
  of disease, 141
  in epidemiology, 141
  for homeless, 460
  for ineffective family coping related to family violence, 339-340
  for ineffective family coping related to hopelessness, 341-342
  for ineffective family coping related to substance abuse, 337-338
  of infant mortality, 452
  involving school-aged children, 227-231
  involving young adults, 244
  involving young children, 203-204
  in Neuman's health care systems model, 40, 44, 224
  of substance abuse, 585
Self-actualization, definition of, 488
Self-care, medical, definition of, 71
Self-efficacy model for wellness, 73-74, 93
Self-evaluation, quality of health care and, 176
Self-responsibility, wellness and, 68-69
Self-transcendence, 251
Seminal emissions in puberty, 213
Senility in older adults, 254
Senior citizen center, 266-269
Sensation, reduced, nutrition in older adults affected by, 529
Sensory disorders, children with, 494-495
Septicemia, death rates in young and middle-aged adults from, 241*t*
Serax; *see* Oxazepam
Setting sun sign, 494

Sewage sludge, 544
Sex, activity in, by developmentally disabled, 496-497
Sexual assaults in correctional institutions, 454
Sexual dysfunction, middle-aged adults affected by, 250
Sexual expression, right of, by developmentally disabled, 501
Sexuality
  of developmentally disabled, 501
  of mentally retarded persons, 501
  of older adults, changes in, 260*t*
Shigellosis, 470*t*
Sick building syndrome, 91
Single-parent family, 277
Sister Callista Roy, development of community health nursing influenced by, 17*t*
Sisters of Charity, nursing and medicine influenced by, 5*t*, 8
Situational crisis, definition of, 280
Skin
  diseases of, occupational illness and, 426-427
  in older adults
    physical assessment of, 263
    physical changes in, 256
Skin, chemical agents absorbed by, 432
Slater nursing competency scale, 159
Sludge, sewage, 544
Smallpox, 465
Smell, in older adults, changes in, 258*t*
Smog, 556, 557-558
Smoke
  sidestream, wellness affected by, 91
  tobacco, home pollution caused by, 563
Snow, John, epidemiology influenced by, 140
Social power, 129, 136
Social Readjustment Rating Scale, 88, 90
Social Security Act of 1935, 23
  amendments to, 23, 25*t*
Social support for wellness behavioral changes, 74, 76
Social system, definition of, 39
Social vulnerability index, 31
Social workers
  home health care planning by, 351-352
  role of, in delivery of high-tech care, 385
Socialization, 302
  of black children, 316
Sodium, reduction of, 517-518
Sore throat, streptococcal, 470*t*
Sound
  definition of, 555
  inharmonic, wellness affected by, 91
Speech pathologists, home health care provided by, 352
Spermatogenesis in boys, 213
Spiritual development
  in middle-aged adults, 250-251
  in school-aged children, 214
Spirituality, definition of, 251

St. Francis of Assisi, nursing and medicine influenced by, 5*t*, 8

St. Thomas Aquinas, nursing and medicine influenced by, 5*t*, 8

St. Vincent de Paul, nursing and medicine influenced by, 8

Staging, definition of, 177

Standards, definition of, 171

Standards of Community Health Nursing Practice, 17, 596, 610-611

Stay Well Plan, 67

Stepfamily, 278

Stereotyping, 303

Stewart, A., occupational health nursing impacted by, 423

Stimson, Julia, army nursing and, 14

Stimulants, abuse of, 577-578

Stimulus-response learning theories, 100

Storming in groups, 126

Strabismus, 230

Streptococcal sore throat, 470*t*

Streptococcus mutans, tooth decay caused by, 519

Stress
  immunity affected by, 465
  inner harmony and, 88
  in middle-aged adults, caused by life position, 247
  occupational, 433-434

Stressors
  affecting family system, 334-335, 345
  in day-care, 202
  family system affected by, 326*t*

Study, analytical, 152-153

Substance abuse, 570-590; *see also* Alcohol, abuse of; Chemical dependency; Drug abuse
  by adolescents, 573
  causes of, 571-572
  client with history of, home parenteral therapy and, 395-396
  cultural aspects of, 572-573
  diagnosis of, 584
  dysfunctional families and, 325, 327
  in families, 573-574
  ineffective family coping related to, nursing care plan for, 337-338
  issues and trends in, 570-571
  by older adults, 575-576
  risk factors for, 572-577
  treatment objective of, 588

Sugars, dietary limitations of, 519-520

Suicide
  death rates in young and middle-aged adults from, 241*t*
  by middle-aged adults, 248
  in school-aged children, 220

Sulfonylureas, effect of, on weight reduction in diabetic, 516

Sulfur dioxide, health affected by, 556*t*

Surgeon General of United States, 25

Surgeon General's Report on Nutrition and Health, summary of, 513-521

Surveys
  descriptive, 151
  epidemiological, for high-risk aggregates, 450, 461
  field, 153

Susto, 312*t*

Swallowing, problems with, nutrition in older adults affected by, 529

Syphyllis, 471*t*

T

Taste, in older adults, changes in, 258*t*

Tax Equity and Fiscal Responsibility Act, 23, 25*t*

Tay-Sachs disease, 411

Teaching
  of adults, guidelines for, 105
  assessing abilities for, 109-110
  definition of, 99, 119
  evaluating effectiveness of, 119
  health; *see* Client teaching; Health teaching
  methods of, 114*t*, 115-116
  plan for
    implementation of, 116-119
    obstacles to implementation of, 120
    preparation of, 111-116
  primary goal of, 103
  principles of, 104*t*
  situation for, 109

Teaching/learning
  principles of, 103-105
  process of
    mistakes in, 118*t*, 119
    nursing process and, 105-119, 120

Teaching/learning theories, 99-100

Teeth, loss of, in children, 213

Television, impact of, on children, 215

Temperature, normal, in primary-school children, 212

Temperature inversion, 555
  definition of, 556

Tertiary prevention, 58
  of chemical dependency, 586-589
  of communicable disease, 472, 483
  in correctional institutions, 456
  of disability in older adults, 258*t*-260*t*
  of disease, 141
  in epidemiology, 141
  for homeless, 461
  for ineffective family coping related to family violence, 340-341
  for ineffective family coping related to hopelessness, 342
  for ineffective family coping related to substance abuse, 337-338
  of infant mortality, 452
  involving school-aged children, 231-232
  involving young adults, 244
    case study on, 244-246
  involving young children with special needs, 204

Tertiary prevention—cont'd
  in Neuman's health care systems model, 40, 44, 224
Testosterone, production of, by older adult male, 257
Tetanus, 471*t*
Tetanus/diphtheria, immunization against, 472
Tetrahydrocannabinol, 581
THC; *see* Tetrahydrocannabinol
The Fundamentals of Good Medical Care, quality of health
    care affected by, 158
The Hazard Communicating Standard, 425
The Wellness Workbook for Helping Professionals, 68
The Worker's Right to Know Act, 425
Thioridazine; *see* Mellaril
Thiothixene, 503
Thorazine; *see* Chlorpromazine
THR; *see* Heart rate, target
Three-generation family, 277
Ticks, Rocky Mountain Spotted Fever transmitted by,
    467
Tine test, 472
Tinea capitis, 471*t*
Tobacco smoke, home pollution caused by, 563
Toddler
  cognitive development of, 188-189
  diet for, 526
Tofranil; *see* Imipramine
Tolerance, drug, 325
TOSCA; *see* Toxic Substances Control Act
Total parenteral nutrition
  initiation of, in home, 395
  medicare coverage of, 396-397
Touch, changes in, in older adults, 258*t*
Toxic Substances Control Act, 425-426, 550
Toxicology, 432
Toys, preschool, 191-192
TPN; *see* Total parenteral nutrition
Tracers, quality of health care evaluated by, 176-177
Tranquilizers, abuse of, 579-580
Transmission of communicable disease
  chain of, 467
  mode of, 466-467
Tranxene; *see* Chlorazepate
Trauma, cumulative, peripheral nervous system affected
    by, 429
Travis, John, wellness movement and, 68
Trichlorethylene, diseases caused by exposure to, 431*t*
Trips, 580
Truth telling, 603, 607
TSCA; *see* Toxic Substance Control Act
Tuberculosis, 473
  screening test for, 472
Twentieth Century, nursing in, 13-16
Typhus, nursing and medicine impacted by, 8

U

Ulcers, stasis, in older adults, 265

Uniform needs assessment instrument, for discharge plan-
    ning, 375, 377-378, 380
United Kingdom, health care delivery system in, 34
United States Public Health Service, 25
Universal blood and body fluid precautions, 477
Unmarried couple/child family, 278
Unmarried parent/child family, 278
UR; *see* Utilization review
Utilitarianism, 604, 608
Utilization review, 178

V

Valium; *see* Diazepam
Value orientation
  of black Americans, 315
  of Eastern Asians, 309
  of Hispanic Americans, 311-312
  implications of, for health care practice, 305*t*, 319
  of native Americans, 313
Values, definition of, 304, 603
Varicella, 471*t*
VDTs; *see* Video display terminals
Vegetarians, iron intake by, 521
Venereal disease, 471*t*
Venous access, peripheral, 391
Veterans Administration, home health care financed by, 356
Video display terminals, radiation emitted from, 429
Vietnam War, influence of, on nursing and medicine, 14
Vinyl chloride
  diseases caused by exposure to, 431*t*
  health affected by, 556*t*
Violence
  in dysfunctional families, 324
  family, 327-331
    aggressive intervention in, 340
    ineffective family coping related to, 339-341
    philosophies about, 340
    policy changes for primary prevention of, 339
    types of, 327*t*
Vision
  disorders in, in children, 494
  in older adults
    changes in, 257, 258*t*-259*t*
    physical assessment of, 263
  testing, in school-aged children, 229-230
Visiting Nurse Association
  home health care provided by, 353
  problems of, in Chicago, 353
Visual acuity, measurement of, in school-aged children,
    230
Vital signs in primary-school children, 212
Vitamin B$_1$2, pernicious anemia treated with, 266
VNA; *see* Visiting Nurse Association

W

Wald, Lillian

Wald, Lillian—cont'd
  contributions of, to nursing profession, 11-12, 19
  school nursing programs and, 221
Waste dumps
  open, 543
  wellness affected by, 91
Wastes
  chemical, 547-552
  hazardous, 546-552, 565
  radioactive, 546-547
  solid
    definition of, 543
    disposal and dispersal of, 543-546, 566
Water, pollution of, 552-553, 566-567
Weight
  body, nutritional status of older adults assessed by, 531, 532
  control of, 515-516
  gain in, during pregnancy, 521
  and height
    nutritional status of children indicated by, 526, 527t
    of primary-school children, 209, 212
    in school-aged children, 227-228
  loss of, evaluating significance of, 531t
  prepregnancy, low birth weight infants and, 522
  reduction program for, 516
Weight-loss programs, 88
Well-being, hallmarks of, 236
Wellness
  achievement of, strategies for, 80, 84
  in community, 65-94
    family and, 274
  components of, 85-93
  definition of, 71, 93
  health belief model for, 71-72
  holistic nursing model for, 79-80
  models of, 71-80
  movement for
    historical development of, 66-68
    prominent individuals in, 68-69
    terms used in, 70-71

Wellness—cont'd
  promotion of, role of nursing in, 93
  school nurse's role in motivating, 227
  self-assessment of, 80
  self-efficacy model for, 73-74
Wellness behavior
  assessment of, 80-85
  social support for, 74, 76
Wellness model, Ardell's, 68-69
Western blot, HIV identified by, 479
Wheel model of human-environmental interactions, 146
Wilkinson windmill model of occupational health nursing, 436
Women, abused, responses to, 332
Work
  effect of chemical dependency on, 576
  right to, for developmentally disabled, 501
Workmen's compensation laws, 425
Workplace
  effect of, on health, 427
  hazards in, categories of, 428-434
  nursing process in, 443
    case study on, 444-445
World War I, nursing impacted by, 13-14
World War II, nursing impacted by, 14

Y

Young adults
  chronic illness involving, 411-413
  common causes of illness in, 242
  developmental stage of intimacy versus isolation in, 236, 251
  developmental tasks for, 236-238
  developmentally disabled, 496
  health promotion activities for, 244
  major causes of mortality in, 236, 237, 239t-241t

Z

Zidovudine, infection during early stages of AIDS treated with, 478

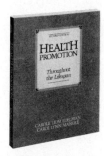
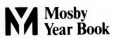